A

SYSTEMATIC TREATISE

ON THE

PRACTICE OF MEDICINE,

106356

BY

A. E. SMALL, A. M., M. D.,

PRESIDENT OF HAHNEMANN MEDICAL COLLEGE AND HOSPITAL OF CHICAGO;
MEMBER OF THE AMERICAN INSTITUTE OF HOMŒOPATHY;
PROFESSOR OF MEDICAL JURISPRUDENCE AND
THE PRACTICE OF MEDICINE IN
THE ABOVE COLLEGE.

CHICAGO:

DUNCAN BROTHERS,

1886.

PREFACE.

In offering to the profession and students of medicine the practical results of over forty years' experience and observation, it has been the author's effort to state in plain language the result of his observations, of the practical advantages of Homœopathic therapeutics, covering a period of active and extensive practice [in the past.] There has been no haste in gathering these into one volume, for the labor of preparing them has not been recent, with many parts of the work, which have been in the course of preparation in the midst of arduous labors for several years, and if he has succeeded in any degree in adding anything, however imperfect, that is valuable in medical literature, his purpose will have been accomplished.

In the introductory chapters the author has endeavored to present a concise view of the predisposing and exciting causes of disease without confusing the mind of the reader by dwelling on the conflicting theories of diseased conditions. He has presented the standard of health and a state of equilibrium of the vital forces and the manner of their preservation, by an orderly reference to the hygienic elements. Water, cold, tepid or hot, has its conspicuous place in the catalogue of hygeia as one of the necessary medicines for promoting health. It is a diluent of solid aliments, and satiates the thirst. It cannot be dispensed with in the preparation of food, nor in promoting cleanliness. He has briefly pointed out the importance of judicious bathing with tepid water, and also the importance of looking out critically the proper time, the proper condition of the system, and the relation of baths to eating and drinking, all of which are practical hints. The hints which will be found concerning the aliments and their

preparation for the promotion of health are also believed to be
practical, as well as those relating to temperature, exercise and
ventilation, clothing, etc., etc. It is as much the duty of the physician to consider well the means and measures to be adopted for
the promotion of health as to restore it when lost.

It has been the purpose and intention of the author to avoid
needless technicalities and synonyms as headings to the various
subjects or diseases treated of, inasmuch as the plainest description
of the phenomena attendant on diseased conditions furnishes a
much better guide to the practitioner in deciding upon measures
for affording relief than the mere classification of diseases, according to the dictation of the most eminent nosologists.

The day for treating diseases by their names has long since
gone by. No two cases of the same disease are sufficiently alike to
warrant an appeal to the same remedial measures. He has therefore recognized the fact that every case of disease has individual
peculiarities, and that a counterpart is susceptible of being found
in the pathogenesis of some specific remedy, and from the obvious
fact that nearly all diseases have primary causes in imponderable
agencies, as from odors escaping from odoriferous bodies, as from
the rose producing erysipelas or *moschus*, which in impressible
subjects provokes syncopy; or invisible agencies in fire, air, earth
and water which, acting on impressible vital forces, provoke derangements and diseases too numerous to individualize. It at once
strikes us as reasonable that imponderable remedial agents, affiliated in accordance with certain conditions and laws, may be
brought into the most successful antagonism to all diseases.

When materials used for medicines are duly prepared for administration, the utility of minute chemical or mechanical divisions turns out to be a necessity, because the size of the effective
surface is so greatly increased that less of the material is needed,
and the system has a more tolerable burden to bear.

Although the author has in many instances spoken of the attenuation prescribed, and the dose and frequency of its repetition,

there is nothing arbitrary for the government of others; he has merely given instances of his experience and observation. The same remedies in different attenuations in the hands of others, when critically affiliated, have undoubtedly been followed by prompt remedial action.

In addition to the simple headings of subjects treated of, with the slight allusion to synonyms, we have omitted long, speculative remarks on various diseases that have long been discussed, as to their nature and primeval origin, because we have verily believed that this kind of literature was unprofitable and tedious, in a practical point of view.

In classifying symptoms, or in other words, grouping them, so as to demand particular medicines, he has found first "the obvious phenomena or signs which belong to the external or visible appearance of the patient, and over which he has little or no control," as the expression of the countenance, color and temperature of the skin, pulsations of the heart and arteries, respiration, breath, condition of the digestive and genito-urinary organs, attitude, appearance of the eyes, nose, lips, tongue, mouth and throat; the secretions and excretions, the surface of the body, swellings, (in relation to size, hardness, softness, elasticity, fluctuation. etc.,) the condition of the muscles, in relation to contractility, strength, debility and motion; the voice, mode of expression, and appearances of discharges from the stomach, intestines, bladder, uterus, vagina, nose, ears, eyes, mouth, and from abscesses, ulcers, etc., all of which, according to Marshall Hall, are included under the head of *physical signs* of disease.

These signs may always be observed without any descriptions from the patient or his friends, and in many instances without the consciousness of the patient, and as he has frequently shown, they often indicate with satisfactory certainty the character of the malady. In infants and children, and even in adults, who either from injury or disease are incapable of describing their sufferings, he has found these observable signs a sufficient guide in the employment of remedies.

In the second place, he has relied on the physical sensations as verbally and truthfully described by the patient, such as pain in any part, and pains of all descriptions, and all other uneasy or unnatural feelings, as well as all circumstances connected with the approach, continuance, aggravation or remission of the patient's suffering.

In the third place, he advocates the strictest attention to the mental and moral symptoms, which include the disposition, temper and all the variations of the intellectual and moral sentiments, which do not accord with the normal standard. The above arrangement is recommended for convenience in ascertaining the patient's true condition, and for the purpose of aiding the practitioner in the selection of remedies.

In prescribing remedies for any and all diseases it will be seen that the author has drawn from the resources of *materia medica* in accordance with the recorded symptoms to be found in the careful provings or pathogenesis of each remedy, for indications of therapeutic properties. He has employed the remedies either in the form of *triturations* or dilutions. He does not discard the use of pellets, disks or tablets properly medicated. A disk or tablet fully saturated with any dilution is an ordinary dose.

So far as the author has been satisfied of the utility of remedies recently introduced, he has given them a liberal consideration. He has avoided as far as possible giving anæsthetic agents any doubtful position as therapeutic agents. As palliatives of pain they have their use. He has given but little attention to the theories and practice of treating bacterial diseases, or those supposed to arise altogether from infusorial agents, spores, fungi, fibrous or other microscopic discoveries in the air or water, for as yet he has found nothing in them superior to the symptoms as a guide to therapeutic measures. He has made no mention of inhalants or treatment by inhalation, yet this mode of administering remedies intended to benefit the respiratory system is by no means discarded. The same remedies selected for administration in the usual way may be placed in an inhaler and be taken by inhalation.

It will be seen that the author has said but little about the employment of accessory treatment in acute diseases, aside from the usual hygienic measures. That such cases may arise when the employment of external agents may be necessary to aid the action of internal remedies is indeed probable, but from many years' observation he can assert his faith in the curative effect of remedies when administered internally, if the conditions of affiliation are duly respected. Well ventilated apartments, in an atmosphere salubrious and pure, and a temperature in no manner deteriorating, with crystal water to drink, and non-medicinal food to satisfy the demands of the appetite and promote recuperation, the remedies acting in the direction of morbific influences which nature is struggling to eliminate from the domain of life, will be all that is required.

The grand proposition, *Similia Similibus Curantur*, he has regarded the corner stone of *therapeutics*. In the treatment of quite a number of the diseases, a brief statement of Allopathic treatment has been given, in order that its objectionable features may be seen in contrast with the Homœopathic treatment which immediately follows. He has not uniformly given the outline of Allopathic treatment in all diseases, but whenever he has it has been either for the purpose of exhibiting its injurious tendency, or insufficiency in producing a speedy cure, while the Homœopathic treatment, which is given more elaborately in striking contrast, promotes a more rapid return to health, without the entailed prostration and debility produced by Allopathic drugs.

With regard to the employment of Homœopathic remedies he has advocated a strict adherence to the "Law of Cure," without any restriction to high or low potencies. In his practice he has relied in most cases on the 3x trit. or 3x dil. His experience in witnessing the salutary effect of this potency in a large proportion of the wide range of diseases described in the following pages has led him to do so.

The critical affiliation of a remedy to any condition of disease is of the utmost importance. It is by no means a commendable practice to give remedies in frequent alternation. If a selected remedy, critically affiliated, in the 3d attenuation, fails to show a beneficial result, he changes to a higher attenuation of the same, and for instance, from 3x to 6x and from 6x to 12x, and so on to 30x, and in nine cases out of ten he has found the one remedy all that is required in any given curable case. High and low potencies he has found serviceable when given in alternation, or in some instances he has recommended an alternation of a psoric with an antipsoric, as in the employment of *Calc. c.* with *Pulsatilla*, in leucorrhœa, or Sulphur with Belladonna in some cases of scarlatina. He has seen the salutary effects of the high and highest potencies in many malignant attacks of some of the diseases mentioned in the book. But in order to be successful he has found it necessary to note the prominent symptoms of the disease and then to seek for a remedy whose pathogenesis presents similar characteristic symptoms, and he has found in such cases that the high and even the highest potencies are prompt in their action.

In preparing the copy for this volume we take pleasure in making honorable mention of the assistance of J. W. Marelius, M. D., M. A. Bowerman, M. D., and for many valuable hints from Prof. Ludlam, M. D., to whom we express our heartfelt thanks, and with the hope that the work, in spite of its incompleteness and imperfections, may be charitably received by the profession, and prove a valuable addition to medical libraries, the volume is most respectfully submitted.

A. E. SMALL.

CONTENTS.

PREFACE 11

INTRODUCTION 33

CHAPTER I.

A GENERAL VIEW OF HEALTH AND DISEASE 40

CHAPTER II.

NATURE AND DIVISION OF THE CAUSES OF DISEASE ETIOLOGY . 45

CHAPTER III.

OBSERVATIONS ON DIET, CLOTHING AND EXERCISE 60

CHAPTER IV.

OBSERVATIONS ON ABLUTIONS, BATHS, INCLUDING THE USE OF WATER AS A THERAPEUTIC AGENT 70

CHAPTER V.

INFLUENCE OF OCCUPATION AND SEDENTARY HABITS AND STUDY 74

CHAPTER VI.

THE SIGNS OF HEALTH AND HOW TO DENOTE ANY DEPARTURE FROM THE STANDARD 81

The Skin—The Pulse—The quality of the Pulse—The Tongue—Urinary Secretions—Perspiration—The Bile—Fæcal Discharges.

CHAPTER VII.

A GENERAL VIEW OF THE STRUCTURE OF THE HUMAN BODY 87

CHAPTER VIII.

A GENERAL VIEW OF PHYSIOLOGY.........................94
Functions of the Living Human Body.

CHAPTER IX.

MATERIA MEDICA AND THERAPEUTICS 101
Remedies and their Antidotes—Remedies which may follow each other.

CHAPTER X.

SPECIAL DISEASES AND THERAPEUTICS — DISEASES OF THE ALIMENTARY CANAL 133

Inflammation of the Mouth — Aphthæ of Children, or Pultaceous
Inflammation of the Mouth — Aphthæ of Adults, Follicular In-
flammation of the Mouth — Gangrenous Inflammation of the
Mouth — Diseases of the Tongue — Inflammation of the Tongue,
Glossitis — Cancer of the Tongue — Diseases of the Teeth —
Toothache — Caries of the Teeth — Causes of Dental Decay —
Nervous Toothache — Exostosis of the Teeth — Tartar on the
Teeth — Diseases of the Gums — Hypertrophy of the Gums —
Shrinking of the Gums — Inflammation of the Vellum and
Uvula.

CHAPTER XI.

DISEASES OF THE THROAT, PHARYNX AND ŒSOPHAGUS....149

Inflammation of the Fauces or Throat — Inflammation of the Tonsils — Inflammation of the Pharynx — Pharyngitis — Mucus in
the Pharynx — Diphtheria — Gangrenous Inflammation of the
Pharynx — Inflammation of the Œsophagus — Stricture of the
Œsophagus — Cancer of the Larynx.

CHAPTER XII.

DISEASES OF THE STOMACH 160

Inflammation of the Stomach — Chronic Inflammation of the Stom-
ach — Gastrorrhœa or Catarrh of the Stomach — Cancer of the
Stomach — Hæmorrhage from the Stomach — Hæmatemesis —
Gastralgia — Heartburn — Cramps in the Stomach — Gastrodynia
— Vomiting.

CHAPTER XIII.

DISEASES OF THE INTESTINES 175

Inflammation of the Small Intestine — Dyspepsia — Inflammation
of the Large Intestine — Typhlitis — Inflammation of the Colon
— Dysentery — Chronic Dysentery.

CHAPTER XIV.

DISEASES OF THE INTESTINES CONTINUED... 190

Perforation of the Intestines — Diarrhœa — Chronic Diarrhœa.

CHAPTER XV.

CHOLERA INFANTUM 196

Constipation — Obstruction of the Intestine — Enteralgic Colic —
Common Colic — Bilious Colic — Painters' Colic — Tympanitis —
Cancer of the Intestines — Hæmorrhage of the Intestines —
Hæmorrhoids — Piles — Prolapsus Ani.

CHAPTER XVI.

INVERMINATION — WORMS 212

CHAPTER XVII.

CHOLERA MORBUS ... .219

Asiatic Cholera — Cholera Asphyxia — Adipous Diarrhœa.

CHAPTER XVIII.

DISEASES OF THE PERITONEUM.......................... 239

Inflammation of the Peritoneum — Chronic Peritonitis — Puerperal
Peritonitis — Puerperal Pelvi-Peritonitis — Cystic Peritonitis —
Morbid Productions in the Peritoneum and Intestines.

CHAPTER XIX.

HYDROPS — DROPSY 260

Hydrothorax — Hydroarchis — Hydrocephalus

CHAPTER XX.

DISEASES OF THE RESPIRATORY ORGANS 269

The Nasal Cavities — Physical Examination of the Chest — What
is Percussion — Directions for Percussing — Auscultation —
Catarrh — Chronic Catarrh — Epistaxis or Nose Bleed — Diseases of the Larynx and Trachea — Inflammation of the Larynx
Chronic Laryngitis — Œdematous Inflammation of the Glottis.

CHAPTER XXI.

CROUP, CYNANCHE TRACHEALIS 302

CHAPTER XXII.

DIPHTHERIA, LARYNGITIS EXUDATIVA........................315

Comparison between Diphtheria and Croup — Period of Life — Char-
acter of the Effusion — Principal Symptoms — Distinction be-
tween Diphtheria and Scarlatina — Liability to a Second Attack
— Eruption of the Angina — Dropsical Affections — Modes of
Termination in Death — Diphtheria and Scarlatina Anginosis —
Diphtheria and Syphilitic Ulcer on the Tonsil — Relation between
Diphtheria and Erysipelas.

CHAPTER XXIII.

SPASM OF THE GLOTTIS 342

Spasm of the Glottis in Adults — Morbid Productions in the Larynx and Trachea — Foreign Bodies in the Larynx and Trachea.

CHAPTER XXIV.

DISEASES OF THE BRONCHIA AND LUNGS..................337

Epidemic Acute Bronchitis or Influenza — Chronic Bronchitis —
Summer Bronchitis or Hay Fever — Whooping Cough, Tussis
Convulsiva — Hæmorrhage into the Bronchia — Hæmoptysis —
Hæmorrhage into the Lungs — Pneumonia — Inflammation of
the Lungs — Spinal Sehlerosis with Intercurrent Pneumonia —
Typhoid Inflammation of the Lungs — Typhoid Pneumonia —
Gangrene of the Lungs — Œdema of the Lungs — Emphysema of
the Lungs — Inter-Lobular Emphysema — Asthma — Tubercles
of the Lungs — Tubercle — Pulmonary Consumption.

CHAPTER XXV.

DISEASES OF THE PLEURA...............................423

Chronic form of Pleurisy — Typhoid Inflammation of the Pleura —
Pleurodynia — Dropsy of the Pleura — Air in the Pleura — As-
phyxia — Asphyxia of New Born Infants during Uterine Life —
Asphyxia from Anæsthesia.

CHAPTER XXVI.

DISEASES OF THE CIRCULATION............................437

Plethora or Fullness of Blood — Paucity of Blood.

CHAPTER XXVII.

DISEASES OF THE CIRCULATORY ORGANS...................442

Dropsy of the Pericardium — Endocarditis — Hypertrophy, or Enlargement of the Heart — Angina Pectoris — Fainting Fits.
Swooning or Syncope — Intermittent Pulse — Aneurism.

CHAPTER XXVIII.

PHLEBITIS — INFLAMMATION OF THE VEINS 455

The Phlegmasia Dolens or Milk Leg — Varicose Veins — Varicose Ulcers — Goitre or Bronchocele.

CHAPTER XXIX.

DISEASES OF THE ARTERIES............. 461

Inflammation of the Arteries — Ossification of the Arteries — Atheroma — Embolism — Thrombosis.

CHAPTER XXX.

DISEASES OF THE CAPILLARY VESSELS.....................464

Hyperæmia — Inflammation — Diseases of the Glandiform Ganglions.

CHAPTER XXXI.

DISEASES OF THE SPLEEN.................................469

Hypertrophy or Enlargement of the Spleen — Atrophy of the Spleen — The Thymus Gland — Thymic Asthma — Diseases of the Mesenteric Glands.

CHAPTER XXXII.

DISEASES OF THE BILIARY SYSTEM.........................476

Hepatitis or Inflammation of the Liver — Enlargement of the Liver — Jaundice — Diseases of the Gall Bladder — Diseases of the Pancreas.

CHAPTER XXXIII.

RENAL DISEASES..484

Nephritis or Inflammation of the Kidneys — Albuminuria· or
Bright's Disease of the Kidneys — Diabetes — Diabetes Mellitus
— Diabetes Isipidus.

CHAPTER XXXIV.

DISEASES OF THE URINARY ORGANS CONTINUED.............495

Chronic Cystitis — Urinary Calculi or Gravel — Renal Calculi —
Hæmaturia.

CHAPTER XXXV.

ACUTE OR INFLAMMATORY RHEUMATISM 503
Gout.

CHAPTER XXXVI.

THE SKIN AND ITS DISEASES 510

Erysipelas — Impetigo — Acne — Erythema — Urticaria or Nettle
Rash — Prurigo — Scabies — Eczema or Herpes — Pemphigus —
Lepra — Psoriasis — Psoriasis Palmaris — Psoriasis Scrotalis —
Furunculi or Boils — Anthrax or Carbuncle — Purpura Hæmor-
rhagica — Scorbutus, Scurvy.

CHAPTER XXXVII.

EXANTHEMATOUS DISEASES................................524

Scarlatina Simplex — Scarlatina Anginosa — Scarlatina Maligna —
Morbilli, Rubeola, Measles — Varicella or Chicken-pox — Variola or Small-pox — Varioloid or Modified Small-pox.

CHAPTER XXXVIII.

FEBRILE DISEASES.................................. 534

Continued Fever — Intermittent Fever — Dumb Ague — Irregular
Ague — Hectic Intermittent — Remittent Fever — Non-malarious
Congestive Fevers — Irritative Fevers — Infantile Remittent Fe-
ver — Inflammatory Continued Fever — Typhus Fever — Typhus
Abdominalis — Typhoid Fever — Relapsing Fever — Yellow
Fever — The Plague — Dengue Fever.

CHAPTER XXXIX.

THE NERVOUS SYSTEM................................563

CHAPTER XL.

DISEASES OF THE NERVOUS CENTRES.....................575

Congestion or Hyperæmia of the Cerebrum.

CHAPTER XLI.

CONGESTION OR HYPERÆMIA OF THE CEREBELLUM 581

Congestion or Hyperæmia of the Spinal Cord.

CHAPTER XLII.

INFLAMMATION OF THE NERVOUS CENTRES 590

Encephalitis — Inflammation of the Spinal Cord — Myelitis — Cerebro-Spinal Meningitis — Spotted Fever.

CHAPTER XLIII.

ANÆMIA OF THE NERVOUS CENTRES 604

Apoplexy — Hæmorrhage in the Nervous Centres — Softening of the Nervous Centres — Induration of the Nervous Centres — Accumulation of Serous Fluid in the Nervous Centres — Morbid formations in the Nervous Centres.

CHAPTER XLIV.

DISEASES SUPPOSED TO HAVE THEIR SEAT IN THE NERVOUS SYSTEM..... 618

Augmentation of Sensibility — Diminution or Deprivation of Sensibility — Perverted Sensibility.

CHAPTER XLV.

CEPHALALGIA — HEADACHE 624

Sick Headache.

CHAPTER XLVI.

ECLAMSIA — EPILEPTIC — SPASMS........................ 635

Convulsions of Children — Eclamsia in Pregnant and Parturient Females — Clonic Spasms — Epilepsy.

CHAPTER XLVII.

CHOREA — ST. VITUS' DANCE 650

Nervous Apoplexy — Catalepsy — Hysteria — Tetanus and Trismus — Opisthotonos — Emprosthotonos.

CHAPTER XLVIII.

RABIES — HYDROPHOBIA 667

Hydrophobia — Delirium and Delirium Tremens — Mental Alienation — Hypochondriasis — Hypochondria.

CHAPTER XLIX.

DISEASES OF THE NERVES............. 693

Neuritis — Inflammation of the Nerves — Neuralgia or Pain in the
Nerves — Odontalgia — Toothache — Partial Paralysis or Paral-
ysis of Certain Muscles — Partial Paralysis — Palpitation of the
Heart — Palpitatio Cordis.

CHAPTER L.

DISEASES OF THE EYE................ ----................707

Simple Ophthalmia — Catarrhal Inflammation of the Eye — Purulent Ophthalmia — Purulent Ophthalmia of Infants — Gonorrhœal
Ophthalmia — Iritis — Rheumatic Iritis — Amblyopia — Amaurosis — Muscæ Volitantes — Cataract — Glaucoma — Strabismus
or Squinting — Inflammation of the Eyelids — Stye on the Eyelids — Inversion and Eversion of the Eyelids — Tarsal Ophthalmia — Granulated Eyelids — Eczema.

CHAPTER LI.

DISEASES OF THE EAR AND NOSE.......................722

Abcesses — Accumulation of Wax — Diseases of the Membrana
Tympani — Perforated Membrana Tympani — Inflammation of
the Mucous Membrane of the Tympanum — Accumulation of

Mucus within the Tympanum — Otorrhœa — Running from the
Ears — Deafness — General Remarks Concerning the Ears —
Diseases of the Nose — Inflammation of the Nose — Nasitis —
Bleeding from the Nose — Epistaxis — Perversion of the Sense
of Smell.

CHAPTER LII.

DISEASES OF THE MALE SEXUAL ORGANS — URETHRITIS 732

Syphilis — Spermatorrhœa.

CHAPTER LIII.

DISEASES OF THE FEMALE GENERATIVE ORGANS............744

Metritis — Amenorrhœa — Suppression of the Menses — Chlorosis
— Cancer of the Mammary Gland — Cancer of the Womb — Dysmenorrhœa — Menorrhagia — Metrorrhagia — Leucorrhœa.

CHAPTER LIV.

CLINICAL NOTES AND OBSERVATIONS 774

Arsenicum in Bright's Disease — Apis Mellifica in Intermittent
Fever — Baryta Carb. in Whooping Cough — Eucalyptus in Hay
Fever — Eucalyptus in Erysipelas — Gelsemium in Hay Fever —
Naphthalin in Hay Fever — Alcohol in Chronic Otorrhœa —
Aconite in Arachnitis — Zizia Aurea in Epileptiform Diseases
— Gambogia in Dysentery — Helleborus Niger in Dropsies —
Hypericum Perforatum for Injury and Laceration of the Nerves
Ignatia in Quotidian Fever — Ignatia in Chorea — Ignatia in Af-
fections of the Heart — Iodine in Goitre — Iodine in Croup — Io-
dine in Indurated Swelling of the Glands — Iris Vers. in Sick
Headache — Iris Vers. in Choleroid Affections — Kali Bich. in
Diphtheritic Croup — Kali Bich. in Membranous Croup — Kali

Carb. in Asthma — Kali Hyd. in Rheumatism — Lachesis in
Chronic Sore Throat — Lachesis in Quinsy — Lachesis in Bron-
chitis and Pneumonia — Lachesis in Heart Disease — Lauro-
cerasus in Phthisis Pulmonalis — Lobelia Inflata in Asthma —
Lycopodium in Pneumonia — Merc. Viv. for Cough — Merc. Cor.
for Sore Throat — Merc. Cor. in Dysentery — Merc. Jod. for
Nasal Catarrh — Merc. Dulc. in Cholera Infantum — Moschus in
Nervous Prostration — Moschus in Hysteria — Natrum Mur. in
Herpes — Sulphate of Nickel in Headache — Nux Juglans in
Noli-me-tangere — Nux Juglans in Scrofulous Consumption —
Nux Mos. for Headache — Nux Vom. in Sleeplessness — Oleum
Jecoris in Rheumatism — Opium in Coma — Petroleum in Hypo-
chondria — Sulphate of Zinc in Dysentery — Sulphur in Chronic
Dysentery — Plumbum in Dysentery — Hamamelis in Dysentery
Cantharis in Dysentery — Colchicum and Iris in Dysentery —
Merc. Viv. in Dysentery — Merc. Cor. in Tenesmus — China
in Dysentery — Iris Vers. in Bilious Diarrhœa — Phos. Acid
in a case of Chronic Diarrhœa — Phosphorus in Chronic Diarrhœa — Iris Vers. in Chronic Diarrhœa — Rheum in the treatment
of Diarrhœa in Teething Children — Dulcamara in Diarrhœa —
Colocynth in Diarrhœa — Veratrum in Diarrhœa — Pulsatilla in
Diarrhœa — China in Cholera Infantum — Chamomilla in Cholera
Infantum — Chamomilla in a case of Protracted Colic — Pneumonia — Phosphorus in Pneumonia — Carbo Animalis in Pneumonia — Aconite in Pneumonia — Stiblum in Pneumonia — Sulphur in Typhoid Fever — Aconite in Chills — Lachesis in Tuber-
culous Deposits — Lycopodium in Pneumonia — Tartar Em. in
Pneumonia — Bituminous coal in Pneumonia — Chelidonium in
Pneumonia — Gelsemium in Pneumonia — Phytolacca Decandra
in Diphtheria — Phytolacca in Rheumatism — Phytolacca in
Swelling, Induration and Abscess of Mammary Glands — Pulsatilla
Nut. in Irregular Menstruation — Polygonum Hyd. in Amenor-
rhœa — Polygonum in the Treatment of Ulcers — Rhus Glab. in
Syphilitic Ulcerations — Rhus Ven. in Erysipelas — Pepsin in
Dyspepsia — Lycopersicum Esculatum in Tetter — Rumex Crisp.
in Diarrhœa — Rumex Crisp. in Cough — Spigelia in Neuralgia of
the Face — Spigelia in Diseases of the Heart — Urtica Urens in
Burns — Veratrum Vir. in Convulsions — Stannum in Chronic
Bronchitis — Sulphur in Chronic Bronchitis — Baryta Carb. in
Asthma — Ferrum Met. in Bronchial Cough — Dioscorea in Chron-
ic Bronchitis — Hamamelis in Pneumonia — Belladonna in Chronic

Laryngitis — Hepar Sul. in Acute Laryngitis — Moschus in Laryngitis — Causticum in Laryngitis — Hepar Sul. in Laryngitis —
Kali Bich. in Laryngitis — Tartar Em. in Croup — Bromine in
Membranous Croup — Bromine in Catarrhal Croup — Argentum
in Chronic Laryngitis — Causticum in Chronic Hoarseness — He-
par Sul. in Laryngitis — Belladonna in Acute Bronchitis — Belladonna in Cough — Nux Vom. in Acute Articular Rheumatism —
Arnica in Rheumatic Fever — Sulphur in Chronic Rheumatism —
Kali Hyd. in Acute Muscular Rheumatism —Nux Vom. in Chron-
ic Rheumatism — Bryonia in Pemphigus — Belladonna in Ery-
sipelas — Belladonna in Chills — Bryonia in Acute Rheumatism
— Change of Climate for Asthma — Kali Hyd. in Asthma — Kali
Hyd. in Congenital Asthma — Rhus in Typhoid Fever — Bry. and
Rhus in Typhoid Fever — Aconite in Typhoid Fever — Arseni-
cum in Typhoid Fever — Phosphorus in Asthma — Merc. Viv. in
Typhoid Fever — Phosphorus in Typhoid Fever — Tartar Em. in
Typhoid Fever — Nux Vom. in Antecedent Heart Disease — Dis-
eases which generate Cardiac Lesions.

INDEX   869

A

SYSTEMATIC TREATISE

ON

THEORY AND PRACTICE.

INTRODUCTION.

In commencing a work of considerable extent and one that necessarily requires much care in arranging the data, we find the retrospect of many years no easy task to chronicle. At the remote period of forty-five years ago our name was entered as a student of medicine with one of the most successful practitioners of medicine in New England. The medical literature at that date was not less voluminous than at present, neither was the standard of preliminary attainments required of the student previous to commencing a course of study for the regular profession at so low a grade as has since been tolerated. A good English education together with a tolerably fair knowledge of the Latin language was the lowest grade of requirement that was regarded indispensable in that locality for those intending to pursue the study of medicine. After passing the ordeal of an examination by our chosen preceptor and being found worthy of the distinguished privilege, we were permitted to enter upon our career as a student under his direction.

The first text book put into our hands was Wistar's Anatomy and an ancient looking medical lexicon and a box containing the detached bones of a human skeleton. We read and reread the department of osteology until we became quite familiar with the mechanism of the skeleton in parts and how by syndesmosis the several parts were joined together. We then went on from ligaments to the muscles, nerves, arteries, and veins; the thoracic and abdominal viscera and the viscus of the cranium and nervous system of the animal and organic functions. All this was for the sake of becoming familiar with the structure of the human body.

Our next task was to go over the whole ground again in order to study structure in relation to function. In this review our preceptor placed in our hands three volumes of Bichat's writings, from which we gained an outline of physiology or rather physiological anatomy and then we devoured two volumes of Bostock; after which we ventured to form some idea of the processes and operations constantly taking place in the human body when in health.

After attaining a general knowledge of the anatomy and physiology of the human system, we turned our attention to works on materia medica of which Coxe's Dispensatory and Paris' Pharmacologia were the principal. We then attempted to gain a knowledge of diseases by reading Gregory and Dewee's Practice of Physics and the writings of Hippocrates, from which we gained more or less information concerning the natural history of diseases and the nosological terms that designate them. We also read the text books on surgery, obstetrics and chemistry. The remainder of the first year (aside from the time we spent in making pills, boluses, powders, etc., for our preceptor) was spent in reviewing the studies we had gone over and the reading of monographs upon phlebotomy, emetics, cathartics, fevers and febrifuges, diaphoretics, diuretics, emenagogues, hydrogogues, sialogogues, etc.

We were particularly interested in polypharmacy as well as the botanical and chemical history of the substances embraced in the materia medica and to make ourselves familiar with the manipulations of preparing and compounding medicines, we were for some time employed at this work under the direction of an experienced pharmaceutist. With Wood and Bache's Dispensatory and the American Pharmacopœa as text books, and in a laboratory where every variety of chemical and compound used in medicine were manufactured and put up in parcels to suit the dispensing apothecary, we became familiar with the medical properties and uses of the vegetable, animal and mineral substances; and also of the tinctures, extracts, powders, mixtures, pills and other products they were made to yield. In this orthodox field of study and research we verily believed we were making rapid strides towards perfection in the healing art.

We had learned the classification of medicines and how to prepare them and how to use them in driving disease from the vital domain. We knew that *emetics* would drive it out of the mouth from the stomach; that *cathartics* would expel it through the bowels; that *diuretics* would send it drifting through the urinary passages, that *diaphoretics* would eliminate it in perspiration from the skin, that *expectorants* would give it an exit from the air passages, *sialogogues* from the salivary glands and *errhines* from the nose; and besides we had learned that what could not be expelled by the above processes, could be made to flow out with the crimson current or be made to escape by counter irritation and blisters.

Furnished with all these weapons we could' but feel certain that we almost had absolute power over disease, therefore we longed for the credentials that would warrant us in risking an engagement, when some pestilence was abroad at noon or some fearful epidemic scourge was decimating the land.

We left the apothecary shop and went to Philadelphia to attend medical lectures, and for three terms we made ourselves familiar with hard benches, dry lectures and tedious experiments; nevertheless we were taught by demonstration how to do it, how and when to bleed, how and when to blister, how and when to write prescriptions for emetics, cathartics, tonics, etc. We were made so familiar with authorities upon all these subjects that we never dreamed of calling in question what any author said. We were admitted into the large hospitals to see the practical workings of the theories with which we had been made familiar.

Our interest in witnessing the skillful handling of the scalpel and knife in the surgical wards was exceedingly great, and equally so were all the mechanical contrivances employed in the art. No student, unacquainted with bandaging or the employment of splints or other mechanical contrivances for reducing fractures and dislocations, can feel himself competent to preside in these matters and then again there is a medical treatment for all surgical cases, which had to be learned.

In the *lying-in* department we were taught how and when to render assistance to the parturient woman and the necessity in all cases of employing a brisk cathartic the third day after confinement.

Suffice it to say; we attended lectures didactic and clinical until nearly every disease in nosological tables covering the practice of medicine, surgery and obstetrics were described and their clinical treatment demonstrated. After this we were duly examined in all the branches and passed as a candidate for the doctorate, which honor was duly received and certified to by a Latin diploma which was a testimonial that gave a passport into the profession, and now we sought a field for entering independently upon a professional career. We soon decided upon one, and armed with the necessary implements and medicines, we hung out our shingle, sent out cards, gave distinguished references and soon after we had an opportunity of measuring our skill in the treatment of the sick.

For several years we endeavored to follow out the principles and practice into which we had been initiated during pupilage. We met with the usual variety of diseased conditions and were often self complacent of success, when our patients recovered. We had been taught to subdue ordinary febrile diseases with saline cathartics or with sudorific drinks and in a majority of mild cases our patients in time recovered. We saw that the cathartics would reduce the system for a while and that forced diaphoresis was generally followed by prostration; but after a time our patients would recover both from the effects of the medicines and the disease. There were however some exceptions. We observed critically that the reducing treatment was often followed by derangement of some of the functions. The stomach would remain in an irritated condition, the bowels would become torpid and constipated, the skin would look sallow, the appetite would be indifferent, etc. All of which we invariably ascribed to the original disease, and to remove which we would resort to moderate doses of calomel and rhubarb or perhaps to blue pills, which we were taught to follow with a dose of castor oil to rid the bowels of the mercury after it had done its work, and by this time our patients would find themselves so weakened as to require building up and so nervous and restless and peevish as to require constant nursing. Mild tonics would then be called into requisition to bring up the strength and there would follow constipation again and then a mild cathartic, which would for a time reduce the strength. This course we found necessary to repeat, even to the discomforture of our patients, until they were manifestly obliged to desist from medication, after which we often noted a rapid recovery, which we ascribed to the faithful manner in which they had been treated.

We found a class of female patients in our *ride* who always seemed in miserable health, dyspeptic, bilious, nervous and dejected, who were all the time seeking relief by taking aperients and tonics which in their estimation they could not live without, and what to do for this class of patients I could not divine. It never once occurred to us that their debility could be attributed to the constant interference of medicines with the efforts of nature. But meeting a physician of forty years experience who had treated many such cases he counseled us to beware of the injurious effects of aperients, tonics and nervines in such cases, because of their interference with the natural recuperative power of the physical system. He added that in one instance many years before, he had attended a lady for three months, exerting his best skill with medicines, vegetable, mineral and animal and yet she remained in the same low debilitated condition and disgusted with his success he abruptly discontinued all medicines as useless. Two or three weeks after he found her very greatly improved and rapidly recovering health and strength. The venerable practitioner remarked further that the study of this case had enabled him to treat such cases more successfully without medication. This experience for the first time impressed us with the important fact that much of the debility and prostration attending the tedious recovery of febrile patients might be occasioned by the medicines given in good faith to promote recovery and in our future practice we were careful to avoid interference with drugs, that only taxed the vital forces farther than was necessary to remove obstructions to a return to health. Following out this idea in the treatment of the class of patients, who were always miserable and always keeping their systems disturbed by medicines, we found our success far more satisfactory provided we could persuade them to rely more upon the natural recuperative power than upon perpetual dosing with drugs.

In the treatment of pleuritis and pneumonia we had been taught the necessity of blood-letting and counter-irritants, accompanied with minute doses of Tartar emetic and we found no difficulty in removing the acute suffering characteristic of these diseases by a resort to these means and for several years we were satisfied with the pursuit of this course. Nevertheless there was frequently if not always a painful sequel to this treatment. Debility and tardy recovery were invariably noticed; while in many cases serous effusion in the pleural cavity would ensue and œdematous swelling of the lower extremities would manifest itself.

In reflecting upon this treatment, which was orthodox according to the highest authority, the query arose, if the protracted debility was not a fault of the treatment, whether the serous effusion did not result from the heroic use of the lancet; and also the œdema of the feet. After discussing the matter for some months and I may say years, we first dispensed with bleeding and then with antimonials and other prostrating agents; but not until we had seen it demonstrated that a few doses of Aconitum napellus would control the inflammatory fever and produce warm perspiration and cause the pain to subside and the recovery of the patient without a long siege of prostration.

In the reducing treatment of inflammatory diseases and especially fevers we discovered a source of derangement not usually taken into account. During an epidemic of inflammatory continued fevers that prevailed in the valley of the Schuylkill, near Philadelphia, in 1840, we came into competition with several older and more experienced practitioners whose practice was to bleed copiously in the first stage and to follow the bleeding with saline purgatives, and in nearly every case as the inflammatory stage passed off, a low nervous fever would follow from which there was an average fatality of one in four. This fearful rate of mortality led us to inquire if there was no way of reducing the arterial excitement, without depriving the patient of strength and all innate power of resisting and throwing off disease. We soon learned that in the outset of an inflammatory fever bleeding was unnecessary, that a few drops of a mild tincture of Aconite in a gill of water, administered in teaspoonful doses at intervals of an hour would reduce the frequency and hardness of the pulse and produce a warm moisture upon the surface and the patient would be greatly relieved.

We found also that our lying-in patients seldom acquired strength rapidly after the usual dose of castor oil was administered on the third or fourth day after delivery, and upon mature reflection we came to the conclusion that the bowels required rest after labor and that the cathartic was an injury. And ever after we waited patiently for the time to come when, in accordance with the demand of nature, the bowels would move safely and without loss of strength to the patient. We have since attended several thousand cases of parturition and our uniform rule has been to never give a cathartic and we have never lost a patient of the kind.

In other classes of diseases both surgical and medical we have instituted a critical inquiry into the predisposing and exciting causes, as well as into the effects of the prevailing practice in their treatment and we came to the conclusion that oftentimes more injury than benefit resulted from the treatment. It is our purpose therefore, to enter somewhat into detail in giving our experience in the treatment of the various diseases. But before proceeding with the subject contemplated, it is incumbent on us to state what observations have been made in a general way concerning health and the predisposing and exciting causes of disease and the general principles of hygiene which must be observed.

CHAPTER I.

A GENERAL VIEW OF HEALTH AND DISEASE.

Health has been defined to be a condition of the body when all the animal and organic functions are exerted in perfect regularity and harmony. It is not absolutely necessary however, that every faculty and sense should be perfect in order to constitute health. Some of the faculties may be imperfect and yet the general organism may be in a healthy condition. Congenital deformities may exist and still the body may be in health. For instance, the sight may be affected or the ears may be imperfect from birth, while the general soundness of the organic functions enables them to operate harmoniously in preserving a healthy condition and an ample provision for sustaining and promoting the growth as well as the restriction of the various tissues.

It cannot be said that one is not in sound health, when he eats, drinks and sleeps according to the demands indicated by a good appetite, perfect digestion and the consequent rest and ease which a healthy or normal state ensures.

When the mind is sound and the animal and organic functions co-operate together in normal harmony, no other impression than that of absolute unity can possibly exist to mar or disturb unreflecting consciousness. Mind and body co-operate together as a complex unit, and when one moves on in all the activities of life with no other sense than that of being a unit, he is evidently in the enjoyment of sound health. And so far as this innate consciousness of being a unit exists, even if some of the senses or the prehensive and locomotive apparatus are congenitally deformed, he may, nevertheless, be accounted healthy. It is therefore manifest that a healthy standard consists in the harmonious activity of the organic functions, a perfect mental manifestation and muscular contractility under the direction of the will.

From this standard we are to judge of the nature of disease. A thorough acquaintance with the anatomy and physiology qualifies one to proceed in fixing in his mind by comparison any departure from normal structure or function. Disease becomes

40

manifest only by comparison with health as a standard and it is anatomy and physiology that present this condition.

"Health," therefore, "consists in a natural and proper condition and proportion in the functions and structures of the several parts of which the body is composed. From physiology we learn that these functions and structures have to each other and external agents certain relations which are most conducive to their well being and permanency; these constitute the condition of health. But the same knowledge also implies that function and structure may be in states not conducive to their permanency and well being; states which disturb the due balance between the several properties or parts of the animal frame and these states are those of disease." (Williams.)

Experience and observations both teach that in health the digestion of food is easy and comfortable. But if the taking of food is followed by pain, sickness or uneasiness, we know that the function of digestion indicates a departure from the healthy standard and *is diseased*. And if in spite of remedies, this diseased condition long remains and affects a change in the structure of the stomach not observable in health, we also know that this is *disease* of *structure*. Disease of function is apparent therefore from a standard furnished by physiology, and *disease of structure* from that of *anatomy*. When both together are taken as standards, disease may be defined *a departure from the condition and proportion furnished by normal anatomy and physiology in one or more parts of the body.*

The standard of health varies in different individuals according to age, sex and temperament. The healthy pulse varies from 70 to 100 in adult males and we have noted a similar variation in children and women, but this variation is in the main attributable to the difference in temperaments. What may be sound health in the sanguine temperament may amount to disease in the nervous. Some are endowed with strong muscular power and others with feeble muscular strength, neither of which can be regarded as morbid conditions. Some persons fatten readily upon quantities of food that would scarcely save others from starvation. The animal functions, the nervous sensibility and sensorial powers vary in a marked degree in different persons without exceeding the bounds of health.

We have noted among individuals a variety of temperaments,

and these proceed from unusual proportions of certain structures or functions scarcely to be regarded as morbid and yet they show certain proclivities in that direction. When the nervous structure prevails predominantly there is a proclivity to nervous affections. When the nutritive temperament prevails which is the case when the nutritive functions are greater in proportion, a person is liable to become stout and bulky and yet in perfect health, he is exposed to the danger of becoming so plethoric and fat as to exceed the bounds of health. And on account of the interference with the well being and order of the bodily functions, this plethora and obesity becomes a disease.

Dr. Meridith Clymer states that "all variations from regularity in the actions performed by living beings constitute the phenomena of disease. The investigation of these phenomena and the reduction of them to general laws, expressive of their conditions, is the object of pathology. Here as in the kindred science of physiology the study of all the conditions is requisite and hence we have to make ourselves acquainted on the one hand with the characters of all the external agents which can produce a deleterious effect upon the living body, whether their operations be mechanical, chemical or vital, as well as the results of the suspension, partial or complete of the conditions by which its healthy action is maintained."

In order to fully comprehend the countless variety of secondary results, which may arise from any disturbance in the body, we find it necessary to investigate the changes of structure or derangement of function, on which these secondary results depend. It is the purpose of pathology to individualize the symptoms of diseased action, so that by induction we can arrive at satisfactory conclusions concerning the nature of the condition that gives rise to them.

The *ars medendi* or practice of the healing art is founded upon a correct interpretation of symptoms and some general law of affiliating the remedies. For instance when the healthy body is assailed by disease in any part thereof, there ensues a natural struggle to get rid of it; this struggle becomes manifest by a corresponding group of symptoms. The symptoms are not the disease. They serve merely to indicate the direction in which nature is struggling to rid herself of the change which has occurred in her economy. When Tartar emetic in a three grain dose is taken into a healthy stomach it becomes an irritant which the stomach aided by all the other functions struggles to expel.

This is shown by pale and sunken countenance, nausea, vomiting, anguish and pressure, great straining and sometimes cramps. These symptoms are not the disease produced by the drug but the phenomena or symptoms, that indicate the struggle aroused in the whole economy to obtain relief. When the same organ becomes the seat of irritation or inflammation from any other cause, known or unknown, a similar struggle becomes manifest in precisely the same phenomena. When any drug that has a specific action upon the bowels, is taken in quantities to have a toxical effect upon the healthy system, a different struggle ensues, the mucous membrane of the alimentary canal becomes irritated and inflamed and enters upon a struggle to get rid of the trouble and this is shown by pain and distension of the abdomen, diarrhœa and sympathetically by nausea, eructations and general debility. Whatever be the cause of the irritation, either known or unknown, nearly the same symptoms show forth the struggle.

In order to base the practice of the healing art on the *ratio medendi* or the laws on which such practice should rest, we have found it necessary to draw a parallel between diseases produced by drugs and those which occur from unknown causes. In this way we are able to come to a satisfactory conclusion concerning the relation of the two to each other.

By studying the natural history of diseases and their symptoms and comparing this with what becomes known of the diseased action produced by drugs, we naturally acquire a knowledge of the facts capable of generalization and from which a theory, principle or law may be inferred. We know of no way of ascertaining how a material used for medicine acts or what influence it will exert, except by ascertaining from observation its range of action upon the animal system when in health and then by noting carefully the resulting changes of structure and function.

In like manner we learn from observation the range of diseases and their characteristic symptoms, when attributed to such exciting causes as cold, heat, malaria, etc. It is by carefully observing the symptoms, purposely called out by drugs to show the nature of their action upon certain tissues or vital functions, and those arising from morbific excitants, which call into vital activity the same class of tissues and vital functions, that we find ourselves able to practically apply the former in antidoting or dissipating the latter.

We cannot proceed rationally in any undertaking without a
knowledge of what we desire to accomplish and of the means we
find it necessary to employ. We must have some practical
knowledge of the principles of relationship between diseases and
their remedies or we cannot proceed intelligently in their treatment. The more accurate our knowledge of the causes of disease,
the less will be our ignorance of the nature of its symptoms.
Therefore, in addition to a thorough knowledge of anatomy and
physiology, which present the standard of health, we require a
knowledge of the agencies that operate to produce either functional or organic changes, and this is comprised under the head
of ETIOLOGY.

That part of PATHOLOGY, which treats of the origin of diseases is termed PATHOGENY. The primary departure from the
healthy standard presents phenomena, effects or symptoms, the
study of which comes under the head of SEMIOLOGY. These phenomena admit of classification and division under different names.
This classification is termed NOSOLOGY. How to discriminate
and interpret the characteristic symptoms of the various classes
of diseases is termed DIAGNOSIS. The results indicated by the
symptoms and vital condition of patients come under the head
of PROGNOSIS. The principles of treatment and the employment
of remedies come under the head of THERAPEUTICS. All the
means or measures called into requisition to prevent the origin,
development or spread of disease come under the head of PROPHY-
LACTICS.

CHAPTER II

NATURE AND DIVISION OF THE CAUSES OF DISEASE.—
ETIOLOGY.

A general knowledge of the causes of disease is what is understood by Etiology. In further delineation of this branch of the subject it will be requisite to keep in mind what has been defined a condition of health, any departure from which is termed disease, and must result from certain agencies that precede it and to which its occurrence is due. In some instances these agencies are not disclosed to observation and sometimes when the true cause is apparent it may be connected with antecedents which have no agency in producing the result and yet it requires careful discrimination to prevent mistake. It is only by careful observation that we can sift out the genuine from the apparent causes. The test to be applied is this; the circumstances that are sometimes present and sometimes absent are non-essential, while those always present are undoubtedly the cause.

The real cause which might otherwise remain in obscurity, may sometimes be disclosed by examining the ultimate nature of the disease in which the cause may be plainly reflected. As for example, the filthy are often victims of scabies and want of cleanliness is looked upon as the cause, but the microscope reveals the acarus or Itch insect as the true cause of the disorder.

We cannot obtain a satisfactory view of this subject without referring to agencies that have their field of operation entirely within the body, as well as those entirely without. Those within the body are termed *intrinsic*, because they exist independently of any external influence, that is, they originate in some constituent or process in the blood or in some functions having either an excess or deficiency of vitality, while those without or external agents that induce disease are termed *extrinsic*.

There are many circumstances attendant on the organic functions or vital processes which may so act upon the body as to induce disease. The most trifling excess or diminution of the healthy processes of absorption and secretion must result in general derangement of the animal system. The same is true of all the vital forces. Either the excess or deficiency of nervous or muscular force, peristaltic or circulatory, if persistent, results in extensive bodily disease, all of which are included among the *intrinsic causes*.

Under the head of *extrinsic* causes may be classified all the variations of external circumstances that can possibly operate on the body or mind, such as heat, cold, moisture, food, poisons, medicines, diluents, etc.

Without consuming time in noting the division that different authors have made in classifying causes of disease, we may proceed to state briefly the results of our observation concerning the general causes, divided into two classes, viz., predisposing and exciting.

The *predisposing causes* of *disease* are within the body and consist of the various circumstances that influence its functions and structures unfavorably and yet do not amount to actual disease, until operated upon by some kind of exciting agency. We will proceed to enumerate the conditions that come under the head of PREDISPOSING CAUSES, debility, excitement, previous disease, inherited constitutions, temperaments, age, sex and occupation.

Under the head of *debility* we find numerous predispositions, for constitutional strength implies power of resistance. Therefore defective nutrition enfeebles the most important functions of the body and renders it liable to disease. A feeble action of the heart and arteries, a feeble nervous system and a want of tone in the general functions of the body render it susceptible to disease. This debility may be constitutional or acquired. When constitutional it is permanent, but when acquired from want of proper nourishment or the effects of an impure atmosphere, the removal of the cause may produce invigoration.

Excitement or *exaltation* or so to speak a redundancy of good living without sufficient exercise, predisposes the system to a variety of disorders. For when the system is stimulated or over-exercised, it invites the action of depressing influences such as cold, malaria, inflammatory diseases and hæmorrhages. Excitement predisposes to congestions or for assault from cold winds and a damp atmosphere, ending in rheumatism. Exaltation from stimulants predisposes to inflammatory diseases and renal disturbances. Alcoholic stimulants predispose the system to the disastrous effects of cold, to biliary difficulties, to inflammatory rheumatism and gout, epileptiform diseases, chorea, hysteria and many other nervous difficulties.

PREVIOUS DISEASE often leaves a predisponent to other attacks as in the case of croup, inflammatory rheumatism, enteritis and numerous affections of the nervous system. *Present disease* is a powerful predisponent as in case of structural disease of the liver, heart, indolent tumors and the like, inviting other disorders.

Inherited or hereditary constitutions are such as often run in families, having a tendency to gout, rheumatism, scrofula, epilepsy, mania, asthma, blindness and deafness. The tendency, however, to these diseases does not render it certain that all or any of the offspring will become affected, for this depends on individual peculiarities transmitted from the parents. Sometimes a whole generation is passed over and in the next the disease will appear. Children born of gouty parents have escaped entirely, but have transmitted it to their offspring. It has been observed that in constitutional syphilis, the first child born of parents, one of whom has been affected, may be tainted with venereal poison, while the second would be perfectly healthy and the third would be diseased and the fourth sound. It must not be supposed that hereditary proclivity of disease commences at birth. In a few instances it is congenital, but in a majority of instances it is developed by growth or other circumstances in life. When a parent has the gout at forty, his son will not be liable to it at an earlier period. Many facts have been collected which serve to prove the transmission of hereditary tendency to disease that only awaits the co-operation of some exciting cause to develop.

TEMPERAMENT is a peculiarity of constitution which often predisposes to particular disease. It consists in a predominance or defect of some function or set of functions. Thus the *sanguine* temperament, by reason of rich proportion of red blood gives a disposition to inflammation, congestion and active hæmorrhage. Opposite to this temperament is the lymphatic, which by reason of deficiency of red blood has the proclivity to watery fluxes, dropsy and other chronic ailments. In the *bilious* or *melancholic* temperament met with in persons of dark complexion, pensive and sad, there is a proclivity to dyspepsia and other biliary and gastric derangements. The *nervous* temperament disposes to hysteria, spasms and nervous sufferings. These temperaments seldom exist in their purity, but generally mixed in the same individual.

The last head of predisponents of disease to be noticed is AGE. We have observed the proclivities of *childhood* to diseases of the digestive organs, to derangements of the stomach and bowels, worms, croup, chorea, etc. And at the *age* of *puberty* we have discovered great susceptibility to disease particularly in females, which deserves particular attention and care.

At the termination of *growth* there is another critical period, which in the robust shows a proclivity to fulness of the vessels and hypertrophy, hæmorrhage and inflammation, and in feeble to tubercules. *Youth* is a susceptible period for moral and physical impressions. *Adult age* is usually a period of settled health and without proclivity to any disease unless brought on by disorderly habits or inheritance. As *age* advances the system undergoes changes and the power of resisting disease becomes lessened.

OLD AGE exhibits changes in the exterior of the body, that indicate the failure of those functions which were active in youth. The body emaciates, the skin shrivels, the fat disappears and the muscles become thin and sinewy, the joints stiffen and there is a general tendency to feebleness and the loss of particular faculties. The morbid tendencies of *old age* are too numerous to particularize and every day is attended with increasing infirmities and liabilities to disease.

During forty years of observation we have noted the difference of constitutions in men and women and the nature of predisposing causes of disease, and so numerous have we found them, that we find it utterly impossible to more than glance at them and this for the purpose of showing how liable various classes of persons are to be assailed by disease when some exciting cause operates with the unconscious proclivity they carry with them. As these predisposing causes become known, great care is required to protect them against development from exciting causes, which we shall next proceed to delineate.

Under the head of EXCITING CAUSES of DISEASE we shall consider those circumstances and agents which operate on the body, when predisposed, in a way to excite disease. These causes are of two classes. One is cognizable and the other is non-cognizable. The former are such as come within the range of observation and embrace physical and mental agents of which we can take cognizance independently of their operation in producing disease. And the latter are such as to elude our senses and we infer their existence from their morbific effects.

THE COGNIZABLE AGENTS are: Chemical, mechanical, ingesta, bodily exertion, mental emotion, excessive evacuation suppressed or defective evacuation, defective cleanliness, ventilation and drainage, temperature and changes.

The non-cognizable agents: Endemic, epidemic and infectious poisons. As both of these classes are too important to pass over hastily we shall proceed to consider them at some length.

Cognizable Agents.

Chemical causes of disease are as numerous as chemical agents. There are chemical irritants, which affect the body whether applied to a part or inhaled in vapor such as acids, alkalies and many salts. Chemical poisons such as Corrosive sublimate or other metallic salts, Oxalic acids and other strong acids, alkalies, Iodine, Chlorine, etc., produce disease by their known chemical affinities which affect decomposition of the tissues and impair the functions.

It is probable that many of the substances that cause disease in the alimentary canal do so by reason of their chemical action. Although the process of digestion is mainly due to superior vital power, yet in part it is carried on by a subservient chemical process. For no sooner does the vital power fail than we have fermentation and putrefaction, which cause eructations of gas or sour liquid from the mouth and there may follow the discharge of ill-colored and fetid matter by stool. Then too, may arise a great many disorders, which in part may be referred to those injurious chemical changes.

Chemical changes may excite disease in the body by *local irritation* produced by dilute acids, alkalies and various salts, the chemical action of which is resisted by increased action excited in the part. Workmen exposed to the vapors of Phosphorus, suffer from caries of the jaw bones and this is due to local irritation. Strong acids, alkalies, some metallic salts and iodine act as *corrosives* and by their powerful chemical affinity, they completely overcome the vital affinities of textures and decompose them and thus destroy the life and change the condition of the part.

Chemical agents also act as septics, promoting the spontaneous decomposition of the fluids or solids of the body in the same way that ferments or putrescent matters act upon dead organic bodies. Chemical agents may also act as *alteratives* and modify the changes that may take place in assimilation, digestion, transformation of textures, secretions, etc., as in counteracting acidity by alkalies, in variously modifying the state of the blood and urine by acids and alkalies. The operation of chemical agents on the whole body will vary according to their intensity and extent. *Irritants* if extensively applied cause feverish excitement, corrosives, if acting widely depress the vital powers, somewhat like the shock of violent mechanical injuries. They act as *irritants* if the vital powers are excited to resist them. *Septics* when very powerful rapidly overwhelm the preserving vital powers of the body and then it passes quickly into a state of corruption, as in the case of gangrene, pestilential diseases, etc. But if there is a paucity of septic matters and the vital powers are strong, an accelerated action of them may rid the system of the offensive matter. Such instances are witnessed in typhoid fevers, dysentery, cholera and diarrhœa.

Mechanical causes of *disease* are those which derange structure by tearing, cutting, pinching, bruising and straining, and at once produce diseases that fall within the province of the surgeon. Aside from these the physician finds many mechanical causes of disease that require treatment at his hands. Long-continued pressure may produce disease. Tight neck-ties may cause headache and even rush of blood to the head impeding the flow of blood in the large vessels. Tight lacing may press on the heart, cause fainting and other derangements such as colic and costiveness by pressure upon the free passage through the large intestine causing an obstruction. Pressure upon the stomach after a meal by sitting at a desk may cause indigestion. Long sitting or standing or a protracted continuance of any one position will partially obstruct circulation and innervation and produce swelling and paralysis of the lower parts or of those beyond the obstruction, and in time may cause inflammation and death of the parts pressed upon.

Mechanical causes also operate within the body. A stone in the bladder irritates and obstructs the passage of the urine. Gall-stones may obstruct the flow of bile. Hardened fæces may mechanically obstruct the passage through the large intestine and cause irritation and inflammation. The stomach is often irritated by its contents and is made to disgorge by vomiting whatever it contains or otherwise the mechanical pressure of undigested masses may provoke inflammation. The air passages of a certain class of mechanics, who work in stone or steel dust, may become mechanically irritated and inflamed from small particles lodging in the mucous membrane of the bronchial tubes. Numerous are the instances of the mechanical pressure of tumors, of urinary calculi and other obstructions that cause inflammation and structural lesions.

The solid and liquid ingesta may cause disease by acting injuriously on account of being innutritious or of defective proportions or in excess of quantity. Salts, pickles, condiments, drugs, intoxicating liquors are frequently exciting causes of disease, because they are all more or less irritating or stimulating to the digestive organs, and if used without prudence may cause inflammation, congestions and functional derangement of the stomach and bowels and thus affect all the processes of nutrition. The long train of diseases which alcoholic stimulants may generate can scarcely be told. They derange the nervous system, disastrously affect the biliary and urinary organs and contribute greatly to the production of an abundant supply of over-heated and ill-assimilated blood, which either finds its vent on the surface and particularly on the face in inflamed eruptions or tubercles of the skin, or in local hæmorrhages or fluxes causing many functional deviations, such as vertigo, stupor, delirium, tremors, palpitation and dyspepsia. Persistent topers are liable to gout and attacks of rheumatism, particularly if they indulge in the sour wines, ale or porter to excess. Sedentary habits and deficient secretions greatly favor the deleterious effects of these beverages. The habitual drunkard loses his appetite for food and the power of digesting it and he then drinks and starves, the victim of delirium tremens, of restless excitement and sleeplessness.

Unwholesome or adulterated food is a fruitful source of disease. Salt provisions too long used produce scurvy. Water impregnated with vegetable and animal matter, pours the stream of deadly poison into the circulation. When impregnated with calcareous matters it is unsafe to drink because it constipates the bowels and contributes to calcareous deposits in the bladder and goitre. Brackish waters bring on dyspepsia, diarrhœa and general derangement. Chalybeate waters containing iron are constipating, while such as contain lead induce colic, constipation, paralysis and great emaciation.

Under the head of non-alimentary matters which may cause disease our observation recognizes the injudicious use of drugs, nostrums and patent medicines. These non-alimentary ingesta, as a common cause of disease, should in this enlightened age be carefully considered. Too much medicine is taken and too many diseases are the result.

Aliments of bad *quality* constitute another condition of the ingesta that may provoke disease. Man is said to be an omnivorous animal and his general health is best maintained by mixed proportions of an animal and vegetable diet. Physiologists have experimented on animals with the simple elements of food supposed to be the most nutritious and found starvation would ensue almost as quick as without any food at all. Thus, dogs fed on sugar, gum, starch, oil or butter, soon became victims of starvation. From a report published in France, in 1841, it appears that animals fed on pure fibrine or albumen or gelatine soon die of starvation. Dogs fed on white bread made of superfine flour would die in fifteen days. Gluten or vegetable albumen is the only simple principle which will alone sustain life. It is therefore a matter of observation that a mixed diet of azotised and non-azotised food is necessary to sustain health and life, or otherwise the simple elementary food becomes a source of disease.

"Nature's common aliment," says Dr. Prout, "is milk, and this is the great type of all kinds of proper nourishment. It contains albumen, oil, sugar and water; and custom sanctions the use of those kinds of food only which contain these elements. Bread contains gluten which is vegetable albumen, and starch is nearly allied to sugar. But bread does not relish without butter or some kind of fat with it. Neither does meat which contains albumen and fat suit the taste without a combination with bread, rice, potatoes or other vegetables containing starch or sugar."

Albumen, gelatine, oil and sugar may be viewed as the chief articles for nourishment and we shall briefly note how a defect or excess of either may operate in causing disease.

Albuminous food such as the lean of meat, fowl, fish, gluten and caseine of milk supplies the abdomen and fibrine of the blood and textures of the body. Therefore a defect of this kind of nourishment will first cause weakness of the heart and other muscles and diminish the richness and quantity of the blood and thus cause general wasting or emaciation. An excess of this kind of food induces plethora, an exalted circulation, feverishness and sometimes hæmorrhage. Protracted living on butcher's meat not only leads to plethora, etc., but to gout and other inflammatory diseases. A bad quality of this kind of food is peculiarly injurious to digestion and assimilation. *Gelatinous* food, soup, broth, isinglass jelly, etc., are not so supporting as albuminous aliments; but when combined with bread they are valuable for nourishing the body and in the opinion of some, gelatine may assist in the formation of albumen. But when used uncombined with bread, rice or lentils, it soon ceases to nourish or prevent emaciation.

Oleaginous food, such as butter, fat of meat, oils, and such containing them not only supplies the material for the adipose tissues, but it assists in the formation of other structures and secretions and it affords the best food for maintaining animal heat. But a defect of fat in the food occasions loss of flesh, causes the eyes to sink in their sockets and a wrinkled condition of the skin soon supercedes the plumpness and smoothness of surface. It also induces a dryness of the mucous surfaces and synovial membranes of the joints, and further it diminishes the biliary secretions and contributes to imperfect digestion and fæcal excretion as well as a diminution of animal heat.

All varieties of oily food if stale or rancid are exceedingly offensive to the digestive organs. They either become solid or undergo changes that result in the formation of butyric or oleic acid which are injurious to the coats of the stomach; starch and sugar although consisting of the same elements, differ materially in their physiological effects. Both are important for nourishing the body when mixed with other aliments, but the former in excess impairs the action of the intestines and the secretions of the liver, whereas the latter often relaxes the bowels and augments the secretion of bile. In excess both are exciting causes of disease, that prey upon the stomach and the bowels. Nevertheless they form the mildest materials of food and serve to dilute the stronger articles such as fibrine and oil and to render them more palatable and digestible. And therefore, when deficient, the food is more apt to disagree and fail to impart its nutritive qualities.

Were it not for the guide which nature furnishes it would require much scientific knowledge to select and mix them to the wants of the body. But happily the appetite and taste indicate the best proportions of the various kinds of food, provided they are not morbid or pampered by condiments and refined cooking.

Excess of *food* to gratify an inordinate appetite may so burden the digestive organs as to cause them to fail in properly appropriating the nourishment, when this is the case they become distended, irritated and otherwise disordered by what they cannot digest. Or if they are strong enough to digest the excess, they send too much chyle into the blood and morbidly distend the vessels and derange the function of assimilation. From this may result plethora, apoplexy, gout, gravel, and inflammatory disorders, according to the predisposition of the subject.

Defective nourishment excites many disorders and fails of replenishing the blood so necessary for the nourishment of the various textures. Extreme deprivation of food begets the cravings of hunger in alternation with nausea and a sense of sinking. These follow extreme depression alternated with transient fever, delirium and general feebleness of body and mind and a marked deficiency of animal heat. Starvation produces inflammation of the stomach, probably from the irritating action of its secretions upon the unrelieved vessels. In less degrees of abstinence, enjoined in the treatment of disease, symptoms of vascular and nervous irritation often arise in the midst of weakness. Insufficient nourishment is fatal to the well-being of the body and sooner or later death will inevitably ensue as a consequence.

Defective nutrition lays the foundation for many diseases. Nearly every famine is attended with a variety of malignant fevers, dysenteries and other disorders of that class. Dr. Clymer says: "The prolonged use of a scanty regimen is the frequent cause of constipation and digestive troubles in those who fast throughout Lent."

Excessive bodily exertion of various kinds is a common exciting cause of disease. The great muscular effort required in running up hill, rowing or lifting, hurrys the circulation of the blood back to the heart and resists its distribution through the arteries in such a degree that the heart, lungs, brain and other organs become subject to great pressure of blood upon them. The greatest bodily exertion often exhausts the vitality and becomes an exciting cause of disease.

Strong mental emotion is a common cause of disease, because both body and mind are so knit together that it is impossible for one to exist without the other. The heart is often affected from mental emotion. A sudden shock whether of grief or surprise, fear or joy may cause a partial suspension of the heart's action. Even death has ensued from sudden fright and convulsions have been quite common. Spasmodic asthma and spasm of the throat, apoplexy, palsy, inflammation of the brain, epilepsy, insanity and other troubles have been caused by sudden mental shock, excessive anger, fear, terror, surprise and joy. Very often fright or anxiety may act upon the bowels or liver and bring on diarrhœa and jaundice and produce other disarrangements in the alimentary canal. The slower emotions are not less likely to act as exciting causes of disease. Long continued depression of spirits or anxiety sometimes induces asthma, dyspepsia, torpidity of the biliary system and other disorders, such as constipation and heart troubles. The urinary function is more or less controlled by mental emotions as well as the periodic function of the uterus and a variety of derangements are traced to this source. Over-exertion of the mind in business or study often affects the cerebral organs and brings on giddiness, stupor, headache and even apoplexy and palsy. Habitual concentration of the mental faculties may result in monomania of some kind or other, either on religion, politics or business and when we consider the various straits through which the mind has to pass in fighting the battle of life, it is by no means surprising to find some smitten with melancholy or monomania and others with dementia or complete insanity.

Excessive evacuations become the exciting cause of disease first by impoverishing the blood and then by leaving predisponents of other diseases. A certain amount of blood is necessary for the performance of health functions and where there is a loss of this vital fluid, all the functions must suffer to a greater or less extent. Other evacuations aside from blood letting have nearly the same effect. Purging, sweating and vomiting, protracted catamenial and seminal discharges, when excessive, are capable of producing syncope and general debility. It is difficult to enumerate all the diseases which excessive evacuations may directly or indirectly occasion.

Deficient evacuation of excrementitious matters from the bowels and from the blood is a fertile source of disease. When either urine or fæces are long retained in the system they become the exciting cause of diseases of a varied character. The sudden suppression of the menses excites a multiplicity of ailments as does habitual constipation and deficient exertion of the kidneys. Inflammation of the bowels may arise from deficient evacuations from the bowels and the most inveterate typhoid symptoms are known to be uremic poisoning from retention of the urine. Deficient perspiration or a sudden check of the same all have observed as the forerunner of serious pulmonary or urinary disorders. Many persons of full habit are relieved by nosebleed which if checked may excite headache or rush of blood into the cranium and hæmorrhage in the cerebral hemispheres. In brief, the diseases excited by deficient evacuations, may vary as persons are differently predisposed, but generally they are of the nature of local or general vascular fulness or some disorder of the secretions or of the nervous system caused by a disturbed circulation, as for examples, congestion of the brain, apoplexy, portal congestion, gout, palsy, hysteria, epilepsy and hypochondria, etc. Suppressed eruptions or discharges from sores, excite rheumatism, gout and other inflammatory difficulties.

Defective cleanliness, ventilation and *drainage* are properly classed among the pernicious influences that excite disease, from which the greatest depopulation of cities occurs. Epidemic and endemic diseases generally arise from this source. A filthy exterior of the body favors the propagation of vermin and the spread of contagious diseases. Cleanliness preserves health and to neglect it is a crime.

Defective ventilation or want of change of air in sleeping apartments, work shops, prisons or nurseries is a fruitful source of disease as varied in its character as there are persons of different predispositions to operate upon. Diseased teeth fill the mouth with filth which may pass into the stomach with food and thus find its way into the circulation. Our observation upon the effect of impure air and filth goes to prove that this exciting cause of disease is quite universal. Badly ventilated houses and tenements, both of the rich and poor are sources of infectious poison, detrimental to health and life. We have on record many examples of the influence of a vitiated atmosphere upon whole neighborhoods and cities, where the drainage was defective, resulting in cholera, yellow fever and other malignant diseases.

Defective drainage is the most pregnant source of foul air and offensive effluvia. When such sewers are opened the stench inhaled from them gives some idea of their deleterious effects, in producing nausea, vomiting and diarrhœa, and instances have occurred where persons have become suddenly suffocated by the gases of cess-pools.

One of the common exciting causes of disease is temperature in extremes or in sudden transition from cold to hot or hot to cold. Both heat and cold have different modes of operation and cause disease in various ways. Heat is a stimulant and cold is a sedative, and while heat expands the tissues, cold contracts them. And from this general law we have observed that cold will drill and prepare the way for a reaction of febrile heat. We have seen this verified in chills and fevers. When the hands or feet have been long exposed to cold, they seem shrivelled and shrunken. When warmed the blood rushes to them and they become swollen with heat. The same is true of the nose and ears. When they become frozen, they appear white and contracted, but as soon as warmed they become swollen and red and this action and reaction in various individuals give rise to a variety of diseases. It is therefore necessary to act from this hint and study the wide range of malignant and ephemeral diseases, that cold and heat or the extremes of temperature may cause.

We have thus alluded briefly to the cognizable agents that may excite disease, and, now we will briefly allude to those which are non-cognizable.

Under the head of non-cognizable agents, we shall first consider *endemic influences*, which induce diseases in particular districts. In low marshy plains we have agues, to which those inhabiting dry highlands are not subject. In certain deep valleys persons become affected with goitre or bronchocele, whereas the neighboring residents of the highlands are not so affected. Various are the opinions concerning the sources of endemic malaria. Some think it emanates from the soil and others from the water. That the cause of disease is peculiar to marshes is proved by the number of persons affected by intermittents, remittents, etc., who reside to the leeward of these districts and receive the influence of the winds that blow across them. It is therefore probable that the air surrounding these districts becomes impregnated with effluvia, miasm and malaria which is an aerial poison and supposed to be inhaled by the breath and absorbed into the system. Neither chemical nor microscopical observation have yet been competent to detect its character, and what it is remains in obscurity. Some have supposed that it is sulphuretted hydrogen in some places, as in western Africa. But this theory has been disproved by others and therefore our only knowledge of miasm and malaria is obtained through its effects. The chief points known are that the malaria is developed through the rays of the sun's heat on marshy ground, or the banks of tideless waters after evaporation has succeeded to a certain extent. The virulence of the malaria is shown by its morbific effects and the severity of the disease excited, and in the number which it affects. There can be but little doubt of the existence of different kinds of malaria, which causes remittent, intermittent, yellow fever and plague.

Nearly allied to endemic causes of disease are the epidemics which affect many persons in the same place and at the same time. Epidemic influences unlike the endemic do not return at stated periods, nor are they confined to any particular localities, and yet they infest some more than others, but they attack a whole district, a whole country and almost a whole hemisphere within a brief period and no obvious cause can be assigned for their appearance. They prevail for some time and disappear for an uncertain period, it may be for a month or for years, or not within the memory. These are called endemics—a blight blowing *on the people*, affecting a whole country at once. The cause is believed to be in the atmosphere, because the atmosphere is the only medium common to all places where they occur.

It is true that some epidemics are faintly traceable to the extremes of temperature — to dryness or moisture of the atmosphere. Those prevailing from cold usually occur in winter, and, those from heat in the summer. But the nature of epidemic influences is still in obscurity. We simply know that they cause disease. Dr. Prout noticed that there was a change in the weight of the atmosphere, immediately preceding epidemic cholera, that it was made heavier by some ponderous gas. At the same time he observed an unusual acidity of the saliva even in healthy persons and the absence of lithic acid in the urine, and he supposes that the inclination to form oxalic acid was referable to the same unknown cause, which produces cholera. Many theories concerning the nature of epidemic influences have been broached. Some maintain with considerable plausibility, that epidemic diseases are caused by infusoria in the atmosphere but the advocates of this theory have failed to show us their presence. Some maintain that infinitesimal parasites preying upon the mucous surfaces cause the cholera, but in like manner they fail to exhibit them. It is all conjecture, as the infusoria and parasites elude discovery.

Infectious causes of disease are which operate to impregnate one person with disease from another, as from wounds, or from inoculation of pustular diseases and syphilis. A disease is contagious where persons take it from coming in contact with it. as in case of the itch, variola, etc. Persons may be infected from inhaling the breath of those suffering from them. Contagious diseases are now regarded conditions of the body, that give off morbid poisons, which may affect others by standing over them or being in the same apartments with them. Some diseases communicate themselves by infection from its products as in case of the excoriated scab of a dried pustule from a person who has recovered from variola.

CHAPTER III.

OBSERVATION ON DIET, CLOTHING AND EXERCISE.

In the preceding chapter we have hinted briefly at the predisposing and exciting causes of disease and now we will state the results of our observation concerning the best regimen to guard against their development or influence. In order to preserve health the laws that govern our well-being should be critically obeyed.

In the first place let us inquire: "What beverages are most conducive to health?" Water takes the first place, pure water is the best diluent that can be taken into the stomach. Large draughts may prove injurious under some circumstances and ice-water when taken into the stomach when the system is over-heated may have an injurious effect. But, in the main, thirst is more easily satiated by moderately cold water, than by any other beverage.

Milk diluted with water may also be used as a diluent and be taken at meals; as an article to quench thirst it is far inferior to pure cold water.

Black tea of moderate strength may be taken at breakfast or at the last meal before retiring. A cup of black tea is for most persons a delicious beverage and a harmless diluent for solid aliments.

Coffee of moderate strength may be taken hot in the morning with sugar and cream by persons in health and not under medical treatment. But a frequent resort to strong coffee is often injurious. It is a nervous stimulant and many of the nervous affections of females are fairly traced to this stimulant. It thickens the blood, constipates the bowels, brings on nervous headaches and frequently deranges the nutritive functions and cannot be taken by those under medical treatment for any diseased condition.

Pure cocoa prepared in moderate strength is a good, nourishing and wholesome beverage, that may be taken with meals in the afterpart of the day. By pure cocoa is meant the shells ground for the purpose of making a decoction. *Prepared cocoa* is composed of the ground shells with other admixtures to render it suitable for an article of nourishment as well as a diluent for stronger food. It is classed among the wholesome beverages.

Cold black tea or iced tea is becoming quite common as a beverage at meals in warm weather and is believed to be a healthy drink for healthy persons.

Warm or *hot* coffee or tea at meals are regarded for the most part healthy beverages and may be indulged with impunity unless they are found to disagree, which is often the case with some persons. Thus, for the sustenance of health, water, cocoa, milk, black tea and coffee form the group of beverages that may be taken with meals.

Beer as a beverage heats the blood and contributes to an abnormal stimulation. Habitual beer drinkers often become fat and unhealthy and subject to biliary and gastric ailments. Beer therefore is not necessary for the preservation of health, neither is it safe for a beverage of common resort for invalids under medical treatment. It often becomes acid and a source of great annoyance to delicate stomachs.

Porter and ale as common beverages for the healthy are by no means commendable. They are the source of many morbid derangements and the habitual use of them will sooner or later prove disastrous to health.

The malt liquors are sometimes useful to individuals of feeble nutrition, but should be prescribed with great caution by competent physicians. From many years observation we are led to the conclusion that the habitual use of them is injurious to health and contributes to the formation of powerful predisponents of malignant diseases.

Wine made of grapes is not commended as a healthy drink, even with meals, and yet the lighter wines have been freely used in grape-growing countries and some persons become so habituated to them that they form a part of their daily healthy regimen. But nevertheless all wines are feverish and heat the blood and sooner or later they affect the kidneys, liver and skin. For enfeebled stomachs the sour wines such as claret or the Rhine wine may sometimes be advantageously prescribed. But the daily habitual use of them produces plethora, rheumatism, gout, etc.

Port-wine is objected to on the ground that it constipates the bowels, heats the blood, unsettles the nerves, produces gastric derangements and liver complaint. It is therefore unsafe as a common beverage. *The brown and pale sherry* are liable to the same objection as common drinks and in fact all wines whether made of the different varieties of grapes, currants, gooseberries or other berries, by reason of the alcohol they contain are unsafe for daily dietetic drinks because they derange the powers of body and mind and beget morbid appetites that may lead to habitual intoxications. They must be prohibited when medicines are prescribed, because they interfere with their action.

Distilled liquors such as brandy, rum, whisky and other alcoholic stimulants are not conducive to health, neither can they be looked upon as preserving it. They are absolutely prohibited when Homœopathic medicines are prescribed, because they interfere with their action or prevent them from having a curative effect. In short, the free use of spirituous liquors destroys health, life and peace. It has been ascertained that all fermented liquors contain alcohol, which does not act as a sudden poison but slowly and very gradually it undermines health and the vital condition of the whole organism.

In regard to the malt liquors it may be said that they are deleterious drinks because they are commonly mixed with a little alcohol and not unfrequently with Quassia, Nux vomica and other poisonous ingredients in small quantities and the persistent use of them must seriously impair the health.

From the foregoing it may be inferred that nearly all the fermented and distilled liquors are hurtful for the healthy and therefore it may be concluded that the sick can seldom profit by them. Always, when used, they should be prescribed by competent physicians who are able to judge accurately of the conditions under which they can be usefully employed.

They are for the most part medicinal, and cannot be allowed when Homœopathic medicines are prescribed; they interfere and prevent their legitimate effects. To insure the action of remedies, no other than non-medicinal beverages should be allowed to the sick when under treatment.

We have thus pointed out the diluent drinks that are necessary for preserving health and life and the injurious ones that are never a necessary resort for the same purpose, and now we will proceed to a consideration of the aliments that are to be commended for the sustenance of the body when in health and when suffering from disease.

Where persons are in good health and their appetites indicate a demand for food, the following rules may contribute greatly to their interest, and:

1. Those of sanguine temperament, which is denoted by red hair, blue eyes and a florid complexion, may be allowed the common cooked *vegetables*, such as potatoes, turnips, onions, tomatoes, squash or parsnips and cooked meats, such as beef, mutton, poultry and game, or a change to salt provisions such as beef, ham, etc. Meals should be regularly taken at stated hours, not hurriedly, but slowly, allowing time for complete mastication.

2. Those of the *bilious* or *melancholic temperament* may partake of vegetables and meat *ad libitum* except pork or other kinds of fat meat. Bread of superfine and unbolted flour may be taken with butter at each meal and also farinaceous puddings and fruits may be taken at dinner with coffee or tea at morning and evening meals.

3. When perfectly well, persons of all temperaments may partake of the various kinds of fresh fish, except eels or other oleaginous varieties and some varieties of salt fish.

4. Those of the *lymphatic temperament*, inclined to obesity or corpulence, should subsist upon the lean of well-fed beef or mutton with a moderate quantity of stale bread, well cooked turnips, hot and cold cabbage according to taste. They must avoid an excess of bread and butter, potatoes and all kinds of starchy food. They must deny themselves of sweet-meats and sugar either in tea or coffee and pastry of every kind.

5. Persons of *nervous temperament* may partake of food more fattening, such as fat beef and mutton and poultry with a plenty of starchy vegetables such as potatoes, sweet potatoes, farinaceous food, puddings and preparations of milk and eggs, and for the reason that the nervous system becomes less active and more inclined to rest when sufficient adipose tissue is provided to furnish bedding for the nerves to rest in. We have observed many instances where men having all the attributes of a nervous temperament, thin in flesh, swift in motion and rapid in speech and evidently inclined to give themselves but little rest, have apparently been worn down by perpetual excitement and in later years,

living generously on rich meats and vegetables and beverages, have become more fleshy, robust, less excitable and lived at greater ease, and had not this change came over them they must have worn out and come to an early grave.

6. It is therefore evident that much depends upon diet and regimen in preserving and promoting health. The demand for nourishing food by all temperaments and constitutions should be judiciously supplied and the food should be as free from medicinal influences as possible, and therefore all irritating and corroding condiments should be dispensed with. Salt being an exception, when used merely for seasoning. But this condiment in excess, persistently used will produce scurvy. Vinegar, pickles, stimulating sauces and rich gravies form no part of healthy diet. *The aliments* then which may be commended for good and wholesome food are as follows:

7. *Meats.*—Beef, mutton, poultry, game, fresh salmon, trout, codfish, halibut, white fish, shad and other varieties of salt and fresh water fish, not oleaginous; butter, cheese, curd, etc.

8. *Vegetables.*—Potatoes, rice, arrowroot, yams, turnips, peas, lentils, beans, beets, parsnips, salsify and onions.

9. *Shell-fish.*—Oysters, clams, lobsters, crabs may under some circumstances constitute a healthy diet if taken moderately and not persisted in.

10. *Beverages.*—Tea, coffee, milk, cocoa, table beer and light wine may be taken with meals.

11. *Soups.*—Among the healthy soups or broths we may enumerate mutton, beef, chicken, beans, peas, rice, barley, and fish chowder.

The above table is sufficient for all classes to select from, each according to his peculiar taste or fancy. But when sick and under medical treatment, the following tables may be consulted:

12. Beef either roasted or broiled or made into soup. Mutton, also quails, chickens, grouse, rabbits with toast, potatoes, arrowroot, cornstarch, farina, eggs and milk, served up in puddings or custard. Fresh shad, white fish, trout, smelts and other delicate fresh water fish, boiled or broiled and served free from condiments except salt.

14. The following diet may sometimes be allowed if the patient, when in health, had been accustomed to them. Ham,

veal, lamb, turnips, beets, cabbage and cauliflower, butter and sugar, salmon, halibut, mackerel, oysters, eggs, clams.

15. *The aliments strictly forbidden* when under treatment are: Pork, fresh or salt, fat meats of every description, pork and beans, sour-krout boiled with fat pork, rancid fish or meats of every kind, rancid butter, rich pastry, highly seasoned soups, such as mock-turtle, pepper pot and minced pies, sausages and all indigestible and acrid condiments and all medicinal substances. Ale, porter, lager beer, hard cider, rum, gin, brandy and all strong drinks of every description.

16. If persons wish to gain in strength, they must subsist mainly on albuminous food such as lean meat of animals, fowl, fish, gluten of bread and casein of milk (cheese). If they wish to get fat let them subsist on that food which contains the most oil and fat, as oleaginous food contributes to the increase of the adipose tissues. If they wish to overcome obesity and get lean, let them subsist on lean meat and those vegetables that contain neither starch nor sugar, such as turnips, cauliflower, cabbage, etc., and if they wish to support the medium between the two extremes let them partake of an admixture of oleaginous and albuminous food; as bread and butter, meat and gravies, turnips and potatoes, etc.

All articles that contain albumen, gluten or fibrin are termed *nitrogenized* and all containing starch, sugar and oil are termed *non-nitrogenized*. The former contribute to the formation of muscle and the fibrous tissues in general, and the latter to the adipose tissue in all those that are benefited by fat and the adipose tissue in general. To keep in mind the distinction between the two kinds of food will enable us to form some definite idea of what is best in prescribing a diet for individual cases.

Next in importance to diet in preserving or contributing to health is *clothing*. As the seasons tread rapidly upon the heels of each other, we have observed that all persons become more or less influenced by the extremes of temperature, and the clothing should accord with the temperature of the weather, whether in midsummer or midwinter or amidst arctic frosts or in tropical heat.

Warm clothing for cold weather is instinctively demanded and for extreme warm weather light clothing only is required.

5

Clothing, manufactured from silk, wool and cotton, is worn next to the skin in cold climates. And it seems necessary to make some discrimination as to which is the best. Some maintain that cotton is the best material for underwear, because it is warmer and healthier to the skin than either silk or woollen, and, besides, cotton is capable of undergoing frequent and repeated washings without shrinking or losing its power to protect from cold. From observation we are led to the conclusion that cotton affords the best protection and contributes to the greatest cleanliness of the skin.

Flannel made of lamb's wool and sufficiently heavy to afford adequate protection is also found to be a non-conductor of heat from the body and to frequently impair the follicles of the skin and render it unhealthy. In order to contribute to good health, all underwear should be frequently changed and kept clean. The body should be clothed by a suitable thickness of flannel and clothing outside of it, to keep from getting chilled from the atmosphere of winter. The coldest days should be provided against, because the sedative action of cold simply provokes a febrile reaction that may end in general derangement of the functions. Much of the sickness which prevails in the winter season is due to a want of good thick warm clothing. In order to relieve from embarassment, it may be stated briefly that in frigid climates

1. Men require thick cotton flannel undershirts and drawers and good thick clothing made of heavy cloth to wear over them and when exposed to extreme cold an overcoat of thick cloth is indispensible.

2. Too much clothing about the neck is not beneficial because our observation assures us that cold and sore throat more frequently happen to those who wear much clothing about the neck, than those who wear little or go with the neck nearly bare.

3. The feet and hands should be well clothed when exposed to cold. It is injurious to the general health to sit in a carriage with cold feet, besides there is great danger of chilling the whole system and provoking a general febrile condition. We have known cold hands to be followed by pain in the stomach and bowels and other derangements. It is therefore necessary to protect the hands and feet with proper clothing in order to promote health as well as comfort.

4. A sufficiency of flannels and clothing to protect the body against cold is as necessary as food, or otherwise malignant and fatal diseases may occur as a consequence. We have known a malignant and typhoid to follow a sleigh-ride on a cold winter's day when not sufficiently protected by warm clothing. Many diseases of the winter season, which are usually mild, when the body is well and warmly clad, become malignant if otherwise. Therefore clothing next to food affords the best protection to health.

5. Bed clothing in abundance in cold weather and in cold sleeping apartments is necessary to promote health. The number of cases of extreme sickness brought on by sleeping under light covering can hardly be told. Too much clothing upon the bed is also detrimental to the health and great care is necessary to avoid either extreme.

6. During the warm season or in warm climates the clothing should be light so as to guard against overheating the body and thus bring on prostration and general derangement of the stomach and bowels. It is nevertheless a source of danger to incautiously throw off the flannels as soon as the warm season approaches.

7. When autumn brings warm days and cool nights critical attention should be paid to the clothing so as to guard against the chill of night, that often proves the source of autumnal dysenteries. When the body is kept warm and in a state of perspiration during the day and falls to sleep at night under insufficient clothing, the perspiration recedes from the surface and falls upon the mucous surface of the bowels or lungs and results in much sickness especially with children. Scarcely a season passes by without much trouble from this source. And to guard against its disasters neither adults nor children should be allowed to fall asleep unconscious of the danger to which a chilling atmosphere before morning might subject them.

8. As the temperature changes from warm to cold great care is necessary to keep the body protected from the extremes of heat and cold, or otherwise a multitude of diseases may follow as a consequence.

Next in importance to food and clothing for the protection of health is a proper attention to *exercise in the open air*. There can be no question concerning the truth of the aphorism that:

"Exercise promotes health." To be confined to sultry heat in warm weather without a sufficient amount of out-door exercise weakens the entire body. An early morning walk before the scorching rays of the sun render it impracticable, fortifies the nutritive functions against deterioration, and evening exercise in the open air prepares the body for invigorating sleep. Of the different kinds of exercise that may be demanded, we will note *walking* to exercise the muscles of locomotion; this exercise diverts the circulation from the upper portion of the trunk and head, and renders it more vigorous in the legs and feet.

Running may sometimes be useful in quickening the respiration and thereby causing the absorption of more oxygen in the lungs. In case of sluggish circulation and general torpor of the nutritive system this exercise is useful.

Lifting has been found useful in promoting the strength of the muscular system, in diverting the blood from the nervous centres to the extremities.

The *health-lift* as it is termed is of great utility in promoting general health and strength of the body. It is so arranged that a certain weight is lifted by the hands and arms by extending the lower extremities, which are flexed, to seize the weight and by extending the lower extremities without relaxing the grasp of the hands, a given weight is raised. At first the weight to be lifted is such as the strength of the patient can lift with ease and when the exercise is practiced daily the weight to be lifted is increased until from fifty pounds there is a gradual increase of power in the hands and knees to lift five hundred pounds or more. And the effect of this lifting upon the general health is sometimes remarkable. Very feeble persons sometimes commence exercising with the health-lift when they are able to lift less than fifty pounds and by daily continuing the exercise, they gradually acquire strength for lifting until they are able to lift six or seven hundred pounds. The changes that sometimes take place during this lifting process are quite remarkable. Those habitually troubled with indigestion have been greatly benefited, headaches have been cured, rheumatism has disappeared and the general tone and vigor of the system have been improved.

Invalids suffering from general debility have tried the health-lift with advantage. We once knew of an individual who suffered much from coldness of the extremities, headache and asthma, who ultimately was relieved of the whole by judicious practice with the *health-lift*. As a useful exercise therefore, as well as a means of easing divers disorders, a resort to this process is commended.

Varied exercises for males and females, whose employments subject them to sedentary habits, are essentially necessary for preserving vigorous health and strength of the muscular system. Such exercises as billiards, tenpins and base-ball as well as moderate dancing and other social plays when indulged in for the sake of relaxation from sterner duties are calculated to refresh and invigorate the powers of mind and body.

In the economy of the circulation, nature supplies blood to invigorate all portions of the muscular tissue, when subjected to useful exercise. She withdraws the vital fluid from such as cease their activity. The solens muscle loses its rotundity when not used for locomotion and so with other muscles dependent on the will for their activity.

CHAPTER IV.

OBSERVATIONS ON ABLUTIONS, BATHS, INCLUDING THE USE OF WATER AS A THERAPEUTIC AGENT.

Cleanliness is a virtue and personal cleanliness promotes health. It is incumbent on all classes to resort to frequent ablutions for the purpose of keeping the face, hands and skin free from filth and other impurities, dangerous to health. Every time soiled clothing is exchanged for clean underwear, the whole body should be washed with a wet towel or sponge and wiped dry, after the soiled linen is removed and before the well aired and dry is put on. This tends to keep the surface of the body in a healthy condition and prevents the exhalent vessels from being obstructed by sebaceous secretions which often render the skin rough, unhealthy and subject to various humors or eruptions.

Pure rain-water is always the best for ablutions and it may be employed daily of such temperature as best comports with health. For those of robust habit and uniformly healthy, common cistern water, if pure, may be employed of the temperature found in its native state.

But for children and those of delicate constitutions, tepid or moderately warm water is best if softened with castile soap as occasion may require.

In fevers warm or tepid water is applied *therapeutically* to reduce febrile heat. A sponge or towel, wet with the same is passed briskly over the surface of the body under the bed clothing and is very refreshing, and often so quieting as to compose the patient to rest. Sometimes washing the feet in warm water is resorted to for the same purpose. Placing the feet in warm water and washing freely the lower extremities below the knees, diverts action from the head and reduces the general febrile heat of the body. In cases of extreme debility of young children, washing them in water medicated with salt, cinchona or malt has been found of great benefit. A male child who had attained the age of twenty-two months without being able to stand on its feet, was subjected to daily salt water ablutions and the effect was remarkably favorable in strengthening the child's muscles, and he soon was able to walk without difficulty.

We know a little girl five years of age, who had not been able to stand or walk alone, who was washed with malt-water as a last resort and the effect was a rapid gaining of strength and ability to walk without aid from her nurse.

We have also observed that water or soap and water would aggravate certain dermic disorders, such as furfuraceous eruptions, while water softened with wheat or corn meal and carefully strained would not only be a valuable wash for cleansing but also for soothing if not healing the surface. Under the head of baths and rules for bathing more will be said upon this subject.

Baths are called into requisition for the purpose of cleansing and refreshing and invigorating the body.

The cold water bath should never be resorted to at a lower temperature than 65° F.

Tepid baths should be of a temperature from 85° to 92° F.

Warm baths may be of a temperature from 92° to 98° F. Each of the above baths may be employed usefully under the guidance of the following rules.

1. In warm weather, when the thermometer ranges from 70° to 80° F., the cold water bath may be employed once a day for persons in health. The time consumed in bathing should not exceed six minutes, and coming from the bath the body should be briskly wiped off with dry towels. The most suitable times for bathing are early in the morning before breakfast and just before retiring at night. Bathing on a full stomach or immediately after a meal is not to be commended.

The cold water bath may be required in cold weather once or twice a week. But the room in which the bath is taken should always be of a higher temperature than that of the water employed and the usual time of six minutes is as long as any one should remain in the bath, and the same rule for briskly wiping off with dry towels should be observed.

The tepid water bath gives rise to a sensation of either heat or cold according to the temperature of the body at the time of bathing. It cleanses the body or the skin, promotes free perspiration and allays thirst. It is sometimes used as a preparation for the cool or cold bath. In persons predisposed to apoplexy the simultaneous immersion in the tepid bath and affusions of cold water over the head have been recommended.

The warm bath causes a sensation of warmth which is more obvious when the body has been previously cooled. It renders the pulse fuller and more frequent, ameliorates respiration and augments perspiration. It causes languor, diminution of muscular power, faintness and tendency to sleep.

As a relaxant the warm bath is employed in reducing dislocations of the larger joints and in hernia. It is used with the greatest advantage in the passage of urinary or biliary calculi and thereby alleviates the pain and facilitates the passage of the concretions. It will be seen therefore that the warm bath is a valuable therapeutic agent for the above and also for gastritis, enteritis, cystitis and nephritis. In exanthematous diseases it greatly assists the manifestation of the eruption and is highly serviceable as a therapeutic agent in chronic cutaneous diseases, rheumatism, amenorrhœa and dysmenorrhœa. Time allowed—ten minutes.

The hip bath is often called into requisition in inflammatory or spasmodic affections of the abdominal and pelvic viscera and also in dysmenorrhœa and amenorrhœa. The hip bath should be tepid or warm water and not to be continued longer than ten minutes at a time. Other partial baths are employed in piles, prolapsed rectum, strangury, etc.

The foot bath of warm water is used therapeutically as a revulsive or counter-irritant in slight colds. It is used also to promote the menstrual and hæmorrhoidal discharges. The partial warm bath may be employed topically for other purposes and may be applied either to the upper or lower extremities.

The hot bath has a temperature from 98 to 112° F and is employed on account of its being a powerful excitant in paralysis, rheumatism, and topically for inflammation of the brain and other local inflammations. Its use is founded on the fact that it causes a sensation of heat, renders the pulse fuller and stronger, acelerates respiration, occasions extreme redness of the skin and subsequently intense and copious perspiration, etc. From several year's observation we are certain that hot humid applications to inflamed surfaces are better than cold ones and are more effective in relieving the suffering.

The topical application of *cold water* is a valuable therapeutic agent when judiciously employed. The most formidable cases of croup are speedily relieved by wetting a towel with cold water and binding around the throat with a dry covering over it. The pain of dislocation is greatly relieved by binding a cold wet towel around the affected joint and a dry towel bound tight around it. In cases of bruises or sprains the topical application of cold wet cloths with dry coverings are known to give efficient relief and the same bound around the bowels with dry coverings have relieved the great torpidity and inveterate constipation, which some persons are prone to suffer from. In chronic febrile conditions of the entire body, with torpid liver and restlessness, a wet sheet wrapped around the entire body with a plenty of outside dry covering will often afford complete and substantial relief.

Many are the therapeutic uses of tepid and cold water and it is impossible to so individualize them as to present a complete view. We have therefore given examples that may suggest a wider range for the employment of this agent.

CHAPTER V.

INFLUENCE OF OCCUPATIONS AND SEDENTARY HABITS AND STUDY.

That men are exposed to particular diseases from the nature of their occupations is a fact well known, but a remedy for such ills is a desideratum. Most people are under the necessity of following such occupations as they have been bred to whether they are favorable to health or not.

Chemists, founders, forgers, glassblowers, and several other artists are the victims of certain diseases in consequence of the kind of air they are obliged to breathe. The noxious exhalations from metals and minerals, together with a perpetually heated atmosphere, subject them to the danger of inhaling poisons that must sooner or later seriously impair the health. To prevent such a consequence as far as possible, it is necessary to provide apartments for carrying on these occupations, that shall be perpetually supplied with pure and invigorating air, a current of which might dissipate the smoke and other metalic exhalations which might prove a source of disease and death. Chemists and artificers in the metals should frequently relieve themselves of surrounding influences in order to preserve health or guard against the inroads of disease. This class of persons includes the miners and all who work under ground. The stagnated air of deep mines contains a poison, which may be inhaled or dermically impregnated, that generates serious disease.

The working classes are generally the most healthy yet they are subject to more or less exposure growing out of the nature of their employments.

Farmers are exposed to vicissitudes and changes of the weather, which in this country, along the sea coast and in the region of the great lakes, are sudden and give rise to colds, coughs, rheumatisms, fevers and other acute sufferings. The labors of the husbandman are such as to require a great expenditure of physical strength and sometimes sprains, distention of the blood vessels, ruptures and pleurisies are the result.

Porters are necessarily obliged to bear heavy burdens for short periods, that cause them to hold the breath and distend the lungs more than is necessary for natural respiration. As a consequence we have often observed asthmatic breathing and, in some instances, expectoration of blood which comes from the bursting of over-stretched vessels in the lungs. All employments that require great exertion of strength are liable to produce serious injuries and to avoid anything of the kind it is necessary to observe the following rules:

1. Never attempt to carry heavy burdens that overtax the strength or to accomplish at once what ought to be done by piece-meal.

2. Never indulge in feats of strength to gratify a vain spirit of emulation.

3. Rest often when doing heavy work, which calls into requisition extreme muscular activity.

4. Avoid as much as possible the lifting of heavy weights, for this exercise frequently causes the blood to be sent to the head with such force as to produce nosebleed and sometimes apoplexy. Such employments as blacksmithing, carpentering and other kindred employments often lead to overtaxing the strength to a degree that brings on disease.

5. When violent muscular exertion causes a copious perspiration, never drink cold water while in this heated condition, for a sudden check of perspiration from anything cold or from wet feet or a draft of cold air. may bring on rheumatism, erysipelas and other inflammatory diseases.

6. Avoid all exposure to the extremes of temperature after violent exercise or hard labor in any employment, because colic and other bowel complaints are liable to be produced from a careless exposure of the kind.

7. When outdoor work necessitates an exposure to severe cold, and the hands and feet, fingers and toes become chilled, avoid coming directly to the fire, for such a proceeding is often the cause of whitlows and other inflammations of a painful character.

8. Laborers in the hot season should never lie down and sleep in the sun. For this is often the source of malignant fevers; neither should they allow themselves to drink freely of cold water.

9. When laborers leave off work, which they ought always

to do during the intense heat of the day, they should seek suitable protection by retiring into shade or to their homes, where they can repose in safety. By so doing they will avoid much sickness and acquire fresh vigor for further laborious pursuits.

10. Laboring people should eat and sleep at regularly appointed times and not go too long between meals, for this is injurious. Three meals a day of good, substantial and nutritious food are absolutely required for field hands and other daily laborers.

11. Bad living or an insufficient amount of good food must be avoided; for hard labor and poor living breeds malignant fevers, diseases of the skin and other disorders. Too great a restriction to salt provisions and a scarcity of vegetables breeds the scurvy, a fact which all laborers should bear in mind.

Soldiers and sailors are often subjected to great hardships and deprivations. The former from the inclemency of seasons, long marches, bad provisions, hunger, watching, bad water, etc. The latter are similarly beset with great inconveniences and exposures. In order to protect the health of soldiers, their commanders should see that they are well fed and clothed, and when their campaign is finished they should be provided with dry, well aired winter quarters, and suitable hospitals should be provided for the sick entirely away from the camp. By following this rule the health of soldiers can be protected. But one great source of sickness among the sailors is the excesses into which they plunge when on shore. After having been' long at sea without regard to climate or their own constitutions, they are apt to plunge headlong into all manner of riot and licentiousness, until they become the victims of fatal diseases. When on duty they are necessarily exposed to all kinds of weather and frequent hardships, but when on land this useful and indispensable class of laborers should find friends to provide them with suitable homes and surroundings to protect them as much as possible from the dangerous excesses in which they are prone to indulge.

The unwholesome food, which sailors subsist upon when at sea, is a serious detriment to health. The salt provisions in constant use influence the blood and other humors and bring on scurvy and other obstinate disorders. To avoid this fresh provisions and vegetables should be supplied when practicable, and no ships should be laden with provisions for a sea voyage without a profusion of canned fruits and vegetables, which modern art and contrivance are able to supply in great abundance.

Sedentary habits are not conducive to health and yet employments of this kind are necessary in every community. The habits of females generally and those of a great proportion of males are decidedly sedentary in our large factories, yet a constant subjection for life to sedentary employments is quite unnecessary. A portion of each day only should be so occupied, for constant confinement is ruinous to health. Males and females may not be injured by confinement for five or six hours a day, but if obliged to sit twelve or fifteen hours they will soon become diseased. It is therefore a want of exercise alone that injures sedentary people. And if due attention is paid to this fact, some practical advantage may grow out of it.

Many who follow sedentary employments are constantly in a bending position as shoe-makers, tailors, cutters and grinders. Such constrained positions if long continued are extremely hurtful and as a consequence we find such complaining of indigestion, flatulence, headache or pain in the chest and disease of the lungs. In order to guard against all these injuries, manufacturers should set their wits to work to devise some provision for frequent change of posture for these useful tradesmen; and a like provision should be made for females to guard them against self-immolation to the altar of mammon, and, then we should have a less number of stooping, ill-shaped specimens of both sexes, and a less number of spinal difficulties to contend with.

A few rules for the sedentary may not be out of place and we therefore venture to give them.

1. Avoid as much as possible all awkward postures when at work, and guard against unstrained positions that may affect or weaken the respiratory and digestive organs.

2. Pay the strictest attention to cleanliness, especially when obliged to labor in apartments where a moiety of filth from each would taint the whole atmosphere and render it unsafe for inhalation.

3. Cherish a conscientious regard for temperance and wholesome food that will not taint the breath and be a serious annoyance by corrupting the air of the room, and also avoid flatulent food hard to digest.

4. Tailors, shoe-makers, seamstresses and all laborers confined to sitting postures when at work should seize every opportunity, when relieved temporarily from work to walk in the open air and not indulge in sedentary games.

5. Let every person, who leads a sedentary life, either male or female, secure the advantage of outdoor pursuits, such as cultivating a patch of soil or nursing and pruning a bed of flowers or plants to which a brief period of time may be devoted every day.

6. And finally let all such be regular at meals and exercise great care in eating slowly, allowing sufficient time for thorough mastication and further to refrain from indulgence in all kinds of liquors that muddle or intoxicate, and all unnecessary condiments, salads and pickles, and with the assurance that exercise out of doors as far as practicable in one shape or another is absolutely necessary to health, we append the advice to neglect no opportunity of indulging in it.

The effects of *too much* or *too intense study* upon the health has been with us a matter of observation for years. Intense thought upon any subject soon proves destructive to health; and as hard study always implies a sedentary life, a double influence of the kind cannot fail of undermining the most robust health. A few months of intense study and neglect of exercise will often ruin an excellent constitution and establish a train of nervous complaints which can never be removed.

So great is the power of the mind over the body that all the physical functions may be accelerated or retarded to an indefinite extent. Cheerfulness and mirth give rapidity to the circulation and activity to the secretions. Sadness has the contrary effect. Profound thought depresses the activity of the vital functions and often produces torpidity of the liver and derangement of the digestion and in order to secure relief and relaxation from perpetual study only a few hours in the day should be devoted to it.

Those who give themselves up to study without regard to the consequences soon become unfitted for the more rational enjoyments and are liable to become afflicted with gout, gravel, jaundice and deterioration of the blood. Numerous are the cases of pulmonary consumption, that have been caused by sedentary studious habits. Long sitting at the desk or table pouring over books will result in organic changes of the circulatory organs. A bending posture over the edge of a plain table while writing has been assigned as the cause of pericardium adhering to the breastbone in some instances. Continuous and profound thought often produces headache, vertigo and apoplexy. And when writing or studying by gas or candlelight is persisted in, the eyes become inflamed and the sight impaired, and, by reason of the excretions being interrupted, dropsy may result, as any one may observe that sitting makes his legs swell and that exercise may cause the swelling to disappear. Overstraining the mind in deep thought, sometimes results in nervous fevers and hypochondria, which seldom fails to accompany the wearing effects of long-continued study. Finally nothing can be more injurious than to make study the sole business.

When it becomes manifest that prolonged study is wearing upon the general health students should give heed to the following rules:

1. Discontinue the habit of constantly reading and writing and engage in pursuits that will occupy the thoughts in the open air and divert them from the business of the closet. Attention to more trivial subjects should supercede thoughts and study upon weightier matters. All work and no play for the mind makes it dull and despondent.

2. Those who read and write much should sit and stand by turns and should make choice of a large airy place for the exercise.

3. So to divide the time that a given number of hours may be allotted to study and then a season of relaxation and bodily exercise should follow. Walking or riding fails to give rest to the student, when he does not withdraw his mind from his pursuits and occupy his hours for relaxation with something mirthful, and even trivial, and this would prepare him to return to study refreshed and invigorated.

4. Students, on rising in the morning, should refrain from immediately entering the closet for study. But go forth with an empty stomach into the open air and indulge in walking, riding or athletic exercises and then return to their books, invigorated and prepared for several hours of thought and study.

5. Those fond of music may find much relaxation from the fatigue of study by playing on some instrument a few strains

or by singing such airs as have a tendency to rouse the spirits and inspire cheerfulness and good humor.

6. Always bear in mind that it is a reproach to students to betake themselves to strong drink to relieve them of the weariness of their toil, for this is a desperate remedy and always proves destructive. When one's spirits are depressed an indulgence in out-door sports will prove a more effectual remedy than any cordial or exhilarating liquor.

7. Good and wholesome food in moderation for students is a *sine qua non* and they should give some thought to a judicious variation of exercises so as to give action to all parts of the body.

8. Cold bathing in warm weather is a valuable substitute for exercise, which should not be neglected.

9. No one should resort to hard study or violent exercise upon a full stomach or immediately after a meal.

It is not to dampen the ardor of students that the evils connected with persistent hard study have thus been pointed out, and the above rules are commended, but to suggest to them the proper way of studying with ease and without permanently endangering the health, or in other words to teach them the art of being studious without foregoing the pleasures of life or seeking a monkish seclusion from outdoor pastimes and sports. It is possible to be serious and not sad, mirthful and not frivolous and cheerful without indulging in levity, all of which should receive proper attention from students.

CHAPTER VI.

THE SIGNS OF HEALTH AND HOW TO DENOTE ANY DEPARTURE FROM THE STANDARD.

The signs of health have already been given to some extent and in a general way in a preceding chapter and therefore we now proceed to note many particulars.

The skin or surface of the body is usually warm, soft and emollient, whereas in an unhealthy condition, it is dry, hot, shrivelled or cold.

The pulse. In a healthy condition the pulse is from 60 to 80 in a minute but in an unhealthy condition it varies materially. In persons of robust health, it varies in frequency from 60 to 80 a minute, but with such in a diseased condition it may be accelerated from eighty to one hundred or an hundred and twenty, thirty or forty. In a febrile condition the pulse may rise to 120 a minute, whereas in health it would be from 65 to 80. Therefore much depends upon the rate and quality of the pulse. But we can better appreciate the true condition of the entire organism by instituting a comparison between that which is normal and that produced by disease, and therefore we submit the following standard: *A healthy pulse in men* beats without irregularity from 60 to 80 times a minute, but in case of disease it may be much accelerated or depressed below the normal standard, and this points to the nature of the abnormal action. The condition of the pulse being ascertained, in order to estimate correctly we may say that in adults of both sexes it ranges from sixty to ninety a minute and any acceleration beyond this standard may indicate a diseased condition. Therefore we are able from the normal standard to form some idea of the nature and extent of certain derangements of the body, which affect the circulation. But to be more definite, the following table may be consulted:

In men of sound health, of the sanguine temperament, the pulse will range from 70 to 80 beats in a minute.

In those of the bilious temperament its average is from 60 to 70 beats in a minute.

In those of the nervous temperament it averages from 80 to 90 beats in a minute.

In those of a lymphatic temperament the average is from 50 to 60 beats in a minute.

In healthy adult women of these different temperaments the average is about ten per cent. more than in men.

In children under three years of age the average number of pulsations in a minute is from 110 to 120. In those from three to seven years of age the average pulsation in a minute is from 100 to 110, and from seven to the age of puberty the average number of pulsations is from 90 to 100 a minute. Thus it will be seen that the standard varies with age. In youth the pulse beats more vigorously and in old age it beats less frequently. And also the beats are more numerous when standing than in the sitting posture, and the sitting is marked by a greater number of beats, than the recumbent. It is necessary to be informed of all these peculiarities to prevent falling into great mistakes.

All practitioners of medicine attach great importance to the arterial pulse. It is expected of them as a matter of course that before prescribing they will feel the pulse and really the information revealed by doing so is often of the most interesting and instructive kind.

In disease the pulse may acquire a frequency, scarcely calculable, and the less so, because as it increases in frequency it beats more and more feebly. It will reach 150 to 160 and even 200 beats in a minute. At other times, in a different class of cases, its number of beats will diminish. In the case of a shock or concussion or in apoplexy or some organic affections of the heart; the pulse will become extremely slow. In a case of heart disease in a man sixty-eight years old attended with dropsy, his pulse sunk to 25 in a minute.

Irregularities of the pulse are full of meaning and interest. In some persons it is natural. We know a man of good sound health whose pulse is habitually irregular. But when we find a pulse that beats rapidly and slowly or is tense and soft in the same minute, we are led to inquire for the cause, and, when we find one that intermits every 6th or 7th or 8th beat, we know that something interrupts the regularity of the circulation. Disease of the head, organic disease of the heart, a simple disorder of the stomach or extreme debility, may cause irregularity;

and how important it must be to ascertain which produces this phenomena, and provided we become satisfied on this point, it suggests a treatment to ward off attendant or prospective difficulties.

The quality of the pulse also reveals the nature of disease. A hard, incompressible pulse denotes inflammation of a vascular kind. That which strikes the finger as a thread or wire, sometimes termed the wiry pulse, indicates a low state of the system such as might occur in nervous fever. Inflammatory continued fevers are revealed in the full, bounding or hard pulse and formerly was the indication for phlebotomy, but latterly for the use of Aconite. The wiry pulse denotes prostration and formerly suggested stimulants or Quinine, but latterly a class of febrifuges that relieve the depressed or excited condition of the nervous system. The full hard pulse may also indicate hypertrophy or enlargement of the left ventricle of the heart and suggests remedies that in some degree affect the heart's action. The full, hard pulse may be the result of excessive stimulation and suggests temperance, if not total abstinence. The quality of the pulse whether dependent on the head, disease of the cardiac organs of circulation or depressed condition of the nerves, always demands the most critical attention.

When we look upon a person in health we recognize unmistakable signs of the vital condition of his body. We find a good normal appetite for food and drink, and a freedom from suffering of any kind. This is kept in mind and when we find him void of appetite, afflicted with nausea and disgust for food and a consequent emaciation, we know that some cause is operating to produce a general derangement of the organic functions and this suggests the employment of remedies that will overcome the inappetency and restore the functions of digestion and nutrition.

When we find *healthy respiration* we find no obstruction to the normal oxidation of the blood; but when we find cough, expectoration and emaciation, we recognize a departure from the healthy standard, that calls for remedial measures for relief.

The tongue of a healthy person is free from every kind of abnormal coating and exhibits a moist and pliable condition for testing the qualities of food and drink. It is also the index of disease and when the stomach is diseased or the bowels disordered or when arterial excitement betrays a febrile condition, the tongue assumes an abnormal condition and therefore a patient would think it the result of carelessness or ignorance if the condition of the tongue was not duly inspected at every visit of his physician as well as the feeling of the pulse.

Urinary secretions.—In a healthy condition of the urinary apparatus a given quantity of urine of a clear amber color is secreted every twenty-four hours and there is no pain or obstruction to its passage into and out of the bladder. But when we find a departure from this condition and the urine is cloudy and deposits in the vessel a quantity of sediment we recognize it as evidence of the presence of disease.

The quantity of urine passed by an adult in good health averages forty ounces in twenty-four hours. This quantity is regarded the standard for a healthy person and its color should be of a citron yellow. Dr. Golding Bird notes three varieties of healthy urine: 1st, that which is passed a short time after drinking freely of fluids and generally pale and of low specific gravity, 1,003 to 1,009, secondly, that which is passed after the digestion of a full meal, sp. gr. 1,026 to 1,028 or even 1,030 and thirdly that which is secreted independently of the immediate stimulus of food and drink, as after a nights rest and of a sp. gr. of 1,015 to 1,025 and presents the essential characteristics of urine. An excessive discharge of urine, far beyond the normal standard is termed diabetes and is of two varieties. The one is an excessive flow of aqueous urine varying but little from that which is passed in health. The other is termed diabetes melitis, because it contains a large proportion of sacharine matters and the effect of this departure from the normal standard is extreme emaciation.

Albuminous urine denotes serious disease of the kidneys and may be ascertained by heating the urine in a test tube over a lamp; the heat will solidify the albumen.

Bloody urine denotes inflammatory disease of the bladder and urethra and is subject to medical treatment.

When there is *pain* in passing urine and a perpetual straining to void it, it may denote inflammation of the neck of the bladder or gravel. The passage of urinary calculi is indicated by severe pain in the region of the kidneys and an intensely severe colic, caused by small concretions passing through the ureters into the bladder.

Other abnormalities of the urinary apparatus are easily noted by taking cognizance of the deviations from the normal standard. The urine is highly colored or odorous or fetid in fevers, rheumatism, erysipelas, etc., all of which goes to prove that a knowledge of the normal function of the kidneys and the normal character of their excretion are essential in making a proper estimate of diseased conditions.

Perspiration is normal when it is inodorous, warm and serves as nature's mode of regulating the temperature of the body, but it denotes a malignant febrile condition when it is extremely odorous and fetid. It is acid in rheumatic diseases and indicates that acetic acid in the blood may cause inflammatory rheumatism or that lithic acid in the urine denotes a gouty diathesis.

When the urine is *scalding* or *acrid*, there must be some impurities in the system, which the kidneys are struggling to eliminate. It is important therefore, for everybody to understand the relation of the urine to the various conditions of health and disease.

The bile.—The liver, when in a healthy state, secretes a normal quantity of bile that aids digestion and is carried off with the innutritious matter separated from the food after it is reduced to chyme in the stomach and is passed into the intestine to become chyle. This healthy process is unattended by pain when the function of the biliary system is in a normal condition. Therefore the color of the skin is one of the means of judging of the normal or abnormal state of the bile. When the skin is ruddy or white, soft and emollient. it indicates that the bile is secreted and excreted by the liver through natural channels to aid the process of nutrition and maintain health. But when the skin is yellow or copper-colored, we at once know that the gall ducts are obstructed and that the bile is diverted from its normal passages and excreted through the pores of the skin, which becomes colored as in jaundice. And also its presence in the fæcal discharges from the bowels is wanting and the fæces are white or ash colored and denote derangement of the biliary system.

Fæcal discharges.—When the body is in health and all the organic functions are acting in harmony, the appetite is good, the stomach is in a healthy condition to digest food, the liver performs its office well in furnishing its product to aid in separating the innutritious matter from that which is nutritious and the former is carried downward through the intestines to be discharged as worthless, and, when the system is in a healthy condition there will be an evacuation of feculent matter duly discharged with bile, every twenty-four hours. But when there is an interruption of these healthy processes, the bowels become constipated or their contents may liquify and pass off in fluxes as in dysentery and diarrhœa. Therefore, a knowledge of healthy evacuations from the bowels is essential in forming a true estimate of diseased conditions. And finally, we must not lose sight of the general appearance of the healthy. In making proper *examinations of patients*, all the changes of sensible qualities must be noted,—the temperature of the body,—the color of the surface and especially of the face,—the diminution or increase in bulk,—emaciation and swelling,—whether general or partial, —the character of the circulation and also of secretions and excretions, that are ever-varying under the influence of disease, to which we shall have occasion to allude hereafter.

CHAPTER VII.

A GENERAL VIEW OF THE STRUCTURE OF THE HUMAN BODY.

Inasmuch as all parts of the human body are subject to disease, it is proper to glance at the various elements, that make up the structure.

1st. The bones form the framework of the body and give it firmness and strength. They form points of attachment for the numerous muscles and give shape to the human form. Each bone and its disposition are always adapted to the office it is designed to fulfil. The natural skeleton is formed of bones and ligaments, which unite them to each other and keep each in its place. It is divided into the *head, trunk, upper and lower extremities.* The head has eight bones, that in the aggregate form the skull and the face have fourteen. The upper extremities have 32 on each side and the lower extremities have 31 on each side. The trunk has 56, viz., 24 vertebræ in the spinal column, one sacrum, four coccygeal, two that form the resting place of the viscera of the abdomen, 12 ribs on each side and one sternum or breastbone. In all, the skeleton exclusive of the teeth and small bones of the ear, contains 200 bones varying in shape, as the long, short, flat and irregular. The long bones are found in the arms and legs, the short in the wrist, ankles, fingers and toes. The flat are found in the skull and the irregular are those of various shapes found in the temples, nose, palate, upper and lower jaws, etc.

The trunk is composed of the spine, thorax or chest, pelvis and abdominal walls. The spine is situated at the back part of the trunk and extends from the head to the lower opening of the pelvis and is a series of 24 movable joints, which rest upon the sacrum and the bones of the pelvis.

The upper extremities are divided on either side into shoulder, arm, forearm and hand.

The lower are divided on either side into the thigh, leg, knee and foot.

The bones are variously united; those of the head by sutures and those of the trunk and extremities by joints.

Cartilage is a pearly white substance, which enters into the structure of the joints, interposed between the bones, that are united together and movable in sockets and also in the immovable unions of the bones of the skull and pelvis. It is also found on the end of the nose, in the eyelids, the ear, windpipe, end of ribs, etc.

There is a dense membrane surrounding the bones, called periosteum and that which surrounds the cartilages is quite similar and is called perichondrium.

Ligaments are composed of white fibrous tissue, very firm and unyielding and generally diffused in the human body. They serve to tie the bones together and hence we find two kinds, one is called capsular, because they envelope the ends of the bones as caps on the head. The other is termed funicular, because they are mere cords that extend from one bone to another.

There are different forms of articulation or joining the bones together. Some are immovably connected with each other, some have a partial movement as the joints of the spine, some have a free movement as the shoulder, elbow, hip, knee and the great number of the joints of the body. All the movable joints are lined by a membranous sac that secretes a kind of watery fluid, which is termed synovial because it resembles the white of an egg and the office of this synovial membrane is to lubricate and prevent friction.

From this it will be seen that bone, cartilage, fibro-cartilage, ligaments and synovial membrane are the structures entering into the composition of joints.

The integuments of the body are the areolar and adipose tissues and the skin or outer covering of the body. *The areolar tissue* is generally disseminated over the whole body and found beneath the skin between the muscles, connecting membranes and other parts, entering into their composition and indispensible to their texture. *The adipose tissue* is found between the skin and the thin membrane that covers the muscles and intermingles with the fibrous tissue in various parts of the body.

The outer integument of the body or the dermoid covering consists of the skin and its sebaceous follicles—the nails and the hair. The skin has two layers, the cuticle and cutis vera. The oily exhalation of the skin that lubricates its surface is from the sebaceous follicles. The nails are simply the direct continuation of the cuticle.

The muscles form the contractile tissue of the body by, or through which the various motions of the joints, limbs, hands, fingers and toes are affected. The muscles are red, soft and irritable and contractile. They are divided into involuntary and voluntary. The latter are subject to the will which proves the most powerful stimulus to muscular contraction. By it the hand is directed in seizing, grasping, nipping, pinching, squeezing, etc., etc. And the muscles of the lower extremities are set to contracting so as to favor locomotion. The involuntary muscles are those not dependent on the will for their contractile force, the heart for example. The intercostal muscles are partly involuntary and partly voluntary as are all the muscles concerned in respiration. Many of the large and long muscles terminate in tendons which have a white shiny appearance and possess no elasticity or power of elongation or contraction.

The digestive organs consist in an uninterrupted canal extending from the lips to the anus. This is usually termed the alimentary canal and is divided into three portions, the upper, middle and lower. The upper is the mouth, pharynx and gullet, —the middle is the stomach and small intestines and the lower is the large intestine.

The glandular bodies in the alimentary canal are the salivary glands, pancreas, liver, spleen and a large number of little glands, extending along the whole course of the canal.

The mouth contains the teeth, tongue, palate, salivary glands and pharynx, which is the opening into the passage to the stomach.

The abdomen contains the digestive organs and those of assimilation, the secretory and excretory apparatus and the organs of reproduction in the female. The abdomen is divided into six distinct regions by drawing one line round the body parallel with the cartilages of the ninth rib and another in the same way on a level with the highest point of the pelvis and subdividing by drawing a line from the cartilage of the eighth rib on each side perpendicularly. The upper central region is called the epigastric, on either side of which we have the right and left hypochondriac. The middle central is the umbilical or region of the navel. On each side of this we have the right and left lumbar. The middle central region is termed the hypogastric with the right and left iliac region on either side.

The pit of the stomach is the hollow in the epigastric regions. The liver occupies nearly the whole of the right hypochondriac and the upper half of the epigastric region.

The spleen is situated in the back part of the left hypochondriac region. The stomach occupies the lower half of the epigastric region and the greater portion of the left hypochondriac. The small intestine is situated in the umbilical and hypogastric regions and a portion of the right and left lumbar.

The large intestine has its beginning in the right iliac and ascends through the right lumbar and passes into the lower part of the epigastric or upper part of the umbilical according to the state of distension of the stomach, thence into the left hypochondriac, left lumbar and left iliac, passes into the pelvis and descending in front of the sacrum terminates in the anus.

The pancreas is situated across the lower back part of the epigastric region extending from the left to the right hypochondriac and is placed behind the stomach which covers it.

The kidneys are situated in the lower portion of the hypochondria and the upper part of the lumbar region on each side of the spine; the bladder and the rectum are in the pelvis and between them in the female are the uterus, ovaries and vagina.

The peritoneum is a serous membrane lining the abdomen and folded over the outer walls of the viscera. Like all the serous membranes it forms a closed sac with no opening in the male, but in the female there is one through the fallopian tubes. The processes of the peritoneum are known under the general name of omenta.

The stomach and intestines which form the alimentary canal are thirty-five feet in length in adults of average growth. The stomach has the greatest capacity and receives immediately, through the œsophagus and cardiac orifice, the food and drink. The pyloric orifice opens into the small intestine, and thus a channel is prepared for the exit of the contents of the stomach. The first twelve inches of the small intestine is called the duodenum or second stomach, the remaining portion is divided into the jejunum and ileum.

The large intestine exceeds the diameter of the small and receives the effete matter therefrom. It commences at the lower portion of the small intestine and terminates at the anus. The entire cavity of the alimentary canal is lined by a mucous membrane which seems to be a continuation of the skin.

The liver secretes the bile. It is situated in the right hypochondrium. It is the largest gland of the body and is supplied with ligaments. It weighs in the adult about five pounds. The upper surface lies in contact with the diaphragm and the gall bladder is situated in a fissure of the under surface and forms a reservoir for the bile.

The spleen is situated in the back part of the left hypochondriac region, contiguous to the diaphragm above and the colon below and has no excretory duct.

The urinary organs are the kidneys, bladder and urethra. The kidneys secrete the urine and pass it through the ureters into the bladder. These are two small bodies one on either side placed upon the top of the kidney and called the suprarenal capsules.

The bladder is the reservoir for the urine, situated in the pelvis just behind the pubic bones. *The urethra* is a canal which extends from the neck of the bladder to the extremity of the glans penis.

The organs of generation in the male are the penis and testicles with their appendages. The penis is formed of the integument, areolar tissue, corpora cavernosa and the corpus spongiosum urethræ. The prostate gland is a body about the size of a horse chesnut fixed on the neck of the bladder and penetrated by the urethra.

The testicles are two glandular bodies one on each side of the scrotum which is a continuation of the skin to form a pouch for them to rest in. They secrete the seminal fluid.

The female organs of generation are the vulva, vagina, uterus and the ovaries. The vagina is the canal leading from the vulva to the womb. The womb or uterus is a compressed pyriform body of great elasticity, attached by ligaments and at its upper extremity to the right and left are the Fallopian tubes. *The ovaries* are two glandular bodies situated on the back side of the broad ligaments of the womb and about half the size of the testicles in the male.

The organs of respiration are the larynx, trachea and lungs. The larynx is an irregular cartilaginous tube forming the upper part of the windpipe and is supplied with muscles and nerves.

The *trachea* is a continuous tube from the larynx. It divides into two parts when it reaches the upper portion of the chest, one part goes to the right and the other to the left, dividing and sub-dividing as they permeate the lungs. They constitute the bronchia.

The lungs are two bodies, divided by the heart into right and left. The thorax or chest is the cavity which they occupy. The right lung has three lobes and the left two. The pleura is a serous membrane, one portion of which lines the cavity of the chest and the other covers the lungs. Like all serous membranes it forms a shut sac and between the portion that covers the walls of the chest and that which covers the lungs is the pleural cavity.

The circulatory system is composed of the heart arteries, veins and capillaries. The heart has four cavities. The course and description of the circulation are as follows: The blood after getting to the right auricle is forced into the right ventricle and from the right ventricle into the lungs whence it is returned to the left auricle and forced from this into the left ventricle from which it is propelled into the arteries. The capillaries are the minute terminations of the arteries which inosculate with the veins. The arteries contain the renovated or red blood sent from the heart to nourish the various organs of the body and the veins convey the dark blood before it is purified and renovated to the heart.

The heart is situated between the sternum and the spine, having the lungs on either side. Its weight is from eight to twelve ounces and about 5 or 5½ inches in length and at its base about 3½ inches in diameter. Its four cavities are named: right auricle, right ventricle, left auricle and left ventricle. The *great trunk* of the *arterial system* is called the *Aorta* and this gives off branches first to the heart and then to the more remote organs and parts of the body. The arteries are variously named to signify the organs and parts to which they convey the blood.

The venous system is composed of the veins that collect the blood from the arteries in all parts of the body and return it to the heart. Two veins accompany each artery whenever the part is intended for locomotion. The great trunk of the venous system is called the vena cava ascendens and descendens.

The absorbent or lymphatic system are the lacteal and lymphatic vessels. The former absorb the chyle and the lymphatics in various parts of the system absorb the lymph, secreted by the lymphatic glands. The main trunk of these vessels is called the thoracic duct through which the lacteal and lymphatic vessels pour their products into the veins.

The nervous system is composed of the brain and spinal marrow and the nerves sent forth into all parts of the body from these centres. There are two distinct systems that operate in the body, the cerebro-spinal and the sympathetic. The former preside over the animal functions and the latter over the organic, and extend from the base of the cranium to the lower extremity of the sacrum in a series of ganglions. The five special senses are supplied by nerves from the brain, as the optic, olfactory, auricular gustatory and tactile and thus the eye, nose, ear, tongue, palate and sense of touch are duly provided with nervous distributions to provide for the special senses of sight, smell, hearing, taste and touch,—while all the functions operating to provide for the nourishment of the body are supplied from the sympathetic system.

This brief view of the salient points in anatomy is intended to give a general outline of the structure of the body and nothing more. The student who desires a thorough knowledge of the anatomy of the human body will find greater satisfaction in learning particulars from works that enter fully into a minute description of the various organs and parts.

CHAPTER VIII.

A GENERAL VIEW OF PHYSIOLOGY.

All bodies or forms of matter are considered under two different heads—the inorganic and the organic. Inorganic bodies possess the common properties of matter, and their elements under ordinary circumstances are fixed. Organic bodies have properties in common with the inorganic, but they also have others controlling the first in a remarkable manner. Their elements are undergoing constant changes and the sciences which give us a knowledge of these changes as well as of their structure and function are called Anatomy and Physiology.

Inorganic forms differ in regard to their origin, shape, size and chemical character. They also differ in texture, mode of preservation, termination and motive forces.

The object of the science of physiology is to explain the mode in which living beings are born, nourished, reproduced and die. The organic bodies are divided into animal and vegetable, and these differ from each other in the composition, texture, sensation, voluntary motion, nutrition and reproduction. The two kinds of elements therefore, which enter into the composition of the human body are the chemical or inorganic and the organic, which are compounds and the results of vital forces.

The chemical or inorganic forces are oxygen, hydrogen, carbon, nitrogen, phosphorus and lime and in smaller proportions, sulphur, iron, manganese, silicum, aluminium, chlorine, etc., etc. The elements of animal bodies are essentially oxygen, hydrogen, carbon and nitrogen as a general principle.

The organic elements are divided into those which contain nitrogen and those which do not. Those which contain nitrogen are albumen, fibrin, casein or the red coloring matter of the blood, hæmatin or the yellow coloring principle of the bile.

Those which do not contain nitrogen are olein, stearin and the fatty matter of the brain and nerves and other elements. The component parts of the animal bodies are solids and fluids. The solids are bone, cartilage, muscle, ligaments, nerves, etc. The membranes are divided into simple and compound, the former are the serous, mucous and fibrous. The latter are the fibro-serous, sero-mucous and fibro-mucous.

The primary tissues are the areolar, the muscular, the nervous and the albugineous. These tissues uniting form the primary order of solids and again by union they give rise to compound solids, from which bones, glands, etc., are formed. The solids are arranged in filaments or fibres, tissues, organs, apparatus and systems.

A number of filaments united together constitutes a *fibre*. *An organ* is a compound of several fibres and tissues. An *apparatus* is an assemblage of organs arranged for a common purpose. *A system* is made up of organs possessing the same or a similar character. For example, all the nerves of the body constitute the nervous system. The same with the muscles and blood vessels; taken collectively they constitute the muscular and vascular system.

The proportion of the solids and fluids by weight in the body is not easy to estimate. *The fluids* have been classified into chyme, chyle, lymph, blood, perspired fluids, follicular and glandular.

The physical properties of the tissues are elasticity, extensibility, flexibility and imbibition.

Functions of the Living Human Body.

There are three classes, viz., animal, nutritive and reproductive.

The animal functions are muscular motion, sensibility and mental manifestation. *The nutritive* are digestion, absorption, respiration, circulation, assimilation, calorification and secretion.

The reproductive function includes generation. The forces that preside over the various functions are either physical or vital. We will proceed to notice the functions in their order.

1st. *The animal functions.* The faculty of feeling or being impressed is what is understood by *sensibility* and this may be either *conscious* or *unconscious*, the former is termed animal and the latter organic sensibility. The whole nervous system is concerned in the function. *Marshall Hall* makes three divisions of the nervous system, viz., the cerebral or the sentient and voluntary, the true spinal or excito-motory and the ganglionic or the nutrient and secretory. The sentient sphere includes sensations and intellectual and moral manifestations. Sensations may be either *external* or *internal*. The external are the impressions or perceptions occasioned by objects entirely external to the part impressed. The external senses are touch, taste, smell, hearing and sight. The sense of touch is located in the skin and is most prominent in the fingers, that of taste in the tongue, that of smell in the nose, that of hearing in the ears and that of sight in the eyes. Each of these organs are adapted to receive impressions from external objects and to convey through their respective nerves the intelligence gained of their qualities to the *sensorium* or brain. Hunger and thirst are examples of *internal sensation*.

Voluntary muscular motion is that which is effected by the muscular system of animal life, under the influence of the will and is shown in the acts of locomotion or prehension. The muscles are excited to action through nerves proceeding from the head and spinal marrow termed excito-motory.

Involuntary muscular motion is connected with the muscular system and the vermicular movements of the stomach and bowels are examples.

There are *seven* of the nutritive functions which effect the composition and decomposition of the body. They are digestion, absorption, respiration, circulation, nutrition, calorification and secretion. Digestion is the process of breaking down the food in the stomach and intestines so as to prepare the nutritive portion for *absorption*. The first product of digestion is *chyme* which is a mixture of the nutritious and innutritious parts of the aliment reduced to a semi-fluid state in the stomach. The next is the *chyle* which consists of the nutritive parts of the aliment separated from the innutritive through the agency of the bile. This fluid, which is milk-like in its appearance is destined to replenish the blood.

Absorption is the process of taking up the chyle from the intestinal canal and passing it into the veins. It is done by a class of vessels called the chyliferous to indicate their office. Absorption also may take place of other extraneous matters from the surface of the body and the mucous membranes and of matters which form a part of the body itself.

Respiration is the function by which venous blood is converted into arterial. But to understand the matter fully we will now revert to the subject of digestion and note the consecutive changes of the solid food, which is first masticated and insalivated in the mouth and then passed into the stomach and changed into chyme, which is passed from the stomach into the small intestine where the process of separating that which is feculent and useless from that which is fit to be made into blood and here called chyle, takes place. The biliary secretion forms a chemical union with the innutritious portion, which is urged onward in the alimentary canal and finally discharged in the form of fæces. The chyle is taken up by the chyliferous vessels and passed through the thoracic duct into the veins and thence to the right auricle of the heart and then to the right ventricle, and from the right ventricle it passes through the pulmonary artery into the lungs and permeates every portion thereof. The act of respiration brings the atmosphere in contact with the impure venous blood thus distributed and imparts to it its oxygen and purifies it. It is now converted into arterial blood and is taken up by the four pulmonary veins and returned to the left auricle of the heart and thence into the left ventricle and from this chamber it is sent forth through the arterial to nourish all the tissues of the body. It will thus be seen that respiration converts the venous blood with all its absorbed matters into arterial blood by a function termed hæmatosis. This conversion takes place in the air vesicles where the blood receives some of the constituents of the atmosphere and yields some of its own in return.

The function of respiration is performed partly by voluntary, partly by involuntary muscles and consists of two acts, which are termed inspiration and expiration. The average number of respirations in a minute is about eighteen. The act of respiration brings air containing oxygen into the lungs and exchanges it for carbonic acid.

The function of circulation is designed to effect an equitable distribution of the blood to the venous parts of the body and its return to the great central organ, the heart.

Nutrition comprises the changes which are constantly taking place in the body, both of absorption and deposition and which renovate each organ or portion of each organized living bodies. The work is carried on by two sets of minute vessels termed exhalants and absorbents.

7

By *the function of colorification* is understood the power to preserve the temperature of bodies independent of surrounding temperature, within certain limits and this is done through the combined influence of respiration, innervation and circulation. The temperature is maintained against cold by these three independent functions. The same is maintained against heat by the elimination of aqueous matter from the system and its evaporation from the surface of the body.

The *function of secretion* separates from the blood the various humors of the body, and this is effected through the follicles of the skin and mucous membrane and the various glands, as the liver, etc. The serous exhalations are secreted by the serous membranes as the pleura, pericardium, peritoneum, arachnoid coat of the brain and the tunica vaginalis testis. In health the serous fluid lubricates these cavities.

The organ upon which the adipose exhalation depends is the vesicle in which the fat is included and is attached to the cellular tissue. The organic elements of fat are olein, stearin, margarin and glycerine. The uses of fat are both local and general. The former serves to diminish the effects of pressure by forming a cushion, by filling up cavities or interstices so as to give a rounded form and contour to the body. The latter serves as a provision in time of need, whether from indisposition or abstinence from food. The *medullary membrane* on which the marrow depends exists in the interior of the bones and serves the general purpose of fat. The synovial membrane secretes the synovial fluid to lubricate the joints.

The *reproductive functions* are included under the head of generation and as peculiar to organized bodies exclusively. The simplest form of generation is where an animal at a certain period of its existence separates into pieces and each forms a new individual. This is called generation by spontaneous division. Gemmiferous generation consists in the formation of buds or germs upon parts of the body, that develop and drop off and form new individuals.

But higher up in the scale, the organs of generation become separate and are divided into male and female and sometimes both exist in the same individual; higher up still they belong to distinct individuals and copulation is the condition of generation. Oviparous generation is that which occurs from eggs out of the body and viviparous generation is when the ovum is detached from the ovary soon after copulation and then is deposited in the uterus or womb, there to be developed until the proper period for its expulsion and after which it may be further nourished by a peculiar and appropriate secretion furnished from the mother, and this is the case with human beings. This viviparous generation and the different acts necessary for reproduction are copulation, conception or fecundation, gestation or pregnancy, delivery or accouchement and lactation or the nourishment of young infants with milk.

The male organs of generation consist of the penis, testicles and their excreting ducts called vasa deferentia, the seminal vesicles and two canals called the ejaculatory ducts. The testicles secrete the sperm. When formed it is passed into the seminal tubes and finally deposited in the seminal vesicles until it is discharged into the urethra during sexual excitement.

The female organs of generation are the vulva, vagina, ovaries, womb and mammary glands.

The periodical discharge of a bloody fluid from the vulva every twenty-eight days is termed *menstruation*, catamenia, flowers, etc., and continues unless interrupted by pregnancy until the critical age or time of its complete cessation.

Its first appearance denotes the capability of becoming pregnant. Conception occurs in the ovary and, in about ten or twelve days after, the impregnated ovum comes into the womb. Conception may take place without any sensible signs of the fact. The period of gestation is about nine calendar months or forty weeks.

The different ages are designated by the terms infancy, childhood, puberty, adolescence, manhood and old age.

Individual differences among mankind have been alluded to under the head of *temperaments, constitutions, habits, idiosyncrases,* etc., all of which require a passing notice. By *temperament* is understood the individual difference produced by the predominance of different functions that exert a controlling influence in the body as for instance an extensive biliary system results in the *bilious* temperament. A large and controlling influence of the blood-vessels indicates the *sanguine* temperament. A large and controlling nervous system is marked by the *nervous* temperament, etc.

By *constitutions* are understood the mode of organization, proper to individuals and by *idiosyncrases* are understood certain peculiar dispositions to be affected by extraneous objects different from the manner in which they affect mankind in general.

We have thus given an outline of physiology far from being complete and yet sufficient for the purposes contemplated in this work; for a more elaborate knowledge of this branch, the specific treatises on this science are commended.

CHAPTER IX.

MATERIA MEDICA AND THERAPEUTICS.

By Materia Medica is understood the materials employed for medicines or remedial agents in curing or palliating disease. Therapeutics signifies a branch of medicine that has for its object the treatment of diseases. With the definitions in mind we will proceed to note the following particulars:

By the term "Materia Medica" in the former schools of medicine the natural history of medicines and their properties and uses as founded upon clinical experience is meant. In *the Homœopathic school* the term means: "the natural history and mode of preparation of each plant, mineral and animal substance used in medicine and also a faithful record of its physiological effect upon persons in health."

In the cure of disease there are but three possible ways in which medicines can act, as derivatives, by counter-irritation, antipathic or by producing symptoms of an opposite nature to those of the disease and Homœopathic by administering remedies capable of producing similar effects to those which are to be removed.

The *antipathic* method was the Hippocratic doctrine expressed in the phrase, *contraria contrariis curantur.*

The *allopathic* method varies in some respects as it implies the employment of agents whose action is neither similar nor exactly opposite to that of the disease. Under this mode of treatment therefore is included that mode of cure effected by counter-irritation, that is, the production of an artificial or secondary disease to remove a primary one. This mode of treatment is professedly derived from observation of the influence of maladies exerting mutually an influence over each other. For instance it has been remarked that a spontaneous diarrhœa will remove the headache or some other internal suffering that primarily existed and therefore this fact suggests the employment of cathartics.

Revulsion and derivation are both cases of counter-irritation. The artificial disease produced by revulsion is produced in a part

101

remote from the seat of the primary malady. For instance leeches or blisters applied to the feet in apoplexy are called revulsives, but the same applications to the head in the same disease would be called derivatives. Although there is this distinction between revulsives and derivatives, there is but little difference.

The Homœopathic method of curing or rather of treating them consists in administering a medicine capable of producing effects similar to the one to be removed and this doctrine is expressed in the phrase "similia similibus curantur." This doctrine was propounded by Hahnemann in 1796 and was afterwards arranged systematically and published in 1810. In proof of the doctrine elucidated by him he cites from Hippocrates a case of cholera cured by Veratrum which several high authorities maintain is capable of producing a kind of cholera itself. He also cites that fearful sweating sickness of A. D. 1415 in England, which was so fearfully fatal and the fact that a cure was found in sudorifics. Dysentery can be produced by Gambogia and Mercurius corrosivus and yet no remedies have been found that will cure the disorder so speedily and effectually. Colchicum will both produce and cure the dropsy. Ipecac will both produce and cure the asthma. Belladonna will both produce and cure the headache. Jalap produces colic and will cure the same in young children. Senna will do the same.

Of the three methods of treating diseases alluded to above we prefer the latter, because from observation we are satisfied that it is the speediest and safest method of cure, and moreover, we think it the most rational and the nearest to nature's demands. Let us look at the subject in the light of reason and facts. Let us suppose a case of fever, produced from cold. At first there is a chill, pain in the bones and a general uneasy aching all over and then there is headache, pain in the back, furred tongue, hot skin, acceleration of the pulse, constipation of the bowels, etc. The cold is the cause of all these symptoms and they simply manifest nature's struggles to get rid of the cause. A certain class of vital tissues have become excited and active in the matter. Now Aconite tincture given to a healthy person will produce a similar struggle marked by very similar symptoms to get rid of it, thus showing its power to excite activity in the same class of vital tissues. This remedy therefore, is Homœopathic to the case and it will effect a speedy cure and why? It travels after the disease, renders aid to that class of organs struggling to throw it off and what can be more reasonable? In asthma the difficult breathing, cough and expectoration are but evidences of nature's struggle to relieve the patient. Ipecac will cause a similar struggle in a healthy person and Ipecac will afford prompt relief in asthma, because the remedy is Homœopathic to the case. Many instances of a similar kind might be cited, where almost every days observation confirms the fact that diseases characterized by a certain group of symptoms are removed by medicines known to act upon the healthy in a way to produce a similar group of symptoms. Thus Senna will produce a colic and will cure a similar one. Opium will produce sopor and stupidity and will remove these symptoms, when produced by disease. Rheum will cause a diarrhœa and will cure a similar diarrhœa when produced by disease and observations apparently confirm the fact, that this law generally prevails in the therapeutic use of medicines.

But only a small or infinitesimal dose of the right remedy is required to effect a cure in all curable diseases and this is attributable to the fact that a diseased and irritable condition is easily impressed. An inflamed eye can bear but little light, an irritable stomach cannot bear much food and this holds good in the consideration of all diseases. A healthy system is capable of resisting the ill effects of noxious agents whereas a diseased and sensitive condition is easily affected by almost inappreciable quantities of them. Therefore to give a concentrated medicine to act on the same tissues, assailed by the disease or excited by it might produce dangerous and unwarrantable aggravations. It will be seen therefore, that small doses are suggested by the fact that they are to aid the struggles of nature and not to increase their violence beyond necessary limits. And besides, remedies are addressed to vital forces already aroused and the way is open for their action in the most attenuated form. It has been observed by several eminent writers that Belladonna will produce all the symptoms of a paroxysm of hydrophobia and these writers assert that they have cured this disease repeatedly by administering small doses of this medicine. Hartlaub and Trinks maintain that Cantharides will also accord with the same description. "Opium," says Pereira, "cures lethargy and stupor by converting it into a natural sleep and constipation is sometimes cured by the same substance. On Homœopathic principles vaccination protects from

the small-pox. Cold is the best application to frost-bitten parts.
Burns and scalds are the soonest relieved by exposing the parts
to heat or to bathing them with heated stimulants containing
turpentine."

It was maintained by Hahnemann that diseases are cured by
similar counter acting diseases produced by medicines as follows:
"The medicine sets up in the suffering part of the organism an
artificial and somewhat stronger disease, which on account of its
great similarity and preponderating influence takes the place of
the former and the organism from this time is only affected by
the artificial complaint, and, this from the minute dose of the
medicine used soon subsides and leaves the patient altogether
free from the disease. The secondary effects of large doses of
medicine are always injurious and it is very necessary to use no
more than is absolutely requisite, for it has been found by experiment that the medicinal effects do not decrease in the proportion
to the diminution of the dose.

Mixtures and compound mixtures of medicines are not used
in Homœopathic practice, because of the great uncertainty of
their precise action. Hence the crude forms of medicines as
found chemically pure in the three kingdoms of nature are employed from which to manufacture the attenuations in use.
Tinctures are made by expressing the juice of the fresh plant,
which is added to an equal proportion of deodorized alcohol.
Mineral medicines are prepared by reducing them to a powder
and by reducing their strength by triturating them in definite
proportions of sugar of milk, until medicinal virtue is developed.
Dilutions are made by reducing tinctures with deodorized alcohol.
The globules are prepared by saturating them with the dilutions.

We have thus alluded to the three methods of cure that have
been continued in use up to the present time, viz., the Antipathic, Allopathic and Homœopathic and it will be necessary
hereafter to illustrate by examples the comparative utility of
each. In order therefore to give some practical idea of the characteristic action of various remedies found in the materia medica,
we will proceed in order:

1. *Aconitum napellus*, wolfsbane. When properly prepared this remedy is the best febrifuge known. It allays vascular excitement, dry burning heat of the skin, restlessness, anxiety,
palpitation of the heart, pleurisy, inflammation of the lungs,

croup, measles, inflammatory rheumatism, asthma, apoplexy, pulmonary hæmorrhage, short and dry cough from a cold, anxious urging to urinate, great thirst, sleeplessness owing to mental anxiety. When fever is present with any of the above symptoms Aconite should initiate the treatment in every case.

2. *Æsculus glabra*, Ohio buckeye, useful in hæmorrhoids, vertigo with nausea, great weakness, etc.

3. *Æsculus hippocastanum*, horse chestnut, useful in spasmodic asthma, hypochondria, constipation, piles and torpor of the liver and also in hæmorrhoidal headaches, coryza, catarrh, waterbrash with pyrosis, in congestive and flatulent colic, chronic affections of the rectum, internal piles, etc.

4. *Agaricus muscarius*, bug agaric. The range of use which this remedy has may be found in those affections which cause the whole body to be very sensitive and especially when the extremities and joints feel lamed and bruised after moderate exercise; itching, burning and redness of the skin in different parts as if frozen; drowsiness in the day time, great chilliness and ailments which break out crosswise as in the left leg and right arm. Epilepsy.

5. *Agnus castus*, chaste tree, is an important remedy for deficiency in milk in the case of lying-in women, sterility, suppressed menses, chronic distortion of the joints, swelling and induration of the spleen, suppression of the sexual instinct and deficient erections, etc.

6. *Alumina* is useful for trembling of the extremities and involuntary motions and twisting of the limbs; herpes and humid scurfs; purulent discharge from the ear; swelling and redness of the nose with discharge of thick yellow mucus, ulceration of the nose; blotches upon the face, sore throat, disposition to catarrh; whooping cough, dry cough early in the morning, short dry cough with stoppage of breath. This remedy for acrid leucorrhœa is highly commended and for tedious constipation in pregnant women and also for constipation in children it is a valuable remedy.

7. *Ambra grisea* addresses itself to cramps in the muscles, twitching and spasm in muscular parts; pains worse in the evening; single parts are prone to go to sleep, vascular excitement and pulsations in the whole body and languor. The whole surface of the body feels numb; chilliness in the morning and flashes of

heat and anxiety in the region of the heart; disconsolate and sad; anxiety in the evening; vertigo when walking, heat of the head, rush of blood to the head; pains in the liver, heaviness and distension of the abdomen, colic, constipation; increase of urine at night; hoarseness, tickling cough at night; oppression of the chest; disposition of the upper and lower extremities to go to sleep.

8. *Ammonium carbonicum*, carbonate of ammonia is indicated in debility, headache and nausea, drowsiness, anxiety, vertigo and pain in the head as if it would split; hardness of hearing, swelling of the parotid glands; bitter taste in the mouth, heartburn, pain in the stomach and nausea, constipation; dryness of the nose and dry coryza; dry cough at night, difficult respiration; palpitation of the heart; the back and nape of the neck feel painful as if sprained or bruised.

9. *Ammonium muriaticum* is indicated for a paralytic weakness and languor, rigidity of the joints with pains in the extremities at night. Coldness and chilliness in the evening and sweat at night; increase of urine at night, pains in the kidneys; pains in the upper and lower extremities.

10. *Anacardium*, malacca bean, for pain in the occiput; dimness of sight as from cobwebs before the eyes; fetid breath; excited or diminished sexual excitement; cough with vomiting of food, trembling of the hand and burning of the soles of the feet.

11. *Antimonium crudum* or crude antimony is indicated for lienteria, nausea and vomiting of bile, heartburn and dyspepsia; indurations of the skin and spongy swelling of the knee.

12. *Apis mellifica*, honey bee, is useful in dropsy after scarlatina or measles, stings of insects, hydrothorax and hydrocephalus; dropsy of the ovaries and urethra; swelling of the knees, nettle rash, etc.

13. *Argentum* is useful for chronic affections of the larnyx, sore throat, clergyman's sore throat and sore throat from singing and speaking, etc.

14. *Argentum nitricum*, nitrate of silver. This remedy is directed against epilepsy with dullness of the head; dropsy dependent on affections of the liver: catarrhal and syphilitic sore eyes; deficient sexual desire; loose spongy gums that easily

bleed; hysteric colic, etc.; cough with or induced by constant titillation of the larynx, nightly palpitation of the heart.

15. *Arsenicum*, arsenious acid, is directed against extreme thirst and all pains characterized by burning whether internal or external; sudden prostration of strength; watery diarrhoea with burning pain in the bowels and anus, fetid diarrhoea with coldness of the surface and sunken countenance, dysentery with discharge of pure blood and violent burning tenesmus; fever with simultaneous chilliness and heat; last stage of Asiatic cholera, when the breath is cold. · It is a valuable remedy in asthma, nocturnal palpitation of the heart, ascites, hydrothorax, anasarca and hydrocephalus. It is indicated in intermittents, when there is absence of thirst during the chill; dropsical bloat of the body after the use of quinine. Extreme emaciation in typhus fever, etc.

16. *Arnica montana*, leopard's bane. The great utility of this remedy is found in mechanical injuries, bruises, sprains, blows, or fevers arising from thence. It may be used internally and externally for all pains characterized by great soreness or sensation as if bruised. It has been found of great utility in renal colic and for gravel. In apoplexy, tetanus, trismus and other nervous diseases it fills an important place. In whooping cough when the victims cry in dread before a paroxysm, or after any violent fit of coughing that has produced soreness of the chest or bowels. It is a valuable remedy for intermittents when the flesh feels sore as if bruised and for dysentery when the tenesmus has the sensation of soreness as if bruised.

17. *Assafœtida* is suitable for nervous restlessness, hysteria, intermittent pains, pulsative, stinging and tearing and bone-pains after the suppression of syphilis and especially when agravated by the warmth of the bed; cough, expectoration.

18. *Aurum foliatum*, goldleaf, is indicated for nightly bone pains, inflammation and caries of the bones, produced by either syphilis or mercury. It is indicated in melancholic temperaments inclined to suicide. It is useful in hernia and prolapsus uteri after Nux vom. Fearful and oppressive anxiety and longing for death, jumping of the heart, better in the open air.

19. *Aurum muriaticum*. Ulceration of the bones of the nose, caries of the bones of the face, head and spine; secondary syphilis, affecting the palate; induration of the testicles, suppuration of

the inguinal glands and also for depression of spirits and for the mania of suicide.

20. *Baptisia tinctoria*, wild indigo, useful in low fevers, whether of a gastric, bilious or nervous character. The keynotes for its use are coma, foul breath, thickly-coated tongue, fetid eructations, diarrhœa. ulceration of the bowels; dysentery.

21. *Baryta carbonica*, carbonate of baryta, useful in affections of old people, scrofulous ailments, atrophy of children with large bowels and glandular swellings; paralysis after apoplexy; humid and dry scaldhead, falling off of the hair; enlarged and inflamed tonsils; weakness of the male organs and in females aversion to sexual intercourse, painful stiffness of the back and nape of the neck; ulcers on the legs, fetid sweat of the feet and pains in the left side of the body while sitting; they pass off during exercise in the open air.

22. *Belladonna*, deadly nightshade. This remedy acts decidedly on the brain and is useful in vertigo and inflammation of the brain, meningeal inflammation, delirium, screaming of children without any apparent cause, headache over the eyes, hemicrania, heat and swelling of the face, erysipelas, neuralgia of the face, toothache; scarlet fever, measles, swelling and induration of the glands, weak sight, rush of blood to the head and chest; apoplexy violent, chilliness; congestions of the chest, bowels and uterus; angina pectoris or neuralgia of the heart; sore eyes, throat and other congestive or inflammatory affections.

23. *Borax.* For ailments arising from taking cold in damp and chilly weather; unhealthy skin, tetter, inflammation of the eyes; toothache in damp weather; aphthæ; premature and profuse menses, chronic and corrosive leucorrhœa, sterility, galactorrhœa; cough with musty expectoration, pains aggravated during the exercise of walking, dancing, etc.

24. *Bovista*, puffball, useful in humid, scurfy tetter; chronic febrile diarrhœa; nosebleed, scurfy nostrils; drawing, boring pains in decayed teeth; chronic backache with stiffness after stooping.

25. *Bromium* is useful for stitching constriction of the larynx, inflammation of the larynx and trachea, hoarseness, feeble low voice, rough hollow dry cough with weariness or with paroxysms of suffocation or with wheezing or rattling respiration

with croupy sound. It is useful in croup even in the last stages; pains worse in the evening and before midnight.

26. *Bryonia*, wild hops, acts chiefly on the joints and is therefore valuable in arthritic rheumatism or for pains in the joints aggravated by motion and relieved by rest; in intermittent fevers with thirst during the cold and hot stage; dry cough with stitches in the chest. Typhoid fevers with burning heat and thirst, dryness of the skin; pleuritic stitches and pneumonia; obstinate constipation, nosebleed in typhoid fevers; toothache aggravated by warm food or drink, the teeth feel loose, toothache temporarily relieved by cold water and worse in a warm room and in cold damp weather.

27. *Cactus grandiflorus*, night-blooming cereus, is a valuable remedy for affections of the heart, angina pectoris. It acts specifically upon the heart and its bloodvessels, dissipating congestions and suppressing irritations without weakening the nervous system; sanguineous congestions in persons of a plethoric habit, injurious consequences of taking cold.

28. *Calcarea carbonica*, carbonate of lime, acts chiefly upon the bones and is therefore a valuable remedy for caries of the bones and rickets; for scrofula, dry tetter, scaldhead, polypus of the nose and uterus; indurations of the mammary glands, swelled neck or goitre; fistula in ano; emaciation with large bowels and good appetite; sensation of cold about the head and constrictive headache; slow closing of the fontanelles; running at the ears and deafness after scarlet fever; leucorrhœa; constipation, cough with copious expectoration as in pulmonary consumption; palpitation of the heart with feeling of coldness. It is useful in diarrhœa of children and cholera infantum, when the stools have a sour smell and are worse at night; toothache of pregnant women with rush of blood to the head, difficulty of first dentition; a morbid sensation as if the body were shrinking, softening of the intestinal organs.

29. *Calcarea phosphorica*, phosphate of lime, for gout with swelling of the joints, curvature of the joints, very painful; is frequently used in consumption.

30. *Camphora*, camphor, meets that febrile condition which renders one susceptible to cold followed by chilliness, colic, diarrhœa and cholera with violent cramps in the calves, coldness of the surface, etc.

31. *Calendula officinalis,* marigold flowers, applied externally and internally for healing large shaggy ulcers or bleeding wounds favors the process of cicatrization.

32. *Cannabis sativa,* hemp. Shuddering and chilliness with thirst and low pulse, general languor; urging to urinate, pain and inflammation of the kidneys; inflammatory swelling of the prepuce; gonorrhœa and strangury.

33. *Cantharis,* Spanish flies. Fever consisting only of coldness; burning in all the cavities of the body; erysipelas; nephritis, retention of urine with spasmodic pains in the bladder, inflammation of the urethra and bladder and secondary gonorrhœa; violent sexual desire, painful erections, etc.

34. *Capsicum annum,* Spanish pepper. Chilliness and coldness of the whole body with lowness of spirits; chill and shuddering every time one drinks. Intermittent fevers, characterized by chilliness and thirst; aching pains, affections of the joints, crampy feeling in the body with stiffness of the limbs, dread of motion; burning in the pit of the stomach after eating; distention of the abdomen as if it would burst; tenesmus of the bladder, burning when urinating, discharge of blood from the urethra; tenesmus of stool, nocturnal diarrhœa with burning at the anus; impotence with coldness of the sexual parts, cough most violent in the evening and at night, disposed to draw a long breath.

35. *Carbo animalis,* animal charcoal is suitable for indurations of the glands especially of the mammæ, cough with greenish expectoration, night-sweats, suppuration of the right lung, hardness and swelling of the axillary glands.

36. *Carbo vegetabilis,* vegetable charcoal. For burning pains in the limbs, bones, ulcers, deafness after measles, cough with soreness of the larynx and chest, chronic hoarseness, low stages of typhus, collapse of the pulse in dysentery and cholera.

37. *Causticum.* Whooping-cough, chronic hoarseness, racking cough with spirting of the urine.

38. *Caulophyllum thalictroides.* Useful in neuralgia and rheumatic headaches, when dependent on uterine disorders, for uterine rheumatism or false pains as they are sometimes termed and for rheumatic affections of the bowels. It is useful in amenorrhœa, dysmenorrhœa and for severe after pains and for any abnormal irritation of the uterus.

39. *Cepa*, common onion. Cold, coryza, hay-fever or summer catarrh, running of the nose, sore eyes and urinary difficulties, coryza with profuse lachrymation and sensitiveness of the eyes, alternate chills and heat, pains more in the warm room and less in the open air.

40. *Chamomilla* is suitable for greenish watery diarrhœa in children and especially when teething, flatulent colic and crying of infants; hoarseness and constriction of the chest from a cold; fever with redness of one cheek and paleness of the other.

41. *China*, Peruvian bark. For general debility when caused by loss of blood and other fluids from onanism, nursing, debilitating emissions, emaciation, atrophy of children, exhausting sweats; debility from fevers; intermittent fever in malarious districts with absence of thirst during the chill and heat; nocturnal wetting of the bed with children, general dropsy, hemorrhages and loss of blood from the womb; toothache of pregnant women; involuntary stools and flow of urine from debility.

42. *Chimaphilla*, pipsisiwa, is suitable for diseases of the mucous membrane of the bladder, discharge of mucous from the urethra; leucorrhœa, etc.; tenesmus of the bladder; scrofulous ulcers; dropsy, etc.

43. *Cicuta virosa*, water-hemlock, is a valuable remedy for pain in the lower portion of the spine, tetanic spasms and convulsions, obscuration of sight, involuntary discharge of urine from paralysis of the bladder.

44. *Cimicifuga racemosa*, black cohosh. Hysteria, uterine irritation, delayed menses, dysmenorrhœa and other female ailments; for nervousness produced by indigestion, etc. Neuralgia of the ovaries, chorea, threatened abortion, after pains, etc., etc.

45. *Cina*, wormseed, a valuable remedy for worms, pinworms, long round worms, spasms of children from worms, epilepsy especially at night.

46. *Cistus canadensis*, rockrose, for swelling and suppuration of the glands, running from the ears, scrofulous ailments; vesicular erysipelas of the face, pains worse towards morning and after an unpleasant emotion.

47. *Clematis erecta*, virgin's bower. Gonorrhœal rheumatism of the joints; chronic red and humid tetter and itching in the warmth of the bed and after washing; scrofulous sore eyes; swelling and induration of the groin, stricture of the urethra,

swelling of the testicles; induration of the breasts and gouty deposits in the fingers.

48. *Cocculus indicus*, seeds of the cocculus, is suitable for seasickness or nausea from riding in a carriage, vomiting worse from raising the head, spinal irritation, sickness of pregnant women, angina pectoris of hysteric females, pains aggravated by riding, driving, walking or smoking.

49. *Coccus cacti*, cochineal, has been advantageously employed in whooping cough with gagging and vomiting and raising a large quantity of albuminous, tenacious, ropy mucus, white or yellowish white, having a saltish taste, cutting pains in the region of the bladder, dull, stinging, spasmodic pains in the kidneys.

50. *Coffea cruda*, raw coffee. This remedy has been employed to obviate the consequences of sudden emotion, for sleeplessness, crying of infants with colic, or when the nerves are much excited from various causes, also for spasms in young children and for the anxiety of lying-in females.

51. *Colchicum autumnale*, meadow saffron. This remedy is employed in gout and rheumatism, especially in warm weather and for wandering pains when the weather is cold; œdema, general dropsy; nocturnal heat of the body and thirst; distension of the abdomen, fall dysentery with discharges of white mucus and tenesmus; scalding urine and tenesmus of the bladder and burning in the urethra; hydrothorax, pains aggravated from motion and worse at night.

52. *Colocynth*, wild bitter cucumber. For colic with violent pains in the umbilical region, pain in one side of the head with vomiting and in the afternoon; morbid craving of hunger; yellow diarrhœa excited by eating or drinking; pains in the hip joint, etc.

53. *Conium maculatum*, spotted hemlock, a successful remedy for indurations of the breasts with violent pains, indurations of the glands generally; spinal irritation, catarrh, chronic obstruction of the nose, tetter on the back of the hands and forearm; cancer of the lip caused by a bruise, cough only at night, immediately after lying down.

54. *Crocus sativa*, saffron, is one of the most valuable remedies for uterine hæmorrhage and for pains occasioned by the violent movements of the fœtus in utero.

55. *Crotalus horridus*, rattle snake poison, has been employed against paralysis of the right side after an attack of apoplexy and for spasms and convulsions with violent cries and delirium, swelling of the whole body; inflammatory fevers with pulse 130, first full and strong and afterwards feeble and scarcely perceptible and also according to Dr. Mure it is a remedy for some cases of traumatic tetanus and for erysipelas in the face.

56. *Cuprum metallicum*, copper, is employed against dry cough which takes away the breath and for whooping cough when children turn blue in the face as if suffocating; spasms preceded by weeping; against *Asiatic cholera* if the vomiting and diarrhœa are attended by pressure at the pit of the stomach and convulsions of the extremities; and epilepsy and epileptiform diseases.

57. *Digitalis purpurea*, fox glove. This remedy is employed in organic diseases of the heart, hydrothorax and ascites or dropsy of the chest and abdomen and also in bleeding from the lungs; blueness of the lips, lids and nails, slow pulse, dilatation of the pupils; amaurosis, hydrocele; cough with expectoration resembling starch gruel.

58. *Drosera*, sundew, is employed in whooping cough with vomiting, better when moving about moderately, warm perspiration, whooping cough with bleeding at the nose and mouth, pains in the right and left side, nosebleed in the morning and also in the evening when stooping; laryngeal phthisis and emaciation, cough aggravated by singing, laughing, crying, smoking and drinking.

59. *Dulcamara*, bittersweet. For diarrhœa and colic from taking cold, swelling and induration of the glands, catarrh, humid tetter on the arms, dropsy of the chest.

60. *Dioscorea villosa*, wild yam root, is employed in bilious colic, flatulent colic, neuralgia of the bowels, diarrhœa, etc.

61. *Erechtites hieracifolia*, fire-weed, has been successfully employed in cholera, mucous dysentery and mucous irritation of the lungs and bowels with satisfactory results.

62. *Erigeron canadense*, Canada fleabane, employed in uterine hæmorrhage, diarrhœa and dysentery, vomiting of blood and piles, urinary difficulties and catarrh of the bladder.

63. *Eryngium aquaticum*, button snakeroot, useful in chronic diseases of the lungs and bladder, prolapsus ani, severe burning

at pit of the stomach; leucorrhœa and gonorrhœa, nocturnal emissions; influenza, hacking cough, etc.

64. *Euonymus atropurpureus*, wahoo, employed in ague, dyspepsia, liver complaint, constipation, dropsy and pulmonary affections, cold sweats, death-like sickness at the stomach, etc.

65. *Eupatorium aromaticum*, white snakeroot, used in pleurisy, inflammation of the lungs, bronchitis, whooping cough, irritation of the bladder, etc.

66. *Eupatorium perfoliatum*, boneset, valuable in intermittents, where there is little or no sweat and violent thirst before the chill, which usually comes on in the morning, distressing headache during the fever, periodical headache in the morning, soreness of the eyelids, rheumatic affections, gouty affections of the joints, etc.

67. *Eupatorium purpureum*, queen of the meadow, in disease of the kidneys, gravel, dropsy, chronic irritation of the bladder, rheumatism and gout, retention of urine, debility of the uterus; a preventive of abortion.

68. *Euphorbium officinale*, spurge, employed against burning pains in the internal organs, rheumatic pains of the limbs and burning in the extremities, urging to urinate, the urine passes off in drops.

69. *Euphrasia officinalis*, eyebright. Inflammation of the eyes from injuries, spots on the cornea and profuse flow of tears· cough in the daytime with phlegm on the chest, difficult to throw off; cramp in the calves while standing.

70. *Ferrum*, iron. For debility, deficiency of red blood, milky leucorrhœa, smarting of the vagina during an embrace, deficient sexual desire, flow of blood from the uterus with bearing-down pains; general dropsy and dropsy of the abdomen, liver complaint and debility arising from loss of fluids.

71. *Gelsemium sempervirens*, yellow jessamine. This remedy has been used with great success in colds of the head, orbital neuralgia, facial neuralgia and toothache; spasmodic croup, "goneness of the stomach," gastralgia and cramps; dysentery, bilious diarrhœa; impotence, seminal weakness; neuralgic dysmenorrhœa; catarrhal fever, influenza; pneumonia and bronchitis. In fevers of a comatose character or having cerebral congestion, nervous fevers characterized by low delirium and other febrile conditions, its range is as extensive as Aconite.

72. *Glonoine*, nitro-glycerine, used against the effect of sunstroke, headache as if the brain were pressed assunder, violent rush of blood to the head, throbbing in the forehead as far as the nape of the neck, headache and acceleration of the pulse, moisture upon the forehead, stitches and pains in the eyes; pain, heat and chills down the back, vertigo when walking.

73. *Graphites*, black lead, in humid tetter, scanty and tardy menses with cutaneous eruptions; chronic costiveness; falling out of the hair.

74. *Helleborus niger*, Christmas rose. Dropsy [after scarlet fever or measles, acute and chronic hydrocephalus, aphthous sore mouth, etc.

75. *Hepar sulphuris calcareum*, sulphuret of lime, for gouty and rheumatic pains with inflammation and swelling of the affected parts; hoarseness, croup; suppurations and ulcers; inflammation with swelling; gathered breasts; erysipelatous inflammation with swelling; fetid running from the ears; inflammation and swelling of the parotid gland, chronic hoarseness and persistent laryngitis, laryngeal phthisis; leucorrhœa with smarting.

76. *Hyoscyamus niger*, black henbane. Employed in night cough, inflammation of the brain; effects of disappointment; squinting, hydrocephalus, etc.

77. *Hypericum perforatum*, St. John's wort. This agent cures punctured wounds, cuts, bruises, lacerations, tetanus, trismus, etc. It is an analogue of Arnica montana, and like it may be used internally and externally in cases of neuritis from injuries or laceration of the nerves. The indication for its use is violent pain proceeding from the injury, resembling toothache and extending along the limb.

78. *Ignatia amara*, St. Ignatius bean. In general prostration and the consequences of grief, mortification or suppressed emotions of every kind and also for convulsions, spasms and fits of crying after disappointment, grief, fright, insults or excitement; also for hysteria, epilepsy, premature menses, etc., from similar causes; for affections of the heart, spine and diseases of the nervous system in general.

79. *Iodine*. For scrofula, swelling and induration of the glands; œdema, general dropsy; fever, alternate chills and flushes of heat with delirium; hectic fever; continual vomiting; induration of the spleen, swelling of the inguinal glands, ovarian

dropsy; flow of blood from the womb when at stool, chronic corrosive leucorrhœa; inflammation of the larynx, hoarseness, croup, chronic hoarseness, cough with white expectoration sometimes tinged with blood, laryngeal and tracheal phthisis; goitre or bronchocele, swelling in the groin, knee and all kinds of inflammatory swellings with violent pain and suppurations.

80. *Ipecacuanha*. In loathing of food and drink, nausea, vomiting, intermittent fever, gastric symptoms, oppression of the chest, asthma, asthmatic croup and wheezing cough, dysentery, uterine hæmorrhage and also hæmorrhage from any cavity of the body.

81. *Kali bichromicum*, bichromate of potash. Secondary syphilitic eruptions, sore mouth, fetid discharge from the nose, sour or bitter taste in the mouth, heartburn, dryness of the throat and bronchial tubes, pain in the larynx, constant titillation and dry cough day and night or croup with expectoration of tenacious mucus, sometimes gray or yellowish; pains in the kidneys and suppression of urine; rheumatic pains in the upper and lower extremities.

82. *Kali carbonicum*, carbonate of potash, is suitable for hoarseness with sensation as if a plug were in the throat, cough with anguish and suffocation or with vomiting, especially in the morning, whooping cough with œdematous countenance, cough with purulent expectoration in old people and also for goitre.

83. *Kreasotum*. Marasmus in children with diarrhœa, swelling and induration of the neck of the uterus, incipient cancer, putrescent stools and fetid ulcers.

84. *Lachesis*, suitable for ailments consequent on change of life in females; paralysis, epilepsy, chorea; ulcers on the legs secreting a fetid pus; sore throat, tubercles and gangrenous ulcers.

85. *Laurocerasus*, cherry laurel. For consumption with expectoration of blood, loss of speech, tetanus, epilepsy; inflammation of the liver; constipation; retention of urine, paralysis of the bladder; profuse uterine hæmorrhage during the critical period with dark clots, cough with copious jelly-like expectoration streaked with blood, slow panting respiration, paralysis of the lungs; pains less in the open air and at night.

86. *Ledum palustre*, marsh tea. Nodous gout, dry itching

herpes, stings of insects, musquito bites, swelling of the feet and legs.

87. *Lycopodium clavatum*, club moss. Tedious constipation; nodous gout; scrofulous and rickety complaints, curvature of the spine and softening of the bones; mercurial bone pains; paralysis; humid tetter and scald head, fistulous ulcers and tuberculous consumption; ulcers on the legs, impotence, ulceration of the membrane of the nose, etc.

88. *Magnesia carbonica*, carbonate of magnesia. Toothache of pregnant women; oppressive pains in the stomach with sour eructations.

89. *Magnesia muriatica*, muriate of magnesia, is employed against scirrhous indurations of the womb and spasm of the broad ligaments.

90. *Manganum*, manganese. In pains in the bones at night; chronic hoarseness of the throat, cough with expectoration of greenish mucus in little lumps, laryngeal consumption.

91. *Mephitis putorius*, skunk, whooping cough or any spasmodic cough.

92. *Mercurius vivus and solubilis*, quicksilver, employed against syphilis, cancerous ulcers; rickets and scrofula, dropsy and swelling and caries of the bone, inflammatory bone-pains, rheumatic or gouty pains in the joints and limbs at night, curvature of the bones and also brittleness, intolerable pains in the joints and limbs at night in a warm bed with perspiration that affords little or no relief; syphilitic tetter; spreading ulcers, spongy and bluish which bleed easily; inflammatory swelling of the glands, mumps and suppurations of various kinds: *inflammatory fevers* with accelerated pulse and excessive sweats of a sour smell; eruptions on the scalp, falling off of the hair; inflammation of the eyes and lids, purulent discharge from the ears; inflammation and swelling of the nose; apthous sore mouth; tearing and jerking toothache at night; inflammation of the tongue; sore throat; enlarged tonsils and profuse flow of saliva; vomiting of bitter bilious matter, *greenish gonorrhœa*, inflammatory conditions of the liver and bowels, bloody urine, falling of the rectum, falling of the vagina and corrosive leucorrhœa; swelling and hardness of the breasts, catarrh, influenza, dry racking cough as if the head and chest would fly to pieces.

93. *Mezereum* is employed against the abuse of mercury such as are chronic and affecting the bones, swelling of the parotid glands; humid scaldhead; excessive vomiting of green and bitter mucous or bloody and chocolate colored; burning pains in the stomach; discharge of blood when urinating, etc.

94. *Millefolium*, yarrow, is chiefly recommended for hæmorrhage from the various orifices of the body.

95. *Moschus*, musk, is daily used in hysteria and hypochondria, for convulsions in males or females; excessive vascular excitement; headache as from a heavy weight on the head with a sensation as if cold compresses were applied; pressure in the stomach increased by drink; throbbing in the region of the stomach; constipation relieved by coffee; violent sexual desire with tittilation of the sexual organs; jerking of the extremities followed by severe pains in these parts, some of the pains abate in the open air.

96. *Muriatic acid* is employed against foul ulcers on the legs, and typhus fever when the patient settles down in bed with fetid breath and aphthous sore mouth, compressible and intermittent pulse.

97. *Natrum carbonicum*, carbonate of soda, is employed against glandular swellings of the neck and groin. Swelling and coldness of the feet.

98. *Natrum muriaticum*, salt. For intermittent fever after the abuse of quinine, where there are pains in the bones and great prostration, bitter taste in the mouth, backache and sallow complexion, ulcerations at the corners of the mouth, loss of appetite, pressure in the pit of the stomach with painful sensitiveness when touched; scurvy; chronic constipation and diarrhœa; falling of the rectum with burning in the anus and discharge of bloody ichor; tetter at the anus, painful hæmorrhoids, scanty and retarded menses, acrid leucorrhœa with sallow complexion; cough, bronchial irritation with chills with tickling in the throat or pit of the stomach, stitches in the chest when drawing a long breath or coughing; palpitation of the heart after the least exercise, irregularity of the beating of the heart; dry and brittle skin on the hands, burning or coldness of the feet, etc.

99. *Nitric acid*, employed against mercurial symptoms, chancre, gonorrhœa, figwarts, ulcerations of the mouth, nursing

sore mouth, bleeding gums; inflammation and swelling of the
testicles, the pain extending upwards along the spermatic chords;
swelling and suppuration of the inguinal glands; affections of the
kidneys, urinary complaints, bleeding piles, ulcerative phthisis,
chilblains, etc.

100. *Nitrum*, nitre. Itching blotches on the body, except the
hands and feet; headache after a meal; throbbing toothache at
night, aggravated by cold drinks, pneumonia, cough with purulent expectoration of bloody mucous; pains appear for the most
part in the afternoon or evening.

101. *Nux moschata*, nutmeg. Consequences of exposure to
dampness and cold, affections accompanied by drowsiness or disposition to faintness; intermittent fever with drowsiness, white,
coated tongue, humid asthma, expectoration of blood and but
little thirst even during febrile heat; diarrhœa after taking
boiled milk.

102. *Nux vomica.* Nausea, heartburn with sour eructations,
acid vomiting, flow of water in the mouth; *bloated bowels and
pain in the back,* tightness round the abdomen, bilious vomiting,
effects of intoxication; excessive use of coffee, wine or brandy,
mental labor, talking or walking at night; *delirium tremens;*
falling of the womb, pain in the bowels after confinement;
obstinate constipation, hæmorrhoids; inflammation of the liver,
soreness of the stomach on pressure, pain in the head as if it
would split aggravated by mental labor, restless sleep, pain in the
occiput, irritable, consequences of chagrin and hypochondria.

103. *Oleander,* for painless paralysis of the lower extremities,
sadness and self-distrust, humid eruptions on the scalp, obscuration of sight when looking sideways; throbbing in the pit of the
stomach, deficiency of the seminal secretion.

104. *Opium.* This remedy is employed in sopor, delirium
tremens, intoxication, torpor of the bowels, coma, stupor after
debauch, dreamy, stupid sleeplessness; consequences of fright,
trembling and jerking convulsions beginning with rigidity of the
whole body; loud cries, epilepsy, tetanus, lockjaw; lead-colic;
torpidity of the bowels in old people; infantile colic with constipation.

105. *Petroleum,* rockoil. This is a valuable remedy for scrofulous ailments, glandular swellings and indurations; scaldhead,
soft tumors on the head painful when touched; deafness caused

by paralysis of the auricular nerves; hypochondria; tetter upon the thighs, humid tetter on the scrotum and extreme itching, chapped hands, obstinate ulcers on the toes.

106. *Phosphoric acid.* Ulcers on the glands that burn, pain in the periosteum as if scraped with a knife; affections of the bones, painless diarrhœa not weakening; diabetes; nocturnal emissions, onanism, debility and emaciation.

107. *Phosphorus* is a valuable remedy in pneumonia with stitches in the chest, rusty sputa, stage of hepatization, chronic hoarseness and loss of voice; loss of blood during pregnancy; smarting leucorrhœa, constant disposition to diarrhœa during cholera; fistula of the mammary glands; affections of the bones and nightly pains; amaurosis, cataract; ardent desire for sexual intercourse with the male and aversion to it in the female, ulceration of the mucous coat of the bowels and pain in the umbilical region in typhoid fevers.

108. *Platina*, is a valuable remedy for unnatural sexual excitement, sterility, profuse and premature menses, induration of the womb and prolapsus and for hysteria.

109. *Plumbum*, lead, is used against paralysis of the extremities; constipation, violent pains in the region of the umbilicus, spasmodic retraction of the abdomen, colic relieved by pressure; vomiting of feculent matter, etc.

110. *Podophyllum peltatum.* Morning diarrhœa, patient driven out of bed with much pain; hepatic affections; hæmorrhoids; pain in the back and loins of weak and feeble women.

111. *Pulsatilla.* A valuable remedy for females for scanty and tardy menstruation, amenorrhœa from cold; green sickness, irregular menstruation, painful cramps in the womb during the menses; leucorrhœa; feeble labor pains, after-pains, retained placenta; unnatural stoppage of the lochia; fainting fits, palpitation of the heart; indigestion; epileptiform diseases, hysteria when caused by menstrual difficulties; measles, consequences of measles; fistula lachrymalis or fistula generally, scrofulous ophthalmia; running from the ears, earache; dry coryza, catarrh with loss of smell; nose-bleed; headache from retarded menses, dry cough or cough with expectoration of yellow, bitter, salt or sweetish mucus streaked with blood; diarrhœa of infants, burning in the rectum, bleeding piles; urging to urinate with involuntary dribbling of the urine, discharge of mucus from the

urethra, diabetes, wetting the bed, especially in the case of little girls, derangement of the stomach from rich or fat food, pastry and the like, heartburn made worse by rapid walking; flatulency and inflammation of the bowels; *angina pectoris*, suffocating paroxysms, constriction across the chest with pain in the chest; wandering gout, rheumatism of the knees; a characteristic symptom is the absence of thirst in all Pulsatilla pains. This remedy is suitable for females of gentle and timid dispositions, pale complexion, blue eyes and blonde hair, pains worse in the evening and during rest in a warm bed or in a warm room and they abate in the open air or when the patient is lying on the back or during moderate exercise.

112 *Ranunculus bulbosus*, crowfoot, is a valuable remedy for scalds, flat spreading ulcers with sharp edges and stinging burning itching; ophthalmic affections with immobility of the pupils; the pains are excited by contact or a change of position.

113. *Rhus toxicodendron*, poison oak, this is a valuable remedy for erysipelas of a vesicular character, pains in the limbs during rest and at night, rigidity and stiffness of the limbs, numbness and tingling of the extremities, pain in the joints as if sprained; nocturnal diarrhœa, preceded by colic, dysenteric diarrhœa alternating with constipation, swelling of the arms and also in typhoid fevers when there is great prostration and incipient paralysis.

114. *Ruta graveolens*, rue, is valuable for sprains of the ankle joint to apply externally, contusions of the bones and periosteum, pains in the limbs during rest, when sitting and relieved by motion; weakness of sight induced by reading and sewing; falling of the rectum, etc.

115. *Sabadilla*, Mexican barley, is suitable for intermittent fever always recurring at the same hour and for vomiting long round worms and tape worms and louse disease.

116. *Sabina*, savin, prevents miscarriage, especially in the third month of pregnancy and is useful for metrorrhagia, the blood being bright red.

117. *Sambucus nigra*, elder, suitable for profuse sweat after midnight; asthma, cough with little expectoration and difficult to raise and for intermittent fevers with exhausting sweats.

118. *Sanguinaria canadensis*, bloodroot. Violent headache, mostly on the right side with nausea and vomiting of food or

bitter substances, recurring periodically, excited by a variety of causes, generally commencing in the morning, increasing during the day, relieved by sleep, aggravated by noise, walking, etc. Consumptive cough, inveterate ulcers and spongy excrescences.

119. *Secale cornutum*, spurred rye. Deficient labor-pains, metrorrhagia ; detached placenta, protracted bloody lochial discharges, miscarriage; exhausting diarrhœa and frequent stools, *Cholera* with ricewater discharges; paralytic weakness in the lower extremities dependent upon spinal debility, and affections of the toes of old people.

120. *Senega*, rattlesnake root, is employed against dry cough or cough with difficult expectoration, wheezing respiration, racking pain through the whole chest; spots on the cornea or dimness or sponginess of the same.

121. *Sepia*, cuttlefish, is especially useful for females who have scanty menstruation and for the ailments incident to the change of life, hysteria, sick headache with nausea and vomiting; lichen, spots upon the face, humid tetter; cough with saltish expectoration, otorrhœa, cataract, etc.

122. *Silicea* for whitlows, corns, fistula, caries of the bones, rickets, hayfever, stoppage of the nose, gangrenous sores, etc.

123. *Spigelia*, pinkroot, for worms, periodic headaches and faceache of the left side, aggravated by noise and motion; organic enlargement of the heart and dropsy of the chest.

124. *Spongia maritima tosta*, burned sponge. Croup, goitre with pressure and tingling, and also when a sense of constriction is felt; hoarseness after singing; laryngeal phthisis.

125. *Squilla maritima*, squills. Fever with internal chilliness and external heat; cough with pleuritic stitches; bloody expectoration; pleurisy and pneumonia.

126. *Stannum*, tin. Mucous consumption with hectic fever and night sweats; spasms during teething; epilepsy in the evening, etc.

127. *Staphysagria*, stavesacre. Scald head; diseases of the kidneys, bladder and urethra, boils on the lids along the edges; excrescences on the gums: toothache in decayed stumps with swelling of the cheeks.

128. *Stramonium*, thorn apple. For asthma; delirium, illusions of the fancy; lascivious mania, proud mania, occasionally

ludicrous gesticulations and sad expression of countenance, with great violence, striking, kicking, etc., catalepsy.

129. *Sulphur* is the chief remedy for the itch, herpes and eruptions of various kinds; constantly recurring erysipelas; dropsy; bone-pains; rheumatism, gout; goitre; intermittent fever of scrofulous patients; leucorrhœa, falling of the womb; chronic diarrhœa and constipation; hernia; piles; pneumonia with hepatization; wetting the bed; burning and itching of the anus; impotence, nocturnal emissions; suppressed chronic eruptions; epilepsy, etc., etc.

130. *Sulphuric acid.* Consequences of bruises, etc., with ecchymosis of the injured part; infants sore mouth; weakness and trembling after smelling coffee; incarcerated hernia; profuse menstruation; metrorrhagia; hæmoptysis; painful chilblains on the fingers.

131. *Symphytum officinale*, common comfrey. This remedy is useful for removing the effects of fractures, contusions or injuries implicating the bones and periosteum and may be used in the form of tincture for external bathing of the injured parts and in dilutions for internal administration.

132. *Tartar emetic*, stibium, is employed against vesicular eruptions, intermittent fever with absence of thirst and sopor; vomiting of sour and acrid substances also with diarrhœa and great debility. It is also useful in catarrh, coryza and croup.

133. *Terebinthina* is useful in tympanites of the abdomen; general dropsy after scarlatina, with discharges of dark urine having the odor of violets; inflammation of the kidneys and discharge of blood from the urethra.

134. *Teucrium marum varum*, wall germander, is sometimes used against polypus of the nose, pinworms and ailments produced by them.

135. *Thuja occidentalis*, arbor vitæ, is employed against fig warts and warts in general, syphilitic ulcers and syphilis, indurations of the abdomen, etc.

136. *Urtica urens*, nettle, is employed in burns and scalds; itching blotches; nettle rash with headache and fever and for general dropsy after the suppression of eruptions of the skin; swelling of the head, etc.

137. *Valeriana officinalis*, valerian, is used against morbid nervousness and pains which set in suddenly with a racking fury in

a state of apparent health; intermittent fever with slight chill followed by constant heat and dullness of the head, especially in the afternoon and attacking children with worms. It is also employed in hysteria, head and face ache, which comes on in paroxysms.

138. *Variolin* is employed as a preventive of small-pox in place of vaccination. It is also employed in curing variola and varioloid.

139. *Veratrum album.* For cramps in the legs, during cholera. It is employed as one of the chief remedies in Asiatic cholera characterized by vomiting and purging, with great prostation and coldness of the surface of the body, ricewater discharges from the bowels; severe pain in the occiput with fever and cold sweat, great thirst, feeble and hurried pulse, pains in the chest, abdomen and groins; whooping cough in feeble children who have cold sweat upon the forehead, chilliness and aversion to talking, sudden prostration of strength with great thirst; coldness of the extremities, numbness and a crawling sensation of the extremities, pain in the extremities aggravated by damp weather; tetanic spasms; intermittent fever with internal heat and coldness of the surface with violent thirst for cold drinks; delirium, loss of memory, confusion of the head; religious mania; unreasonable amorousness; short paroxysms of delirium from fright and other causes.

140. *Viola tricolor*, pansy, has been found useful in milk-crust attended with burning and itching at night and discharge of tenacious, yellow pus; urine smells like cow's urine.

141. *Zincum metallicum* is employed against paralysis of the brain, various kinds of chronic eruptions such as tetter and seminal weakness; discharge of blood from the urethra after urinating; St. Vitus dance and pain in the chest when riding in a carriage.

In the range of all pointed out in the foregoing list it will be seen that nearly every diseased condition has in the materia medica an appropriate remedy. The list might be greatly enlarged, but a sufficient number have been cited to give some idea of the wide range of remedial action, and we therefore conclude the chapter on materia medica. In addition we simply note the fact, which has been made apparent to the observation of experienced practitioners that some remedies are noted for acting more especially on diseases that affect the right side of the body and others for those which affect the left side.

Those that act more especially on the right side are: Agaricus, Alumina, Belladonna, Cantharis, Causticum, Crotalus, Drosera, Hepar sulph., Ignatia, Moschus, Plumbum, Rhus tox., Ruta, Sabadilla, Sabina, Sanguinaria and Staphysagria.

Those which act more especially on the left side are Aconite, Apis, Arnica, Asarum., Calcarea carb., China, Colchicum, Colocynthis, Crocus, Iodine, Lachesis, Mercurius, Nitric acid, Nux vomica, Spigelia, Sulphur and Sulphuric acid.

A critical attention to the above will materially aid in the affiliation of remedies in the treatment of diseases which will be noted in the following pages. Before we proceed in this department we will call attention to the various forms in which remedies are prepared and the manner of preserving them in a pure state. Medicines are prepared in the following forms: First, by triturations; second, tinctures; third, dilutions; fourth, saturated globules, and fifth, saturated wafers, etc.

Minerals, earths, and many of the salts are taken in the pure state and prepared for use by triturating them with a neutral medicine in certain fixed proportions, as for example: one grain of the pure metal, earth or salt is triturated in a porcelain or glass mortar with nine grains of sugar of milk until the whole is thoroughly mixed and intimately united. This is termed the first decimal trituration; the second is made by triturating one grain of the first with nine grains of pure sugar of milk; the third in like manner with one grain of the second and nine grains of the medium and so on with successive attenuations on the decimal scale. On the centesimal scale one grain of the crude material is triturated with ninety-nine grains of the medium for the first and one grain of this to ninety-nine grains of the medium for the second and so on with the higher triturations on the centesimal scale.

Tinctures are made either by mixing equal parts of the expressed juice of fresh plants and pure alcohol or by 1-20 by weight of the material with nineteen parts of alcohol. The dilutions are prepared by adding one drop of the tincture to nine of the alcohol for the first decimal and one drop of this to nine of the alcohol for the second and so on in the decimal scale. The centesimal scale requires one drop to ninety-nine of the alcohol and so on with each succeeding attenuation. Each dilution requires an indefinite number of shakes or succussions in order to sustain the true character of dilutions. Each remedy thus prepared should be triturated or succussed by itself alone and should be preserved in thoroughly cleaned and well corked vials, and should be kept in a cool place, secluded from· light and entirely away from all odors or perfumes that might influence, modify or deteriorate its purity. Most of the remedies are easily antidoted if, on their administration, their effect should require it, as follows:

Remedies and their Antidotes.

1. Aconitum napellus, Wolfsbane, is antidoted by Belladonna, Camphor.
2. Æsculus glabra, Buckeye, is antidoted by Aconite, Sulphur.
3. Æsculus hippocastanum, Horse chestnut, is antidoted by Aloes, Sulphur.
4. Agaricus, Agaric, is antidoted by Camphor, Pulsatilla.
5. Agnus castus, Chaste tree, is antidoted by Camphor.
6. Alumina is antidoted by Bryonia, Chamomilla.
7. Ambra grisea is antidoted by Camph., Nux vom.
8. Ammonium carb. Carb. of Ammonia, is antidoted by Arnica, Camph.
9. Ammonium mur., Muriate of Ammonia, is antidoted by Arsenicum, Camph.
10. Anacardium, Malacca bean, is antidoted by Camph., Coffea.
11. Antimonium crud., Crude antimony, is antidoted by Hep. sulph., Merc.
12. Apis mellifica, Honey bee, is antidoted by
13. Argentum metallicum, Silver, is antidoted by Mercurius, Pulsat.
14. Argentum nitricum, Nitrate of Silver, is antidoted by Merc. Natr. mur.
15. Arsenicum album, Arsenious acid, is antidoted by Iodine, Ipec.
16. Arnica montana, Leopard's bane, is antidoted by Camph. Caps.
17. Assafœtida is antidoted by Camph., China.

18. Aurum foliatum, Goldleaf, is antidoted by Bell., Mercurius.

19. Aurum muriaticum, Chloride of Gold, is antidoted by Bell., Mercurius.

20. Baptisia tinctoria, Wild indigo, is antidoted by Bryonia, Gels.

21. Baryta carbonica, Carbonate of Baryta, is antidoted by Bell., Camph.

22. Belladonna, Deadly nightshade, is antidoted by Black coffee, Camph.

23. Borax is antidoted by Camph., Coffea.

24. Bovista, Puffball, is antidoted by Camphora.

25. Bromine is antidoted by Opium, Camph.

26. Bryonia, Wild hops, is antidoted by Aconite, Nux v.

27. Cactus grandiflorus, Night-blooming cereus, is antidoted by Aconite.

28. Calcarea carb., Carbonate of Lime, is antidoted by Camph., Nitr. ac.

29. Calcarea phosph., Phosphate of Lime, is antidoted by

30. Camphora, Camphor, is antidoted by Opium, Wine.

31. Calendula officinalis, Marigold, is antidoted by Arnica.

32. Cannabis sativa, Hemp, is antidoted by Camphor.

33. Cantharis, Spanish flies, is antidoted by Camphor.

34. Capsicum annuum, Spanish pepper, is antidoted by Camphor.

35. Carbo animale, Animal charcoal, is antidoted by Lachesis.

36. Carbo vegetabilis, Vegetable charcoal, is antidoted by Arsenicum, Lachesis.

37. Causticum, is antidoted by Coff., Nux vom.

38. Caulophyllum thalictroides, Blue cohosh, is antidoted by Puls., Secale.

39. Cepa, common Onion, is antidoted by Camphor.

40. Chamomilla, is antidoted by Acon. Coffea.

41. China, Peruvian bark, is antidoted by Ars., Ipec., Puls.

42. Chimaphilla umbellata, Pipsissewa, is antidoted by Cham.

43. Cicuta virosa, Water hemlock, is antidoted by Arnica.

44. Cimicifuga racemosa, Black cohosh, is antidoted by Secale.

45. Cina, Wormseed, is antidoted by Bryonia.

46. Cistus canadensis, Rockrose, is antidoted by Belladonna.

47. Clematis erecta, Virgin's bower, is antidoted by Bry., Camph.

48. Cocculus indicus, Coccle seeds, is antidoted by Camph., Nux vom.

49. Coccus cacti, Cochineal, is antidoted by Chamomilla.

50. Coffea cruda, Raw coffee, is antidoted by Aconite.

51. Colchicum autumnale, Meadow saffron, is antidoted by Cocculus, Puls.

52. Colocynthis, Wild bitter cucumber, is antidoted by Caust., Cham.

53. Conium maculatum, Spotted hemlock, is antidoted by Coffea, Nitr. spir.

54. Crocus sativa, Saffron, is antidoted by Acon., Bell.

55. Crotalus horridus, Rattlesnake poison, is antidoted by Phosphorus.

56. Cuprum metallicum, Copper, is antidoted by Bell., Ipec.

57. Digitalis purpurea, Foxglove, is antidoted by Nux v., Opium.

58. Drosera rotundifolia, Sundew, is antidoted by Camphor.

59. Dulcamara, Bittersweet, is antidoted by Camph., Ipec.

60. Dioscorea villosa, Wild yamroot, is antidoted by Cham., Coloc.

61. Erechthitis hieralifolius, Fireweed, is antidoted by Causticum.

62. Erigeron canadense, Canada fleabane, is antidoted by Secale.

63. Eryngium aquaticum, Button snake root, is antidoted by Camphor.

64. Enonymus atropurpureus, Wahoo, is antidoted by Ipecac.

65. Eupatorium aromat., White snake root, is antidoted by Camphor.

66. Eupatorium perfoliat., Boneset, is antidoted by Puls.

67. Eupatorium purpur., Queen of the Meadow, is antidoted by Bryonia.

68. Euphorbium officinarum, Spurge, is antidoted by Camphor.

69. Euphrasia officinalis, Eyebright, is antidoted by Pulsatilla.

70. Ferrum, Iron, is antidoted by Ars., China.

71. Gelsemium sempervir., Yellow jessamine, is antidoted by Acon., Bell.

72. Glonoine, Nitro-glycerine, is antidoted by Bell., Opium.

73. Graphites, Black lead, is antidoted by Ars., Nux v.

74. Helleborus niger, Black hellebore, is antidoted by Camph , China.

75. Hepar sulph. calc., Sulphuret of Lime, is antidoted by Belladonna.

76. Hyoscyamus niger, Black henbane, is antidoted hy Bell., Camph.

77. Hypericum perforatum. St. John's wort, is antidoted by Arnica.

78. Ignatia amara, St. Ignatius bean, is antidoted by Puls., Cham.

79. Iodine, is antidoted by Ars., Sulph.

80. Ipecacuanha, is antidoted by Arn., Ars.

81. Kali bichromic., Bichromate of Potash, is antidoted by Hep. s.

82. Kali carb., Carbonate of Potash, is antidoted by Camphor.

83. Kreasot, is antidoted by Aconite.

84. Lachesis, is antidoted by Ars., Bell.

85. Laurocerasus, Cherry laurel, is antidoted by Camphor.

86. Ledum palustre, Marsh tea, is antidoted by Camphor.

87. Lycopodium clavatum, Clubmoss, is antidoted by Camph., Puls.

88. Magnesia carbonica, Carbonate of Magnesia, is antidoted by Cham., Puls.

89. Magnesia muriatica, Muriate of Magnesia, is antidoted by Arsenicum.

90. Manganum, Manganese, is antidoted by Coff., Merc. sol.

91. Mephitis putorius, Skunk, is antidoted by Camphor.

92. Mercurius viv. et solub., Quicksilver, is antidoted by Nitric acid.

93. Mezereum, is antidoted by Mercurius.

94. Millifolium, Yarrow, is antidoted by Puls.

95. Moschus, Musk, is antidoted by Camphor.

96. Muriatic acid, is antidoted by Bryonia.

97. Natrum carb., Carbonate of Soda, is antidoted by Ars., Camphor.

9

98. Natrum mur., Salt, is antidoted by Spir. nitr. dulc.
99. Nitric acid, is antidoted by Calc. c., Merc.
100. Nitrum, Nitre, is antidoted by Merc.
101. Nux moschata, Nutmeg, is antidoted by Camphor.
102. Nux vomica, is antidoted by Bell., Opium.
103. Oleander, Laurel Rose, is antidoted by Camphor.
104. Opium, is antidoted by Bell., Nux v.
105. Petroleum, Rock oil, is antidoted by Acon., Nux v.
106. Phosphoric acid, is antidoted by Camphor.
107. Phosphorus, is antidoted by. Camphor, Nux v.
108. Platina, is antidoted by Pulsatilla.
109. Plumbum, Lead, is antidoted by Bell., Opium.
110. Podophyllum peltatum, is antidoted by Nux vom.
111. Pulsatilla, is antidoted by Cham., Ign.
112. Ranunculus bulb., Crowfoot, is antidoted by Pulsatilla.
113. Rhus tox, Poison Oak, is antidoted by Bry., Camph.
114. Ruta graveolens, Rue, is antidoted by Camphor.
115. Sabadilla, Mexican barley, is antidoted by Camphor, Puls.
116. Sabina, Savin, is antidoted by Camph., Puls.
117. Sambucus, Elder, is antidoted by Ars., Camphor.
118. Sanguinaria canadensis, Bloodroot, is antidoted by
119. Secale cornutum, Spurred rye, is antidoted by Camph., Solan. nigr.
120. Senega, Rattle snake root, is antidoted by Arnica, Bell.
121. Sepia, Cuttlefish, is antidoted by Aconite.
122. Silicea, is antidoted by Hepar sulph.
123. Spigelia, Pinkroot, is antidoted by Aurum, Camph.
124. Spongia tosta, Burned sponge, is antidoted by Camphor.
125. Squilla maritima, Squills, is antidoted by Camphor.
126. Stannum, Tin, is antidoted by Pulsatilla.
127. Staphysagria, Staves acre, is antidoted by Camphor.
128. Stramonium, Thornapple, is antidoted by Nux vom., Opium.
129. Sulphur, is antidoted by Acon., Camph.
130. Sulphuric acid, is antidoted by Pulsatilla.
131. Symphytum officinale, Common comfrey, is antidoted by Camphor.
132. Tartar emetic, Stibium, is antidoted by Ipecac.

133. Terebinthina is antidoted by Camph., Canth.

134. Teucrium marium verum, Wall germander is antidoted by Camph., Ignat.

135. Thuja occidentalis, Arbor Vitæ, is antidoted by Cham., Cocculus.

136. Urtica urens, Nettle, is antidoted by Opium.

137. Valeriana officinalis, Valerian, is antidoted by Camph., Coffea.

138. Variolin, is antidoted by Pulsatilla.

139. Veratrum album, is antidoted by Acon., Camph.

140. Viola tricolor, Pansy, is andtidoted by Camphor.

141. Zincum metallicum, is antidoted by Camph., Hep. s.

Remedies which may follow each other.

In most all the works on therapeutics great stress is laid upon the importance of selecting suitable remedies to follow those which have already been employed in given cases. How far this principle should be observed, or to what extent it is useful, no one has recorded a specific rule.

In our practice we have been governed by the following considerations, viz.:

1st. If called to subdue a fever of an inflammatory character we give Aconite, if this fail we give Gelsemium, Bryonia or any other remedy which the symptoms indicate.

2. If the Aconite does not fail, after the fever is reduced we also select such remedies as the symptoms indicate.

3. When called on to treat any acute disease, as for instance pneumonia, our first remedy is such as the case demands and when the disease passes from one stage to another, we select such remedies as the symptoms call for; we try to exercise reason and common sense. When from a cold a febrile reaction occurs, Aconite is called for, and if the throat inflames, Belladonna is suitable to follow Aconite and to follow with other remedies to meet corresponding developments. It is not necessary to name the remedies which are suitable to follow inasmuch as our great repository—the materia medica explicitly states under the head of each remedy, what are its analogies and what its antidotes.

That each polychrest may form the centre of a group, more or less extensive, in which may be embraced those which have a parallel action.

It is certainly desirable to possess an extensive knowledge of materia medica. But a careful study in reference to specific cases, will not admit of too many comparatives, on account of the liability of becoming confused. A thorough knowledge of the old polychrest, as laid down by Hahnemann and the early Homœopathists, who apparently made better and more successful practitioners then, than any who have come after them, though long before the highest potencies, as well as before a very great proportion of our materia medica provings were unknown. The question of potencies is an open question, although it must, we think, be conceded that from the lowest crude form of drugs, to the highest attenuation claimed—that the law "similia similibus curantur" is alike applicable and should not be overlooked. Medical properties are not more susceptible of measurement by weights and measures than other imponderabilia.

CHAPTER X.

Diseases of the organs of digestion are among the most common that command every day attention. Derangement of function cannot long continue without greater or less derangement of structure, involving the functions of the alimentary canal. The alimentary tube is liable to diversified affections, serious and generally the occasion of considerable discomfort, and even when other apparatus proves to be the seat of irritations, the functions of the alimentary canal are more or less affected, and particularly the stomach, which has been termed " the center of sympathies." On the other hand the derangement of the digestive system reacts upon other organs that pour their secretions into the alimentary canal, which is lined with a mucous membrane from the mouth to the anus. We will proceed to consider the diseases incident to this locality, beginning with:

1. Inflammation of the Mouth.

The mucous membrane of the mouth is subject, 1st, to *simple inflammation*, which becomes red, hot and sensitive to the touch of foreign bodies and even of the tongue. This is termed *simple stomatitis*, and may affect young and old. It is usually of brief duration, though occasionally it terminates in ulceration or gangrene. It is caused by taking hot or acrid substances into the mouth, or by mechanical injuries, or from the process of teething in young children.

TREATMENT.—This form of stomatitis has been looked upon as a light form of disease that may pass off spontaneously in a little time, and formerly washes of flaxseed tea or infusion of slippery elm were the chief remedies employed. Under Homœopathic treatment the washes may be dispensed with, and a dose or two of *Mercurius solubilis* or *Nux vomica* will prove sufficient.

2. Aphthæ of Children, or Pultaceous Inflammation of the Mouth.

This disease is usually known under the name of *thrush*, which attacks the new-born infant chiefly, although adults sometimes suffer from it in the course of certain diseases as in phthisis.

DIAGNOSIS.—The surface of the tongue exhibits unusual redness, with here and there small, curd-like exudations. These gradually increase and coalesce so as to form irregular patches, which are thrown off and renewed, leaving the mucous membrane of a vivid red color. In slight cases the exudations are distinct, while in severer cases they run together, and the whole mucous membrane of the mouth and throat becomes implicated. The skin is usually hot and dry and the thirst quite apparent. Some writers attach but little importance to the disease, which they allege terminates in health in a few days. But we have seen the milder cases that occur in private practice extend down the digestive tube and develop into a diarrhœa of an exceedingly irritative and dangerous character, occasioning redness and excoriation of the anus and extending to the nates.

CAUSES.—Predisposed condition of the mucous membrane in new-born infants with defective nutrition and lack of fresh and invigorating air.

TREATMENT.—The old school treatment is expectant in mild cases; simple washes of milk and water or other emollient liquids are mainly relied on. But in those cases affecting the mucus lining of the bowels and resulting in excoriations around the anus an occasional dose of calcined Magnesia associated with rhubarb is advised. This latter device is objectionable because even the mildest aperient is liable to aggravate the difficulty and our observation is that Homœopathic remedies are the most efficient and less dangerous. *Mercurius* is for the most part indicated when the thrush extends downward and produces burning diarrhœa and excoriations. Two globules night and morning will generally cure, and, also in case of great weakness and diarrhœa, *Arsenicum*, especially if the aphthæ assume a livid and bluish appearance attended with great prostration, diarrhœa and inflamed excoriations around the anus, and thirst. *Borax* is indicated when the child frequently lets go the nipple, showing signs of pains in the mouth from nursing. Apthæ in the mouth or on the tongue, acrid, fetid'urine. Dose, three globules put in the child's mouth three times a day.

3. Aphthæ of Adults, Follicular Inflammation of the Mouth.

The precise nature of aphthæ is not so sufficiently known as to dispel all doubt concerning it. One thing is certain, it manifests itself either in the form of follicular ulcerations, vesicles, or papular eruptions.

This aphthous stomatitis may be distinct or confluent. It attacks the parts especially where the mucous membrane is most exposed. The distinct form is often preceded by some degree of fever and signs of derangement of the stomach. This is of short duration and confined exclusively to the mouth.

The confluent form is rarely confined to the mouth like the distinct, but extends to the throat and at times even to the lower portion of the digestive tube. It is accompanied by general disturbance of the organism, headache, vertigo, and gastric derangement and at times the eruption extends to the intestinal canal giving rise to severe suffering in the abdomen, diarrhœa and low fever, under which the patient may sink. In the discrete or distinct form the mucous membrane of the mouth presents the appearance at first of simple stomatitis or thrush. Afterwards, small, grayish or whitish vesicles are perceptible and at the base of each vesicle there is a raised ring which is resisting and of a white color. After this stage appears, the vesicles break at the top so as to allow the fluid to escape from it; then it is transformed into an ulcer, which spreads, surrounded by a red circle which is the raised border that surrounded the base of the vesicle, which gradually disappears and then the ulcer heals rapidly leaving only a slight trace of redness which soon passes off.

TREATMENT.—As an external wash for the sores, dilute Muriatic acid has been employed and sometimes Nitrate of Silver. When the aphthous sores manifest themselves in women when nursing their babes, it becomes necessary to wean them and then the following remedies may be employed:

Arsenicum, when the margin of the tongue is ulcerated and aphthous with violent burning pains.

Baptisia, when the aphthæ affects the gums and there is an oozing of blood from them; nursing sore mouth, deep fissures in the tongue, which is inflamed and swollen; mercurial sore mouth and profuse salivation.

Borax, when the mouth and tongue are inflamed from aphthous sores.

Bryonia, when the mouth is unusually dry with thirst.

Capsicum, suitable for plethoric persons who lead a sedentary life and especially for burning vesicles in the mouth and on the tongue with swelling of the gums.

Carbo veg., when the mouth is very hot and the tongue stiff and the ulcers have a bad smell.

Dulcamara, when the least cold causes the disease with swelling of the glands of the neck.

Hamamelis virginica, when the gums are spongy and bleeding, burnt sensation on the tongue and blisters on the sides of the mouth and tongue.

Hydrastis for nursing sore mouth, excessive secretion of mucous, a peppery taste, dark red appearance of the tongue with raised papillæ.

Mercurius. Burning pains in the mouth, ulcerated gums which discharge a fetid matter, loose teeth; inflamed, sore, ulcerated mouth and tongue sometimes covered with apthæ; fetid and bloody saliva and burning, acrid diarrhœa.

Natrum muriaticum. Profuse flow of saliva with swollen, sensitive gums, ulcers and blisters of the mouth, etc.

Nitric acid. Mercurial sore mouth with profuse flow of saliva and fetid smell, sore mouth with stinging pains, bleeding, white and swollen gums and loose teeth.

Nux vomica, Phytolacca, Podophyllum, Rhus tox. and Sulphur are remedies which may also be consulted in the treatment of aphthous sore mouth and Sulphuric acid when the disease extends to the mucous coat of the intestines as in the confluent form of the disease.

DOSE AND ADMINISTRATION.—Any of the above remedies may be given in drop doses and repeated every hour or two hours; prepare the remedies in water, one drop to a dessertspoonful. When the triturations are used give one or two grains for a dose.

Gangrenous Inflammation of the Mouth.

All the forms of stomatitis described before may be followed by those more severe until a gangrenous inflammation sets in, which does not always present the same appearance or symptoms. The most terrific form is commonly known under the name of canker of the mouth. At times there appear, on the inside of the lips and cheeks, small vesicles of a grayish or livid red or even of a black color, without much pain or swelling, but surrounded by a red base, generally preceded by a strong fetid odor from the mouth and profuse salivary secretion. They speedily pass into a state of gangrene. The pain and swelling increase sometimes to an alarming extent and the teeth drop out and the whole face becomes gangrenous. At other times the disease commences at the edge of the gums opposite the incisors, progresses in a similar manner and the discharge is very acrid and produces excoriation of the parts unaffected when it comes in contact.

CAUSES.—A vitiated atmosphere is looked upon as one of the predisposing causes of the difficulty. Imperfect nourishment is another. It seldom attacks children at the breast. Its greatest havoc is among children from two to seven years of age, who possess a feeble constitution and have been subjected to illy ventilated apartments where they have been compelled to breathe a stagnated air. As the disease sometimes manifests itself in the form of an epidemic, it may be contagious and those affected should be separated from those who are not. This is a judicious precaution even if, instead of contagious, the same cause operates to produce the malady, in asylums filled with children and subject to the same influences.

TREATMENT.—It must be obvious that gangrenous inflammation of the mouth results from extreme deterioration of the vital powers and calls for a treatment directed against this condition. As an external agent with which to wash the mouth a weak solution of *Carbolic acid* may be useful. It has been the prevailing practice to administer Quinine in half grain doses every three hours mixed with chlorine or sulphuric acid. Chloride of soda and Chloride of lime have also been employed as internal remedies. But this practice has proved far less advantageous than well selected Homœopathic remedies. Arsenicum, China, Mercurius, Nitric acid, Muriatic acid and Carbo vegetabilis are remedies that have been employed with great success. They may be employed in dilutions.

DOSE.—Ten drops of either in half a tumbler of water may be given in teaspoonful doses every two hours. But as a condition the windows and doors of the apartments in which they dwell should be thrown widely open to obtain the purest and most invigorating atmosphere. Pure soft water should be employed for cleansing the surface and good food in the form of unseasoned soups should be supplied them at regular periods. Beef tea or essence, wine whey, gruels made of arrowroot, sago, tapioca and farina or corn starch are severally useful for the food of these little sufferers.

Diseases of the Tongue.

The condition of the tongue is universally regarded as an index of disease. It indicates the degree in the function of secretion elsewhere modified and also the morbid condition of the mucous membrane that lines the alimentary canal at a distance from it and morbific conditions generally. Its state of moisture and dryness has likewise to be noted in disease.

1. Inflammation of the Tongue, Glossitis.

We have already considered the superficial inflammation of this organ under the head of stomatitis, but it is the deep seated inflammation that we now have under consideration.

DIAGNOSIS.—The first thing noted is pain, heat, redness and swelling of the organ, which render its movements painful in the extreme. In the onset only a limited part of the organ may be implicated, but gradually the inflammation extends, the pain becomes acute, burning and lancinating, and so sensitive that the contact of any foreign body, however trivial, is almost insupportable and any attempt to swallow or speak or move the tongue excites the most excruciating torment. Occasionally it is enormously swollen and protrudes from the mouth or threatens suffocation and at times indentations are made by the teeth and livid or black appearances presented on the protruded surface seem to threaten mortification. When in this condition a thick fur covers the surface and a copious saliva flows from the mouth and during the stage of inflammation the general symptoms are such as are present in all inflammatory processes and proportionally severe.

Ulceration sometimes occurs on the upper surface which comes on slowly at first from an induration slightly painful on pressure and forms a deep ulcer. The edges of the tongue may be ulcerated from the contact of the teeth.

CAUSES.—Acrid substances taken into the mouth, mechanical injuries from the teeth or by external bodies, mercurial salivation and spontaneous diseases.

TREATMENT.—Allopathic, requires general depletion, leeches applied to the under surface and scarifications on the upper surface and from the application of ice and a blister applied to the throat and neck, active cathartics or cathartic enemas. If gangrene supervenes the actual cautery is applied to the mortified portion and the mouth, which is washed by chloride of lime, soda or other antiseptic applications. Or, in case of induration and slow process of ulceration, emetics and cathartics are the revulsive treatment recommended. This treatment is objected to as being unnecessarily harsh and debilitating.

Homœopathic treatment consists in the administration of internal remedies usually directed against inflammation.

Aconite, if there is general inflammatory fever, full bounding pulse and particularly if there is a hot dry skin.

Arnica, if occasioned by mechanical injuries, soreness of the tongue, etc.

Arsenicum, burning inflammation of the tongue.

Cantharis, if the inflammation is of a burning and painful character or when there is suppuration or when caused by scalding liquids.

Conium maculatum, when there is swelling of the tongue and when there are indurations or inflammation from mechanical injuries.

Mercurius vivus is indicated for most cases of inflammation of the tongue and particularly when caused by syphilis.

Nitric acid, when the inflammation emanates from ulcers in the lining membrane and also *Muriatic acid.*

Sulphur, in chronic inflammation of the tongue has a salutary effect.

Silicea in protracted cases will be found useful.

DOSE AND ADMINISTRATION.—Aconite, Arnica, Cantharis, Conium, Nitric and Muriatic acid may be administered by dropping five drops of any of the dilutions in half a glass of water to be given in teaspoonful doses repeated every two hours. Arsenicum, Mercurius, Sulphur and Silicea may be given in the 3d trituration, one or two grains of the powder and repeated once or twice a day.

Cancer of the Tongue.

Near the tip of the tongue and sometimes at the edge cancer of rare occurrence may be developed.

DIAGNOSIS.—Tumefaction and induration are the first symptoms (unless there has been some preceding inflammation) after which painful shootings are experienced in the further progress of the disease. The mobility of the tongue is interfered with and it becomes painful to move it. Mastication and deglutition are also difficult and painful. The indurated tissue in time passes into a state of ulceration. The ulcers are irregular, red and hard and a sanious bloody matter, which is exceedingly fetid, flows from the mouth along with an increased secretion of saliva. The suffering as in other cancerous affections becomes severe and almost insupportable and the victim gradually sinks from an irritative fever.

CAUSES.—The predisponent is a cancerous diathesis, and injuries to the tongue operate as exciting causes.

TREATMENT.—In Allopathic practice as soon as the indurations are seen an attempt is made to modify the condition of the system by agents that induce a new action in the nutritive system, such as Arsenic and Iodine, and if these agents produce no change extirpation of the affected part is recommended and this is often accomplished without much difficulty. But little or no benefit results to the patient, because the diathesis remains and the injury produced by the operation acts as an exciting cause for new indurations and a more formidable reappearance of the cancer.

THE HOMŒOPATHIC TREATMENT is sometimes more effectual in changing or modifying the diathesis. The remedies employed in the stage of tumefaction and induration are: *Arsenicum*, *Belladonna*, *Carbo animalis*, *Conium*, *Hydrastis canadensis*, *Kreasotum*, *Nux vom.* and *Sepia*. Hartman says: "The employment of some one of these remedies has sometimes proved beneficial." They are administered internally in the form of dilutions and triturations. The former in drop doses that may be repeated several times a day. The latter in the third trituration may be given in powders of one or two grains twice a day under a generous diet.

Diseases of the Teeth.

The process of cutting the teeth is altogether natural and cannot be classed among pathological conditions, nevertheless this sensitive period of an infant's life renders its system so impressible that the irritation caused by the pressure of the teeth upon the nerves of the gum is so manifest that attention is frequently called for.

Dentition is accompanied by a certain class of symptoms which indicates to a greater or less extent a common suffering, such as pain, heat and swelling of the gums induced by the pressure of teeth on them, a constant flow of saliva with a desire to bite objects, unless the soreness of the gums is so great as to prevent it. The child at the same time is fretful, restless, often disturbed in its sleep, and the digestive organs are to a greater or less extent affected by the irritation. These symptoms are so generally present in teething children that they are scarcely looked upon otherwise than as the necessary result of dentition. But in children whose nervous system is unusually impressible, the irritation from the teeth extends to the nervous centres and induces spasms or convulsions. It is therefore important to observe critically the condition of the gums when any derangement occurs at the period of cutting the teeth.

TREATMENT.—When the child is desirous of conveying everything to its mouth, care should be exercised to prevent it from biting hard substances capable of producing a mechanical injury. Rings of ivory or India rubber are the least objectionable. When the gums are much swollen and an implication of the nervous centres is threatened, scarification of the gums with a lancet is advisable, and even after convulsions have ensued, a free division of the gums has often proved a valuable resort. The medical treatment that directs the employment of soothing syrup or soporific doses of paregoric is positively injurious and frequently results in the greatest injury.

HOMŒOPATHIC TREATMENT.—For the ailments which usually attend dentition, *Chamomilla* is a valuable remedy, and especially for convulsions, weeping, moaning and starting in sleep. *Coffea* or *Amber grisea* if there is no fever. *Aconite* and *Gelsemium* where there is a feverish state or where there is a dullness and stupor. *Dose* from two to four globules of the remedy selected three or four times a day.

Toothache.

The membranous lining of the socket of the tooth sometimes becomes inflamed and occasions much suffering. The symptoms which indicate such inflammation are an uneasy feeling in the sockets of the teeth, which is aggravated when the jaws are pressed together, by reason of the teeth being slightly forced outwards so that they cannot be accurately brought in contact. The sensation is painful, pulsative and constant and may last a few days and then subside or in severe forms the inflammation may extend to the gums and the teeth may become loose and sometimes pus may secrete in the sockets and their walls may become carious and a fistulous ulcer kept up.

CAUSES.—Cold and hot fluids taken into the mouth and exposure to heat and cold and moisture are generally regarded as exciting causes. When the fangs of the teeth become carious, the investing membrane usually becomes the seat of painful inflammation.

TREATMENT.—For periodontitis when there is great excitement and excessive pain, the Allopathic treatment consists in scarifying the gums and in the application of leeches externally, while an effective dose of Opium or Morphine is given internally. But this treatment is merely palliative and often proves worse for the patient than his suffering.

HOMŒOPATHIC TREATMEMT.—The inflammatory stage *requires Aconite, Belladonna, Gelsemium* and *Mercurius viv.* For suppuration *Hepar sulph.*, and in case of burning pains and fistula *Arsenicum. Kali hydriodicum* is indicated when the inflammation is followed by the secretion of morbid matter and especially in scrofulous persons.

DOSE.—Of the remedy selected mix five drops of any of the dilutions in half a tumbler of water and give a teaspoonful every two or three hours.

Caries of the Teeth.

This is a common disease and consists in the destruction of sound teeth by decay.

DIAGNOSIS.—When hot or cold liquids are taken into the mouth and produce pain in one or more of the teeth it denotes the presence of a cavity or cavities opening externally in some part of the tooth or teeth affected, or that an internal process of decay has been established which leaves but a shell of bone between the cavity of the tooth and the open air so that the nerve of the tooth is readily impressed by the action of external agents. The precise locality in which the decay commences varies considerably. It is generally supposed that the starting point is immediately under the enamel in the bony crown of the tooth. At first a dark point is observed that gradually spreads until a considerable portion of the tooth becomes gangrenous and opens a cavity with which the external air may come in direct contact. And in this way the whole crown may be destroyed leaving the fangs in their socket to excite inflammation and pain, and when foreign substances come in contact during mastication, that most excruciating of all mortal sufferings—the toothache ensues.

CAUSES OF DENTAL DECAY are commonly ascribed to the action of external agents. Hot liquids taken into the mouth may cause an expansion of the bony crown that sometimes bursts the enamel and leaves fissures in which corrosive matters may lodge and thus be the exciting cause of decay. Cold liquids may also produce a sudden contraction that operates in a similar manner. Aside from these causes a vitiated saliva may have a chemical action upon the teeth and subject them to early decay and one decayed tooth may so act upon those adjoining until the whole set becomes implicated. The destruction of the enamel alone is not the cause of decay but it may open the way for the action of acrid matters upon the bony structure and thus excite the first beginning of caries. It is a common belief that acids and sweetmeats are to be classed among the causes of decay, but unless there is some predisposing cause, this assumption is not verified; nevertheless they may act as excitants where there is an inherent or constitutional predisposition.

TREATMENT.—In order to arrest the process of decay when practicable, the cavities should be cleansed and plugged with some metallic or other substance. When not practicable, relief from pain may be procured by destroying the affected nerves by caustics introduced into the cavities. *The allopathic* treatment is to deaden the pain by the different preparations of Opium or essential oils and stimulants. But this treatment is fraught with evil consequences.

HOMŒOPATHIC TREATMENT.—This consists in the direction of remedies to remove irritation, inflammation and pain, not to supercede the mechanical work of the dentist but to cure the sufferings and obviate the derangement of diseased conditions.

Aconite, when there are feverish symptoms, nervousness and throbbing pain with vascular excitement.

Belladonna, when several teeth on the same side are affected so that it is impossible to point out the precise tooth affected, and when the teeth feel elongated as if they would start from their sockets; when the pain is aggravated by the contact of warm or cold substances; when there is a determination of blood to the head; when there is erysipelatous swelling of the cheek; glandular swellings, simultaneous neuralgic pains, etc.

Chamomilla, when the pain is caused by a draft of air or by a sudden interruption of perspiration, or when the decayed tooth affects the ear; when the pain is augmented by warm drinks and when the cheek and gums are swollen with no redness ot the skin.

China, when the toothache sets in as a consequence of great weakness after loss of blood or when decayed teeth are painful during pregnancy or after parturition and while nursing; when decayed teeth become painful from debilitating losses of blood or from diarrhœa, leucorrhœa, etc.

Causticum, when the toothache is accompanied by stiffness of the jaws and when cold air is inhaled, or when the whole side of the face is affected and especially the right side.

Hepar sulphuris, when the pain is produced by an incipient gumboil, looseness of the teeth after the abuse of mercury; dental fistula and fully developed gumboils.

Mercurius, when the toothache is not produced by the abuse of mercury but is accompanied with ptyalism; violent scraping pain in the cheekbones, toothache caused by syphilis, pains worse after midnight with profuse perspiration.

Nux vomica.—Drawing and boring pain in a decayed tooth as if wrenched out, caused by excessive use of coffee, wine or alcoholic stimulants; especially adapted to all persons who lead a sedentary life and troubled with obstinate constipation; toothache from a severe cold, etc.

Pulsatilla, when the decayed tooth becomes painful at the menstrual period, and when too feeble or suppressed, and the pains are worse in the evening in a warm room or in bed. Cold air relieves the pain, and also when throbbing, as digging pains extend from a decayed tooth to the eye.

Sulphur, for chronic toothache either with or without swelling of the cheek, when the pain is tearing, jerking or stitching and jumping, worse at night, when toothache supervenes upon the suppression of cutaneous eruptions. *Sulphur* with *Mercurius,* when the teeth become detached from the gums, which are diseased and prone to bleed.

To the above we will add the following remedies:

Arnica, for rheumatic toothache when caused by sudden cold or from a blow or contusion, or when it is accompanied by pale and hard swelling of the cheek, or when produced by filling or extracting the teeth. An Arnica lotion held in the mouth is exceedingly useful under such circumstances. It is important to avoid all exposure that may check perspiration when using this remedy.

Bryonia when there is stinging and throbbing toothache, which yields for a time to the application of cold water.

Kreasotum when there are drawing pains in decayed teeth extending to the temples and inner ear, or towards the eye.

Sepia succus for toothache of pregnant women, with China or Belladonna, and for sudden exfoliation of the teeth with Staphisagria.

Staphysagria when the pains proceed from decayed teeth or from stumps, and the head and ears are involved, the cheek swollen, without heat, and the pain is worse after eating or when inhaling cold air, or in case of the teeth becoming suddenly black or decayed and exfoliated (compare Sulphur.)

The above fifteen remedies will be found sufficient to cure almost every form of toothache, provided the proper care and discrimination is exercised in the selection.

DOSE AND ADMINISTRATION.—The medicines may be given in dilutions or globules;—ten drops in half a tumbler of water; of this mixture a teaspoonful may be given every hour or two hours, or twice or thrice a day, according to the acuteness of the suffering, or four or six globules may be given with the same frequency.

While under treatment, coffee, tea, ale, porter, spirits, acids and spices are forbidden and persons afflicted with frequent attacks of toothache and headache should abstain from the use of

10

coffee altogether. The best substances for cleaning the teeth are sugar of milk and charcoal, which remove all impurities without injury. Perfumed toothpowders and acid preparations should never be used for cleansing the teeth as they injure the enamel. It is well to rinse the mouth morning and evening and after each meal with fresh water not too cold. This will prevent the decay of animal matter between the teeth and the formation of tartar.

NERVOUS TOOTHACHE as it is termed is simply a form of neuralgia and requires nearly the same treatment. The neuralgia of the teeth, however, may be mistaken for ordinary toothache and therefore we will state our method of distinguishing the difference. We first inquire into the history of the case and try to ascertain if the pain occurs periodically and whether there is a shooting with extreme violence along the branches of the nerves distributed to the jaws.

TREATMENT.—Allopathic treatment consists in the employment of narcotics to be taken internally in large doses and to be applied locally, and blisters behind the ears. Sometimes the tincture of opium or kreasote are conveyed into the cavity inserting a little cotton thoroughly imbued by them for the purpose of allaying pain. Stimulating liniments composed of strong liquor of ammonia 1 oz., spirits of rosemary ¼ oz. and spirits of camphor 2 oz. have also been employed topically.

HOMŒOPATHIC TREATMENT.—*Aconite, Belladonna, Bryonia, Gelsemium, Calcarea* and *Sulphur* have been called into requisition and each when properly affiliated has produced relief. Pregnant women are liable to suffer from neuralgia of the teeth and *Belladonna* is an excellent remedy.

DOSE AND ADMINISTRATION.—*Calcarea* and *Sulphur* may be given in powder of the third trituration twice a day and the other remedies may be administered in solution, ten drops of either in half a tumbler of water—in teaspoonful doses every hour or less frequently according to the severity of the suffering.

TOOTHACHE of violent, deep-seated pain, which remedies fail to relieve drives the patient to the expedient of having them extracted and then it becomes revealed that the fangs have been the seat of a bony deposit. When from the nature of the pain this deposit is suspected it is well to give Calcarea or Mercurius two or three times a day. Pathologically this affection is termed "*exostosis of the teeth*" and is an organic affection of the fangs.

TARTAR OF THE TEETH.—A calcareous matter sometimes accumulates around the crowns of the teeth at the margin of the gums and is deposited from the saliva. This derangement simply requires strict attention to cleansing the teeth by the daily use of the toothbrush with sugar of milk or finely powdered charcoal for a dentifrice. The condition of the saliva that favors the deposit of tartar may be changed by appropriate remedies such as Nitric acid or Mercurius given three or four times a week. But the accumulation does not always yield to the brush and remedies often fail, then the skill of the dentist is required to remove it with suitable instruments.

Diseases of the Gums.

When we considered the inflammation of the mucous membrane, investing every part of the mouth, under the head of stomatitis, we did not include the affections of the substance of the gum, which require especial attention. Inflammation of the gums is a common occurrence and is denoted by soreness, pain, heat and swelling which may pass off by resolution or pass on to suppuration, constituting the *gumboil*. The cause is not always apparent, but is supposed to result from a morbid condition of the lining membrane of the socket, produced by decayed teeth; when very much inflamed, the *allopathic* treatment is to scarify the gums or to apply leeches to arrest it. But in Homœopathic practice this is regarded unnecessary and from observation we have found *Hepar sulph.*, or *Mercurius* administered twice a day amply sufficient to cure the affection. The use of the lancet is seldom required.

Hypertrophy of the Gums.

Is a disease sometimes encountered and it consists of a morbid growth of hard substance like that of the gum itself covering the molar teeth, at times so as to interfere with the closing of the jaws. It has been recommended to remove these excrescences with the knife but our objection to this is the liability of their immediate recurrence and more formidable than before. From observation of the effects of *Thuja* and *Calcarea*, we have no doubt of favorable effects being derived from these remedies. For that condition of the gums, frequently called "scurvy," *Carbo vegetabilis*, Mercurius iodatus and Nitric acid have been given with good effect and we know from experience that either of the foregoing remedies when otherwise indicated will speedily result in a cure. For polypus of the gums, *Calcarea carbonica* may be given twice a day.

Shrinking of the Gums.

This affection consists in the shrinking away of the gums from the teeth so that they become loose in their sockets.

CAUSES.—Mercurial preparations exercise a marked influence over the gums, and cause them to recede from the teeth; the accumulation of tartar around the teeth encroaching upon the teeth is another cause.

TREATMENT.—*Nitric acid* will generally arrest the affection when produced by *Mercury*, and *Staphisagria* when caused by the incrustations of tartar.

Inflammation of the Velum and Uvula.

This affection produces swelling and infiltration of these parts, so that it interferes with deglutition and respiration, and sometimes to a degree that the patient is almost suffocated.

THE ALLOPATHIC TREATMENT consists in scarifying the swollen parts and the use of gargles of different powers of stimulation and astringency, and in case of this treatment being insufficient and the uvula is much elongated, a portion of it is excised. But this treatment fails to change the condition of the system, and is therefore objectionable.

HOMŒOPATHIC TREATMENT.—This consists of the internal use of *Aconite* when there is fever, furred tongue, dry and hot skin. *Belladonna* when the parts are red, congested and painful. *Mercurius* when much swollen, sore and exceedingly sensitive. *Hepar sulphur* when there is a threatening of suppuration with much throbbing.

DOSE.—Four globules repeated every hour or at longer intervals to meet the requirements of the case.

CHAPTER XI.

1. Inflammation of the Fauces or Throat.

In its simplest form this differs but little from what was described under the head of stomatitis. It consists of an inflammation of the mucous membrane covering the throat and its *diagnosis* is easy, as the symptoms are unequivocal. The mucous membrane of the throat is red, glossy and dry, and interferes with deglutition, subsequently a ropy mucous is secreted which greatly interferes with the act of swallowing. This is one of the forms of quinsy which may implicate the uvula and cause its elongation, which together with the ropy mucous, hanging down into the pharynx, may cause violent retching. The inflammation at times extends to the posterior nares, the upper portion of the larynx and the tubes of the ears, and impairs the sense of smell, the passage of air into the lungs and the sense of hearing.

In a majority of instances inflammation of the fauces passes off by resolution, but sometimes it goes on to suppuration, and the pain of swallowing which had been exceedingly acute during the incipient or inflammatory stage becomes dull after suppuration has become established.

CAUSES.—From the fact that all persons, predisposed to suffer from sore throat find themselves the victims of this disorder during the dampness, changes and winds of the early spring or later in the fall, it is safe to reckon these among the exciting causes. Incidental or irregular exposure to the extremes of temperature, as in the extreme coldness of the winter and the heat of the summer, may operate in the same way.

TREATMENT.—It has been customary to give mild cathartics and to employ astringent gargles to dissipate this form of disease. But such treatment is by no means necessary.

THE HOMŒOPATHIC TREATMENT is altogether best. *Aconite* when the inflammation is attended with fever, hot and dry skin. After *Aconite*, *Belladonna* when there is redness and soreness that interferes with deglutition.

149

DOSE.—Four globules dry on the tongue, repeated every two hours.

Hepar sulph. when the suppuration process has commenced. *Mercurius* when soreness and difficult deglutition remain after suppuration.

DOSE.—Four globules three times a day.

2. Inflammation of the Tonsils.

This is another form of quinsy which consists in the inflammation and swelling of the tonsils, and like inflammation of the fauces it renders deglutition extremely difficult and painful and produces the sensation of a foreign body in the throat during the effort.

In order to inspect the throat in this as in other diseases the patient should be directed to open his mouth widely while, with a flat depressor, the tongue is pressed down so that the tonsils can be seen without difficulty; at first the membrane covering the inflamed part is dry, and at times is diphtheritic. Sometimes only one of the tonsils is affected and it has been observed that the left is most frequently implicated. Tonsillitis often terminates by resolution and frequently it ends in suppuration or in permanent enlargement of the tonsils.

TREATMENT.—In allopathic practice counterirritation is applied to the throat and sometimes leeches. Saline cathartics are employed to operate on the bowels while the feet are subjected to a warm mustard bath. Liniments or sinapisms are applied externally to the throat and cooling gargles or the inhalations of steam are employed to soften the tumefaction.

HOMŒOPATHIC TREATMENT.—*Aconite,* when there is considerable fever, full pulse, dry skin and thirst.

Belladonna, when there is much congestion and swelling with difficulty in swallowing, great sensitiveness in the throat and copious secretion of ropy mucus.

Hepar sulph., when suppuration is threatened and when there is constant throbbing and pain in the swollen tonsil.

Mercurius, when the inflammation continues after suppuration and when the tonsils have a deep red or bluish tint and diphtheritic exudations, tenacious and slimy saliva and the breath a foul odor.

THE DOSE AND ADMINISTRATION of these remedies in an acute

attack of tonsillitis is as follows: When the disease comes on with a chill followed by fever Aconite may be given in doses of four globules every hour until the fever abates. Belladonna may then be given in the same way until the disease terminates by resolution or is observed to be on the point of suppuration, then Hepar sulph. may be given and under certain indications Mercurius sol. in the lower triturations. This latter remedy may be given when Belladonna fails of bringing about a resolution and when the tonsils have a bluish red tint.

Lachesis deserves particular attention when the inflammation has reached a very high grade of intensity and there is a threatening of gangrene.

Ignatia, when there is stinging in the throat between the acts of deglutition and a sensation when swallowing as if a plug or bone were in the throat, a sensation of swelling in the throat with painful soreness when swallowing.

FOR CHRONIC ENLARGEMENT OF THE TONSILS, *Baryta carb.* may be given in daily doses of the third trituration. This remedy has proved singularly efficacious when the tonsils have been so enormously enlarged as to nearly meet and be the cause of much difficulty in respiration.

Iodine. For scrofulous subjects when the tonsils are chronically swollen and when they are the cause of stertorous breathing.

The above treatment will be found efficacious and altogether preferable to the use of the powerful stimulants and burning with Nitrate of Silver so frequently resorted to.

Inflammation of the Pharynx—Pharyngitis.

This affection differs from tonsillitis only in the seat of the inflammation. It is induced by the same causes and generally passes off by resolution or otherwise some degree of suppuration will follow. This disease has been treated successfully with nearly the same remedies as are required in tonsillitis, *Aconite, Belladonna, Hepar sulph.* and *Mercurius* are the remedies to be employed and they have been found effectual in curing the malady, while the usual resort of emetics to relax the pharynx is liable to many objections.

In common parlance, inflammation of the fauces or isthmitis, tonsillitis and pharyngitis are included in what is termed the "quinsy sore throat" and nearly the same treatment is required in each. Sometimes pharyngitis appears to be of a rheumatic character and seated in the pharyngeal muscles and for this variety, which exhibits pain on pressure made on the sides of the neck, very severe, and when fluids are taken, owing to irregular and spasmodic action of the muscles it is liable to a partial return through the mouth and nose, the Allopathic treatment is in general antiphlogistic with the application of leeches. But with Homœopathic remedies such a resort has been dispensed with. *Aconite*, *Bryonia* and *Mercurius* may be employed in succession.

Aconite when there is fever. *Bryonia* when every act of swallowing gives intense pain and *Mercurius* when there is profuse flow of saliva.

DOSE.—Four globules every two hours or five drops of the dilutions in two table-spoonfuls of water may be given in tea-spoonful doses and repeated every two hours.

The pharynx is also liable to disease by reason of accumulation of mucus in the follicles of the throat which can be seen on inspection as so many granulated points varying in size from a pins head to a pea; not unlike the pimples or acne of the skin produced by disease of the sebaceous follicles. This disease is somewhat dependent on an impaired constitution and frequently assumes a chronic form. The granulations sometimes break and discharge small masses of matter which often creates anxiety in the patient who is led to apprehend serious pulmonary mischief.

THE TREATMENT of this affection, allopathically, has been the local application of creosote lotion or a solution of the nitrate of silver. A nutritious diet and the administration of aromatic and tonic medicines such as Iodide of Iron 24 grains in an ounce of water. Dose—a teaspoonful in water three times a day.

THE HOMŒOPATHIC TREATMENT which generally proves competent to affect a cure is as follows:

Causticum.—At first when there is huskiness of the voice with more or less coughing and hawking, sore pain, roughness, scraping and burning in the throat, a copious accumulation of mucus in the fauces and behind the palate; derangement of the stomach, nausea and heartburn.

Sepia, when the follicles are swollen and a sensation as if a plug were in the throat, dryness and disposition to hawk, hawking up phlegm tinged with blood; when on inspection the follicles discharge a cheesy matter; sour or bitter eructations from the stomach, pressure in the stomach after eating, burning or throbbing in the stomach.

Stannum is also a valuable remedy in follicular inflammation of the pharyngeal mucous membrane, when there is a feeling of dryness and stinging in the throat with a desire to hawk. When at the same time hawking makes the throat sore *Hepar sulph.*, and *Sulphur* are remedies to be consulted.

Dose.—The Causticum may be administered twice a day, five drops in a gill of water, a dessert spoonful at a dose. *Sepia, Stannum, Hepar sulph.*, and *Sulphur* may be given in two grain doses of the trituration, morning and evening, or in the higher attenuations in liquid form, the same as directed for Causticum.

Another form of pharyngitis partakes of the character of *diphtheria*. As it will be seen that isthmitis and tonsillitis are usually subject to the same characteristics as pharyngitis we will here include the throat in general. It is a pseudo-membranous inflammation and may be described as follows: In the outset it is insidious and deglutition is not so difficult, at other times an uncomfortable feeling of dryness and heat is experienced in the throat with fever, difficult swallowing and pain on moving the neck which in most cases is slightly swollen. After this the cervical and submaxillary glands may become enlarged and the difficulty of swallowing increased. At times the parotid glands enlarge and as has been observed this enlargement frequently precedes or accompanies the formation of false membranes. At this stage the pharynx may exhibit more or less redness and tumefaction and the same may be the case with one or both tonsils, but it rarely happens that the throat is seen in this early stage as the patient apprehends nothing serious, but as the soreness augments, a full description reveals the character of the disease. The entire mucous lining of the throat, including that of the fauces, uvula and pharynx exhibits small white or yellowish patches irregularly circumscribed and having a curdy appearance. And as these exudations are thrown out the glandular swellings make their appearance. The patches are at first small and discrete but they gradually spread so as to coalesce and become confounded and cover the whole of the pharynx extending into the nasal cavities and air passages.

When the velum and uvula are covered by the patches of false membrane which is semi-transparent, they appear infiltrated and where these pellicles are thickest the tumefaction is the most marked. They are bounded by an elevated red circle which gives them the appearance of ulceration or depression. In a little while they project and become partially loose and a slight oozing of blood from the parts beneath give a slight coloring to the saliva, and the exposed mucous membrane appears red, clotted and injected. It is sometimes of a gray color and dry as if it had been subjected to the action of an acid. When the nasal ducts participate in the disease there is usually a copious discharge of sanious and fetid fluid both from the nose and mouth. The shreds of false membrane thrown off are soon succeeded by others of a thinner and whitish appearance. Large quantities of false membrane are thrown off in this way and from the fact that an offensive odor exhales from the mouth especially in adults, their nature was at one time mistaken for sloughs. Sometimes the false membrane instead of being thrown off in shreds becomes softened and mixes with the saliva and is absorbed.

The general symptoms that usually attend this condition are paleness and puffiness of the face with alteration of the features, tumefaction of the tongue which commonly has a red margin and a thick coat covering the surface. An effort to get rid of the membrane sometimes causes vomiting. The bowels are sometimes constipated while at others a diarrhœa accompanies the disease. At the same time the throat is implicated. There is a singular tendency to the same kind of exudation from all surfaces divested of the cuticle, the lips, nostrils, behind the ears and from the surface of blisters and leechbites and this should warn of the danger of applying blisters to the throat externally to relieve inflammation.

CAUSES.—Diphtheritis is believed to be the result of exciting causes acting in conjunction with a state of deterioration of the blood. It appears in all climates and seasons but chiefly in moist countries. It often occurs endemically where persons are crowded together in restricted spaces. It sometimes occurs epidemically in districts where there is much moisture, dirt and filth, and where many persons are crowded together in illy ventilated workshops. Without due regard to cleanliness the disease seems to partake of the character of an epidemic. It has been maintained by some that it is a specific poison, but this requires confirmation. Shreds of false membrane have been inoculated into the arm without effect and this would seem to indicate with some certainty that it is not contagious. We have seen that the diphtheritic form of pharyngitis is inflammation differing from the simple inflammatory affections of the mucous membrane. We have seen also that a predisposition exists in the system to the formation of false membranes and they may appear on any surface, denuded of the epidermis or cuticle and the inevitable conclusion is that some changes or abnormal condition of the circulating fluid must be the predisposing cause.

ALLOPATHIC TREATMENT.—Emetics are recommended in all stages of the disease and cathartics sufficient to keep the bowels open to carry off the morbid secretions.

HOMŒOPATHIC TREATMENT.—*Belladonna* is indicated when the disease sets in with severe febrile symptoms and marked inflammation of the tonsils. It is of little use after exudation has taken place.

Kali bichromicum is particularly adapted if the exudation is composed of loosely adhering shreds. *Bromium*, when the membrane firmly adheres and is tenacious and when the patient has great debility and nervous prostration for a long time after all the other morbid symptoms have disappeared.

Mercurius iodatus.—After Belladonna and after the exudation becomes apparent and when the patient complains of great soreness and difficulty in swallowing.

Muriatic acid.—When there is an exceedingly low fever with marked lassitude and weariness. *Arsenicum* may be addressed to that general condition of the system that favors gangrenous disorganization.

Phytolacca decandra is indicated in every stage of the disease except when gangrene sets in. It is particularly useful in diphtheritic croup.

The treatment would then stand in the following order: *Belladonna* must be given at the commencement and before the membrane is formed. *Mercurius iodatus* should be given after, followed by *Kali bichromicum* and *Bromine*. *Arsenicum* and *Kreasotum* are employed in case of several gangrenous disorganizations; *Muriatic acid* if the case progresses slowly, and, for debility after the disease has left, *China*.

DOSE AND ADMINISTRATION.—Belladonna may be given drop doses of the dilution in water repeated every hour, Mercurius iod.

in trituration two grains every hour; Kali bichromicum, dissolve a powder in one third of a glass of water and give a teaspoonful every half hour; Muriatic acid, 2d dilution in drop doses every hour; Arsenicum in trituration, a two grain powder every two hours; Kreasotum, 5 drops in half a tumbler of water,—a teaspoonful every two hours. Other liquids and powders to be given in the same way.

DIET.—No invariable rule can be laid down for diet. It may consist in general of farinaceous aliments, but varied to meet the different stages of the disease.

Gangrenous Inflammation of the Pharynx.

This disease is known as putrid or malignant sore throat. It is seen in the malignant form of scarlet fever. The symptoms from the first are of a malignant character and eminently typhous. The prognosis is unfavorable as it generally runs a rapid course and terminates fatally and at times suddenly on the third or fourth day of the disease.

The symptoms from the first are of an appalling character such as are seen in malignant scarlet fever. After considerable indisposition there is chilliness, headache, vertigo, nausea and faintness with slight pain in the throat and occasionally with swelling of the neck which impedes its movements. Then follows a redness and slight tumefaction of the neck, face and chest and also of the upper extremities. The fever is usually characterized by pungent heat, with great restlessness and delirium or with stupor and coma. The tongue is dry and covered with soot like crusts as well as the lips which crack and appear as if burnt. The parotid glands swell, the nose bleeds or some other form of hæmorrhage supervenes with spots on the skin, and the symptoms in all respects are those of typhus. On inspecting the throat the mucous membrane is found to be of a deep red or purple hue upon which patches of a pulpy character and of the color of ashes, which soon changes to brown or black, are perceptible. The parts soon begin to slough and a putrid odor is exhaled from the mouth, and from the nose an ichorous discharge of offensive sanious matter, and the lips and corners of the mouth become implicated in the morbid condition.

THE ALLOPATHIC TREATMENT for this disease consists in the administration of stimulants and the topical application of antiseptic washes.

THE HOMŒOPATHIC TREATMENT requires *Arsenicum, Krea-sotum, Lachesis, Rhus tox.*, etc., while at the same time topical applications of the fluid chlorides of lime and soda are made use of. Of the remedies selected four globules may be given and repeated every hour.

DIET.—The diet should consist of sago and tapioca, gruels, wine whey and delicate broths.

Inflammation of the Œsophagus.

This is a rare affection which differs only in its seat from inflammation of the pharynx. The chief symptoms are local pain with difficult swallowing and hiccough after alimentary substances have passed the pharynx and reached the seat of inflammation. The disease commonly terminates by resolution and differs in no way from ordinary inflammation of the mucous membranes.

CAUSES.—The swallowing of sharp or pointed bodies, pieces of bone or hot and acrid substances, are reckoned among the common causes. But the disease may occur from organic changes, difficult to appreciate.

TREATMENT.—As the disease is rarely severe the restriction of the patient to emollient drinks and allowing them but rarely and the application of sinapisms to the neck and feet with laxative enemata have been found sufficient. *Aconite* may be given in case of fever and *Belladonna* if there is much local pain; Moschus will generally overcome the hiccough. Drop doses of the dilutions may be employed and repeated every hour until the patient is better. In the violent form of the disease, general depletion has been recommended with application of leeches along the course of the pain. But this is unnecessary as well as objectionable, since a few doses of Aconite are sufficient to work a speedy cure.

Sometimes ŒSOPHAGITIS may produce a STRICTURE of the tube but more frequently this trouble is brought on by some malignant affection of the walls of the passage. THE STRICTURE is more commonly formed in the upper portion of the tube and may take place insidiously without the patient suspecting the gradual diminution of the same until it is found to interfere with the swallowing of solids and until nothing but liquids can reach the stomach.

A case of the kind came under my observation several years

ago, where the submucous tissue became so thickened as to form a kind of ring that materially lessened the calibre of the tubes and obstructed the passage of food into the stomach and the patient finally died for the want of sustenance. Previous to this fatal event he would often swallow solids that remained in the tube above the point of the stricture for some little time and then would be returned by regurgitation.

TREATMENT.—In the incipient stage of stricture, internal remedies may be of some avail especially when the stricture consists of a mere thickening of the mucous lining of the tube.

Sulphur, Iodium, Mercurius iodatus or *vivus, Hepar sulph.* and *Arsenicum* have been advantageously employed. But in case of a cicatrice or cul de sac, little advantage can be derived from remedies. The mechanical operation of the graduated sound has sometimes produced excellent effects and may be employed with internal remedies. *Aconite, Nux vomica* and *Tartar emetic* are remedies that may prove salutary in spasmodic stricture.

The sound is almost the only measure resorted to by physicians of the Allopathic school although medicines are sometimes given to modify nutrition.

The ŒSOPHÁGUS as well as the LARYNX are sometimes the seat of cancer which encroaches upon the tube and interrupts the passage the same as stricture. A young man aged 24 first felt a slight uneasiness in the throat in the form of a tickling sensation that afterwards became gradually painful until it assumed a lancinating character and deglutition became more and more difficult. These symptoms are those of cancer, developing in the tube. This case in spite of remedies proved fatal; an autopsy revealed the cause to be a cancerous growth in the tube below the pharynx. When these symptoms manifest themselves it is manifestly proper to try the effects of internal remedies. Arsenicum iodatus, Iodium, Conium and Mercurius are remedies to be consulted.

ALLOPATHIC TREATMENT consists in the use of the bougies in connection with the internal administration of Iodine in doses of ten drops of the tincture and full doses of opium or other narcotics to allay the pain. This treatment at best is only palliative.

In all cases of stricture whether the result of wounds, cancer or morbid growths, that interfere with or interrupt the passage of food into the stomach, both medicine and food may for a time be conveyed into the stomach by means of an elastic tube provided for the purpose, or life may be prolonged by throwing soups, milk and other nutritive solutions into the colon.   But there is scarcely any chance of the patient deriving permanent advantage.

For paralysis of the œsophagus which is usually a symptom of general paralysis much benefit may be derived from the use of Geiger's voltaic battery.   The zincpole to the feet and the copper to the larynx, sides and base of the tongue, three or four times a day a few minutes at a time.   The application may be continued for several weeks.

CHAPTER XII.

DISEASES OF THE STOMACH.

The stomach and intestines are lined by a mucous membrane the same as the œsophagus and fauces but their muscular coat is much thinner and in addition they have a reflection of the peritoneum, which lines the cavity of the abdomen. In consequence of the arrangement of these coats their diseases are somewhat different from those of the mouth and passage to the stomach. The coats of the stomach and intestines are severally liable to be implicated by disease. The more prominent affections however are restricted to the peritoneal and mucous coats. The muscular coat may be more or less influenced, but not liable to any serious implication unless organically deranged.

Inflammation of the Stomach.

Through constant exposure of the stomach to the action of irritants, sometimes though not frequently, the chronic form is met with. It is therefore proper to give each a consideration.

ACUTE INFLAMMATION OF THE STOMACH according to various authors may occur in the mucous coat and sometimes though rarely in the muscular. The former, according to *Broussais* never occurs except in connection with a similar state of the small intestines. *Stokes* on the contrary admits that they often exist together, but can exist alone.

The symptoms manifest in the acute form are first shivering followed by heat of the skin, languor and lassitude and other evidences of internal inflammation; a severe pain in the pit of the stomach which extends to the back, along the course of the adjoining small intestine and upward along the course of the œsophagus and between the shoulders. The pain at the pit of the stomach is augmented by the slightest pressure and by the depression of the diaphragm, so that inspiration becomes intensely distressing. There is also a constant retching and pain, which either solid or liquid aliments, when taken, produce a palpable aggravation of. Burning heat in the stomach and the nausea and retching are superlatively painful. The matters ejected consist of the fluids taken into the stomach, with mucus and bile and blood, and their discharge affords no relief. The thirst is intense and unquenchable and the desire for cold drinks unlimited; and yet no fluid reaches the stomach that is not instantly ejected. The pulse is usually small and frequent, when the gastritis is severe. This severe form of the disease generally progresses rapidly to a fatal termination, which may be in a few hours or not until the lapse of two or three days, and especially when produced by acrid or corrosive poison.

In the milder form of the disease the symptoms are much less marked. A dull pain aggravated by the slightest pressure or when food is taken or when any shock is experienced is felt at the pit of the stomach. The pain is not always continuous, there may be occasional intervals, or if continuous there may be occasional aggravations with uneasy sense of pulsation and tension in the region of the stomach. The appetite is generally impaired but at times it is morbid and craving. Considerable thirst, dryness of the mouth and redness of the tongue are almost always present in all forms of the disease. The appearance of the tongue in endogastritis affords a guide in discriminating between inflammation of the mucous coat and that of the peritoneal, the whole surface at times is vividly red, at other times this vivid redness is confined to the sides and tip, while papillæ at the middle of the tongue protrude through the white coating like red points. This form of acute inflammation of the stomach generally terminates by resolution or it may pass into the chronic form.

The causes that commonly operate in the production of acute inflammation of the stomach are mechanical injuries or wounds produced by taking sharp and pointed substances into the stomach or by swallowing corrosive and acrid poisons.

Treatment.—*Aconite* when there is an active and violent inflammation of the stomach with full and rapid pulse, shivering and bilious vomiting.

Arsenicum, when there is great soreness and burning at the pit of the stomach, continual vomiting and thirst, a dry and cracked tongue and continual shivering and heat at the same time and also a white coating over the middle of the tongue with red margins.

Belladonna, when the gastritis is attended with severe throb-

11

bing frontal headache and also when there is a succession of rigors passing down the spine.

Bryonia alba, when the pain of the stomach is aggravated by turning or moving or when there is continual vomiting of glairy mucus.

Merc. corr. may be suitable for removing certain kinds of inflammation of the stomach characterized by painful burning in the epigastric region and vomiting of acrid matters and considerable thirst.

Nux vomica, suitable for mild cases of gastritis where there is dull pain and nausea but no active vomiting; gastritis of drunkards. *Veratrum album,* when there is coldness of the surface and extremities. All the above remedies should be given in water two or three drops, a small powder or six globules may be dissolved in a cup of water and a teaspoonful every thirty minutes. *Aconite,* when there is much heat with a hard, full and bounding pulse. If there is violent vomiting and altered features and cold extremities *Arsenicum* or *Veratrum; Nux vomica* for the gastritis of drunkards; *Belladonna,* for burning pains in the stomach with delirium and dread of liquids; *Bryonia,* when the burning pains in the stomach are aggravated by motion or when vomiting occurs immediately after drinking; *Cantharis,* for stinging, burning pains in the stomach with pains in the bowels, kidneys or bladder; *Hyoscyamus,* for vomiting blood, dread of liquid and spasms after drinking. *Phosphorus* is sometimes useful after *Arsenicum* and for feeble pulse, violent thirst, anxiety, and coldness of the extremities. When corrosive poisons are the cause of the inflammation of the stomach, they must be got rid of or antidoted, and afterward a few drops of *Camphor* given in a spoonful of tepid water. During treatment the patient should take but little water or barley water or thin gruel.

THE ALLOPATHIC TREATMENT when the inflammation is severe is blood-letting pushed to a degree that makes a decided impression upon the system or by the application of leeches to the epigastric region. Small quantities of cold soda water are given to allay the vomiting and small pieces of ice are allowed in the mouth and enemas are given to operate on the lower portion of the alimentary canal and even cold water is thrown up into the colon. But all this may be unnecessary when Homœopathic remedies are at hand with a careful farinaceous diet. Relapses from error in diet are apt to occur.

Chronic Inflammation of the Stomach.

Some authors have included under this head all the forms of dyspepsia. But it is by no means certain that endogastritis or inflammation of the mucous coat is present in many cases of this disorder and a careful discrimination is necessary in order to institute a proper treatment. Chronic inflammation of the mucous coat may supervene upon the acute form but often when there has been no sign of the latter. The *symptoms* of the chronic form are unlike those of the acute as for instance, in place of acute pain increased on the slightest pressure, the most marked symptom may be a sense of weight, as if some solid substance was in the stomach. This feeling is often persistent and distressing on this account, but not so much from its severity. The appetite is impaired and a nauseous bitter taste in the mouth, which is clammy; a foul tongue especially in the morning on rising, a morbid digestion, flatulence and a sense of distension with occasional distension with occasional nausea and vomiting, torpid bowels, hot skin and frequent pulse, usually attend chronic gastritis, though sometimes there may be a looseness of the bowels, when the mucous lining of the intestines participates with that of the stomach. These symptoms may continue a long time without materially disabling the patient or injuring the general health. But sooner or later unless the inflammation is removed, the entire nutritive system becomes involved owing to the defective condition of the chyle, and the constant irritation and depression of spirits and loss of mental and corporeal energy and emaciation may so operate upon the patient as to cause his death and frequently with all the symptoms of pulmonary consumption.

The most common cause of chronic gastritis is the intemperate use of alcoholic and malt liquors or other stimulants and aliments that disagree with the patient and when the cause is known it must be obviated before any treatment will prove effectual in bringing about a cure.

TREATMENT.—When there is burning in the stomach and acrid eructations, intense thirst, a thick white coating upon the tongue, *Arsenicum* may be given three times a day. This remedy is especially useful when emaciation has progressed to a considerable degree and when there is perpetual inclination to vomit as in acute gastritis.

Nux vomica when the inflammation has come on gradually from the use of stimulants such as malt liquors and wine or alcoholic stimulants of any kind.

Arsenicum in the morning and *Nux* in the evening, we have found the most effectual in the treatment of these cases.

We have alluded to the difference between chronic gastritis and dyspepsia. The former being a chronic inflammation of the mucous coat that may in rare instances result in ulceration, while the latter presenting many of the symptoms in common is nevertheless a functional disorder and embraces all the forms of difficult digestion.

Dyspepsia is difficult digestion often attended by much pain and may accompany chronic gastritis or may exist alone from mere functional weakness of the stomach.

The chief therapeutic agents in simple dyspepsia are *China, Hepar sulph., Ignatia, Mercurius, Nux vom., Pulsatilla* and *Sulphur*.

China when the condition of the stomach is such the lightest kind of nourishment is not digested and when there is great bodily weakness.

Hepar sulph., when the dyspepsia has been caused by mercurial cathartics prescribed in the old way.

Ignatia for dyspepsia in nervous persons brought on by grief or in persons exceedingly sensitive and inclined to weep.

Mercurius viv. when there is cardialgia and water brash or acrid regurgitations.

Nux vomica.—Dyspepsia caused by intemperance or inability of the stomach to digest food from other causes.

Pulsatilla when rich food is taken into the stomach and is difficult to digest, such as fat meat, cake, etc. It is suitable for females suffering from indigestion in connection with menstrual difficulties or hysteria.

Sulphur is suitable for chronic weakness of the digestive organs accompanied by torpidity of the liver.

Pepsin is a valuable remedy for dyspepsia in feeble persons, who suffer after each meal from weight and distress in the stomach.

In selecting the appropriate remedy reference must be had to the symptoms which afford the surest indication to their employment.

DOSE AND ADMINISTRATION.—Of the remedy selected when dilutions are used a few drops may be mixed in half a glass of water and a dessert-spoonful may be given after each meal. Four globules may be given as a dose in the same manner or if triturations are employed give a two grain powder either half an hour before or half an hour after each meal.

THE ALLOPATHIC TREATMENT for *chronic gastritis* is mainly with revulsives accompanied by a light diet—cups and leeches are occasionally applied to the pit of the stomach, or blisters, ointment of Tartar emetic or a few drops of Croton oil, rubbed on the epigastrium. This resort to counter-irritation is chiefly relied on to divert the inflammation from the coat of the stomach. For *transient dyspepsia*, caused by over-eating and drinking, the treatment consists in obviating it by drafts of bitter infusion such as that of *Gentian, Columbo, Chamomile flowers*, etc.—whereas in *chronic dyspepsia* the treatment is mainly dietetic or if there is pretty generally a foul stomach, pulverized charcoal or chloride of lime are administered internally or if constipation is a prominent condition mild laxatives are recommended.

ECLECTIC TREATMENT consists of tonics to improve the tone of the stomach and mild aperients to promote the activity of the bowels. But experience proves that a disabled condition of the stomach is not permanently relieved by these agents. They afford but a temporary relief, whereas a strictly Homœopathic treatment acts with the vital struggle of nature to overcome the weakness, without producing new struggles to be borne up against by the vital economy and in this respect it has shown itself the most competent and reliable for permanent relief. But in all cases of dyspepsia whether transient or chronic, a well regulated diet is essential in order to favor the prompt action of remedies.

Gastrorrhœa or Catarrh of the Stomach.

The mucous membrane of the stomach like that which lines other cavities may be affected with catarrh, although not dependent on inflammation. The cause of this affection is obscure and on this account some have maintained that it is the sequel of gastritis, not unlike the gleet that follows a previous inflammation. This however, is conjecture. The stomachal catarrh as described by *Andral* is a disease separate and distinct from gas-

tritis, though it may exist along with it. There appears to be
two forms of this disorder, one is a simple flux of the mucous
coat and the other takes the form of *pyrosis* or *water brash*.
Both of these forms are associated with dyspepsia and simply indicate a disordered stomach, that interferes with nutrition.

Mucous gastrorrhœa may be cured by the following remedies:
Bryonia, Ipecac, Nux vomica and Tartar emetic.

Bryonia when there are constant regurgitations and vomiting of mucus with sensation of heat.

Ipecac, when there is considerable nausea and occasional
vomiting of mucus, tinged with biliary matters.

Nux vomica, when the mucous membrane has been stimulated by acrid matters or intoxicating drinks taken into the
stomach and especially if there is nausea, vertigo or distress in
the stomach previous to vomiting.

Tartar emetic is perhaps the best and most effectual remedy
in the treatment of this affection and especially when there is an
inappetency and a constant disposition to spit up mucus of a
whitish semi-transparent character having an almost neutral taste
and smell.

THE ALLOPATHIC TREATMENT of this form of catarrh is to
drench the stomach with emetics. Massive doses of *Ipecac* and
Tartar emetic are employed for the purpose and these are followed
by brisk cathartics and after this purgatorial resort, tonics are
given at regular intervals during the day. The objection to this
treatment is the tax it inflicts upon the vital condition of the
stomach, while only a palliation of the difficulty is experienced.

For pyrosis or waterbrash which is the other form of gastrorrhœa, *Mercurius vivus* or *Mercurius solubilis*, taken several
times a day, will generally effect a cure. A few drops of the
third aqueous dilution of *Nitric acid* taken three or four times a
day is also a valuable remedy. In some cases pyrosis is difficult
to cure and in some instances a glass of hard cider has changed
the condition of the stomach and produced a cure, when other
remedies have failed. In all cases of gastrorrhœa the diet should
be light, consisting in part of mucilaginous drinks.

Cancer of the Stomach.

The pyloric orifice of the stomach is in most cases the seat of
cancer. It may, however, attack both the anterior and exterior
surface of the organ.

The symptoms that indicate cancer of the stomach are at first those of ordinary dyspepsia or chronic gastritis; a shooting pain is subsequently felt in the epigastric region or otherwise a sensation of extreme weight. Digestion is always impaired. There is more or less distention of the abdomen after eating even the smallest quantities and the patient is distressed by acid eructations. Vomiting soon after eating is a common symptom of carcinoma seated in the cardiac portion of the stomach or if seated near the pylorus it may not occur for an hour after the aliment is taken. When vomiting occurs on an empty stomach it usually consists of mucous and blood. At a later stage a dark colored discharge from the stomach resembling chocolate or coffee grounds is vomited or spit up continually and often in enormous quantities. But in all cases the rejection of the contents of the stomach affords but temporary relief. There is but little light thrown on the disease by an external examination. In a very few instances a movable tumor has been felt through the walls of the abdomen. We have seen two fatal cases which went through all stages, where no tumor whatever could be felt in any part of the stomach externally. In many cases the patient presents a sallow countenance with the corners of the mouth drawn down, presenting a cadaverous expression. Some authors assert that true cancer of the stomach has been cured, but generally it must be regarded as a fatal disease.

CAUSES.—It is presumed that the causes of cancer of the stomach are the same as those of cancer in general. A cancerous diathesis constitutes the predisposition which may be developed by various exciting causes, among which may be reckoned intense anxiety of mind, a multitude of business cares and disappointments, the habit of drinking ardent spirits on an empty stomach. It is believed that cancerous tumors have existed in a quiescent state for years. The disease is not common between the ages of thirty-five and sixty years.

TREATMENT.—Even in cases of well defined cancer of the stomach, a strict attention to diet with appropriate treatment may prolong the life of the patient for years. The remedies employed in Homœopathic treatment are *Arsenicum, Lycopodium, Nux vomica.*

Arsenicum when the patient is beset with intense anxiety and depression of spirits with constant burning in the stomach with inclination to vomit blood and mucous or dark acrid matters, a constant regurgitation and spitting of chocolate colored matter.

Lycopodium when there is a griping and tearing sensation in the stomach and flatulent distension of the abdomen and tedious constipation.

Nux vomica when instead of sharp shooting pains in the stomach there is a perpetual sensation of a heavy weight and when there is much anxiety and vomiting of acrid matter, dark and resembling coffee grounds and also when the patient is troubled with constipation. A case came under our observation ten years ago where the patient had been long troubled with the above symptoms and had been pronounced by several physicians incurable. *Nux vomica*, 6th decimal attenuation was prescribed and the patient began to improve. The remedy was continued for several weeks in connection with a diet of mutton broth and farinaceous gruels. The Nux was administered every night. The appearance of the patient improved continually until all the symptoms disappeared and he felt quite well. He soon regained his strength and until the present time has remained quite well.

Hartman records several cases of cure with this remedy and in the hands of other practitioners it has been employed with like effect. Lutze records a case of a lady which had been abandoned as hopeless by all her physicians. She threw up nothing but a chocolate colored ichor and fæces. She was completely restored by the alternate use of Nux vomica and Arsenicum every two hours and the lady was living five years after in perfect health.

Conium when the disease is caused by a blow or fall upon the stomach.

Plumbum has likewise been employed for excessive vomiting and constipation when the matters ejected had the appearance of verdigris or black, bilious and bitter matter with periodical paroxysms of burning distress with anxiety and cold perspiration.

THE ALLOPATHIC TREATMENT consists of the administration of iodine and other agents in palpable doses for the purpose of modifying the condition of the blood and through it that of the system of nutrition. Antacids are recommended for acid eructations and mild aperients and enemas to overcome constipation while the severe pain is palliated by the preparations of opium. It will be seen that the treatment is merely palliative and not calculated to effect a cure and besides its weakening effect upon the entire organism rather hastens than retards a fatal termination and especially is this so, when blisters, cups and leeches applied to the epigastrium are employed as adjuvants.

A milk diet as a general rule is the most appropriate, but should this disagree the farinaceous preparations as arrow root or sago or animal broths may be substituted.

Hæmorrhage from the Stomach—Hæmatemesis.

This occurrence is not unfrequent, and when independent of disease in some other organ, it is not usually regarded a very serious affection.   It is generally a symptom of some other disturbance which sooner or later discloses itself.

The premonitory symptoms before any blood is discharged from the stomach, the patient experiences signs of concentration of action towards some internal organ with others peculiar to the stomach itself.   Usually the first sensation felt is chilliness, and a feeling of heat and distention of the stomach, at the same time the face is pale and the extremities cold.   The upper portion of the stomach now becomes distended with a sense of weight.   A sweetish taste is perceived in the mouth, followed by nausea and vomiting, in most cases, of a large quantity of blood, which by reason of its gradual accumulation in the stomach is mixed with the gastric fluids and other contents of the organ, and is always black and often grumous.   Vomiting of blood may be a mere symptom of softening, of perforation or of cancer, in which vessels may be perforated or ruptured, and thus a copious discharge of blood may ensue.

THE CAUSES of hæmorrhage from the stomach may be mechanical injuries either from blows or the passing of sharp substances into the stomach, or it may take place from active gastritis or even from inappreciable circumstances.   In females whose menses have never appeared, it may prove to be a vicarious discharge and attended with less danger.   It is a symptom of purpura and typhus.   When caused by chronic gastritis or cancer the previous symptoms may throw some light upon the pathology of the disease.   Whatever impedes the return of the blood along the portal system towards the heart, may result in hæmorrhage from the stomach.

TREATMENT.—The remedies employed in the treatment of hæmatemesis are *Arnica, Belladonna, Chamomilla, China, Ipecac, Millefolium, Nux vomica, Opium, Phosphorus.*

Arnica when the hæmorrhage results from mechanical injuries and when there is soreness of the stomach as if bruised.

Belladonna is suitable at the commencement when the patient complains of chilliness, and also when there is a discharge of blood from the mouth and from the rectum at the same time.

Chamomilla if chagrin has caused an exudation and vomiting of blood from the stomach.

China when the patient has been suffering from extreme debility.

Millefolium may be given after *China* and for similar symptoms.

Nux vomica when brought on by drunkenness and debauch. *Opium* also for cases of this kind.

Pulsatilla may be given for vomiting of blood at the menstrual period, or in cases where the menstruation has not appeared.

Phosphorus in case of great debility when there is much heat in the stomach.

Ipecac for painless vomiting of blood from unknown causes.

DOSE.—*Six globules* of the selected remedy may be given every hour or two hours according to the severity of the case or a few drops of the dilution in a cup of water, may be given, a teaspoonful at a time every two hours.

THE ALLOPATHIC TREATMENT is not uniform for this disease. In plethoric persons when there is no evidence of gastritis a full antiphlogistic treatment is recommended in connection with phlebotomy and where it arises in consequence of obstructed catamenia the same treatment is advised. When from amenorrhœa saline cathartics are commended. In other cases astringents are recommended as follows: Equal proportions of diluted Sulphuric acid and tincture of Opium in doses of twelve drops every three hours.

Gastralgia.—Heartburn.

This affection consists of a gnawing or burning uneasiness at the cardiac portion of the stomach. It is a common symptom of dyspepsia as well as of chronic gastritis and cancer of the stomach. Simple heartburn is characterized by acid eructations, violent burning and marked effervescence when Carbonate of lime and soda or Magnesia are taken into the stomach. The remedies employed are chiefly *Mercurius* and *Nux vomica*.

Mercurius, when the heartburn is attended with acrid or burning regurgitations and considerable distress in the cardiac region.

Nux vomica, when the heartburn is caused by an acid stomach and the regurgitation of acid matters.

The effect of these remedies is to restore normal vitality to the stomach and thereby promote healthy digestion.

THE ALLOPATHIC TREATMENT consists mainly in the administration of ant-acids which have only a temporary effect in chemically neutralizing the acids of the stomach. *Carbonate* of *magnesia*, Carbonate of soda or Carbonate of lime and soda are the chief agents advised. But the Homœopathic treatment is altogether preferable.

Cramps in the Stomach.—Gastrodynia.

There are different degrees of this affection along with other signs of dyspepsia. It is only the most severe form that is usually designated " cramps in the stomach." We have observed that many dyspeptics are prone to suffer from neuralgia pain resembling colic, which at times occurs before food is received into the stomach and other times during the digestion of the same. It is often extremely violent at the epigastrium and may in some instances be accompanied by vomiting. Pressure seldom aggravates the pain but on the contrary pressure relieves it. Its occurrence may be frequent for years without resulting in organic disease, coming on at times rapidly and violently attains its extreme point and as rapidly passes off to be reproduced by like causes. A crust of bread will often relieve slight attacks and sometimes a severe attack be mitigated by resorting to this expedient early in the morning on an empty stomach. Many cases of this kind are upon record. In certain cases the spasm of the stomach is excessively severe and is accompanied by anxiety, nausea, eructations and coldness of the extremities, failure of strength and inclination to faint. It is then termed "*cramp in the stomach*" and like every other form of gastrodynia it is relieved by regurgitation. It is sometimes induced by cold drinks and in all probability it may be an attack of gout, transferred to this region. It is believed that in general this distress is more persistent than dangerous. Some authors affirm that it is wholly devoid of danger in all cases and after it occurs it never leaves behind any traces of its existence.   But, in as much as colic may induce inflammation, we dissent from this opinion.

TREATMENT.—The remedies employed in the treatment of gastrodynia are *Arnica, Belladonna, Bryonia, Chamomilla. China, Carbo vegetabilis, Cocculus, Calc. carb., Graphites, Ignatia. Nux vomica, Pulsatilla, Stannum, Staphysagria, Sepia* and *Sulphur.*

Arnica when spasmodic pains are produced in the stomach by lifting heavy weights or doing hard work and when there is a digging pain in the pit of the stomach with bitter and foul eructations.

Belladonna.—For pressure and cramp in the stomach returning every day at dinner, also at night with trembling and even with loss of consciousness on account of intense pain, which is relieved by stretching the trunk backwards and holding the breath, and, when there is vertigo, vomiting of bile or mucus, intense thirst and the pains are aggravated by drinking.

Bryonia.—Oppression after eating, soreness, crampy stitch when making a wrong step.

Carbo vegetabilis.—Painful pressure at the pit of the stomach and cramp with burning after the use of fat and flatulent food.

Chamomilla.—When chagrin is the exciting cause of painful pressure at the stomach as from a stone; painful bloating at the pit of the stomach with shortness of breath, anxiety and throbbing headache. Aggravations at night relieved by bending double.

China for oppression of the stomach after eating ever so little; bitter eructations tasting the ingesta.   Cramps set in after the loss of blood or from diarrhœa, or any exhaustion after excesses or from nursing or spermatorrhœa; pains worse when the patient lies on the side, or relieved when turning on the back or rising from his seat and feels better in the morning before breakfast.

Cocculus.—Constrictive pains in the stomach and abdomen relieved by passing off flatus.

Graphites for cramps of the stomach attendant on scanty menses.

Ignatia when caused by care or grief, feeling of weakness and qualmishness in the pit of the stomach or a sense of emptiness and pricking in this region.

Ipecac.—Intense distress at the pit of the stomach and vomiting greenish and gelatinous matter.

Nux vomica.—Suitable for drunkards and for those who indulge in excessive use of coffee, violent cramps and tearing sensation in the stomach or as if flatulence had become incarcerated under the ribs; burning in the pit of the stomach, distention, vomiting and heartburn. This remedy occupies the first place for persons of a sedentary habit and inclined to be irritable.

Pulsatilla.—Especially adapted to females having a pale complexion with gentle, desponding dispositions, scanty or suppressed menses, pressure in the stomach after taking fat food, pastry, warm bread. Bitter taste, no thirst, flatulence in the evening and during motion.

Sepia.—Pain in the stomach with sour and empty eructations; pressure in the stomach as from a stone with stinging and burning. Especially adapted for the critical period, when the menses are scanty or intermittent.

Stannum, for pains in the stomach with retching and griping, short breath and vomiting of food.

Staphysagria, pressure in the stomach as from load, made worse by eating.

Sulphur is especially suited in cases where the patient has been or is affected with chronic eruptions and has pain in the stomach with empty or sour eructations, as in heartburn.

These medicines may be administered in water or globules of the remedy indicated, four globules may be given every hour in severe cases or a few drops of the dilution may be given in half a glass of water, a teaspoonful every hour or two hours, according to the nature of the case. No treatment for this distressing malady has afforded more prompt and decided relief than the Homœopathic and it is to be commended in all cases.

THE ALLOPATHIC TREATMENT for cramps of the stomach is the employment of stimulants and opiates with hot applications to the epigastrium. The following formulæ is the one approved in Allopathic practice for severe colic.

℞. Tinct. Opii   ʒij   For inveterate cramps.
   Æther Sulph ʒiss   ℞. Kreasoti m iv.
   Mist. Camphor. ℥iij   Mist. Camphoræ.
M. Half to be taken and   Infus. Gentian aa f ʒvj.
   repeated in an hour.   M. fiat haustus. Teaspoonful every hour.

The additional disorder of the stomach which this treatment imparts renders it objectionable.

Vomiting.

Although vomiting is a symptom which accompanies all the affections of the stomach we have considered, yet there can be no question, but that at times it is the main feature of the disease or a purely nervous phenomena. When of this character it may be cured by *Ipecac, Nux vomica* or *Tartar emetic*. Drop doses of the dilution, each in a spoonful of water given at each paroxysm, will soon change the condition and obviate the difficulty and this will supercede the deleterious use of *Magnesia, Hydrocyanic acid, Alum* and *Kreasote* and *Peppermint water*, generally resorted to in Allopathic treatment and given in an atmosphere impregnated with camphor, musk, valerian, ammonia, etc. But, to be explicit, we will recommend for acid vomiting, *Nux vom.;* for bilious vomiting Ipecac, for vomiting from atony of the stomach, Tartar emetic. For vomiting in sea sickness or riding in a carriage, *Cocculus* given as above.

CHAPTER XIII.

DISEASES OF THE INTESTINES.

It will be borne in mind that the small intestine is simply a continuation from the stomach of similar coats and membranes, and, with the exception of the gastric acid like secretions take place from the mucous lining of the tube. In addition, however, the liver and pancreas pour the materials of their secretion into the upper portion of the small intestine and influence more or less the execution of its functions, and the varying condition of the small intestine cannot fail to react upon these glands. Nevertheless the diseases of the small intestine bear a close resemblance to those which assail the stomach.

The larger portion of the abdominal cavity is occupied by the small intestines, while the large intestine occupies the sides, crossing over beneath the stomach and inclosing them. The duodenum or second stomach commences at the pylorus and terminates in the jejunum. The remainder of the small intestine constitutes the ileum which is the portion chiefly implicated when violent pain is felt in the umbilical region.

In studying the diseases of the large intestine it is essential to keep in mind its position in the abdomen as well as the location of the three divisions—the cæcum, colon and rectum. The cæcum commences at the termination of the small intestine and extends to the point where the colon commences, at the posterior and left side of which is the vermiform appendix. The colon extends along the right flank as far as the under surface of the liver, crosses over the abdomen to gain the left flank, along which it descends into the left iliac region to form the sigmoid flexure and terminates in the rectum.

The coats of the large intestine are the same in number and structure as those of the small but they are not so thick and not so easily separated on dissection. The most marked difference between them are the pouches of the large intestine which serve as reservoirs for the excrement, in which it becomes hardened by the absorption of the fluid portion.

The rectum differs somewhat from the other portions of the

large intestine in being possessed of thicker walls and a more powerful muscular coat. The lower portion of the rectum, just before it reaches the anus, is wide and capacious enough to admit of enormous quantities of indurated fæces, which sometimes takes place, as the expulsive power is lessened, as in aged people.

The large intestine is a reservoir for the fæces, which, when expelled, have the shape of the intestine or aperture through which they are evacuated. They do not pass into the rectum in large quantities, unless in a fluid state, but are retained in the colon until an instinctive desire for an evacuation occurs, and then they descend into the rectum to be evacuated.

The structure of the alimentary canal is so similar throughout that diseases which affect one portion are apt to extend to others, hence gastritis and enteritis are often found to exist at the same time, and also ileitis and colitis. The former is termed gastro-enteritis, the latter ileo-colitis, and as such they have generally been described.

Inflammation of the Small Intestines.

As there are two coats of the small intestines that may be attacked with either the acute or chronic form of inflammation, it may be proper to consider them separately. The *peritoneal coat* is subject to acute inflammation in any portion of the intestine. It announces itself with the following symptoms: violent burning, cutting or stitching pain in the abdomen, proceeding from a given point it spreads over the whole abdomen. The pain is continuous, increasing from time to time without any intermission as in colic. The abdomen is hot, distended and extremely sensitive to touch or pressure. There is usually an increase of pain after eating or drinking the smallest quantities. Accompanying these symptoms there are unceasing eructations, frequent vomitings of greenish matters and sometimes of fæces and urine and constant hiccough. The bowels are often constipated, though at other times a greenish diarrhœa sets in with intense suffering and anxiety and violent urging to stool, retention of urine, which is only voided in drops and has a fiery red appearance. The patient is tormented with internal heat, dry tongue, intense thirst, excessive anxiety, restlessness and sleeplessness, continuous fever, with small, soft, frequent, intermittent

and but rarely full and hard pulse. Delirium generally supervenes upon these symptoms with wild looks, spasmodic twitchings of the facial muscles, contraction of the pupils, obscuration
of sight, sopor, stupor, coldness of the extremities, violent burning in the bowels, strength fails rapidly, fainting fits, etc., etc.

The pains are most violent in the region of the umbilicus.

The inflammation of the mucous coat has a great variety of
symptoms, but not so intensely severe as in the inflammation of
the peritoneal. It may be seated in any portion or in various
portions of the small intestine, and the first effect, as in every
inflammation of mucous membrane, is to arrest the secretion
which in a normal condition flows from them. Unless the
inflammation is soon subdued a reaction occurs and the secretion
becomes greatly increased in quantity and morbid in quality. If
the inflammation is seated in the mucous membrane of the duodenum the pancreatic and biliary ducts become implicated so that
a similar action and reaction may occur with them. The upper
portion of the small intestine is therefore the seat of many
of these affections termed " bilious," for which bilious pills
and chologogue nostrums or bile expellers have been called into
requisition.

Dyspepsia, or biliousness as it is termed in common parlance,
is often associated with inflammation of the upper portion of the
small intestine.

The prominent symptoms of mucous enteritis are pain, if the
inflammation is violent, but absent where the inflammation is less,
and may always be detected by careful pressure with the tips of
the fingers during a deep inspiration of the patient. There is
thirst but no particular preference for cold drinks; the bowels
are moderately loose; the tongue is red at the tip and sides and
sometimes in the center and large quantities of mucus are passed
from the bowels. Sometimes there is nausea and vomiting. In
inflammation of the mucous coat of the intestines the abdomen
is usually flat and this constitutes the most important means of
diagnosis of the mucus from the peritoneal inflammation. The
latter being always attended by distention of the abdomen.

The chronic form of enteritis of the peritoneal coat is not a
very common disease and yet it is sometimes met with and may
be known by the following symptoms: The patient feels pain in

12

some part of the abdomen by pressing firmly upon it and moving the body or coughing or sneezing. Sometimes fever exists and at others it is wholly absent. The patient is subject to frequent attacks of colic and various evidences of indigestion. Alternate constipation and diarrhœa are often met with in these cases. When the disease is of long standing the intestines are apt to become glued together by the effusion of plastic lymph from the inflamed surfaces and occasionally knotty irregularities can be felt by carefully pressing upon the relaxed abdomen.

These morbid formations often end in suppuration, the pus being discharged into the bowels or the peritoneal cavity and the patient dies worn out by hectic fever, or, at other times a general serous effusion may occur and the patient may sink from ascites or from peritoneal dropsy. The causes of the chronic form of enteritis are repeated attacks of colic or other intestinal diseases or it may be the signal of acute enteritis.

TREATMENT.—For the therapeutic treatment of the various forms of enteritis much will depend upon a knowledge of the causes. In acute enteritis, at the commencement of the attack if caused by sudden check of the perspiration, *Aconite* will generally control the disease. Especially if there is heat of the skin, dry tongue, and acute soreness of the exterior of the abdomen and full pulse.

Arsenicum, when there are cutting, tearing, burning pains in the bowels, restlessness and anxiety, vomiting, sunken features, coldness of the extremities, small quick pulse, often intermittent, and discharges of blood from the bowels.

Arnica mont., when caused by blows upon the abdomen or other mechanical injuries and particularly if the pain is of a sore unbearable character.

Belladonna, when the ordinary symptoms of enteritis are accompanied by delirium or spasms.

Bryonia, after Aconite if the fever is less, but the abdominal integuments continue very sore and sensitive, the pains are aggravated by the least motion or if a typhoid character develops itself.

Chamomilla for enteritis in children during dentition, with foul diarrhœa, slimy or watery evacuations.

Mercurius, cutting pains in the bowels and burning sensitiveness to pressure, quick pulse, rheumatic pains in the limbs, chiefly indicated in the fall when dysentery, violent colics or rheumatic pains in the extremities prevail.

Nux vomica, when enteritis is caused by sudden suppression of hæmorrhoids, with stinging tension and burning in the bowels, also with eructations and disposition to vomit. When drunkenness is the cause this remedy is also extremely useful.

Pulsatilla, when menstrual suppression is the cause, tearing pains in the bowels, coming on in paroxysms and being attended with chilly creepings.

Rhus tox. when caused by keeping on wet clothes after exposure to rain, and when there is pressure, stinging, tearing and burning in the bowels, worse after drinking or when the disease assumes a typhoid form.

Sulphur, if caused by the suppression of cutaneous diseases.

DOSE AND ADMINISTRATION.—From six to ten globules may be put in a cupful of water and a teaspoonful may be given every hour until relief or change.

For the chronic form, *Arsenicum* and *Sulphur* together with *Nux* and *Calcarea* may be given in the form of a trituration a two grain powder of the sixth centesimal twice a day.

Arsenicum and *Belladonna* or *Arsenicum* and *Pulsatilla* in the hands of some practitioners have been wonderfully commended, when given in the thirtieth potency and the dose repeated every three hours alternately. According to the observations, which have been made by me personally, I would recommend *Aconite, Bryonia, Arsenicum* and *Belladonna* in the thirtieth potency as sufficient for the successful treatment of most cases, if early attention is given to them. But I would recommend the use of each remedy by itself according to the indications afforded.

It is well known that acute inflammation of the bowels is a formidable disease and under allopathic treatment many recover and many cases terminate fatally. The sheet-anchor of treatment, as in other cases of inflammation of serous membranes, is bloodletting pushed even to syncope, which is always followed by reaction and immediately after a full sedative dose of *Opium* two and one-half grains. This, says Dr. Armstrong, is superior to bloodletting. The repetition of both remedies is recommended according to the urgency of the case. More confidence is reposed in the Opium than in the lancet. Poultices of flaxseed are ap-

plied over the abdomen and other derivative means found in sinapisms, blisters, etc. Saline purgatives are recommended to follow these and if the disease becomes extinguished or the patient
recovers, it is either a miraculous escape or a miraculous cure.

Inflammation of the Large Intestines.

This disease is termed typhlitis when confined to the cæcum
and vermiform appendix and consists of an inflammation of the
lining membrane of this portion of the large intestine either with
or without an implication with that of the colon. The most
marked symptom indicating inflammation of the mucous membrane of the cæcum is pain in the right iliac fossa which pressure aggravates and renders sharp and lancinating. The pain is
constant and often proceeds in the direction of the ascending
colon. The evacuations are copious and frequent, sometimes from
ten to twenty a day and are mucous or bloody or both and along
with these symptoms some fever and gastric disturbance generally
occurs, the pulse being accelerated and hard, the skin hot and
dry and the urine highly colored. In some cases of typhlitis the
peritoneal coat may be attacked or otherwise, all the coats of the
intestines may be involved in the inflammation. Much attention
has been paid to this form of the disease of late as cases of this
kind are attended with more or less tumefaction in the iliac region,
owing to some mechanical impediment in the cæcum. When the
peritoneal coat is particularly the seat of the disease, the ordinary
signs of peritoneal inflammation are manifest, of which constipation is one. The inflammation may extend to the cellular tissue
investigating the cæcum (*perityphlitis,*) and is indicated by an
inflammatory pain in the iliac region with a distinct hardness and
constipation.

THE CAUSES of typhlitis may be mechanical and are denoted
by very decided evidences of local inflammation. It is seldom
that the disease originates from the ordinary causes as from
exposure to changes of weather although cases occasionally are
met with where no other causes can be assigned. Peach stones as
well as those of other fruits are frequently lodged in the cæcum
and are the cause of typhlitis. Hardened fæces may also collect
in this locality and cause inflammation.

TREATMENT.—*Aconite* when there is considerable fever, thirst, redness of the tip and margin of the tongue and particularly when the pulse is full and bounding, and considerable heat and dryness of the skin. Aconite 6th may be given every two hours until its effect is perceived on the skin, which usually becomes moist.

Arsenicum 6th, drop doses every two hours, when the patient has retching, vomiting and intense thirst, great prostration, very restless, dark colored stools; tympanitis and more or less pain in the right iliac region and soreness on pressure, skin warm, looks anxious, tosses about in bed and complains of excessive cramps and pains in the right iliac region. *Veratrum album* 6th may follow Arsenicum.

Mercurius vivus when the stools are green and watery with masses of mucus floating on the discharges like fat.

Nux vomica when the bowels are constipated and there is severe pain in the right iliac fossa, extending into the back and also when the patient complains of acidity of the stomach and nausea.

In a case of typhlitis with the following symptoms: Pains in the right iliac fossa, distension and tympanitis and great soreness on pressure, loose discharges of bloody mucus, eight stools every twenty-four hours, much thirst, glassy redness of the tongue, great restlessness and prostration, variable appetite and some fever, pulse not much accelerated, skin at times unnaturally warm, Mercurius, Nux vom., Arsenicum, Sulphur, Sulphate of Zinc, Phosphorus and Phosphoric acid and many other remedies were selected with great care and administered in various potencies and still all the prominent symptoms were persistent and the patient becoming emaciated more and more until his life was despaired of. It was finally concluded to give him Calomel in grain doses once in three hours until five grains were taken, after which he passed enormous quantities of fæces and the diarrhœa ceased and convalescence followed.

TYPHLO-ENTERITIS presents nearly the same characteristics as if the cæcum only were involved and the remedies employed are Aconite, Arsenicum, Bell., Bry., Ipec., Mercurius, Nux vom.,Phosphoric acid, Sulphur and Veratrum. The remedy selected may be given in drop doses of any dilution from the 6th to the 30th, repeated every hour or two hours according to the severity of the case.

THE ALLOPATHIC TREATMENT FOR TYPHLITIS or typhlo-enteritis is half an ounce of castor oil and forty drops of laudanum repeated every two hours until satisfactory evacuations take place, or infusion of senna, two ounces with two drachms of Sulphate of magnesia, every two hours until the effect is produced. In addition warm enemas and warm baths are commended as adjuvants. This treatment detracts from the normal vitality of the system and as a matter of course weakens the reactive power of the organism against the disease and the sequel may be suppuration or abscess.

THE VERMIFORM APPENDIX is liable to be affected in the same way as the cæcum, which is by no means easy to determine. Nevertheless the treatment according to the indications will require the same class of remedies.

Inflammation of the Colon.

Like the rest of the intestinal canal, inflammation may affect either the peritoneal or mucous coat. When the former is the seat of inflammation there may be constipation, considerable pain on pressure with more or less distension of the colon, vomiting and great restlessness. When the disease becomes chronic, the colon is subject to adhesion to the other viscera or thickening of its walls and diminution of its calibre to a degree that fatal obstruction may be occasioned.

TREATMENT.—Nearly the same remedies are indicated for this affection as are required in the treatment of peritoneal inflammation in general.

Dysentery.

Inflammation of the mucous coat of the colon which with that of the peritoneal, usually come under the head of colitis is also denominated dysentery and may be either acute or chronic.

Acute dysentery is denoted by pain and tenesmus in the rectum and being an inflammation of the mucous coat of the colon it is characterized by frequent discharges of membraneous matter, white mucus, bile and even blood mostly without any fæcal matter, with violent straining and cutting pains in the bowels. In catarrhal form white mucus is expelled; in the bilious form a mixture of bile and mucus and in the inflammatory form blood or

mucus and blood. In typhoid dysentery the discharges are blackish and decomposed with palpable febrile signs and great prostration.   Dysentery at some seasons of the year assumes an epidemic type.

THE CAUSES of acute dysentery may be exposure to the
extremes of temperature, as for instance when the temperature
of the nights change from exceedingly warm to comparatively
cold, the free perspiration of a warm day may be suddenly
checkèd at night, and its retrocession may befall the mucous
lining of the colon and this produce afflux from the bowels that
soon becomes a dysentery.   As climate and seasons may unquestionably be regarded as predisponents, the use of unripe fruits
and of indigestible aliments of all kinds may prove to be exciting causes of dysentery.   Malarious influences are supposed by
some to be prevalent in epidemic dysentery in hot climates.   In
hot and moist seasons in tropical climates the disease prevails the
most.   Of fifty epidemics that have occurred at different times in
Europe, thirty-six occurred during the heat of the summer,
twelve in autumn, while but one occurred in winter and one in
spring.   Putrid emanations, hardened fæces, scybala, moral emotions, excessive fatigue and the heat and moisture of warm
climates are reckoned among the causes of this disease.

The question has been raised whether dysentery under any
circumstances is contagious, notwithstanding it is generally admitted that it may be associated with contagious typhus.   In
sporadic cases it is difficult to always divine the cause.   Inflammation of the mucous membrane of the colon and rectum may
occur from any irritating influence that happens to affect the intestinal canal.

TREATMENT.—In as much as dysentery is conceded to be an
inflammable affection of the mucous membrane of the colon and
rectum, *Aconite* in the third decimal attenuation may be given in
drop doses every hour in water with general good effect and in
case of a failure to effect a cure, *Mercurius viv.* or *Mercurius solubilis* is a suitable remedy when the days are warm and the nights
cool and when there is heat, thirst and chills.   It may be
given in the third trituration, a two grain powder every two
hours, and especially when there is much tenesmus and frequent
discharges of blood from the rectum, or greenish mucus.

Mercurius corrosivus, when there are cold face and hands with small and feeble pulse, when the pains of the rectum are aggravated by motion and the patient is weak and trembling and complains of hard, tense abdomen, sensitive to pressure, especially about the navel, continuation of severe pains in the rectum after the discharge, suppression of urine.

Ipecacuanha is suitable for fall dysentery of a bilious character with violent tenesmus and colic and stools of bloody mucus, worse in the evening.

We have prescribed *Arsenicum* when the patient was intensely restless and inclined to toss about in bed and where the stools had a cadaverous odor and when a warm bath would afford relief, and also when there was severe burning tenesmus, and small discharges of blood, after which there was great exhaustion and relief from pain. A few drop doses of the 6th dilution in water would afford relief. *Aloes* cured a case of dysentery in an adult male who had frequent stools with violent tenesmus, low down, at each stool he was inclined to faint. *Arnica* has also been found useful when the patient complained of nausea and fullness of the stomach and when the pains were like those of a wound, when touched, and when relieved by passing off wind; or when the stools were a mixture of blood and fæces and where at the same time there was tenesmus of the bladder, offensive flatulence and putrid breath. *Cantharis* has proved curative when the patient has complained of a fiery burning in the anus and the stools had the appearance of scrapings of the intestines. When the stools consist of profuse discharges of blood, *Hamamelis* is usually a certain remedy. When the patient has cramps in the legs and prolapsus ani with swelling of the lower portion of the abdomen, and discharges of jelly-like, white or bloody mucus, *Colchicum* has had a curative effect. When dysentery is accompanied by fruitless efforts to vomit and great feebleness after a stool, severe colicky pains, accompanied by retching and bending the body forward, and when pressure relieves, Colocynth has been found exceedingly effective. Any of the above remedies may be used in the 3d or 6th dilution. five drops or even ten drops in half a tumbler of water may be given a teaspoonful at a time, every hour.

ECLECTIC TREATMENT consists of " emptying the stomach and

bowels by a free Lobelia emetic, followed by one fluid ounce of
equal parts of compound syrup of Rhubarb and Potassa and the
fluid extract of Leptandria Virginica every half hour or hour
until a free evacuation has taken place; at the same time a large
hot pack should be applied to the abdomen and changed frequently. Immediately after the purge from ten to twenty grains
of sulphate of Quinine and one drachm of Leptandrin should be
divided into five or six powders and one given every hour until
all are taken. During this treatment, if the patient be suffering
much from the discharges and tenesmus, fifteen or twenty drops
of the tincture of Opium should be added to five or six ounces of
starch water and injected into the rectum. These injections
should be repeated as frequently as required to arrest pain. As
soon as the patient is thus prepared for the specific medication,
from ten to twenty grains of the triturated Gelsemin should be
added to a tumblerful of pure water and one teaspoonful administered every fifteen or twenty minutes. At the same time
Aconite or Veratrin should be given to control the fever and the
body frequently sponged in warm soda water. During the entire
treatment the patient should be in bed and observe the recumbent
position as nearly as possible. The diet should consist of grapes,
baked apples, bread, rice, coffee, beef tea and ripe fruits. In
bilious dysentery the only additional treatment is to administer
small doses of Leptandrin and Leontodin to increase the secretion
of bile. In the intermittent or remittent forms quinine and iron
should be administered every two or three days until the malarial
poison is neutralized. When the disease assumes a typhoid
character, Capsicum and cream in the proportion of three grains
of the former to a wineglassful of the latter, taken every two or
three hours will relieve that symptom. In case the dysentery
assumes a putrid or malignant form, as it does in camps and certain epidemics, then in addition to the above treatment, two
or three drops of Sulphuric acid should be given in a wineglass
of water every hour or two; and the Gelsemin may be combined
with Baptisin and made into twenty powders and one given every
half hour or hour; Hydrocyanic acid in the proportion of ten
drops to six ounces of water and one teaspoonful given every
half hour in case of nausea and vomiting until controlled. Pills
of one tenth of a grain of Nitrate of silver with pulverized Gum
Arabic, may be given in case of ulceration of the mucous mem-

brane every hour until all are taken. Brandy and wine should be given in case of great prostration when Capsicum and cream are not sufficient." Paine's Eclectic Practice pp. 335 and 336.

ALLOPATHIC TREATMENT.—In ordinary cases the bowels are kept free with small doses of castor oil, and, to render the pain and tenesmus less, ten drops of laudanum are added to each dose, after which the albumen of eggs is freely given. Some recommend opium alone in doses of one, two or three grains every three, four or six hours; others have recommended mild astringents with opium. In severe and prostrating cases, where there is much inflammation, blood letting has been recommended to be followed with calomel in dose to affect the salivary glands. Marshall Hall says that he has watched a severe epidemic dysentery in three successive years and that all violent remedies appeared to him to do harm, and this has generally been our experience.

For the last thirty years a greater or less number of cases have been treated by the writer and any departure from a critical application of Homœopathic remedies has only tended to complicate and protract the disease. In comparison, therefore, with Eclectic treatment, which appears to be too complicated for ordinary use, and Allopathic treatment which often multiplies the chances of a fatal termination, the Homœopathic treatment is the mildest and most certain and is, therefore, the treatment to be commended. While under treatment the patient should be allowed barley water, mutton broths and mucilaginous drinks, together with beef-tea, milk toast and farinaceous gruel, and every resort to any agencies that deteriorate the strength or vitality of the patient is attended with danger.

Chronic Dysentery.

A badly treated case of acute dysentery may assume the chronic form and therefore we regard the latter as a sequel of the former. In such cases the tenesmus gradually passes off,— the pains are less violent, but the evacuations are nevertheless frequent and numerous, preceded by obscure pain and flatulency and consist of mucus mixed with some feculent matter and not unfrequently with a purulent secretion. In a majority of cases the nutritive system is greatly impaired and emaciation becomes apparent and in many cases the patients sink from what, in common parlance, is termed consumption of the bowels. Andral maintains that chronic dysentery is rarely cured, but quite generally has a fatal termination. Under the ordinary mode of treatment this may be the case, but, from much experience and observation, our opinion is the reverse of his. Some cases indeed terminated fatally, but we have witnessed beneficial treatment with remedies in by far greater proportion and have known many to recover entirely.

TREATMENT.—When the inflammation of the mucous coat of the colon becomes chronic, we have found Arsenicum, Calcarea carb., Ferrum, Hepar sulph., Kreasotum, Lachesis, Nitric acid, Sepia, Sulphur and Zincum useful.

Arsenicum, when there is great prostration, thirst and disposition to change place continually, emaciation, worse after midnight, acrid burning stools, offensive and watery or else with tenesmus and discharges of bloody mucus, or, black hæmorrhoidal tumors with burning pain and prolapsus ani.

Calcarea carbonica when the patient has an aversion to the open air and is worse in wet weather or after washing in cold water and has discharge of blood from the rectum, prolapsus ani, cramplike pains in the abdomen, nausea in the morning and eructations and belching of wind, soreness and distension of the bowels. (Also Arnica.)

Ferrum metallicum, when chronic dysentery has followed an acute attack of intermittent, that has been badly treated with Quinine and there are frequent stools of blood and mucus. A lady of bilious temperament after suffering constantly for many months in this way and whose face was bleached white and bloated was cured by taking a few powders of the third trituration.

Hepar sulphuris, when the discharges from the rectum were of a bloody mucus with tenesmus, or at times soft stools and difficult evacuations, and particularly when this condition has been entailed from an attack of epidemic dysentery.

Kreasotum, the 2nd attenuation, ten drops, in half a tumbler and a dessertspoonful three times a day, cured a case of chronic dysentery of more than two years standing in a lady thirty-nine years of age. She was pale and emaciated and suffered much from burning pain in the descending colon and frequent discharges of mucus mixed with bile from the rectum.

She complained of great heat in the abdomen and was constantly beset with acid and offensive eructations. She had been treated Allopathically for a long time, after which she had taken many Homœopathic remedies that seemed to be indicated without effect. The first trial with *Kreasotum* 2nd completely removed the disease and since she has enjoyed comparatively good health.

Lachesis, when from the habitual use of alchoholic stimulants a diarrhœa is contracted that settles into a chronic dysentery and especially when the stools are offensive and there is a sense of constriction after each evacuation, and, especially if the patient is afflicted with large hæmorrhoidal tumors.

Nitric acid cured a case of chronic dysentery when the discharges from the bowels were bloody mucus and pus. The patient had four or five stools of this description every twenty-four hours and for more than seven months had been trying different remedies without relief.

SEPIA.—A lady near the climacteric period, had been troubled with dysenteric diarrhœa for many months and at every stool she passed a greater or less quantity of blood after which she suffered from prolapsion of the anus and pain in the rectum as if constricted. Six powders of the 3d trituration were first prescribed to be taken morning and evening; relief was afforded from these and she continued to improve until her health was restored.

Sulphur.—For chronic bilious dysentery, when the patient had an attack of the colic every night, and before each evacuation and tenesmus after. A case of this kind of long standing was cured by the Tincture of Sulphur, ten drops in a cup of water, a teaspoonful every 24 hours.

Zincum metallicum in the 3d trituration cured a case of six months standing where the patient passed four or five times a day a quantity of bloody water, exceedingly pale, from the rectum, sometimes involuntary. She was pale, emaciated and was subject to flashes of heat with trembling and frequent perspirations.

The remedies we have employed were mostly of the third attenuation, although there can be no doubt of the efficacy of other attenuations, if the remedies are well chosen.

THE ALLOPATHIC TREATMENT of chronic dysentery is the

same as laid down for chronic inflammation of the small intestine, which consists of revulsives and starch and laudanum injections. The objection to this treatment is found in the fact that whatever taxes or depresses the vital condition of the organism is seldom if ever curative, but an additional infliction upon the patient.

CHAPTER XIV.

Perforation of the Intestines.

The symptoms of this occurrence are deathlike from the commencement. During the course of some acute disease and under unexpected circumstances, violent pains in the abdomen supervene suddenly, and this suffering becomes very greatly augmented by pressure. The features change at once, and a deathlike nausea and pinched expression severely indicate perforation, and the disease terminates fatally in a few hours. An autopsy has revealed the fact that the perforations occur in the ileum and the pain usually commences in the locality of the cæcum or near the right iliac fossa.

THE CAUSE may be from softening and ulceration of the mucous membrane or from cancer or strangulation. Some authors ascribe the whole difficulty to the pressure of intestinal worms.

THE TREATMENT of a malady of this kind consists of the administration of remedies to relieve the acute suffering—Aconite, Arnica, Arsenicum, and other remedies may be given freely to ameliorate the pains, which are inclined to lessen as the torpor of death comes over the patient. It has been ascertained that the perforations take place in the center of ulcers which invade the mucous membrane and then the parietes of the intestinal tube, which becomes perforated. Cures of this kind are rare, and yet they are liable to occur in many acute diseases in which the bowels become implicated.

Diarrhœa.

Some pathologists do not admit that diarrhœa is a distinct disease, and yet there is no question that it may arise from morbid disturbance different from inflammation. Therefore diarrhœa may be defined an augmented secretion from the mucous membrane of the intestines increased by peristaltic action of the canal, unattended by any evidence of positive inflammation. It may supervene upon mental anxiety or emotion, such as may produce a free perspiration when no signs of inflammation are present.

DIAGNOSIS.—The acute form of diarrhœa cannot be mistaken. The number of evacuations from the bowels is greater than usual and they are often putrescent, thin and watery. They vary in character, being sometimes acid, especially in children, at other times they are composed mostly of bile, or a mixture of both as may be inferred when the stools are somewhat acid and tinged with a greenish hue. Sometimes mucus may be mixed in considerable quantities with the evacuations, but pain and tenesmus are rarely present.

PROGNOSIS.—The simple form of acute diarrhœa is by no means a dangerous disease, and seldom lasts beyond a period of from two to five days. When complicated with other derangements it is more persistent, which we shall note particularly under the head of treatment.

TREATMENT.—In Allopathic practice it is not regarded necessary to individualize symptoms, with reference to treatment. In ordinary cases of acute diarrhœa they give no medicine, thinking that the disease will pass off in a day or two, without demanding much attention. If it has arisen from errors of diet, they sometimes give an *emetic* to turn the current of things. Generally, however, some astringent tonic is recommended. This is a pernicious practice and mischievous in its consequences. In acrid diarrhœa of children, Soda, Lime water and milk are recommended, as well as powdered Rhubarb and Magnesia, dealt out in small powders but no form of Allopathic practice can claim so direct a utility as the Homœòpathic.

HOMŒOPATHIC TREATMENT with references to causes and symptoms. When dentition is the cause, Chamomilla will generally allay the fever, as well as correct the derangement of the bowels. The indications for its use are red cheeks, feverish breath and thin . or watery stools, sometimes accompanied by colic.

Ipecac is indicated when there is a tinge of blood in the stools and also when the stomach is irritable and the child frequently vomits.

Dulcamara is indicated when the diarrhœa is caused from colic and is generally a good remedy in colic weather.

Mercurius is indicated when the stools are tinged with bile and when the diarrhœa has been of several days standing.

Calcarea carb. for acid stools and when the teeth are slow in making their appearance.

When caused by eating rich food and the diarrhœa consists of pultaceous discharges, *Pulsatilla* is indicated, and also for fetid discharges.

Arsenicum where there is great prostration, thirst and acrid discharges.

Veratrum alb. is indicated when the child cries with pain and appears to suffer from cramps.

Coffea crud. is also indicated when the discharges are frequent and the child appears to be very restless and cries frequently.

In the treatment of diarrhœa in adults we have to consider the cause and characteristics of the trouble.

Feculent diarrhœa, without pain, which is but a mere looseness of the bowels, requires no specific treatment. When accompanied with pain *Colocynthis* is indicated; when there are griping pains and considerable flatulency, Dulcamara or Iris versicolor will afford relief. If there is persistent griping, *Jalapa* will generally cure.

Bilious diarrhœa which is brought on by the intemperate use of fruit and particularly unripe fruit, requires *Nux vom.*, Mercurius, Podophyllin. For dysenteric diarrhœa with no discharges of blood, *Gambogia*.

When there are feculent discharges from the bowels accompanied by loss of appetite and pain in the bowels and there is distention of the stomach and much rumbling in the bowels and a cold dry skin and much thirst, we shall find *Arsenicum* indicated and this remedy may be succeeded by Nux vomica.

For great prostration and weakness, even unto fainting, with dark colored discharges, *Rhus tox.* may be consulted and also *China.* For *involuntary diarrhœa* and painless, *Phos. ac.*

In all cases of diarrhœa it is necessary to place the patient in a warm and comfortable condition and supply him with a suitable farinaceous diet. When the diarrhœa is severe, quiet and rest are indispensible.

The remedies indicated as above may be given in the 3d attenuation, although higher preparations may not prove less

effectual. We have learned from experience that more depends
upon the selection of the right remedy than upon the degree of
attenuation.

When fatigue has brought on diarrhœa, a dose or two of
Arnica and rest may obviate the derangement.

If caused by anger, *Aconite;* by fright, Ignatia. If the
discharges are black, Rhus tox. or China. If brown and offensive,
Carbo veg. If white, Mercurius sol. If gray, Podophyllin.
The doses of four or six pellets may be repeated every hour or
two according to the severity of the case.

The chronic form of diarrhœa is that which succeeds the
acute form, when prolonged until the mucous membrane becomes
unduly excited and subject to an increased discharge. An acute
attack of diarrhœa may end in the continuation of a gleet which
succeeds inflammation of the mucous tissues in general. At other
times the symptoms from the first are those of chronic diarrhœa
and not subject to control within a very limited period. In such
cases the whole digestive tube is irritable, impressible and easily
excited. Any error of the diet, however trifling, may provoke
a return of the diarrhœa after it has been apparently cured.

As in chronic dysentery, the patient may lose flesh and
strength and suffer from distention and soreness of the abdomen.
The small intestine is liable to become involved and in some
instances the discharges are kept up by ulceration of the mucous
lining of the tube.

There is a chronic diarrhœa which in many instances follows
the weaning of children. It is characterized by loss of flesh,
pevishness and the passage of undigested food and great thirst.
If not arrested in time a stupor comes over these children and
they gradually sink away and die.

Chronic diarrhœa is often an attendant on tubercular and
glandular difficulties, and must be treated accordingly.

PROGNOSIS.—The chronic diarrhœa which general debility
inaugurates, as well as that which is but a supervening gleet
upon the acute form requires a diet and strengthening remedies
to insure speedy relief. Boiled milk thickened with superfine
flour, mutton broth, toast and black tea and occasionally a
broiled steak or mutton chop is allowable. Such cases are

13

curable. The diarrhœa which attends glandular affections such
as diseases of the liver and mesenteric glands, in some instances
may be cured, and in others there is little prospect of returning
health. That which attends tubercular affections is rarely curable
but often the reverse, and at best can only be palliated.

TREATMENT.—For mild forms of chronic diarrhœa the Allopathic treatment consists in the free administration of astringent
tonics, such as decoction of wild cherry bark and elixir vitriol,
and other astringent and anodyne mixtures. This treatment is
only palliative while an unfavorable influence is thrown back upon
the stomach and other organs.

HOMŒOPATHIC TREATMENT is attended with the best results.

Arsenicum, when there is great prostration and the stools
are dark and offensive. *China*, when attended with debility and
pain. *Sulphur*, when the diarrhœa is entailed from some eruptive
disease and when it is attributed to the presence of worms, also
when invermination is the cause of chronic diarrhœa; *Aloes,
Cina, Spigelia, Santonin, Mercurius* and *Terebinthina*.

For painless *chronic diarrhœa*, Phos. ac., Phos., Secale cor-
nut., Sulph., China, Arsenicum, Natrum muriaticum. For diarrhœa
brought on by grief, trouble, over exercise of the brain, *Ignatia*.
If from mental exertion, *Nux vom. Chamomilla*, if persistent
after vigilance, or sleeplessness; *Pulsatilla*, if caused from deranged catamenia, and violent emotional excitement.

A lady aged 51 had been suffering from chronic diarrhœa for
fifteen months. She was of a bilious temperament. The trouble
was caused by a cold which terminated in a cough and hectic
fever and chronic diarrhœa. She had been under Allopathic
treatment at first, but received no benefit. She took various
Homœopathic remedies under the direction of a physician and
still received no benefit. At last she took *Sulphate of Zinc* internally 3x and at the same time employed an enema of a solution
of the same in tepid water. Under this treatment she recovered
her health, strength and flesh. She weighed 157 lbs. when she
took the cold and lost during her illness about fifty. For the
diarrhœa which occurs in hectic forms and especially those of a
scrofulous, *Calcarea carb., Arsenicum, Sulphur, Acid nitric,
Sodium, Sepia*, and *Calmia*.

Some cures have resulted from the employment of *Subnitrate of Bismuth* in the watery diarrhœa of phthisis. But when patients suffer from any form of chronic diarrhœa, if their appetite and digestion will permit, they can be allowed any non-medicinal nutritive diet.

CHAPTER XV.

CHOLERA INFANTUM.

In the large cities of this country children are quite liable to fall victims to this fatal disease, as but little if anything is recorded concerning the existence of it in Europe, it is probably owing to the influence of climate in this country. Although there prevails at certain seasons in London, a similar affection called watery gripes, nothing is known of the disease in Paris.

DIAGNOSIS.—There are no uniform symptoms that would indicate the beginning of an attack. The disease in some cases begins with a diarrhœa, but in others it begins with vomiting or purging simultaneously or there may have been previous gastric or intestinal derangement. In most cases there are febrile symptoms, tense and rapid pulse. The discharges are exceedingly thin and often frothy, of a greenish hue or more of a mucous character. In cases of great severity we always find great prostration; often indicating danger. The disease may continue a few days, either before convalescence or death becomes evident. There is intense pain at times in the bowels, which may be increased by pressure, and from the apparent contractions of the muscles of the abdomen and limbs, spasmodically, it would seem that children have cramps, as well as adults in this and kindred diseases; rapid and frightful emaciation indicate a fatal case, the death being generally preceded by convulsions.

Other symptoms indicate a paralytic condition of the alimentary canal. Food passes directly without having undergone digestion, and also putrid discharges take place. In protracted cases apthous sore mouth is apt to accompany the putrid discharges. The appearance of feculent matter indicates the recovery of the patient as well as a restoration of the normal secretions in the evacuations.

CAUSES.—Excessive heat is evidently one of the exciting causes and yet this alone is not sufficient to induce it, as is apparent from the fact that heat in the country is as great as in the cities and yet comparatively few cases occur. Physicians who practice in the country meet with scarcely a case a year and not unfrequently, not to exceed two or three cases in ten years. It would therefore seem probable that defective sewerage or poorly ventilated districts in conjunction with heat, may be a fruitful source of disease. The bills of mortality in cities during the summer months are greatly swelled by the fatal cases of this disease. Teething is second among the causes, which excite in warm weather considerable irritation in the intestines; a common idea prevails that the second summer is not only a critical period, but vastly more so than the first.

TREATMENT.—The Allopathic treatment consists of *Spiced rhubarb elixir proprietatis*, given in half teaspoonful doses, Calomel in small doses is recommended to be given quite often, in order to produce a new action.

HOMŒOPATHIC TREATMENT.—Complete rest for the child, and in the early stage take it carefully into the shade by the side of some large body of water if practical; or on a steamboat to breathe a cool air from the water.

Ipecac is indicated when the child vomits and has a watery diarrhœa. Give 3 to 5 drops in half a cup of water, a teaspoonful every hour.

Veratrum alb. when the stools are watery and frequent or when the stools are greenish or brownish, and the attack has been violent and attended with great exhaustion, or when there are paroxysms of vomiting and when moving the child causes vomiting, when the face is pale, eyes sunken, and great thirst.

Chamomilla is very suitable for the disease when the child is teething and is very restless and the vomiting of sour mucus takes place occasionally and the child has frequent greenish stools, attended with colic and flatulency. It is also suitable for diarrhœa that resembles stirred eggs.

Mercurius.—Suitable for diarrhœa and mucous discharges; when the child strains and seems very weak after each passage and also when the stools are sour and mixed with small particles of blood.

Rheum, when the stools are frequent and of an acid odor.

Iris vers., when the stools are thin and watery and the child is disinclined to take food and seems to fail rapidly.

Podophyllin, when the stools are frothy, slimy and attended with cramp-like pains; child rolls its head and moans in its sleep. ,

Arsenicum.—For great thirst, severe prostration and weakness and when emaciation appears to be taking place rapidly and when the stools are brown, black and of a sickening odor.

Calcarea.—For protracted cases; where emaciation has gradually taken place and when the abdomen is distended and hard and when the stools are clay-colored and putrescent. Skin dry and withered.

DOSE AND ADMINISTRATION.—Ten drops of the 6th dilution dissolved in half a tumbler of water, of any of the above remedies and then give half or a whole teaspoonful every twenty minutes in sudden and severe cases and every half hour or hour in those less severe.

DIET.—Feed the child on mutton broth, toast-water and rice-water.

Constipation.

By some this derangement is regarded a distinct disease and by others only a condition produced by disease. It argues a want of vitality in the rectum, or an inactive condition of the mucous membrane of the large intestine.

DIAGNOSIS.—Fæces retained in the rectum longer than is customary with the individual.

Normal evacuations take place in health every twenty-four hours as a rule, but there are exceptions. Some require a movement of the bowels every day—others only every two days, and some even are very healthy who have their bowels move only twice a week and any departure from the customary time of the individual, indicates derangement or abnormality. It is constipation if the bowels do not habitually move at a given period, even if that period occurs at longer or shorter intervals.

CAUSES.—Torpor of the intestinal functions may be induced in various ways—by change of diet, eating less food than customary, long-protracted study, fever, a shock upon the nerves or whatever interferes with the customary regimen. This torpor is more apparent in old age, when the intestinal tube in common with all the organs, lose in a greater or less degree this vitality.

TREATMENT.—Allopathic consists in the employment of cathartics when the constipation has existed for some time, and laxatives to gradually lubricate, injections of warm water, and to carry and nibble a piece of Turkey rhubarb every day to keep the bowels regular.

HOMŒOPATHIC TREATMENT consists of directing the patient to a simple diet that would have a lubricating effect on the bowels, cracked wheat, apples, pears and bran bread. Vegetables, such as potatoes, squash and regular attention to stools.

Bryonia for tedious constipation, to be given every evening.
Nux vom., to be given every night.
Lycopodium I think should be taken three times a day, and until relief is obtained 6x, drop doses.

Obstruction of the Intestine.

Obstructions may arise from various causes, which will require separate consideration. The symptoms, however, bear a close resemblance in all. Obstinate constipation may result in a mechanical obstruction—strangulated hernia, which must be reduced either by pressure, or by surgical relief the effects of which may afterwards be relieved by Arnica taken internally. Impacted fæces often become an obstruction that must be relieved either by injections of warm water or by sweet oil or castor oil taken into the stomach. The caliber of the tube may diminish from some cause so as to be an obstruction. This may occur from tumors affecting the parietes of the tube or from chronic inflammation. It is impossible to enumerate all of the sources of obstruction. As but few of them can be removed by remedial agents, we leave the consideration of them entirely to the surgeon.

Enteralgic Colic.

The term enteralgia or colic is employed to designate any acute pain in the bowels, and particularly any severe griping pain, which accompanies most of the morbid conditions of the digestive tube. The term colic is used also to denote pain in the uterus, or that which sometimes accompanies menstruation. The principal forms of this peculiar suffering may be embraced under the heads of common colic, bilious colic and painters' colic.

Common Colic.

SYMPTOMS.—Violent pains occurring suddenly in some part of the abdomen, with some sense of twisting about the umbilicus, or along the track of the colon. The pain is usually severe and not increased by pressure, as in enteritis. On the contrary, pressure often relieves and causes a remission, which is often followed by a spasmodic return. On this account it is sometimes termed spasmodic colic. It is usually attended with flatulence, borborygmus and constipation. The discharge of flatus from the bowels often affords relief. When the pain is severe and persistent there is an expression of anxiety and suffering. This is the natural physiognomy of the disease. Vomiting sometimes accompanies the pain and aggravates the suffering.

CAUSES.—Any aliment that disagrees with the stomach of the patient is liable to become acid and productive of colic as it passes down the tube. Any indigestible substance may do the same. When the mother's milk disagrees with the stomach of the child, it may become acid and flatulent, and exert a constipation upon the bowels; incarcerated flatus is the cause of some colic.

TREATMENT.—The Allopathic treatment is by *carminatives* which are a class of excitants calculated to stimulate the intestinal tube, and relieve the local distention and diffuse the flatus. Ginger wine or tea is a favorite resort, as well as camphor and camphorated tincture of opium. Spiced tincture of rhubarb and linseed tea are often prescribed. This treatment is liable to promote a further derangement and therefore the HOMŒOPATHIC TREATMENT is preferred. The remedies are *Chamomilla*, Colocynthis, Coffea, Ignatia, Nux vom. and Pulsatilla.

Chamomilla, when the colic seems to be confined to the gastric region and is caused by adulterated food and when the face is flushed, the breath feverish, and also during dentition of children.

Colocynthis is the principal remedy for colic, especially when the pains are cutting, pinching and crampy, as if the bowels were pierced with knives, and also when the pain is in the umbilical region accompanied with shivering.

Coffea, indicated when the pain is great and the child grinds its teeth and suffers from great agitation and coldness of the extremities.

Dulcamara, when the colic is caused by a cold.

Ignatia, when caused by anxiety and grief and inability to sleep with shooting pains in the sides and chest, and worse at night.

Pulsatilla, shooting and biting pains in the pit of the stomach, a sense of heaviness and fulness in the abdomen with tenderness and pain as if from a bruise. Colic caused by indigestion or from eating fatty substances, worse when sitting or lying down, or when the patient is relieved by going out of doors and also when the colic is accompanied by diarrhœa.

Lycopodium is suitable after Pulsatilla, when there are borborygmus and swelling, with hardness of the abdomen.

Nux vomica, when there is constipation and pressure in the abdomen and when there is an acid stomach, and when the pain is pinching and drawing. Distension and tenderness of the abdomen when touched, cold hands and feet and much griping.

Veratrum, for colic with burning and cramps in the abdomen and a rumbling of wind.

Dose and Administration.—Of the selected remedy, drop ten drops of the sixth dilution in a goblet of water and give a teaspoonful every 15 or 20 minutes, if the case is severe, or in every 30 or 40 minutes if otherwise. Each remedy should be tried at least for five or six doses before a change. Children may take the remedy selected in pellets, two or three at a dose.

Those who are prone to suffer much from colic must keep dry and warm feet, and avoid green vegetables and all acid drinks, and during convalescence from an attack, only spare diet is allowable, and this should consist of mutton broth or other light soups.

Bilious Colic.

This affection is owing to a vitiated condition of the bile, if not primarily, at least as a secondary result. The disease consists in the main of neuralgic suffering of the digestive tube. The impressibility of the mucous lining of the tube is apt to cause a neuropathic condition which extends to the liver, and induces an excess of secretion.

Diagnosis.—The first indication of this affection is a disordered stomach and intestines, bitter taste, fur on the tongue, nausea and vomiting, want of appetite, and sensation of weight at the epigastrium. When the colic sets in the pain is intensely severe, cutting and screwing. Often it is first experienced in the stomach and reaches to the duodenum. At other times it affects the intestines generally, and twists around the umbilicus as in common colic. There is great heat, and in most cases the patient is anxious and restless. Bilious vomiting generally succeeds and the bowels, which before had been constipated become relaxed, and subject to free evacuations of fæculent and bilious matters. The symptoms then abate and health returns. Fever frequently attends the disease and the severer forms are apt to end in inflammation of the bowels, with a fatal result. The disease occurs periodically in summer and autumn, seasons which favor the erythism of the mucous membrane.

TREATMENT.—The treatment in Allopathic practice was formerly sedative. Bleeding from the arm, rubefacents over the abdomen. Terebinth clysters and Epsom salts, and moderate doses of Opium. We need not state that this practice is objectionable as well as injurious, and adds severity to the disease.

HOMŒOPATHIC TREATMENT is less dangerous and more effective. The remedies employed are Arsenicum, Aconite, Bryonia, Colocynth, Elaterium, Ipecac, Mercurius, Nux vomica, Podophyllin and Sulphur.

Aconite when there is fever and great tenderness of the abdomen, restlessness and twisting, retraction of the bowels and a desire to urinate, with unsuccessful attempts.

Arsenicum.—Great pain and burning in the stomach and a sense of chilliness at the same time, inclination to vomit, vomiting of watery and bilious matter, diarrhœa with thirst, shivering and great weakness.

Bryonia.—Fullness and pressure in the stomach and abdomen after eating the most trifling amount of food, followed by cutting pains in the bowels.

Colocynth.—Great pain in the region of the umbilicus and vomiting bile, cutting in the bowels and cramps in the limbs; abdomen swollen and empty.

Elaterium.—Much vomiting and extreme pain and cutting like knives in the abdomen and profuse bilious diarrhœa, much thirst, anxiety and restlessness, with retching.

Ipecac.—Colic with bilious vomitings continually or retching with great desire to vomit and some diarrhœa.

Mercurius.—When the colic extends to the right hypochondrium and the patient vomits much bile and has a diarrhœa both bilious and fecal with some tenesmus.

Nux vomica.—In case the bowels are constipated and the abdomen is hard and distended and very sore to the touch. Nux vom. is also the remedy when indigestion provokes the colic and when there are cramps.

Podophyllin.—When the liver is too active and furnishes a surplus of bile and when the colic is constantly aggravated by profuse bilious vomitings and when there is a jaundiced skin, bitter taste in the mouth and constipation and hæmorrhoids.

The selection of any of the above remedies may be prepared for administration by dropping ten drops of the 3x dilution in half a tumbler of water and given in teaspoonful doses repeated every thirty minutes until some relief or change.

Painter's Colic.

This affection is better known by the name of lead colic, or *Colera pictonum*, and is brought on by working among the preparations of lead.

DIAGNOSIS—The evidences of the effects of lead upon the system precedes the colic in the shape of a peculiar bluish gray tinge of the gums, which sometimes extends over the entire mucous lining of the mouth. This has been regarded an infallible proof, that there is the presence of lead oxide in the system. The teeth also become affected, and there is a styptic sweetish taste in the mouth, fœtor of the breath, sallowness of the skin, general emaciation, small soft compressible pulse. These symptoms are so common with those who are poisoned with lead it is not well to neglect them.

The pain of painter's colic is so severe that it is almost unbearable by the strongest and most resolute persons. When the lead poison takes effect and the disease is fully formed, the pain is so excruciating that the most robust writhe about, break down and cry like children. Sometimes it comes on suddenly, and is attended by scanty evacuations. The pain is subject to remissions and exacerbations, and may be relieved by pressure sometimes, but not always. Then the bowels are almost always constipated and when evacuated in any degree the fæces are in the form of scyballæ.

The pains are not always restricted to the abdomen. The limbs also suffer much, especially the arms, from great weakness of the muscles. Paralysis of the muscles is often a result of poisoning with lead, and the nerves of sense sometimes partake of the debility and become powerless. The pulse is slow, skin natural, but there is a striking change in the expression of the countenance, which is anxious and indicative of indescribable suffering. The duration of the disease varies from one to two weeks.

CAUSES.—Working in lead and among its oxides. The makers and grinders of colors, painters, plumbers, potters, etc., are those liable to suffer in this excruciating way.

TREATMENT.—The Allopathic is calomel and opium in powders of four grains of the former and two of the latter, six times a day. This treatment palliates the suffering, but does not antidote the cause, and also a combination of emetics and cathartics.

THE HOMŒOPATHIC TREATMENT requires Platina, Belladonna, Cuprum acet. and Opium, Atropine and Codein.

Platina is indicated for lead colic when a morbid fear or anger aggravates the suffering.

Belladonna, when the bowels feel constricted or grasped by the finger nails. Cuprum acet., when there is inclination to vomit and the head feels heavy.

Atropine for extreme excruciating pain and a dullness and stupor.

Opium, when there is obstinate constipation, hardness of the abdomen with intense pain, griping and pinching.

It would seem that the deleterious effects of lead are chiefly from the carbonates. The acetate or sugar of lead rarely produces colic. When it does, it is supposed to have become converted into the carbonate. To avoid this conversion a little Acetic acid is advised, when the acetate is administered in Allopathic practice. In Homœopathic practice painter's colic has been successfully treated with the same remedies administered in the same manner as in bilious colic.

Tympanitis.

This is a pathological condition fairly ascribed to the presence of gases in the intestinal canal. It has been ascertained that oxygen gas will distend the stomach and give to the gastric region the appearance of a drum and when percussed a sound is elicited which indicates the character of the distension and also carbonic acid gas when incarcerated gives rise to the same in the small intestine and the same is predicated of hydrogen and carborated hydrogen.

DIAGNOSIS.—Distension of any portion of the digestive tube from pent-up air. But the colon is most commonly the location where the greatest accumulation occurs and it is attended by some pain whether there is any inflammation or not and if the abdomen be percussed there is the same sonorousness as if a drum were struck; this gives the disease its name.

CAUSES.—The generating gases from certain kinds of food and from the lining membrane of the canal, as is frequently the case in typhoid fever. Peas, beans, green corn, sweet potatoes and many other kinds of food contribute to the generation of much flatus, either by the reaction of their elements upon each other or by the increased secretion of air which they occasion.

TREATMENT.—A favorite prescription for tympanitis by the Allopathic physicians is, Ol.Terebinth ℥ss. vitelli ovi, aqua menthœ ℥ iij Misce et fiat Mistura and Sig. Dose ½ and repeat if necessary.

HOMŒOPATHIC TREATMENT.—The entire condition of the patient is taken into account in making an intelligent selection of remedies. For ordinary flatulency and tympanitis, Nux vomica, Colocynth and Pulsatilla. If the distension is accompanied by fever, the face flushed, the pulse rapid and full, Aconite is the remedy. If from subsisting on a flatulent diet, Pulsatilla. If from an acidity of the stomach and burning in the bowels with thirst, Arsenicum. For the distention which occurs in nervous fevers, Terebinthina 3x Arsenicum and Baptisia tinctoria. Any of the remedies selected may be given in drop doses every hour in a dessert spoonful of water.

Cancer of the Intestines.

Cancer of either the small or large intestine is seldom cured and yet a judicious medical treatment will secure much immunity from suffering and possibly may prolong life. It is manifestly proper for us to be able to diagnose the trouble and to administer palliatives if we can do no better.

DIAGNOSIS.—The symptoms of cancer within the small or large intestine do not differ materially from those of chronic inflammation of the bowels. Dull pain is generally present between the intervals of lancinating or shooting pains. These are felt some time after eating, when the ingesta, or perhaps the excrementitious part of the food reaches the disorganized part. As the disease augments the pain returns in paroxysms, attended with vomiting and signs of obstruction of the bowels. When the progress of the cancer reaches ulceration, the discharges from the bowels become quite offensive and repulsive in their odor. The abdomen, when critically examined, shows a hard and painful tumor from whence sharp shooting pains irradiate. If we have in addition to these local signs evidence of a cancerous diathesis, there is not much doubt about the nature of the disease. Nevertheless, it is not easy to make an absolutely certain diagnosis at the commencement of the disease. Sooner or later cancer of the intestines proves fatal either from obstructing the passage of the excrement or by causing inflammation of the mucous or peritoneal coat, or from causing a protracted irritation like all cancerous diseases.

CAUSES.—The same as detailed for cancer of the stomach.

ALLOPATHIC TREATMENT consists in a free resort to any or all the non-constipating narcotics, such as *Hyoscyamus Ext.*, *Belladonna Ext.*, Stramonium and Lactucarium and in very severe and unbearable suffering, Opium, Morphine, Lupuline are given freely, even if inveterate constipation follows. A combination of Opium and Rhubarb, or Opium and Calomel is a favorite resort.

HOMŒOPATHIC TREATMENT.—This is frequently palliative and secures more relief for the patient. *Arsenicum* 3x, will palliate the suffering when the patient vomits blackish matter and complains of much burning. *Conium maculatum* has seemingly prolonged life, after the confirmed stage destroyed all hopes of becoming better.

Nux vomica 3d decimal attenuation was given to a lady who was complaining of much burning pain in the small intestine and at the same time was vomiting matters from the stomach resembling coffee grounds. There was great tenderness of the abdomen and at a single point there was a small hard tumor which her physician pronounced a cancer. The medicine after 24 hours was so palpably beneficial that she could not wait for the interval to pass between the doses. We were called to counsel in this case and from the most critical examination we could make, we confirmed the diagnosis which had been made. The patient improved under the use of Nux vomica and apparently recovered and remained quite well for more than two years, when some fresh exciting cause brought on the same symptoms again. Nux vomica in a lower attenuation was again resorted to, and she after a longer perseverance than before found decided relief and was made comparatively comfortable. She lived many months, while the disease progressed. The Nux vom. kept her bowels in good order until ulceration and inflammation created a mechanical obstruction for which there was no help. From this and other similar cases it is evident that well selected Homœopathic remedies will palliate the sufferings and prolong the lives of patients when affected with cancer of the intestines. In addition to Arsenicum and Conium, Belladonna, Carbolic acid and other remedies, which the symptoms may indicate as useful, may be employed to palliate the pain if not to cure the malady.

Hæmorrhage of the Intestines.

An engorged condition of the bloodvessels of the intestines in some cases of continued fever may ripen into hæmorrhage into the intestines and large quantities of blood will often pass from the rectum. Cancerous tumors or ulcers by destroying the continuity of the vessels are often the cause of the same difficulty.

IN ALLOPATHIC TREATMENT the same as recommended in hæmatamesis is carried out.

THE HOMŒOPATHIC TREATMENT calls for Nitric acid, Arsenicum, Ipecacuanha, Hamamelis virginica, which are remedies to select from to meet different cases.

Nitric acid is particularly the remedy when the hæmorrhage occurs in an abdominal typhus. Arsenicum is an excellent remedy to follow when there is great prostration and also China. These remedies may be administered by dropping of the 6x dilution ten drops in half a tumbler of water. Teaspoonful doses may be given every half hour or hour until a fair trial of the remedy is had. We have many times witnessed a favorable change in a few hours.

Hæmorrhoids—Piles.

The symptoms of this distressing complaint are quite uniform. Nearly every subject experiences at first certain signs denoting "a concentration of the vital activity inwards, a chilliness, cold extremities, heat and pain in the rectum and anus and sense of weight in the loins and we may add gastric disturbance. Then follows in many cases, after a time, a discharge of blood from the anus. Tumors varying in size fill with blood and discharge their contents at intervals, or inflame for a time and become absorbed. These tumors may be *internal or external.* The internal are situated in the rectum above the anus, and can rarely be seen though distinctly felt by an examination. The external protrude and form, sometimes in great numbers, around the margin of the anus. Sometimes they are small, not larger than a pea, at others they are the size of a walnut, of oval shape, darkish red color and when numerous bear a close resemblance to a bunch of grapes. They are hot and painful, the pain being lancinating and pulsatory. When the tumors are attended with a discharge of blood, they are termed *open piles* and when not they are termed *blind piles.*

CAUSES.—Hereditary conformation is thought to be the predisposing cause, and the exciting causes may be any influence which interferes with the venous circulation as hepatitis, sedentary habits and pregnancy. The external piles may supervene on dysentery, or parturition or from constipation and straining to evacuate the bowels, etc. Those who are always taking aperient medicine to keep the bowels open are inclined to suffer from this trouble.

TREATMENT.—The Allopathic treatment consists mainly of local applications, of electuaries and ointments made of lard and tannin and opium or lard and powdered nutgalls,—powdered alum and lard. These applications may have a styptic effect upon the bleeding piles and throw back upon the general system a morbific influence detrimental to the patient.

THE HOMŒOPATHIC TREATMENT admits of a warm sitz bath if the tumors are hard and extend below the anus.

Æsculus hippocastanum in the 3d trituration, a powder of two grains may be given three times a day, half an hour before eating and also an ointment strongly medicated with the same remedy.

Aconite is called for when there is great pain and fever with a full pulse and great heat in the rectum. Ten drops of the first decimal dilution in half a tumbler of water. A teaspoonful of this mixture may be given every two hours until the patient perspires freely or until the throbbing pain subsides.

Nux vom., 3d trituration, in doses of two grains, may be given after each meal, and just before retiring, when there is pain in the back, and when there is a dull aching pain in the lower part of the rectum, and the piles protrude and manifest great soreness, and the patient suffers from constipation.

Aloes generally have a salutary effect in removing the pain of hæmorrhoids, when the suffering is circumscribed to the anus ' and the patient feels all the time like forcing something away ' that is already on the verge of the anus.

Belladonna.—We have found this remedy to exert a beneficial effect in painfully congested hæmorrhoids, and when the pain in the tumors themselves are stinging, shooting and neuralgic.

Hamamelis virginica.—We have used this remedy with good success in the bleeding piles, and when the bleeding was very profuse and when the pain was less severe. Ten drops of the tincture in half a tumbler of water, and a teaspoonful dose every hour. Twenty drops in a cup of water will form a mixture for external use. Wet compresses of soft linen rags and apply them to the protruding piles.

Sulphur.—We cannot say too much in favor of this old standard remedy. When the victim of hæmorrhoids is somewhat under the control of the hæmorrhagic diathesis, there is no remedy in the materia medica more likely to effect a favorable change. A single dose of *Sulphur* in the morning and a dose of Nux vom. in the evening, has undoubtedly cured a vast number of cases.

Persons liable to the piles, should select a diet by no means spare, but such as is slightly laxative. Meat and potatoes without condiments except salt. Bread of unbolted wheat or rye flour, is regarded a good prophylactic. We have heard the remark several times from old friends who had suffered much from the piles, that they had ceased to suffer from them because they use coarse bread and much fruit at their meals.

Prolapsus Ani.

Writers have made two divisions of prolapsus ani, the one being a prolapsus of the rectum, and the other a prolapsus of the

14

lining membrane. The character of the two affections is sufficiently indicated by their names. In both forms of the disease the sphincter ani embraces the protruding portion and thus prevents the return of the blood and causes considerable pain.

DIAGNOSIS.—The slightest prolapsion of the mucous membrane of the rectum is indicated by a pressure or bearing down and smarting, especially when the bowels are moved, and more when the fæces are dry and hard. As soon as the rectum is emptied, the protruding portion will soon return, with little or no assistance. It is by no means safe to neglect the slightest prolapsion, for the longer it is neglected the worse it becomes and the more difficult to replace the gut, and a chronic trouble is entailed. The intestine being exposed may be irritated by the clothing and by other exposure until it takes on an inflammation difficult to subdue and ulceration takes place, and now the health suffers, digestion is impaired, and hectic fever may set in and wear out the patient. This, however, is a rare occurrence.

CAUSES.—Atony of the vascular and other tissues, most likely to occur with very young children and persons advanced in life, is believed to be the predisposing cause of the trouble. The exciting causes are harder to place, and straining to evacuate the bowels and the abuse of aperients, clysters and suppositories, dysentery, worms, parturition and strangury are reckoned among the causes.

TREATMENT—Both Allopathic and Homœopathic practitioners resort to gentle pressure in order to replace if possible the protruding intestine. But little difficulty attends the operation in children, but it is different with adults and especially in chronic cases. *Allopathy* gives astringents, such as Quercus cortex and Alum mixed in water, or alum and water alone to be used as injections, and cold water is also recommended in addition.

THE HOMŒOPATHIC TREATMENT requires *Ignatia* if the protrusion is of a child given to crying.

Mercurius when the atony is caused by looseness or diarrhœa.

Mercurius corrosivus when caused by dysentery. Adults and aged persons should always sit on cushioned stools, if inclined to be constipated and find it difficult to evacuate hardened fæces.

Æsculus ointment and also cold cream may be employed to lubricate the prolapsion. *Cina may* cure the prolapsion in children troubled with worms. So may Santonin. The former in the 3rd dilution, the latter in the 2nd trituration; ten drops of the former in a half a tumbler of water, teaspoonful doses, repeated every three hours. What will lie on the point of a pen-knife of the latter, night and morning.

CHAPTER XVI.

INVERMINATION—WORMS.

The meaning of the term is *worm disease*, and denotes the existence of parasites somewhere in the primæ viæ in sufficient numbers to derange the animal system. In the human body more than twenty different kinds infest various parts of the system. We can name but a few.

1. *The Tœnia or Tape Worm.*—We have encountered in several patients a struggle to rid the system of this parasite, and frequently with satisfactory results. We can, therefore, describe its appearance as it was before our eyes. It is a long, tape-like worm, formed of chain-like flat articulations united together by a membranous border varying in breadth and thickness. Each of the links are actually endowed with the ability of sustaining an independent vitality and capable of becoming a distinct worm. These parasites often attain great length, varying from ten to one hundred feet or more. It is said that they have been seen two hundred, three hundred and even eight hundred feet long.

The species called armed tape worm is found no where but in the human subject, and to dislodge it, is attended with great difficulty, on account of its being armed with two small fangs which it plunges into the mucous membrane of the intestine and holds on fast.

The *tœnia lata* has no fangs and is more easily destroyed, but the armed tape worm is dislodged in joints which resemble the seeds of pumpkin.

2. *Tricocephalus.*—This is a small parasite, very seldom met with, varying in length from one to two inches. The external surface is marked by transverse lines resembling rings. "One part of the body," says *Bresa*, "terminates in a filamentous elongation, as fine as a hair, and curled up in a very singular manner. Another portion ends in a broad obtuse hook resembling the pistil of a leguminous flower. From this extremity the

worm can put forth a sort of a tube enveloped with a sheath. They are found in the ileum and cæcum.

3. *Ascaris Vermicularis* or pin worms are not uncommon. They are frequently discharged in great numbers, and are round and like slender threads, from one-fourth of an inch to an inch in length. They move with great activity and when touched they contract one-half in length. They are most abundant in the rectum and near the anus. They are found in the large intestine but rarely in the stomach.

4. *Lumbricoides*, or large round worms, shaped much like the common earth worm and of the size of a goose-quill. They are either of a yellow color, or transparent, from three to twelve inches in length. They inhabit the small intestine, though they are sometimes found in the colon and rectum, but seldom in the stomach. Young children are more subject to them than adults. They are sometimes rolled together in balls, obstructing the passage and not unfrequently they are discharged in great numbers.

The signs or symptoms of *tœnia* are sense of weight in the abdomen, with burning and a sense of something alive in the bowels "pricking or rather bitings are felt in the region of the stomach. At intervals the abdomen swells and then subsides, sense of cold in the abdomen, voracious appetite, livid complexion, dilated pupils, vomiting and vertigo. The legs and body tremble convulsively and in the discharges from the bowels small substances resembling the seeds of a lemon or of a gourd which are portions of these worms are passed with the fæces. Many of the symptoms detailed above may arise from other causes, but the presentation to the sight, of portions of the worm is sufficient to indicate its presence in the system.

The signs or symptoms of the presence of lumbricoides are pricking and rending pain in the region of the umbilicus, colic with rumbling noise in the abdomen caused by the worm irritating the mucous membrane with its sharp cutting point of its head.

The signs of ascarides are itching of anus, with a stretching and swelling of the lower extremity of the rectum. They sometimes produce inflammation of the rectum, discharges of blood and tenesmus.

The general symptoms of the presence of worms in the in-

testinal canal are a tendency to spasms or convulsions. I have
observed that chorea, catalepsy, tetanus, paralysis, mania and
convulsions have been produced by the irritation of the nerves of
the primæ viæ.   Other affections such as pleuro-rheumatic
pains, dysentery, fever, hydrocephalus, cough, etc., etc. When I
have met a pale leaden-colored face occasionally flushed with
fever, I have suspected worms. Always when I see a child picking its nose, with a blue streak under its eyes which are dull and
heavy, or find him constantly grating his teeth when asleep, or
frequently startled and frightened suddenly out of his sleep, I
suspect worms, and here let me say that nervous restlessness produced by worms may provoke almost any kind of suffering.

Nymphomania in *females* and seminal weakness in males
may be brought on entirely by worms. I have seen both sexes
in this unhappy predicament and I have relieved them by
Cantharis and Terebinth. I have saturated sugar globules about
the size of bird shot with Terebinth and also with the 1st dilution of Cantharis and have administered two at a time and every
two hours for a day at a time and then wait several days, and if
there is no favorable change in the mean time, I begin again and
continue for another day and keep on with this treatment until
the cause, that is the *Ascarides* are made to disappear. Were I to
attempt to record all the sympathetic effects which I have seen
produced by worms it would surpass belief. I have seen that an
old man who was addicted for more than a year to boisterous fits
of laughter, was cured by vermifuge medicines.   I can record
the same of hysteria and other nervous affections. But it is
quite as common to attribute too much to worms as to overlook
their existence.   An indiscriminate use of vermifuges and anthelmintics I have observed to be exceedingly dangerous, and yet
our means of judging whether or not worms are the exciting
cause of sickness are not reliable when we suspect this is the
case. The following test rule has been to me a partial guide, "a
pearly whiteness of the schlerotic coat of the eye,—a brilliant
shining carmine tinge of the lips, particularly the upper, and a
peculiarly indescribable expression of the *alæ nasi* much like
that of the *facies Hippocratica.*"

CAUSES.—The origin of intestinal worms has always been a
question for doctors to settle. It has been generally supposed
that they enter the body in the form of eggs and hatch and grow

to the maturity which they attain and that they feed on the animal tissues, or on the food taken into the stomach, and then into the intestines while undergoing digestion. Some say they are fed by the air we breathe, and others by the water we drink. It is said by naturalists that 15,000 species have been examined in the cabinet of *Vienna*, and that each species belonging to the human intestines could be distinguished. As the process of disorganization and reorganization is constantly going on, effete portions of disorganized mucous membrane may furnish the soil for the generation of worms, even as disorganization of the external skin may furnish the bed for the *Pediculus* to originate and repose in. A healthy child, man or woman never suffers from invermination. There is always some taint or effete exfoliation of tissue that is behind the difficulty. The conclusion that worms originate within the body appears to us to be the most rational, and we base our conclusion on such considerations as follows:

1. They have a characteristic structure differing from that found in worms from other sources.

2. The worms found in various animals are marked by their own peculiarities.

3. They are found in various tissues, in different parts of the body. They are found in the liver, the gall bladder, the spleen, lungs, brain, and cellular tissue. It is the opinion of eminent physiologists that these parasites originate in the places where they are found and must be regarded as a symptom of some prior disease. Broussais taught "that worms are always associated with a chronic inflammation of the gastro intestinal surface and Andral says, they are most always found in a quantity of mucus."

It has always been my observation that feeble scrofulous children are more liable to worms than those of more robust constitutions. Any unhealthy condition of the mucous lining of the intestines that interferes with digestion, furnishes an opportunity for the developement of worms. When the tongue is thickly coated, with swollen papillæ protruding through the thick coating, and also when this papillary exhibition is in the form of oval or round spots, varying in color from a pale to a deep red, there is probability of an irritable condition of the digestive organs favorable to the generation of intestinal worms. "The only certain proof, however, of the presence of worms is

the detection of the parasites themselves, or the ova in the stools
or matter vomited.

TREATMENT.—In Allopathy, anthelmintics, in the form of
vermifuges, or mixed tonic cathartics, as Spigelia (pink root),
and Senna or Dolichos administered in the form of a syrup, or
Turpentine dropped on lumps of sugar, or moderate doses of Calomel. I have observed an apparently disastrous effect from this
treatment.

HOMŒOPATHIC TREATMENT in general requires the administration of remedies according to the manifest symptoms; even the
manifest presence of worms must be regarded a symptom of intestinal disease. We have seen much suffering from ascarides
and even from the lumbricoides in the rectum, and I have recommended enemas of tepid water well saturated with salt, and this
has afforded speedy relief. But the cure of all diseased conditions
of the intestinal canal which favor invermination is the most to
be desired, and this requires the internal use of remedies. I will,
therefore give my experiences in order.

The remedies for *tænia* are Filix Mas or Male Fern which
has been highly commended by the widow of a Swiss surgeon
who had been unusually successful in removing *tænia.*

Kameela is another remedy claimed to possess specific power
in removing parasites. Dr. Burt mentions Curcurbita. Dr.
Baehr recommends Kousso, and this remedy employed in Abys-
sinia is a quick and good vermifuge for *tænia.*

There are different modes of administration. The Male
Fern is given in the form of an emulsion morning and evening for
two or three days, or otherwise in the form of a pill, 3 grs.
morning and evening, or in the form of a cold infusion 1 oz. to a pint
of water. Dose, two tablespoonfuls morning and evening on an
empty stomach. The symptoms which follow the use of this remedy
indicate the 3d trit. of Nux vom., and from personal observation
it operates well. A cold infusion of half an ounce of Kousso in
a pint of pure cold water may be administered in tablespoonful
doses, once in two hours, for two days.

The Lumbricoides and Tricocephalus, Santonin. Cina in the 3rd
attenuation are known to have a salutary effect. The symptoms
for the use of *Cina* are boring of the nose, livid semi-circle under the eyes, tossing about, starting, convulsions, chorea, etc. By
many *Santonin* is regarded a positive specific for the long round
worms.

Mercurus cor. for fetid breath, greenish or pulpy discharges sometimes attended with tenesmus and discharges of blood. For ascarides or thread worms in adults, *Ignatia* for children, three or four doses a day.

Urtica urens and Terebinth for excessive itching in children and also adults, Sulphur and Nux in any attenuations are always useful in removing ascarides.

For the constitutional condition attendant on invermination we have relied on Ant. c., Arsenicum, Calc. carb., Silicea, Sulphur, Mercurius and other remedies.

Hygienic measures should conform to the usages, such as bathing, clothing and food.

In conclusion it may be said that the human body furnishes a habitation for parasites of various descriptions. Some crawl over the skin and burrow beneath its surface. Some find nests in the entrails and breed and propagate their kind. So numerous are these creatures that they explore and find resting places in the various tissues of the body. Some have even invaded the heart and others the arteries and the kidneys, while myriads of minute worms lie coiled up in the voluntary muscles and areola tissue that connects the sarcous elements. More than a score of animals have already been discovered and described, as having their dwelling place in the human body. Each species has its favorite domicile. But in the foregoing chapter we have for practical reasons dwelt chiefly on intestinal worms because of their prominence in diseases of the alimentary canal. In this locality we have seen the different species before described. In order to complete the therapeutics of worm diseases we will detail our experience with some of the anthelmintics that many years ago were in great repute. The first of these is Terebinth, administered in pills or globules of sugar about the size of a buck-shot. Saturate these globules with the turpentine and in ordinary cases of invermination give two of these pills and repeat every two hours until four doses are given. In the case of tape worm, this remedy, from all accounts, has wrought wonders in promoting the discharge of tape worms; in young and old persons it has had the desired effect. There is still another remedy for this parasite that has seldom failed, viz., the decoction of the bark taken from the root of the pomegranate tree. Two ounces of the bark put into a pint of cold water and left for twenty-four hours, may be given in tablespoonful doses every two hours. Many cases of absolute cure are recorded of this remedy. The Kousso also enjoys a great reputation in these annoying cases. These remedies, as ordinarily prescribed, have done good service. Nevertheless in the expression of worm affections there are symptoms connected with the suffering that will point accurately to the remedies to be employed. Santonine, Spigelia, Cina, Dolichos, Sulphur, Mercurius dulcis, and other Homœopathic remedies are always worthy of being consulted.

CHAPTER XVII.

CHOLERA MORBUS.

This disease has been known from early ages and has been regarded as sudden vomiting and diarrhœa caused by an overflow of bile, errors of diet, etc.

DIAGNOSIS.—Sometimes violent purging and vomiting begin suddenly and almost simultaneously, but usually before these decided symptoms declare themselves there is more or less evidence of general derangement of the stomach and bowels. Sometimes there is shivering, headache, pain in the abdomen and nausea.

The contents of the stomach are first thrown up and this consists of undigested aliment with a copious secretion of the mucus membrane, but as the struggle continues the duodenum, and thence the liver, become implicated, an unusual quantity of bile becomes secreted and forced through the pylorus into the stomach as is observed in the ejected matters. This is the simplest and mildest form of cholera morbus. In the severe forms of the disease much pain is felt in the abdomen and especially in the stomach, and violent cramps are frequently felt in the abdominal muscles and also those of the lower extremeties. When improper articles of diet have induced the suffering the pulse becomes accelerated, with more or less heat upon the surface and intense thirst. When the vomitings and purgings and cramps are unusually severe, the surface is pale, the features pinched, the eyes seem to be sunken and the skin is covered with a cold, clammy perspiration. The anxiety and depression somewhat alarming. During the revulsion the urine is suppressed. The disease is generally of short duration in temperate climates.

CAUSES.—Heat of the weather during the summer, improper diet, both as to quantity and quality. Cucumbers, green fruit and nuts are examples. The free use of cold drinks and ices are reckoned among the causes and yet where there is much thirst, small pieces of ice in the mouth are often refreshing and prevents erythisom of the mucus membrane.

TREATMENT.—In Allopathic practice great use is made of opiates in soda water, and sometimes simply soda water and at other times opium or opium and camphor. Observation has taught us that the employment of opiates is objectionable because they depress the vitality of the entire system and prolong, rather than obviate, the disease.

THE HOMŒOPATHIC TREATMENT, briefly stated, is as follows: When the attack comes on with chills, Camphor; with severe griping, Colocynth; with vomiting and diarrhœa, *Veratrum album;* for bilious diarrhœa from the bowels with colicky pains, *Iris versicolar; Nux vom.* when vomiting and cramps in the stomach; Arsenicum when the patient has much thirst, and Aconite if feverish.

Asiatic Cholera—Cholera Asphyxia.

This disease has prevailed epidemically and to a fearful extent at various times. The origin and history of the disease have so frequently been in print that we do not find it necessary to dwell long upon this point. It is sufficient to state that it has been prevalent in Asiatic countries and also in the first cities of Europe.

DIAGNOSIS.—In nearly all the visitations of cholera certain premonitory signs of its approach have attracted attention. These consist in more or less derangement of the digestive system, and attended with more or less diarrhœa. The severity of the disease is liable to follow, characterized by coldness of the surface, spasms and cramps, vomiting, profuse serous purging and collapse. It may be distinguished from cholera morbus in this way: the latter comes on suddenly, cholera is preceded by diarrhœa and then followed by pains down the hips and rapid prostration, rapid reduction of temperature over the surface of the body, cramp and rice water discharges, while *cholera morbus* has simply colicky pains, gradual prostration and reduction of heat upon the surface with vomiting and purging of undigested matter.

CAUSES AND TREATMENT.—The specific cause is said to be septic influences in the atmosphere and therefore a critical prophylactic treatment is worthy of being noted.

As the reapproach of cholera in this country begins to be looked upon as an event likely to occur, it unavoidably serves to awaken an interest concerning the surest and most reliable protection against its inroads. "In knowledge there is power" applies as readily to this subject as to any other, and in order to institute a rational defense against the inroads of disease, or to conquer it when present, our efforts must be based upon the most rational considerations of causes and effects.

It was beautifully expressed by Dr. Benj. Rush, of Philadelphia, who died in 1818, that "Life is a temporary victory over the causes that induce death." This physiological definition of life must be our starting point in quest of knowledge on the subject of protection against disease. The continual conflict between vitality and dust, to which it must ultimately surrender, goes to show that life maintains its power and performs its functions in opposition to the ordinary laws of inorganic matter, and while its power is paramount it resists the operation of these laws. This may be seen in the seeds of vegetables deprived of life. How soon they decay and become subject to the laws of inorganic matter. These laws are resisted only so long as vitality exists in the seeds, and their structure and form are preserved together with the vital endowment of every part. Were the vitality of a seed to be preserved for centuries it would germinate and develop its legitimate form of plant stock or tree as readily as if but the yield of the preceding season. But if placed in a situation and surrounded by influences that overpower the vitality possessed within itself, it would soon change and pass into other forms and become subject to the affinities of inorganic matter.

A certain class of animals lie in a torpid state for days, months, and even years, without nourishment because their inherent vitality resists dissolution and decay; waits for a new combination of influences to develop its activity and gift them with the phenomena of life and the powers of locomotion. It is by the same kind of life and power that the temperature of the body is preserved in all climates and seasons, with little variation, and with ability to convert foreign materials into our own substance, and to dispose of the various materials of which itself consists with the utmost integrity and precision.

In order for the vitality of the body in general to resist the causes that induce disease and death, the various processes concerned in nutrition must be in a perfect state of integrity, for all the victory accorded to organic life is founded on this considera-

tion. The various aliments taken into the stomach for the sustenance of the body would ferment or become putrescent and pass
entirely into other forms of inorganic matter were the vitality of
the stomach destroyed. This tendency to fermentation and
putrefaction can be overcome only by a healthy vitality of the
organ which counteracts the affinities of dead matter and siezes
the nutritious portions of the aliments and transforms it into
chyme.

Were vitality destroyed or depressed at this stage of the
process, digestion would cease in the one case and be seriously
interfered with in the other. When the unimpaired vitality of
the stomach and other portions of the alimentary canal is kept
up so as to carry on the process of digestion and elaboration of
the chyle, and when the chylifrous vessels' are in a suitable vital
condition to perform their tributary work for the blood vessels,
and the heart and lungs take up the process and carry it forward
for the nutrition of the various tissues, a victory to some extent is
maintained over the " causes that induce death " and the victory,
though temporary, is the more complete and prolonged when the
processes of depuration and defecation are carried on harmoniously
with those of assimilation and nutrition.

By the functions of the skin, lungs and kidneys the impurities of the venous blood are extracted and cast off while
the renovated portion becomes fitted for arterial circulation.

It becomes apparent, then, from the very onset of digestion
in the stomach to the last office of the excretory organs in throwing off the worn out, useless and offensive matter of the system,
that some conservative force must exert a constant resistance,
or continuous warfare against deteriorating agencies, for if the
vital power concerned in the process of nutrition and excretion
should be overcome the body could no longer maintain its resistance to dissolution. The causes that induce death would become
supremely victorious.

In brief, the vitality of the animal system must exert its conservative influence over every process, as well as over every part
and particle of its organization, even that of restraining the
particles of effete and worn out matter from taking on the action
of inorganic affinities until conducted from the sphere of its
dominion.

It is generally conceded by physiologists that there is one

tissue entering into the structure of the living organism, in which
vitality seems more particularly to be present, for the purpose of
sending forth its conservative power even to the periphery of the
body. This tissue is the entire nervous system, which seems to
admit of natural division into two distinct parts, one of which is
termed by Bichet, "The nervous system of animal life" and the
other of organic life. The former is connected with the brain
and medulla spinalis and presides over the organs of sensation,
volition and muscular motion. The latter forms what is termed
the ganglionic system and presides over digestion, absorption, circulation, assimilation and nutrition, as well as over the secretory
and excretory processes. As all the animal functions, such as
sensation, volition and voluntary muscular motion are bound together in sympathy by the cerebro-spinal system of nerves, so all
the organic functions are brought into a common sympathy by
the ganglionic system which contributes branches impartially to
the stomach, heart, lungs, kidneys and all the other organs concerned in the grand function of nutrition.

The cerebro-spinal or nervous system of animal life is indis-
solubly united with that of the ganglionic and the preservation
of both depends upon mutual sympathy and reciprocity of favors.
While the former by its inherent vitality generates the *vis nervosa*
for the whole body, the latter returns through the circulation the
products of nutrition. Both labor for the good of the whole and
become sharers of the common stock of vitality that belongs to
the whole economy.

All the nerves of organic life are woven together into a common web of sympathy. They send forth branches which entwine
themselves around the arterial trunks in a kind of lace-work and
follow them in all their numerous ramifications to their capillary
terminations in the skin which invests the body and the mucous
membrane which lines all its open cavities. They pervade all the
organs concerned in the general function of nourishing the body,
and bring them into general and specific relations by conveying
to them the vitality that enables them to perform their respective
uses.

The stomach and intestines, the lacteals and lymphatics, the
arteries and veins, the heart and lungs, the liver and kidneys, the
capilliaries and skin, etc., etc., are all dependent upon the nervous
system of organic life for the vital power of carrying on their

respective functions, chymification and chylification, absorption
and secretion, respiration and calorification, circulation and organization, etc., etc., by or through which the food is transformed
into chyme—the chyme into chyle the chyle into venous blood
and the venous into arterial blood, which is sent forth in its
fluidity and vitality to lay open its bosom to supply the necessi-
ties of the bones and cartilages, muscles and nerves, and every
other tissue of which the body is composed; while the depuratory
organs separate and excrete or throw off the impurities unsuited
to the wants of vital structures. It is therefore manifest that it
is the general vitality of the body, as well as the special vitality
of every organ and tissue that exists, counteracts and subdues
chemical affinities and noxious agents. It is this that for a time
wages a successful warfare and acquires a temporary victory over
the causes that induce death.

We have remarked that a common sympathy pervades the
whole organic system. It may be remarked still further, that
its common centre is the inner surface of the stomach. Supplied
as it is with nerves of various plexuses and from the base of the
brain—by which it is brought into direct relation with the heart,
lungs, brain, etc. The mucous membrane that lines the stomach
and whole alimentary canal from the mouth to the opposite
extremity, forms an extended sympathetic surface that may
become impressed disastrously if any assault is made upon the
stomach. Although this organ does not supply nervous energy
to the system, it may nevertheless, by means of its nervous supply and constitutional relations, be regarded the common index
of the whole economy of nutrition; for the common conservative
resistance to the influence of noxious agents depends upon the
healthy condition of the stomach, properly supplied with health-
ful aliments. Upon the vigor of digestion all the vital functions
depend, and the entire system becomes fitted for the greatest
achievements and power of endurance, and its life wages the
most successful warfare against cholera and other malignant diseases calculated to over power and destroy it. Where the stomach
is in full possession of its vitality and performs its office well,
then man has the greatest power of resistance to the extremes of
temperature and dampness of the atmosphere—then he is the
most fortified against the subtle breath of pestilence that stalks
abroad at noon-day or at night.

On the contrary, when the vital condition of the stomach is so depressed and disordered as to be the victim of preternatural excitability its energies are not equal to the task of performing its legitimate functions; and, as a matter of course, all the other functions languish—respiration becomes impaired and less oxygen is imbibed by inhaling the atmosphere and the blood fails of being replenished and renovated, the circulation becomes feeble, the blood diminished and the tissues deprived of support, while at the same time the excretions and secretions are likely to become morbidly increased or diminished. The whole system, therefore, becomes unfitted for the regulation of its own temperature as well as for successful resistance of lethal influences. It is less able to endure fatigue and consequently less able to resist the effects of humidity and frost, deteriorated atmosphere, infectious and pestilential causes.

In all this we behold the necessity of preserving a healthy condition of the vital functions by guarding against excesses of every description. This course will ensure attention to the support which the susceptibility of the nerves of organic life constantly requires.

Since it becomes so apparent that the greatest security against morbific influences is in the maintainance of the normal vitality of all the organs concerued in nutrition and excretion, what means are necessary to secure this result? What counsel is necessary upon the subject? What advice can the medical profession give that will entitle its members to the respect and confidence of the community? These questions involve grave considerations. The present physical condition of mankind cannot be overlooked. We have seen that when the human system is fortified by the resistance which a perfect integrity of the organic functions can supply, there is comparatively but little danger of contracting disease. But the facility afforded to malignant malaria for makimg inroads into populous cities and towns would argue the existence of circumstances that tend to develop preternatural susceptibilities on the part of those who become the victims, and this seems to have been unmistakably the case with reference to the *cholera*.

Undue excitement of either a physical or mental character has its influence upon the stomach and is likely to disturb its functions and to establish in it a diseased irritability that acts as

15

a powerful predisponent of more serious disease, and if such an excitant as that of *cholera miasm* were to meet it, in all probability the joint action of the predisposing and exciting cause would become manifest in all the fearful attributes of the disease which we term Asiatic cholera.

Food and drink adapted to the capacity and wants of the animal system excite pleasurable instead of painful stimulation of the sympathetic nerves. A very trifling excess or deviation in quality from that which is normally required becomes either a burden or a source of suffering that results in that loss of vital or conservative resistance to disease which is ever necessary to secure a continuance of health, and there is nothing more malignant or painful that can assail the human economy than those maladies invited by predisponents in the *primæ viæ*. The invasion of cholera upon this domain is because the predisposing cause is there.

Before we attempt a solution of the problem, what is cholera and from whence does it come, let the attention be directed to avoidable agencies that mark out a pathway for the disease.

The question may be asked, what agencies are avoidable? The reply is, everything that impairs the vital energies of the nerves of organic life, for if the whole system of these nerves become morbidly irritable the gastro-intestinal irritation may become overwhelmingly powerful of itself and consequently liable to choleroid disease.

There are agencies innumerable that tend to unsettle the condition of the entire nutritive system and render it an easy prey to cholera. An even course of living, upon nutritious aliments to which the various processes concerned in digestion and assimilation have become habituated cannot be looked upon as one of these agencies. Aliments, either vegetable or animal, can be disposed of by the digestive system without becoming irritable on account of their presence provided they are of the kind and quality to which the digestive organs have from habit become affiliated. Therefore, when an epidemic of any description is abroad, there should be no sudden change from what has been demonstrated to be in accordance with health.

The doctrine broached by some, that a rigid course of diet must be pursued as the surest mode of defense against cholera, is entirely set aside by observation and experience. A better rule

to observe is to make no change in diet provided it has been long
fixed by habit and known to have been a course of agreeable support to the vitality of the organic functions. When cholera was
prevailing in one of the eastern cities in 1849, a gentleman who
had been in robust health seized upon the idea that his safety
against cholera might be provided for by inaugurating himself
into a low diet, but the enterprise was no sooner accomplished
than he was assailed by the disease in its most malignant form.
The sudden change of diet served to unsettle and depress the gastro-intestinal vitality, and thus an abnormal irritation followed
which, through the agency of exciting causes from without,
speedily ripened into fatal cholera. It seems to be well settled,
from observations, that a sudden and radical change from a regimen known to be consistent with health must be attended with
great uncertainty in its result. In view of such facts as these
we will commend the following principles as the safest to observe
where a threatened epidemic of cholera is at hand:

1. Avoid excesses of every kind—excessive abstemiousness,
excessive indulgence of the appetite, excessive use of stimulants,
excessive fatigue, excessive indolence, excessive fear and excessive
mental excitement of any kind.

2. Be regular at meals, indulge in the usual variety of aliments known to be nutritious from habitual indulgence in them;
be industrious, cheerful, calm and hopeful. Banish fearful foreboding of evil, whether in the shape of cholera or any other pestilence. Attend calmly to the duties of life. Cherish a love of
usefulness toward mankind. Trust in Divine Providence and
keep the conscience clear.

It is believed that a strict observance of the foregoing rules
will tend to preserve a normal vitality in all the organs and
functions of the body and render them capable of resisting the
effects of any subtle or malignant miasm that may be in the air,
or any infection that may be brought in ships or clothing. On
the contrary, if they are unheeded, the entire organism becomes
exposed to the action of predisposing and exciting causes of
disease. Excessive *eating and drinking* impose a tax upon the
vitality of the stomach and frequently incite a rebellion that
interferes with the process of digestion, the entire apparatus enters
into a struggle that manifests itself in diarrhœa and vomiting
that betokens a form of cholera, although it is simply the result

of an effort to rid the system of agents which have made an assault upon the vitality of the organic functions.

The *filth* that poisons the atmosphere we breathe or leaves its impress upon the water we drink, is unquestionably a fruitful source of disease, and when a cholera epidemic is abroad its ravages have been the most apparent in filthy districts. This would lead to the conclusion that cleanliness is one of the important safeguards against this disease and that the most critical attention to the cleaning of sewers and all other places where filth accumulates should be regarded the imperative duty of private individuals and municipal authorities.

Excessive abstemiousness, as well as excessive indulgence of the appetite, has a disastrous effect upon the process of nutrition. A very low diet fails of yielding the necessary support to the vitality of the organic functions, inasmuch as the blood is deprived of its competent source of supply. The theory that "a low diet and total abstinence from a generous living is a protection against cholera" is fearfully fallacious. The surest protection consists in a rational supply of such food and drink to the digestive organs as have been known from the habitual use of them to satisfy the healthy demands of the system. Any sudden change from the usual dietetic habit when in sound health is attended with danger. Were those who always enjoy good health and in open toleration of the habit of indulging in a glass of wine at dinner to suddenly change to a less generous fare, *omitting the wine,* the stomach might not respond favorably to the new order of regimen imposed, and as a consequence it becomes the central source of irritation to all the organic functions, and if lethal influences are abroad the nervous vitality of the entire chain of organic processes is in a condition to be impressed by them; and again, were those who enjoy good health, upon a regimen which does not include wine, to suddenly include it when cholera is infesting the community, they would incur a serious risk. In all communities where cholera has committed its ravages, it has been observed that the intemperate are the most liable to sudden and fatal attacks of the disease, and those who attempt to shelter themselves from the storm by resorting to alcoholic stimulation are the surest to be overtaken. A resort to Opium, Laudanum and Morphine as protective measures simply multiply the chances of assault, for their influence is to depress the vital powers of resistance, and so derange the process of nutrition, that the door is opened for the entrance of the cholera miasm, armed with its deadly influence, to operate disastrously, because all vital resistance is held in check or depressed by these narcotics. It cannot be otherwise than disastrous to attack even the commencement of diarrhœa with opiates. It accords with experience fully that scarcely any recover from cholera when Laudanum or any other form of anodyne is employed in the stage of invasion. It is better to advise rest as soon as a sense of prostration, accompanied by diarrhœa occurs. Lying quietly upon a couch will often accomplish more in the way of prevention than any of the thousand prophylactics advertised among the nostrums. We have thus far avoided mentioning medicinal prophylactics of any kind. It is yet undecided whether the impressible organism can be guarded by medicinal agents so as to defend it against exciting causes. Some authors have advised the propriety of taking various medicines, which in their estimation give a resisting force against the invasions of cholera; such as Veratrum, Cuprum and Secale, and without doubt they have their use.

We have thus far referred only to the preventi n of the vis. med. naturæ, as the surest and most reliable safeguard. But there are medicinal measures to be called into requisition to correct diseases already existing that act as predisponents when the cholera is abroad. There are certain mixtures or panaceas, sold by the nostrum mongers, professedly universal in their effects in toning up debilitated systems. These pernicious drugs are various combinations of narcotics, disguised with other ingredients, and as disastrous in their effects as any poison that ever came from the Delta of the Ganges. Every physician's face should be set against them as firmly as against cholera itself, for they impose additional burdens upon the stomach and bowels and open up a highway for the invasion of the disease. Those afflicted with predisposing disorders are, nevertheless, subjects for Homœopathic treatment, which, if well directed, will do away with these predisponent difficulties.

Having stated the case physiologically, by endeavoring to illustrate how predisposing influences get the ascendency in the living system, we may allude briefly to what has been said concerning exciting causes. Learned writers have advanced several theories. Some have ascribed the exciting cause of epidemic cholera to the sun and moon. (1) This is what is termed the sol. lunar hypothesis. Some have maintained that the approach of a comet always produces the epidemic. (2) This is termed by some writers the cometary influence. Some say the exciting causes exhale from the bowels of the earth through volcanic craters or are hurled suddenly by earthquakes upon certain localities. (3) This is termed the geological theory. Another theory is that the exciting cause is a malaria in the air, that falls like seed into whatever soil is prepared for it. (4) This is termed the miasmatic theory. Prof. Smith, of New York University, stated what he termed (5) the meteor-attraction theory, which consists in a disturbance of the gaseous and electric elements of the atmosphere or in their mode of union. (6) Then there is the theory of contagion, which has had many advocates, and lastly (7) the animalculæ theory, which is founded upon an elaborate natural history of insects and their proneness to accumulate in stagnated waters, pits and ponds, holes and gutters, tops of houses and steeples. Much that is plausible has been said in favor of all these theories, but yet nothing definite is learned beyond the fact that cholera is a poisonous influence which at times exists in the air, operating upon all who are predisposed to its assaults.

Whatever may be the specific nature of the exciting cause, its fatal energy must be admitted. The suddenness of the attack, the extreme prostration of the vital forces, the universal overthrow of the functions, the speedy termination in death, and the accumulation of blood in the great central organs, as found afte that event, manifest the impress of a most desolating poison. It may, like electricity, penetrate our organs; it may stamp itself upon the dermoid and mucous surfaces and from them find its way to the nervous centres. It may be inhaled through the lungs and passed directly into the circulation. It matters not which If it meets no predisposing influence to open the door to its inroads, it seldom proves overpowering. In this, as in all kinds of desolating disorders, it will be found that "an ounce of prevention is worth a pound of cure."

ALLOPATHIC TREATMENT is various because there are so many theories concerning the disease. By some it has been considered an inflammatory disease and subject to antiphlogistic treatment, such as bleeding from the arm, soda water, chloride of soda in solution mixed with cinnamon water in the proportion 1 oz. sol. chloride of soda to 6 oz. of the water; a large spoonful of pounded mustard seed to be given at once in oft repeated doses of a table spoonful; also, calomel and opium are given in the first stage, and likewise sulphuric ether and opium. But it is now believed that this treatment in the first stage deprives the system of its power of resistance and forebodes evil to the patient. In the second stage, which is characterized by purging and vomiting, rice-water discharges, cramps—opium, camphor and various heating stimulants are employed. In the stage of collapse, cupping, rubefacients and hot drinks are resorted to with the hope of effecting a vital reaction. The above treatment has not proved very successful in either stage of the disease and therefore not to be relied on.

HOMŒOPATHIC TREATMENT—After all the prophylactic and hygienic means have been employed against the invasion of Asiatic cholera and yet we find that it must be encountered, let it be understood that the disease has different stages and requires the Homœopathic affiliation of remedies in each stage.

The first or premonitory stage may come on insidiously, creating no alarm. It consists in a painless, watery diarrhœa, lassitude, giddiness, nausea, and these symptoms are followed by vomiting. The patient should be required to lie down quietly at rest, and for this stage *Aconite either* in the 1st dilution or mother tincture has proved a safe and effectual remedy. Ten drops in half a goblet of water may be given in tea-spoonful doses every thirty minutes. Phos. acid is also a competent remedy when the diarrhœa is painless. Drop doses of the saturated tincture of Camphor should be an immediate resort when the disease first shows itself.

The second stage of the disease, which is denoted by rapid prostration, fainting, vomiting, and purging, thin, rice-water discharges, violent cramps. This stage comes on suddenly, and frequently in the latter part of the night, and is characterized by an intermittent pulse, great thirst, severe burning in stomach, cramps down the thighs and spasms in different parts of the body, coldness and dampness of the whole surface of the body, cold breath and tongue, vomiting incessantly. In this stage I have found the following remedies to prove useful and curative:

Strong tincture of Camphor in drop doses, repeated every fifteen
minutes for awhile, and when no specially good results have
been obtained I have had recourse to Arsenicum, Veratrum alb.,
Iris vers., Ipecac, Cuprum met., Secale cornutum, and Aconite.
I have prescribed all these remedies and with uniform good
results.

The third stage, that of collapse, the pulse is scarcely perceptible, the lips purple, the tongue cold, sunken expression of
the whole countenance, pupils of the eyes dilated and laborious
breathing, every feature sharp and pinched and the entire surface
of a bluish appearance. To overcome this stage of collapse I
have resorted to Muriatic acid, Carbo veg. and Arsenicum, and
with greater encouragement than I have ever known under this
treatment.

Aconite in 1x, ten drops in a cup of water, according to
Professor Hempel and also Dr. Ruddock, in teaspoonful doses
and repeated every fifteen minutes.

Arsenicum, for cramps, suppressed urine and sudden prostration and collapse, 3x in dilution I can recommend from personal experience as being quite a reliable remedy. Ten drops in
a half cup of water; give a teaspoonful every fifteen minutes and
keep the surface warm with blankets wrung out of hot water.
We once knew a lady, aged 35 years, when the cholera was prevailing in Philadelphia, in 1849, who was brought successfully
out of a collapse by this treatment after two physicians had
exhausted their skill and abandoned the case as hopeless.

The *favorable stage*, or stage of convalescence, requires
China, Ars., Canchalagua.

Sometimes typhoid conditions become manifest, which
require Phosphorus, Rhus tox. Ars., Carbo veg., Nit. ac. and other
remedies.

Certain remedies are believed by some to possess prophylactic
powers, these are Cuprum, Veratrum alb. and Camphor. But
after all nothing can take the place of regular habits, good food
and drink and the avoidance of excesses and irregularities of
every kind.

The following is from Dr. P. Jousset, of Paris:

" When diarrhœa appears as the first symptom of cholera,
which is the rule in mild cases, it is not stopped with a few drops
of laudanum, because cholera in evolution is not stopped any

more than variola or typhoid fever in evolution. If M. Jules Guerin has said that diarrhœa in time of cholera epidemic must be treated severely, he has only expressed ordinary opinions by reason of their truth. As to the story of premonitory diarrhœa as described by him, it is a mere romance.

I. *Treatment of the benign form.*—The mild form or *cholerine*, is usually characterized by a watery, pale, rice-water diarrhœa. In a higher degree, vomiting and cramps, but never any signs of asphyxia.

1. The principal drug is *Phosphori acidum;* it is indicated by the character of the diarrhœa; it should be prescribed in the third dilution, a dose every two hours.

2. *Ipecac* will be alternated with Phosphori acidum if the diarrhœa is complicated with vomiting; the dose is the first decimal dilution, one dose every two hours.

3. Finally, should the case be more serious, with cramps, *Veratrum* or Cuprum would be indicated.

II. *Treatment of the common form of cholera.*—The common form shows evacuations upwards and downwards, cramps and asphyxic symptoms. But it is characterized by the regular succession of two periods: *coldness* and *reaction.*

A. *Treatment in the cold period.*—Quite at the outset, if the diarrhœa exists alone, *Phosphori acidum* will be the principal drug to administer, as in the benign form; if vomiting accompany the diarrhœa, unless the coldness be already pronounced, *Ipecac*, 1st to the 10th trit. should be prescribed every half hour. But if the general symptoms precede the evacuations, *Camphora* is a heroic drug.

1. *Camphora* quite at the outset; coldness, great weakness, lipothymic condition, cramps, commencing lividness, no evacuations or very few in number. Camphor is prescribed in the form of spirit, a few drops on some sugar, a dose every ten minutes.

2. *Veratrum* is the principal drug for the completely developed cold stage. It is specially indicated by very copious rice-water evacuations; by decided coldness, violent cramps, and sometimes absence of pulse. In the Charroux epidemic, with globules of the sixth dilution only, we had remarkable success. Generally the third dilution is used in preference; some physi-

cians prefer the mother tincture; the doses should be given every half hour.

3. *Arsenicum.*—Acute poisoning by arsenic shows a perfect picture of cholera in the cold stage, as in the case of the Duke de Praslin, who poisoned herself with arsenic. Louis diagnosed a case of cholera. I. P. Tessier, towards the end of the epidemic of 1849, preferred Arsenic to Veratrum, in serious cases, without having it preceded by Veratrum.

The symptoms specializing the indication of Arsenic are restlessness, agony, and a more decided fear of death than usual, *sensation of internal burning,* with most violent thirst, completely suppressed pulse, pronounced asphyxic symptoms.

The third trituration is generally prescribed, two or three doses in the space of an hour; we may descend to the 2d and 1st centesimal trituration. In the latter case, the drug being much repeated, not more than twenty centigrammes must be put in two grammes of water, a spoonful every twenty minutes.

4. *Cuprum* is specially indicated by violence and persistence of the cramps; by the predominance of the vomitings, which are violent and painful. Hahnemann preferred it even to Veratrum. The 3d and even the 6th trituration have always seemed to me sufficient. Allopaths have used enormous doses of Acetate of Copper without much success.

5. *Aconitum.*—Aconite is a drug suitable to the cold stage of completely developed cholera. The picture of choleraic indication is met with in poisoning by Aconite and Aconitine; even coldness of the tongue, cyanosis, imperceptible and irregular pulse, cramps and suppression of urine. Dr. Hempel, thirty years ago, called attention to Aconite in the treatment of cholera. Dr. Cramoisy presented a paper to the Academy of Medicine on the efficacy of Aconite in cholera; he published numerous observations of cure. Strong doses of the mother tincture have been prescribed by Hempel and Cramoisy.

We would remark that Aconite does not respond so well as Veratrum and especially Arsenic to the suppression of the pulse and urine, in short it has not that notoriety for it like the three drugs used by the generality of the followers of Hahnemann, and that it will need further observation to fix its real worth.

6. *Carbo vegetabilis.*—When the collapse is near to agony and resists other drugs; when asphyxia is advanced and pulse

absent, we have still one resource in the use of Carbo vegetabilis, and English physicians are wrong in not using this drug. We must not expect this or any other drug to bring the dead to life; but it is sufficient that in certain apparently desperate cases Carbo has arrested the collapse and brought on reaction, that it should be looked upon as a very energetic and very certain medicament. We have always used it in globules of the thirtieth dilution, dose every quarter of an hour.

B. *Treatment in the reactionary stage.*—Febrile movements, inflammations, and visceral congestions; suppression of urine will fix the indications.

1. *Aconitum* is indicated by a clearly established febrile motion; pulse strong and full; redness of the face; general heat and thirst; continuation of the diarrhœa is a further sign for the prescription of Aconite.

2. *Belladonna.*—Belladonna should be prescribed if the brain is affected during reaction. Congestion of the face, throbbing of the carotids, eyes brilliant and protuberant; dilatation of the pupils, delirium, pronounced albuminuria.

3. *Opium* on the contrary will be indicated when somnolence prevails, and especially if the coma is complete with stertor and dilated pupil these two drugs are prescribed in the 6th or 3d dilution; a dose every two hours. If the diarrhœa is persistent during the period of reaction, Arsenic will be still the principal drug unless the diarrhœa continues in spite of the use of this drug during the cold stage.

4. *Mercurius corrosivus* is prescribed if the stools are small, green, sanguineous, slow, with colic and tenesmus; the 3d dilution is usually sufficient.

5. *Secale cornutum* is extolled by Drysdale and Russell for watery, abundant and painless stools, (Richard Hughes, *Manual of Therapeutics*, p. 105.)

6. *Phosphorus and Phosphori acidum* are used when the diarrhœa is persistent after the disappearance of other symptoms. For absence of urine after the cessation of the cold stage, Richard Hughes thinks highly of *Cantharis, Terebinthina* and *Kali bichromicum.* To which I would add *Digitalis*—a precious medicament of true anuria.

III. *Treatment of the ataxic form.*—This form also called the typhoid is characterized by the apparent mildness of the cold stage, by the length and gravity of the following reaction, in cases of death by a terminal cold period.

Treatment of the cold stage is the same as in the preceding form, with this difference that Camphor is more often indicated. Independent of Aconite, Belladonna and Opium, whose indications have been formulated as to the common form, and which would often find their use in the reactionary stage of the ataxic form, we would notice three remedies, *Lachesis, Secale cornutum* and *Nux vomica.*

1. *Lachesis*, like Secale cornutum, suits the treatment of visceral inflammations, progressive and terminal chilliness, which is the pathological characteristic of the ataxic form. Lachesis is more particularly indicated by the inequality of the reaction, whether the warmth reappears only in one part of the body, whether having reappeared, it disappears again to still reappear. The lipothymic state and tendency to syncope is again an indication for Lachesis; as it is also the same for the predominance of cerebral affection and for the comatose condition mingled with asphyxia resulting therefrom.

2. *Secale cornutum* is chiefly indicated by cold and other symptoms of collapse and principally by the continuance of a copious diarrhœa, rice-watery and painless.

3. *Nux vomica* has often been used by I. P. Tessier, in the reactionary period of the ataxic form against persistent vomiting, but this drug would not be suitable if collapse had commenced.

IV. *Treatment of the foudroyant form.*—This asphyxic form, *black cholera* of authors, is characterized by culminating asphyxia. In the common form the symptoms of asphyxia show themselves successively; in the culminating form, cyanosis is present from the outset at the same time as the cramps and evacuations. Let us add that the cyanosis acquires from the first hour a great intensity and that the pulse weakens and disappears from the beginning.

This form is nearly always mortal. This fatal ending is due as much at the same time to the violence of the disease and to the want of absorption preventing the action of the medicines. I have not succeded with inhalation, pulmonary absorption being suppressed as it is at the stomach. Dr. Drysdale has administered arseniated hydrogen by inhalation. I do not know if he was thus successful. Medicines administered by the hypodermic method might, perhaps be more successful.

Hydrocyanic acid.—This drug is indicated when patients are suddenly struck down, the pupil dilated, the eyes prominent, sight diminished or gone, breathing weak, intermittent, insensible, pulse small or insensible in one arm or completely disappeared; general coldness; involuntary evacuation.

Dr. Sircar, who practiced in India, speaks in these terms of Hydrocyanic acid: "And in fact, it is the only remedy when the pulse disappears, the breathing is slow, deep, painful or difficult and spasmodic, separated by long intervals during which the patient appears dead. If any drug deserves to be spoken of as a charm it is certainly this one; it seems sometimes to resuscitate a corpse." (Richard Hughes loc. cit. p. 105.) The dose is not mentioned. We have used the fifth dilution; we think a stronger dose might be used, the second dilution, for instance. As to ponderable doses, it must be remembered that in patients struck with foudroyant cholera absorption is suspended and consequently medicamental doses may accumulate in the stomach and become toxic at the reactionary period.

Veratrum, Arsenic, Camphor and *Carbon* may be prescribed according to the indications named in regard to the treatment of the common form.

V. *Regimen and hygienic rules.*—During the cold period every effort should be made to warm the patient by dry friction and especially by accumulation of heat to the exterior; rubbing the limbs to lessen the cramps; giving iced and gassy drinks to satisfy thirst and prevent vomiting. In certain cases very hot alcoholic drinks are desirable and comfort more than cold drinks. During the period of reaction, broth in very small quantity as food is given, and a strict regime must be observed during convalescence."

Adipous Diarrhœa.

Some pathologists have described a diarrhœa which consists in the discharge of fatty matter from the bowels. From my own observation this never occurs except when patients have taken either castor or olive oil in such quantities as to commingle with the secretions of mucous membrane of the intestinal tube. A lady who took much olive oil to favor the passage of gall stones and to relieve the pain always attendant on the passage of biliary calculi, was surprised to find that fatty matter was discharged from the bowels in large quantities which was kept up daily for many weeks. The matter passed was in the form of globules, varying in size from that of a pea to that of a moderate sized grape, and of the color of cream and sufficiently consistent to retain its form and bear being cut with a knife like soft wax. This accords fully with the theory that oleaginous substances taken into the stomach must be the cause of this form of diarrhœa. But Stokes and Good have given examples of this disease when no oily substances have been swallowed, and from this fact it would seem that the fat must have been formed at the expense of the system.

The quantity evacuated differs materially with different subjects. Dr. Jackson, of Boston, cites a case where about eight ounces were evacuated every twenty-four hours for a period of four months. An analysis of the matter, by G. Melin, gave 74 parts of acid fatty matter, in which stearine predominated, and 21 parts of something analogous to fibrine, and four parts of phosphates of lime.

TREATMENT.—The Allopathic treatment consists in revulsives and a complete change of diet and other hygienic influences.

The Homœopathic treatment is believed to be the most effectual. The remedies that have been successfully employed are *Arsenicum*, China, Podophyllin, together with a generous nutritious diet, well ventilated apartments. Other remedies, such as *Murcury*, Iris versicolor, Secale and Dulcamara, may be consulted.

CHAPTER XVIII.

DISEASES OF THE PERITONEUM.

The peritoneum lines the parieties of the abdomen and provides a coat for a great proportion of the viscera. It is a serous membrane and like all membranes of this class is kept moist by a thin albuminous fluid of its own secreting. In the cavity of the abdomen it forms a closed sac containing no viscus. It extends from the diaphragm over the abdominal muscles, over the bladder and in the female, over the uterus, from thence over the rectum, the kidneys, enveloping the intestines, and constituting by its own lamina the mesentery, giving a coat to the liver and receiving the stomach between its duplicatures. Its physiological use is to yield a support and fix the different viscera and by means of its secretion to enable the intestines to move more readily upon each other. The cavity of the peritoneum is its shut sac, which when it fills with fluid and greatly extends, is termed abdominal dropsy or ascites. What is termed the omenta or epifloa, are fatty reflections of the peritoneum after it has covered the stomach and the intestines.

The peritoneum is susceptible of general disease or only a small portion may become implicated; and the symptoms will be modified to accord with the particular viscus invested by it. We have already treated of parietal peritonitis, under the head of enteritis of the peritoneal coat, and also under the head of other peritoneal viscera invested by it. We will, as occasion now offers, treat of those affections which appertain to the peritoneum generally.

Inflammation of the Peritoneum.

This affection may be considered under three heads. First, the acute form, second the chronic, third the puerperal.

Acute Peritonitis.—The symptoms are essentially the same as those of acute enteritis of the peritoneal coat. An acute pain is experienced in some portion of the abdomen, which may be circumscribed, or it may extend over the entire abdomen. It is

severe when the peritoneal lining of the abdominal cavity is extensively involved, and so sensitive that the slightest pressure is unsup-
portable.   The weight of a blanket excites intolerable suffering.
" The parietes of the abdomen are tense and tumid, the countenance has at times a peculiar expression, the upper lip being
drawn upwards and bound tightly over the teeth."   The respiration is not aided by the depression of the diaphragm, more than
the patient is obliged to permit, on account of the intense pain
produced by the pressure; therefore costal respiration is almost
wholly relied on to keep the lungs in motion.   The patient lies
on the back with the knees drawn up to relieve the pressure of .
the bed clothes.   The pulse is unusually quick and feeble and the
skin hot and dry, and almost always there is pain in the pubic
region.   We have been observing the characteristic peculiarities
of acute peritoneal inflammations for more than thirty-five years,
and we have observed the above symptoms as a uniform rule.   In
addition, we have known patients to complain of the unpleasantness of the slightest touch upon the great trochanter.   This fact
has been confirmed by the clinical observation of others.   The
relation of the nerves of the parts in which the pain is felt to
the peritoneum and by its connection with the fascia and muscles
about them, is offered as explanation.

Attendant upon these local signs there is always derangement of the stomach and bowels, even if there is no vomiting or
constipation.   The great use of the clinical thermometer in
making a prognosis of this disease cannot be doubted.   The disease may terminate unfavorably in a few days, or when its course
is more protracted there may be a sero-purulent effusion into the
peritoneal cavity.   This condition admits of a more favorable
prognosis, as the effusion may absorb or form an opening into
the intestines from the cavity.   The signs indicative of the termination of the inflammation in this way are: a measurable dis-
sipation of the pain and swelling, with a soft or doughy feel of
the abdomen and infiltration of the parieties of the abdomen and
the lower extremities.   The pressure of the fluid is easily detected
by percussion.

It has been maintained that by oscultation the dryness of the
membrane can be detected even before effusion takes place, as the
sound of friction can be distinctly heard by the aid of the stethoscope; inflammation of the serous membranes causes their sur-

faces to become dry, and as a consequence they emit the sound of friction when rubbing against each other.

CAUSES.—Exposure to the extremes of temperature without being well protected, as well as excessive fatigue, irregularity of the bowels. The effects or after-effects of surgical operations may be included among the causes of internal inflammation.

TREATMENT.—The Allopathic treatment of acute peritonitis appears to have been antiphlogistic and sedative. Blood-letting was formerly the *sheet anchor*, followed by sedative doses of Opium and then by laxative doses of Castor oil, and in addition, Calomel and Opium were formerly advised as follows: Three grains of Calomel, half grain of Opium mixed with Conserve of roses, formed into a pill, to be taken every three or four hours. At the same time Mercurial ointment was applied externally over the abdomen by friction until a profuse ptyalism was produced. This treatment was recommended by Marshall Hall and is substantially the same as obtains at the present day; to which warm enemas and fomentations are added.

This treatment is liable to many objections because it does but little to mitigate the suffering of the patient and far less in multiplying the chances for recovery.

HOMŒOPATHIC TREATMENT.—In the uncomplicated form of acute peritonitis an early resort to Homœopathic remedies is likely to be rewarded with success.

Aconite when the disease is produced by a cold and comes on with shivering and a predominance of febrile symptoms. We have seen the action of this remedy when given in the early manifestations of the disease to be decidedly favorable and rapidly curative.

Arsenicum.—We have also witnessed the apparent actions of this remedy when the patient complained of great thirst, such as cold water could not satiate, and have been agreeably surprised at its prompt action in giving relief. A dose every hour of the above remedies may be given until relief is obtained.

Arnica.—We were once called to see a gentleman who had been kicked by a horse in the abdomen and who had peritoneal inflammation as a consequence. We prescribed *Arnica*, a dose every hour, and he soon experienced relief.

Bryonia.—When the patient complains of stinging, burning pains, which are greatly aggravated by movement, and when the bowels are much constipated, and there is general uneasiness and unwillingness to be disturbed, even by the weight of the bed clothes, *Bryonia*, in hourly doses, will soon give relief.

Mercurius corrosivus is a well chosen remedy for acute peritonitis in a scrofulous subject, when the skin is sallow, and also when the tongue has upon it a yellow coating and the abdomen is tympanitic and abscess is threatening. Two grains of the third decimal trituration may be administered every two hours. In a case of this kind where constipation was followed by dysenteric diarrhœa, we gave this remedy and it was soon followed by complete recovery.

We have found many cases where *Arsenicum* was indicated and was given with only partial success, and *Bryonia* was substituted with the best of results; and where there was intense thirst and a metastasis of the disease to the brain, and where the face was flushed and the eyes were fiery red, we have given *Belladonna* after the *Arsenicum* with satisfactory results.

In the treatment of this disease we have allowed the patients frequent sups of cold water, and even small pieces of ice in the mouth, and warm water fomentations to the abdomen. We have found those of tepid water better than hot, and sometimes the cold has answered an equally valuable purpose.

Acute peritonitis is a formidable disease and if not subject to early treatment, and subdued thereby, it is liable to prove fatal. We would recommend the use of the clinical thermometer, applied in the axilla, before every change of remedy, that the temperature of the patient may be ascertained, and rational judgment be formed of his true condition.

Chronic Peritonitis.

Acute peritonitis may terminate in the chronic, or may have been insidiously of the chronic form from the first and difficult to diagnose. The symptoms are not so severe, the abdominal pain not acute, sometimes not detected until by a careful pressure. Marshall Hall says there may be no pain, tenderness or tumor in the abdomen, which as in the acute form may be tense and doughy, and even more so, and fluctuations of the effusion in the peritoneal sac more perceptible. This may appear to be the case, because a more careful percussion can be practiced. Every afternoon and evening the pulse is small and more frequent than natural. Seldom, if ever, the patients vomit or are subject to purgation. They may retain a fair appetite, but emaciation progresses and the fever appears to be of a hectic character. We have encountered many of these cases in our long practice and have regarded them in the light of a phthisis abdominalis.

CAUSES.—Defective nutrition, or protracted drain upon the bowels, or perhaps circulation, and tubercular deposits in the mesenteric glands.

TREATMENT.—The Allopathic treatment is derivative cups and leeches are applied to the abdomen, repellants of various forms are called into requisition. But this treatment is liable to the same objection as that prescribed for acute peritonitis.

We have seen cases of chronic peritonitis among children of a scrofulous diathesis. The inflammation of the mucous membrane induced a similar condition of the mesenteric glands and lays the foundation for what is termed *tabes mesenterica*, for which a similar Allopathic treatment is recommended.

HOMŒOPATHIC TREATMENT.—*Arsenicum* where there is distention of the abdomen and great prostration, and a muco-purulent diarrhœa.

Calcarea carbonica for the general scrofulous diathesis, for pain in the head, acid stomach, and mal-assimilation of food.

Lycopodium in those cases where there is a tedious constipation.

Mercurius corrosivus for burning pain in the lower abdomen and fetid discharge from the bowels, and also for dysenteric tenesmus.

Sulphur for the general condition of the peritoneal coat when chronically inflamed. The above remedies need not be administered oftener than morning and evening.

Accessory means.—Good food, beef tea and even fish, cheese and oysters, particularly oyster broth, tepid fomentations and sometimes a cold compress worn over the abdomen, are a source of great relief. As emaciation seems gradually to progress, in both children and adults, we must infer that chronic peritonitis is a form of consumption and dropsy rarely cured when ascites becomes apparent. In those cases much temporary relief may be obtained from the use of *Arsenicum, Apis mel. Apocynum, Helleborus niger* and *Digitalis.*

Puerperal Peritonitis.

There has been much warm controversy on this topic in former times, if not recently; but there can be no hesitancy in referring it to inflammation of the peritoneum, modified by the existing condition of the female or, some maintain, by a prevailing epidemic.

In modern times more attention has been given to the disease, more critical observation has been made upon the nature of the same. From one who has made a *specialty* of *Diseases of Women* for years, and one who is entitled to our highest respect as an *Author*, I give the following extracts from the lectures of my respected friend and colleague Professor Reuben Ludlam. These extracts are taken from a special course of twenty lectures on the *Puerperal Diseases* delivered by Prof. Ludlam in the Hahnemann Medical College and Hospital of Chicago.

Puerperal peritonitis may be epidemic or sporadic, primary or secondary, diffuse or local, simple septic or pyæmic. In its onset it may suddenly attack and involve the whole peritoneal surface, or it may begin in the local form and successively extend to other parts of that structure.

The epidemic variety, which is most apt to be septic, generally sets in within a few hours, or a day or two after delivery. It has few, if any, premonitory symptoms, but comes on abruptly, and it is evident that the patient is desperately ill from the first. In this case it is manifest that the inflammation has seized upon the membrane throughout its whole extent, and that the lesion is a primary and not a secondary one.

The more common or non-epidemic form of puerperal peritonitis comes later, after some days, or when the child is from one to two weeks old, and is almost always preceded by signs, either of endo-metritis or metro-salpingitis or some form of pelvic or abdominal inflammation. It is more apt to be pyæmic than septicæmic, although in exceptional cases, if the mother has been exposed to the causes of common peritonitis prior to the birth of the child, it may develop directly after labor, in which case the symptoms of putrid infection would be more likely to complicate the case. This variety of peritonitis is usually local, regional and circumscribed and not diffuse, and hence it has been treated as an ovarian, iliac or hypogastric, intra-pelvic, epiploic, cystic and diaphragmatic.   *   *   *   *   *

SYMPTOMS.—Most authors insist that the disease begins with an initial *chill*, just as in peritonitis outside the puerperal state. Exceptionally, however, it is conceded that the *chill* may be lacking altogether. In one or two severe epidemics Drs. John Clarke, 1793, Leake, 1792, and others, did not observe a single case of this disease in which there was a chill at any period.

If we except very nervous persons (in whom the non-severity of the chill will be detected by the thermometer) the degree and duration of the chill, or chills, will afford a pretty good criterion of the gravity of the attack. It is important to remember that as a rule, if the case is septicæmic, there will probably not be more than one chill, while if it is pyæmic there may be several of them. In the latter case the period of their recurrence will not be regular.   *   *   *   *   *

The severity of the chill can best be measured by taking the degree of the patient's temperature at its close. If it exceeds 103 deg. F., the case is a dangerous one. Other things being equal, if with the general symptoms of puerperal peritonitis the patient has a prolonged chill after the fourth day when the flow of milk has already been established, the case is a more serious one than if the chill had come earlier.

After all that we have said of the *temperature* of *patients in the puerperal state*, see an essay on the *Temperature and the Pulse in Puerperality*, being an *Analysis of Fifty Cases Treated in the Puerperal Ward of the Hahnemann Hospital*. Transactions of American Institute of Homœopathy for 1878, page 149. And also a report on a *Second Series of fifty cases treated in the same hospital;* contained in the North American Journal of Homœopathy, Vol. X (new series), p 230.

I beg you not to forget that apart from its power to detect the septic or pyæmic complications, and to measure the severity of the fever, the thermometer is of no especial use or significance in puerperal peritonitis, for by it alone we cannot distinguish between this and any other form of inflammation to which lying-in women are liable.

The *pulse*, however, is peculiar, for it is always frequent. And although this acceleration of the pulse has its remissions and exacerbations, which are usually of the diurnal type, although it may and does become more frequent with each accession of the disease in the local form of it, still this marked and ever-present frequency does not entirely disappear until the disease has run its course. It may be modified by accidental complications; as, for example, an attack of pleurisy, but it does not lose this peculiar character until the peritonitis has been cured. •

Sometimes the pulse is full and bounding, with evidence of strong arterial tension, but more often it is small, thread-like, weak and compressible. These peculiarities, and more especially its marked frequency, are in strong contrast with the ante-partum pulse of the patient and also with the restoration of the pulse in puerperal cases that are normal.   •   •   •   •

But this frequency of the pulse is not pathognomonic of puerperal peritonitis, for we may also find it in other puerperal inflammations, more especially in puerperal phthisis and endometritis.

The perspiration is more free and abundant in those cases in which there is either putrid or purulent infection. The pain is identical in character with that which accompanies the non-puerperal variety of peritonitis, and is usually in proportion to the severity of the attack. The exceptions to the latter rule occur in low forms of secondary peritonitis which are typhoid in type and which are accompanied by what Trousseau very properly styled "colliquative suppuration." In the circumscribed form of the disease the suffering is renewed with the extension of the lesion. *There is a spurious peritonitis, as there is a false pleurisy, in which the suffering is self limited.*

Either vomiting or diarrhœa, and sometimes both, are present in most cases. The latter is often critical and salutary, particularly in septic peritonitis. Either of these modes of discharge may furnish the means of escape for the extraordinary escape of bile which *Hervieux* has noted as one of the accompaniments of peritonitis in lying-in women.

We had one case in the puerperal ward of the Hahnemann Hospital within a year in which very large quantities of orange-colored bile were vomited on the third and fourth days. She, however, made a good recovery. In some cases, and in some epidemics, it is said, the *abdominal tympanitis* bears a close relation to the nervous systems. It may, indeed, be more nervous than inflammatory, and hence its degree is not always a reliable criterion either of the extent or of the severity of the peritoneal lesion, and it is very apt to be reproduced by a nervous shock, or it may arise from the transmission of the utero-vaginal tissues; from the enteric lesions that are incident to a co-existing typhoid fever, from typhilitis, from septic inflammation and ulceration of the intestinal mucous membrane, or from puerperal metritis with the decomposition of the lochial and placental *debris*. But whatever its cause, it is almost always present in puerperal peritonitis.

The respiration, like the pulse, is hurried and frequent. In bad cases it is not very rare to find the patient breathing as often as from forty to fifty and even sixty times in the minute. The relative proportion between the number of respirations, the temperature and the frequency of the pulse is preserved in many, perhaps in most cases. But if there are cardiac or pleuritic complications, especially the breathing disproportionately rapid, as well as anxious and panting, usually, but not always, this symptom is more marked when the meteorism of the abdomen is most pronounced. From this cause alone the patient may find it as difficult to lie down as it is in cardiac affections and in asthma. I have already told you that this rapidity of respiration invalidates the record of the thermometer in puerperal peritonitis when the temperature is taken by putting the bulb of the instrument beneath the tongue.   *   *   *   *   *   *

The two last symptoms modify the patient's expression, which is always one of anxiety, if not of anguish. If the case has progressed, more especially if there has been an extensive or exhausting effusion of serum, of pus, or of blood into the peritoneal cavity, the features are pinched and almost hippocratic. The complexion is often jaundiced, sometimes it has a dull, earthy hue, as in the copræmia of Dr. Barnes, and again the puerperal tint of M. Bourdon.

If the case is septic there will be more or less *delirium*, and so also if the tympanitis is very considerable, or if there is anæmic intoxication. But if there is purulent infection, pyæmia, she will be dull, stupid, apathetic, indifferent and perhaps comatose.

Neither the *lochia* nor the *milk* are especially affected in puerperal peritonitis. When the former is suppressed it is the consequence and not the cause of the accompanying fever. In simple sporadic and non-malignant cases the lacteal flow may continue to be as free and of as good quality (if we may judge of its effect upon the infant) as in health, which is a very unusual circumstance in puerperal endo-metritis.   *   *   *

In the spring of 1879 I called the attention of my sub-classes to three cases of puerperal peritonitis which began in a peculiar way. In each of them the first abnormal symptom noticed by our house physician, Dr. Spring, was an inability to urinate without great pain *after the flow*. In every case and for several consecutive days these patients had passed the urine voluntarily and without any suffering; but without any known cause there came on a sharp pain, which was referred behind the symphysis pubis to the organ of the bladder, and an indisposition to urinate because of it. Directly following there was a circumscribed peritonitis which passed through all the stages of the disease when it occurs elsewhere.

CAUSES.—Puerperal peritonitis may arise (1) from traumatic injury of the peritoneum about the lower segment of the womb in tedious or violent labor, in case of deformed pelvis, and from the operation of version or the use of forceps or other instruments; (2) from laceration of the cervix and consequent injury to the uterine lymphatics; (3) from the ordinary causes of peritonitis, as a chilly or damp atmosphere, or from an excess of heat, especially in rheumatic or scrofulous subjects, and (4) in a secondary way, either by an extension of inflammation from the cavity of the womb through the Fallopian tube (metro-salpingitis), by the escape of pus or other fluids through the oviduct into the peritoneal cavity; by the spreading of the inflammation from the lining membrane of the uterus so as finally to involve all of its tissues and thus to reach the enveloping peritoneum (metro-peritonitis), or in consequence of the ulceration of the bowel in a co-existent typhoid fever, typhilitis or septicæmia.   *

TREATMENT.—The treatment is local and general; the topical use of hot applications, either wet or dry, as a means of assuaging the pain, is almost always necessary.

Dry heat is the best. A dry poultice of wheat bran or hops, or corn meal heated very thoroughly and frequently renewed has the advantage of being available, light and inoffensive. Hot flannel or cotton batting may answer in mild cases. The objection to wet applications is that they are heavy, and that in consequence of their cooling so rapidly the patient is liable to take cold.

In the ovarian and cystic forms of this affection, when the disease is of limited extent, I often direct the application of the oleaginous collodion, from which, in the puerperal wards especially, we have excellent results.

The old turpentine stupes were often efficacious, partly because the terebinth had a specific action and curative relation to the peritonitis; but they are too nasty for use among decent people.

In case either of septic or pyæmic complications the internal treatment of this disease should be preceded by the use of means that are designed to combat the puerperal infection. If the temperature is at or above 103 deg. our plan in the Hospital and, in private practice also, is to give Veratrum viride, in the second or third dilution, every half hour or hour until it falls to 100 or thereabouts.

If this fails, or the patient is very weak or exhausted, milk punch may be taken every hour with Veratrum.

If there are pyæmic and recurrent chills with colliquative sweats, with torpor of the intellect, with stolidity and indifference, grain doses of Quinine, repeated hourly, will do good service in advance of the more specific internal treatment.

When these preliminary essentials are disposed of we come to the treatment of peritonitis proper.

Under these conditions the indications that call for *Belladonna*, Bryonia, Rhus tox. and Cantharis are as useful as in the ordinary form of peritonitis.

If the attack of peritonitis is secondary upon puerperal endo-metritis, I think you will do well not to forget the excellent virtues of *Arsenicum* and of *Mercurius* especially. The character of the pains and of the lochial discharge, as well as the constitutional symptoms, must decide between them.

If the inflammation has extended to the ovary, *Aconite, Belladonna, Colocynth* and Terebinth are the principal remedies. In puerperal ovaritis *Lillium tig.* has not been successful in my hands as it has in the non-puerperal form of the disease.

Dr. Jousset's observation, that while Cantharis is a very useful remedy in pleurisy, it has almost no effect in inflammation of the pelvic peritoneum, is undoubtedly true; but this remark does not apply to lesion of the abdominal peritoneum, more especially, I think, to diffuse puerperal peritonitis.

Puerperal Pelvi-Peritonitis.

For an account of this form of pelvic-peritonitis we extract note to Joussett's Clinical Medicine, American Edition, as follow :

"There is one form of pelvi-peritonitis occurring in lying-in women that sometimes gives the physician a great deal of trouble. It is that in which there is an inflammation of the portion of the pelvic peritoneum which covers the bladder. Outside of the puerperal state, this disease is variously denominated *peri-cystitis*, *epi-cystitis*, and *ante-uterine pelvi-peritonitis*.

"This is a local or circumscribed peritonitis, which is not usually septic, pyæmic or symptomatic, and which sets in some days after delivery. The flow of milk is apt to be arrested, but not so with the lochia. The liability to an attack seems to bear no special relation to the severity of the labor, although it may follow a traumatic injury and irritation of the lower segment of the womb and of the cervix uteri. It occurs both in primiparæ and in pluriparæ. One of my private patients has had it in her three successive labors.

"The commonly received view that peri-cystit is always follows general peritonitis, cystic, uterine, or cellular inflammation, will answer for the ordinary form of the disease; but it is not true of the puerperal variety,—nor is it often due in childbed to an extension of endo-metritis, or of salpingitis, to the peritoneal cavity. It is almost always an idiopathic affection. It may develop in such a manner as to involve the remaining coats of the bladder, and finally result in chronic cystitis. It is not a dangerous affection, providing it does not end in the perforation of the bladder, and in the extravasation of the urine, in which case it might cause death from diffuse peritonitis, or from urinæmia and septicæmia.

"Its most common cause is the accumulation of urine in the bladder during the early period of the lying-in. Naturally enough the vesico-uterine excavation is more shallow in puerperal than in non-puerperal women. This is especially true for the first week or ten days after delivery, when its depth and situation are very much changed. Under these circumstances a comparatively small quantity of urine, retained in the bladder, may produce a mechanical effect that would not otherwise be felt, or be capable of doing the least mischief.

"If this accumulation continues, whether it be through the oversight of the doctor, the carelessness of the nurse, or because the semi-anæsthetic condition of the soft parts after labor renders them more tolerant than usual, and makes the patient indifferent thereto, the effect is the same. The fundus uteri is forced away from the symphysis pubis, and the angle of its lateral deviation is very much increased. Its involution is arrested, and this is the prime condition for inflammation, either in the womb itself or in some of the neighboring organs.

"In a considerable share of cases the uterus and its appendages escape, and the bladder becomes the seat of the difficulty. One of the first symptoms is an inability of the patient to void her urine. The labor might have been natural, and she may have done well in every respect for four or five days, or even for a week, after her delivery. Being able to pass the urine voluntarily, meanwhile, attention has not been directed to the bladder. Then, the physician and the nurse may have neglected to make any further inquiries concerning it, and if the patient has not had the usual desire to urinate for some hours, or even for a day and night, there will be an over-distension that may act both as a cause and an effect.

"The attack usually begins with a chill, which is not always so severe in degree as in the onset of the other forms of peritonitis. This chill is very apt to repeat itself. It is not usually followed by a very high fever, for, unless there are some septic complications, the patient's temperature averages about 100°, the highest figure being 102° or 102.5°. The chill, partaking more of the nature of a rigor, does not produce so profound an impression as it does in the case of the non-puerperal variety of pelvi-peritonitis. The pulse is not so slow as in the normal retardation during the puerperal convalescence, nor is it usually so rapid as in the diffuse form of peritonitis, or of metro-peritonitis of childbed. In this respect its distinctive diagnostic quality may be lost.

"The kind and degree of pain varies in different cases. Sometimes it is brought on and increased by the inaction of the bladder and the retention of a considerable amount of urine. In this case it is sharp and lancinating, and is accompanied by an irresistible desire to urinate. Exceptionally this may be followed by involuntary urination. Again there is no suffering until the bladder has been emptied with the catheter, when its contraction causes a pain that may continue for some time after the water has been discharged. One of my hospital patients described this pain as very similar to that which is sometimes felt in cases of stone, when the bladder has closed firmly upon the calculus. These pains may change their location from time to time, or they may radiate, like a neuralgia, to either inguinal region, or upward toward the umbilicus. They are very much increased by motion, by downward pressure over the pubic region, and by upward pressure toward the symphysis, when the index finger is passed *per vaginam*. They are generally relieved by having the limbs drawn up. The meteorism is usually not so pronounced as in other cases of pelvi-peritonitis.

"As a rule, there is no exudation, and consequently there is no intra-pelvic tumor, in this circumscribed form of puerperal peritonitis. The roof of the vagina is natural, or nearly so, unless it may happen that the womb has dropped very low on account of its faulty involution. In extremely rare cases, however, it is possible that an effusion which might be poured out from the inflamed peritoneum around the bladder and above the anterior cul-de-sac, might float backward, and be found in the lowest part of the peritoneal cavity, at Douglas's pouch, and behind the cervix uteri.

"TREATMENT.—The first indication is to direct that the urine shall be drawn regularly every four hours during the day and night. This should be carefully and not roughly done. The patient should not be allowed to strain in the attempt to force the flow, nor to worry about passing it naturally now and then without the instrument. Nor should she be teased or disgusted with diluent drinks and such expedients as are designed to stimulate a free secretion of urine, for the fault is not with the kidneys. The bowels also should be kept open, or in a laxative state, for, if she has difficulty at stool, or with constipation, the worst results may happen to the bladder.

"The more recent the date of the labor, if there are no septic or pyæmic complications, the better the indications for *Aconite* and *Arnica*, the good effects of which remedies are shown every day in our puerperal clinic.

"Dr. Jousset's recommendation of *Cantharis*, 3d dil., in pleurisy is a very valuable one; but in this form of peritonitis we, also, have sometimes found the Cantharis to have very little effect.

"For the best of clinical reasons, we have great confidence in the internal employment of *Terebinthina* in puerperal peritonitis. It is closely related in its effects upon the urinary organs to Cantharis, and, like it, is also possessed of a wonderful influence upon the serous membranes. But, in our judgment, it is far better adapted to the peculiar condition of the blood, and to the state of vitality of lying-in women, which modifies the puerperal inflammation (even when there is no septic or pyæmic infection), than Cantharis. This condition is very analogous to that which is met with in typhoid and low hæmorrhagic states, as in typhilitis and dysentery. And we have prescribed it in this puerperal peri-cystitis with the same excellent results that we have several times had from its employment in peri-typhilitis. The abdominal and vesical symptoms given in the provings confirm its indication. Our habit is to order it in the second trituration.

"*Bry., Bell., Rhus tox., Thlaspi, Collinsonia can.*, are useful remedies under the indications already given."

Cystic Peritonitis.

If the case develops into one of cystic peritonitis and the bladder becomes directly or indirectly involved, there is no remedy that compares with *Terebinth* in the second or third dilution. Under these circumstances great care should be taken not to allow the urine to accumulate or the patient to strain very severely in passing it. The best rule of procedure is to have it drawn off by the catheter at regular intervals, just as we do after operations for vesico-vaginal fistulæ. The patient complains continually of weight in the lower part of the abdomen, and when the accumulation becomes so great as to crowd the abdominal viscera from its normal resting place and cause it to crowd upon the diaphragm, it may produce a fainting sensation or laborious breathing. Under all such circumstances the kidneys are by no means disposed to be sufficiently active to produce their ordinary amount of urine and there is evidently a less transpiration from the cutaneous surface.

When diagnosis is difficult, the greatest facility for detecting the fluid is by placing the tips of one or two fingers on the iliac fossa and tapping the opposite iliac region slightly but briskly with a finger of the other hand.

As ascites, like dropsy in general, is in most cases rather the evidence of a pathological condition than a pathological condition itself, the visceral derangement which gives rise to dropsy may be extensive or limited, just in the ratio that dropsy is dependent of visceral mischief, we witness the distension of the abdomen. Sometimes there is an enormous distension; so great, even, and so inconvenient, that the operation of paracentesis is a necessity.

But relief obtained by this remedy is but temporary. The water reaccumulates readily and the operation has to be performed again and again until in some cases it has been repeated twenty times or more, and at each operation a quantity of fluid amounting to several gallons has been removed. It almost surpasses belief when we say that some subjects are tapped three times a week and at each operation they part with from four to six gallons of fluid. It is recorded of one case that the operation was performed ninety-six times within a few years and that the aggregate amount of fluid taken from this patient was two hundred and seventy-five gallons and a half.

Encysted dropsy is sometimes confounded with *ascites*, but an accurate history of the case will readily determine the difference.

The swelling is not equable as in ascites; it will be partial or more prominent in some part of the abdomen than the other. It is barely possible to confound dropsy with pregnancy when the abdominal enlargement is very great, owing to the amount of liquor amnni, the fluctuation being very great.

The most distinguished of the profession have sometimes been mistaken. Two or three of the most eminent of the profession have met with cases in which it proved to be impossible to discriminate either for or against pregnancy. A young lady in Philadelphia who asserted her innocence of any sexual intercourse began to experience enlargement of the abdomen, which had been gradually increasing for more than five months. A physician and a celebrated accoucheur was called upon to diagnose her case and he at once pronounced it pregnancy. The young lady being unmarried and a member of one of the most respectable families in the city, treated the physician's opinion with great indignation. He questioned the young lady closely and she said she had never kept the company of a man, nor was she ever alone with a man in her life, and that she never had slept in bed with any person but her maiden aunt. The story was believed by her friends and family, and finally the doctor said, on further examination, that it was a bad case of ascites and recommended paracentesis and appointed a day for the operation. He had stated the case to one of his professional friends, who had promised to be present when he drew the water; and the evening previous to the time of the fulfillment of the appointment she went into labor and soon became a mother. The young lady still declared that she had stated the facts, but when severely rebuked for the deception she had practiced, she repeated again that she had never cohabited with a man or had never been in bed with one. To the question " how did you become a mother?" she very blushingly replied that she supposed a boy about thirteen years old must be the father of her child. The round assertion that she had never copulated with any man, in her estimation, was true, inasmuch as she had only *kept company with a boy.* Another one came under my observation where a highly esteemed servant girl, who had been employed for several years, began to be suspected of pregnancy, as her abdomen became distended enormously and had the appearance of a woman in the seventh month of gestation. When charged with being pregnant she was very indignant.

Several physicians saw her and decided that she was pregnant. The poor girl told them that she could prove her innocence, and sure enough, such was the case. She went under medical treatment for ascites, and so great had been the confidence in her by the head of the household where she lived she was not discharged, although the enlargement of the abdomen had so encroached upon the stomach that her breathing was much affected and terribly labored.

Not long after a vigorous treatment was commenced with appropriate remedies; her kidneys and bladder resumed their normal condition, and the signs of pregnancy began to disappear and but a few weeks elapsed before she felt quite relieved, and was finally able to resume her domestic duties in the household. She happily escaped from any unjust suspicion of her character and the doctors were forced to the opinion that they had been mistaken.

CAUSES.—Ascites results mainly from the want of balance between the organs of absorption and secretion; the loss of balance depends upon visceral disease, or perhaps on inflammation of the spleen induced by protracted intermittents.

It has been observed that ascites is not an uncommon disease among the intemperate users of alcoholic stimulants, and especially of those who drink intemperately of gin. It is the office of the secreting surface to furnish the lubricating fluid for the peritoneum, and when the exhalent vessels furnish it in excess of that which is disposed of by the absorbent vessels, accumulation will go on from day to day indefinitely. On the other hand, if only a normal amount of secretion is furnished by the absorbents, there will be no accumulation of serum in the peritoneal sac unless the absorbent vessels fail of doing their normal work; and it must be seen that wherever the absorbent or exhalent vessels fail, there must arise serious derangement; and, moreover, if the exhalents secrete too much and the absorbents remain healthy, there will be an accumulation; and a like result will follow if the exhalents perform their normal functions and the absorbents become obstructed, then there will also be an effusion.

It matters but little whether the ascites be the result of active exhalation of serous fluid, and beyond the capacity of healthy absorption, or whether it results passively, because the absorbent vessels, if obstructed, cannot perform their normal functions. When the liver becomes so diseased that the blood of the portal system cannot circulate freely through it, congestion of the abdominal venous system will supervene, and transudation, or increased secretion of the more watery parts of the blood, takes place in the cavity of the peritoneum.

Whatever interferes with the regularity of the circulation may induce a loss of balance between the absorbent and exhalent vessels. Sometimes it takes place without any cognizable cause, and frequently after a miserable debauch.

PROGNOSIS.—When this disease is dependent on serious mischief in the organs, the prognosis merges in that of those affections—the issue will in most cases be unfavorable.

Being frequently relieved of the fluid by surgical operations affords but a temporary palliation—the system gradually wears out. The degeneracy of the blood becomes more and more apparent, till a stupor and signs of central pressure indicate that the end is near.

TREATMENT.—Forty or fifty years ago great reliance was placed upon blood-letting, by Allopathic practitioners, and if the disease was active, with brisk hydragogues, cathartics, diuretics and local revulsions. This practice, with some modifications, obtains at the present time. Diuretics, when the kidneys are diseased, are much relied on for carrying off the serous accumulation. *Quinine* is given freely in those cases of acute ascites which are believed to be the sequel of intermittent fever.

HOMŒOPATHIC TREATMENT.—The remedies which have the most marked effect in ascites are *Apocynum, Apis mel., Arsenicum, China, Croton tig., Helleborus niger. Apocynum,* given in the tincture, cured a case of ascites in a woman passing the menopausical period. She suffered from an enormous accumulation of fluid in the peritoneal cavity, which gave to her the appearance of an advanced stage of pregnancy. She urinated but little, the kidneys seemed inactive, and her bowels were generally constipated; her appetite was fair at times. Drop doses of Apocynum, repeated every two hours, restored the normal function of the absorbent vessels and she gradually recovered.

Arsenicum.—We have seen the good effects of Arsenicum in peritoneal dropsy when the patient complained much of thirst and difficulty of breathing, and was so prostrated as to compel the sitting posture. We have given Arsenicum from the 3d to the 30th potency in such cases with satisfactory effect, and when there has been decided derangement of the kidneys we followed Arsenicum with *Galium aperine* and always with benefit to the patient.

Apis mellifica.—This remedy has a decided action on the kidneys and the absorbent system. The author cured a case of ascites with this remedy in the case of a little girl six years of age; he has also employed it in other cases of peritoneal dropsy with satisfactory results. The particular symptoms which indicate its use are acute febrile action from a chill, and strangury or suppression of the urinary functions.

China is particularly indicated when the spleen is implicated and when the ascites has supervened on intermittent fever, or after any inflammatory disease, when the system has been depleted. The particular indications are: pain in the left side, a sensation of great debility, pain in the head from weakness, and particularly after exposure to malaria.

Croton tiglium—According to the author's observation, is a remedy which acts with great force upon the absorbent vessels and in curing some cases of ascites; he has observed that persons given to diarrhœic complaints, and when the evacuations come by a spurt, and who are at the same time suffering from effusion into the peritoneal cavity, this remedy will have good effect.

Digitalis is indicated when the central source of the circulation manifests great activity and when the accumulation passes upwards to the lungs so as to obstruct free respiration. We have given this remedy with good effect.

Helleborus niger in our hands has proved a valuable remedy when in addition to ascites there has also been some indication of hydrocephalus. In children of a dropsical diathesis this may occur, and . particularly when constipation is a prominent symptom.

Accessory means in the way of a soft and moderately warm atmosphere, and also in case climate has been a powerful agent in producing the dropsy, a change of residence has been recommended. A damp climate is unfavorable. In acute ascites the diet should be about the same as in acute fever. But in the chronic form follow the indications of the appetite for a nutritious non-medicinal diet. Drink but little and never in excess of what thirst requires. Warm baths to promote perspiration, and where the kidneys are torpid small quantities of Holland gin is allowable.

Morbid Productions in the Peritoneum and Intestines.

1. Tubercles are sometimes met with in the peritoneum, accompanied with inflammation, and at other times they are without inflammation. " They are found in the form of granulations more or less thickly dispersed over parts." When a tubercular diathesis is present in the individual, peritonitis may be associated with tubercles. It is seldom that tubercles are found in any part of the body except in cases of pulmonary tuberculosis.

Louis says they never occur after the age of fifteen. Other pathologists say they may be present in the peritoneum, when not found in the lungs, varying in size from that of a pin head to a small pea. Tubercles may also be found towards the terminus of the small intestines. They may exist insidiously or they may present symptoms resembling chronic enteritis. They are generally attended with emaciation.

2. Another morbid production is in the shape of a black, hard substance called *melanosis*, near which ulcers and cavities may form. This black, hard substance is mostly observed in the great omentum or the epiploic appendages of the colon. A modulated variety is sometimes seen, the tumors, whether isolated or agglomerated, being generally adherent by small pedicles and enveloped in cysts of fine cellular tissue.

Fibrous tumors of enormous size sometimes form on or under the peritoneum and increase in size until they fill the abdomen. The late Washington Atlee and Dr. Pennock give interesting details of cases of this kind, as well as Professor R. Ludlam, now of Hahnemann Medical College and Hospital of Chicago.

There are other morbid productions of the peritoneum which become manifest by swelling of the abdomen, such as encephaloid or cancerous tumors.

These morbid productions in the peritoneum are worthy of some consideration in reference to treatment.

Tubercular deposits, with inflammation, may be benefited by *Calcarea* 30x, and also by *Sulphur* 30x. Melanosis requires *Kreasotum* 30x, *Conium* 30x, *Arsenicum* 30x and also *Lachesis* 30x.

The *fibrous tumors*, in their incipient state, may be cured. We have seen Thuja and Rhus employed in these cases with good effect, also *Baryta carb.*, *Kali hydriodicum* and *Jodium*. But if in spite of remedies they augment in size, and become a serious burthen, they should receive attention from a skillful gynæcologist.

CHAPTER XIX.

HYDROPS—DROPSY.

Having treated many cases of dropsy, originating from a variety of causes, it has occurred to me that a clinical review of the treatment might be interesting and practical. It is hardly necessary to describe the dyscrasia, for nosologically it is generally understood to be a preternatural collection of fluid, either in the areolar tissue or some cavity of the body which has for its lining a serous membrane. When the areolar or cellular tissue is generally filled with water we have anasarca; when confined to the lower extremities or feet, or infra-orbital tissue, it is termed *œdema*. When the pleural cavity is wholly or partially filled with water we have hydro thorax. When there is an accumulation of serum in consequence of inflammation of the spinal membranes we have hydroarchis, or dropsy of the spinal cord, sometimes in the form of a protruding sac filled with fluid, *spina-bifida;* when the pericardium becomes the seat of dropsy we have hydro-pericarditis; the arachnoid cavity filled with water is hydrocephalus; in the peritoneal sac an accumulation of water is termed *ascites*, and besides, we sometimes meet with dropsy of the womb and the testes, which, for practical purposes, must be separately considered. We may here remark that pathologists have noted two conditions from which dropsy may occur, one of which is an excited condition of the exhalent vessels, which pour out more fluid than is absorbed; the other arises from a weakness of the absorbent vessels, which favors an accumulation of fluid.

The medical treatment necessary to obviate either the active or passive diathesis must depend greatly on the cause, locality and symptoms. *Anasarca*, or dropsy of the cellular tissue, may manifest itself in general or local swelling. When in the most general form and non-inflammatory, and especially if it is the sequel of acute or inflammatory rheumatism, we have found Apocynum can. in the 3d decimal dilution an effective remedy. If localized in the feet or ankles, *Arsenicum* 3d attenuation may soon produce absorption and the œdema will subside. Anasarca, after scarlatina, will generally yield to Helleborus. We can assert positively that this condition, associated with albuminuria, has been cured by Helleborus alone. In some cases *Arsenicum*, after the use of Helleborus, has proved a valuable adjuvant. The symptoms which particularly indicate Arsenicum are paleness of the face, great prostration, dry and red tongue and great thirst. When this dropsy is associated with asthma, and symptoms of suffocation when lying on the back, we have found in our protracted experience no remedy that can take the place of Arsenicum. When anasarca supervenes on a cold, we have for several years relied on Apis. In some instances, where exposu e to cold has caused retrocession of some eruption, followed by anasarca, we have been satisfied with the therapeutic action of Dulcamara. We seldom fail of procuring complete relief from the suffering of our patient by the administration of Apis when dropsy sets in after the suppression of an exanthem. We call to mind many instances of successful treatment of this affection with Apis, Arsenicum and Helleborus. For the anasarca that frequently follows intermittent and remittent fevers we have been rewarded with satisfactory success by the use of Arsenicum, Ferrum and Sulphur. And in all cases of anasarca caused by the loss of blood, or by prostration, diarrhœa or dysentery, our experience leads us to point to China, Ferrum and Apocynum.

The anasarca that supervenes on protracted inebriation, in view of the fact that all the vital forces have been abused, promises but little from treatment. Yet, in some cases, we have known Arsen. Nux vomica and other remedies to greatly relieve suffering. In cases of recent development, having much thirst with asthmatic or labored respiration, swelling of the lower extremities, etc., Arsenicum, 3d and 6th decimal, given alternately, at intervals of three hours, has greatly relieved. In case of gastric irritability and occasional vomitings, swelling of the lower extremities, etc., Nux vomica relieves.

TREATMENT.—In the treatment of dropsical inebriates whose intemperance has been the cause of the serious derangement of the absorbent and secretive organs, we have found good results from Sulphur followed by Rhus tox: Dose of Sulphur at night, Rhus at morning and noon—patient required to observe total abstinence. In those cases of hæmorhage brought on by intemperance attended with excessive weakness, China has had good effect, and also Arsenicum.

We have treated various cases of dropsy, evidently caused by excessive dosing with mercury, or calomel. Phytolacca from the 3d to the 6th dilution, given in drop doses alternately, has invariably been followed with beneficial results; and when dropsy appears to have originated from diseased conditions of the liver and spleen, Chimaphilla will generally cure.

Acute anasarca may be caused by a severe cold. Apis, Arsenicum, and Apocynum have each in different cases proved signally useful. We have experienced great satisfaction in using these remedies. *Apis* works like a charm in those cases of œdema attendant on menstrual irregularities—and when the circulation is so obstructed and deranged by diseases of the heart as to cause œdema of the lower extremities, we have found no remedies that can take the place of Arsenicum and Lycopodium. Wherever the filling of the areolar tissue with water occurs, it is a form of anasarca and the usual remedies are called into requisition. In the local dropsies the serous membranes instead of areolar tissue are the most seriously implicated. We will now relate our experience in the treatment of some of these serous effusions in different cavities. We will first call attention to *ascites* or dropsy of the abdomen. This consists of a collection of fluid in the peritoneal sac, causing an increase in the size of the abdomen and may be distinguished from any other cause of enlargement by fluctuations. Ascites is rarely a primary disease. It is always dangerous and difficult to cure. A lady aged 41 was cured of ascites by Apocynum, 1st dec. 20 drops in a goblet of water, a teaspoonful every hour. Her case had been in charge of a distinguished physician who informed her that paracentesis was the only thing he could propose, and it would afford only temporary relief. She declined this, and came under our supervision. She first took Arsenicum without much effect. This remedy was followed by Apis and Asclep tuber. but no improvement. Apocynum was then prescribed, as above, and a gradual improvement from day to day was noted. Under the use of this remedy the absorbent vessels became active, the ascites disappeared.

A female child 4 years old, was the victim of ascites and her abdomen was so enormously swollen that her respiration was exceedingly labored and her stomach very irritable. She was pale, peevish and fretful. Arsenicum cured this case. We have had many cases of ascites in adults and children not primarily the disease with them. In some cases we could obtain no relief from remedies, and by reason of the accumulation being so much that the greatest discomfiture and distress was observed. We resorted to the use of the trocar or aspirator to draw off the fluid. In a case where the sac was emptied by tapping, the patient recovered under the administration of Helleborus niger, 6th decimal attenuation. We once had a case of ascites complicated with albuminuria, which was apparently cured with Terebinth, 3d. A case of ascites occuring after a severe metrorrhagia recovered entirely under the use of China. In all cases when the exciting cause is known as well as the pathological character of the disease and the general symptoms are noted the selection of the right remedy depends on the care of making a correct affiliation.

Hydrothorax, or dropsy of the chest in a certain cl as of subjects may be idiopathic and may be associated with that of hydropericardium, for which there is no assignable cause except that the disease may be inherited and the tendency to its development congenital. Positive measures afford some relief to patients of this kind, but such organic trouble is seldom if ever cured. When hydrothorax is not idiopathic, it is symptomatic of some other disease. This may be first some organic trouble of the heart, or pleuritic inflammation. The symptoms of hydrothorax complicated with disease of the heart are irregularity and feebleness of the pulse and after the patient has remained some time in a recumbent posture the breathing becomes rapid, laborious and frequent sighing as if distressed, face pale and waxlike, sometimes puffy, fullness of the chest, dull sound on percussion, scanty urine of a high color. The slightest exercise or lying down produces dyspnœa,—sudden starting up with fright during sleep and irregular pulsations of the heart will enable us to diagnose this affection with certainty. From the fact that it accompanies many acute diseases, as well as those of chronic form, its presence says Laennec, announces the near approach of death. Nevertheless, in more modern times our therapeutics have greatly lessened the fatality. In 1874, a gentleman aged 45, was under medical treatment for a chest trouble which was believed to be aneurism of the ascending aorta. There was no swelling of the cardiac region, neither irregular action of the heart, but a constant sensation of some obstruction to respiration in the left side of the chest, and like that of a foreign body pressing on the superior portion of

the lung in the clavicular region. He was first under the
treatment of the regular school with no satisfactory result. He
then came under our care for a while and we confess we were unable to make a satisfactory diagnosis. He then placed himself
under the care of Dr. Hammond, who after much trouble diagnosed a cystic accumulation of water high up in the cavity of the
pleura, and after applying all the tests he introduced the needle
of the aspirator; he drew off thirty-five ounces of water and
afterwards, under the employment of Homœopathic remedies, he
recovered his health, strength and normal condition, and what is
more satisfactory he has remained a healthy, robust and active
business man until now. We unhesitatingly give to Dr. Hammond the credit of arriving at a correct diagnosis of this case and
also for the skill of resorting to a surgical measure so eminently
successful. But for the constitutional change in the diathesis we
must give credit to such remedies as Apis, Apocynum and
Lachesis.

CASE II. We had a case of hydrothorax, a young lady aged
23, after a severe attack of measles; at first she suffered from
pleuritic stitches and was feverish and thirsty and afflicted with a
distressing cough; her respiration was labored and her face pale.
She complained of a sense of suffocation and had alarming attacks
of dyspnœa. Her pulse was variable and her heart at times
beat vehemently. She came under my treatment after a siege of
thorough orthodox medication and the 1st trituration of Apis
mel., two grain powders every three hours, worked like magic in
affecting a cure.

CASE III. Miss S. aged 21, after an attack of scarlatina began to suffer from difficult respiration and dull pains in the sides of
the chest. When in a recumbent position she experienced the
sense of suffocation and her heart would immediately beat, and
yet with no irregularity. She voided but little urine and yet she
was very thirsty. She was pale about the mouth. She frequently sighed and grunted when lying down. The mother said
she had lost two daughters similarly affected after typhoid fever
and she was completely discouraged about this one. Arsenicum
6th dilution was prescribed in drop doses every hour. She soon
began to improve and much to the satisfaction of her mother and
other friends it was regarded a triumph over the Allopathic treatment, which had ever before been the resort of the family in sick-

ness. The appropriate remedies for dropsy of the pleural cavity
are Apis, Arsenicum, Apocynum and Asclepias tuberosa. When
complicated with dropsy of the heart we find Digitalis and Veratrum viride must be added to the group. A greater percentage of
cures have taken place since these remedies have been brought
into use. Hydrothorax, hydro-pericardium and ascites are so
closely allied in pathological characteristics that nearly the same
remedies may be required in each affection. Ruckert mentions
the case of hydrothorax complicated with ascites and œdema,
which was cured by the third decimal trituration of Apis. A case
of hydro-pericardium in our practice of a man aged about fifty,
was cured by Digitalis, 3d decimal trituration.

We have treated cases of hydrothorax after a siege of low
fever where the pulse was irregular, skin dry with desquamation,
scanty urine and very red, which Apocynum c. twenty drops of
the tincture in half a goblet of water and a desert spoonful every
three hours have cured. A man aged sixty-seven was cured of hydrothorax by Apocynum. Hydrothorax complicated with Bright's
disease, we have never cured, neither have we seen a case that
was cured, yet we have seen in our practice several cases relieved
by Kali hydroiodicum, given in solution twenty drops at a dose.
Among the important remedies which Homœopathy has brought
to light as palliatives in hydrothorax, ascites and anasarca complicated with Bright's disease of the kidneys is *Elaterium*. As a
palliative. Eupatorium purpura is well calculated to relieve and
mitigate the suffering arising from such organic derangement.
We have treated many cases of hydrothorax, and have been
familiar with the action of many remedies, but our selection has
depended on these considerations. Is the disease idiopathic? Is
it the sequel of typhus? Is it the sequel of scarlatina or measles?
Is it complicated with rheumatism and heart trouble? Is it associated with *hob nail* liver or disease of the spleen? or is it the
sequel of pleuritis or pneumonia. These are important considerations and pave the way for a judicious affiliation of remedies.

Hydroarchis, or dropsy of the spine, is simply a soft, semi-
transparent tumor or sac filled with serum and supposed to be
caused by inflammation of the spinal membranes, and seems to
be constituted of the membranes of the spinal marrow. These
are supposed to distend and project backwards from the vertebral
canal, the posterior wall of which, when the affection is congen-

ital to a certain extent, is wanting. This affection is often complicated with paralysis of the lower extremities. Except in a
few instances this trouble has terminated fatally. It is, however, in
the province of therapeutics to prolong life, and certain remedies
may have this effect. We have usually treated such cases as we
would rachitis. If the head is large and the fontanelles had
been or are remaining open, we have given Calcarea c. and
Silicea. In dwarfs with spinabifida, Baryta carb. may be consulted. But in spite of all remedies, such cases being congenital,
are apt to terminate fatally.

Hydrocephalus is one and the same as tuberculous meningitis, generally seated in the meninges and surface of the enceph-
alus, and is not an uncommon disease of childhood. It generally
admits of division into three stages. The first stage is that of headache and general febrile irritation, sensitive to light and sound, and
subsequently delirium. The second stage succeeds that of the
inflammatory and exhibits signs of effusion, which are great slow-
ness of the pulse, crying out as if in distress, moaning, dilated
pupils, strabismus, etc. The third stage is indicated by profound
stupor, paralysis; convulsions, involuntary evacuations, quick
pulse, and the *facies hippocratica*. The prognosis is extremely
unfavorable. Therapeutic measures in the first stage may ward
off the second, and then again the second stage does not always
merge into the third when vigorous treatment is persevered in.
We once had a case in this city that an eminent physician (since
deceased) pronounced hopeless at 11 P. M. and at 1. A. M. we
took charge of the case; our prognosis was unfavorable because
there could be no mistake about effusion having actually taken
place, and yet under the action of Arsenicum and Hyoscyamus
given in alternation this child recovered. We had a child aged
one year and seven months that had great heat in the head and a
swollen condition of the anterior fontanelle, its convexity repre-
senting the appearance of half of an orange, plastically stuck to
the scalp. The child was intensely thirsty and craved bits of ice
all the while. Arsenicum was indicated but a fair trial yielded
no success either in satiating the thirst or relieving in any way,
and in order to obviate the constant use of bits of ice, a tumbler
filled with ice water and medicated with Aconite was directed as
a wash for the mouth, the child was crazy after the swab wet
with this water and for twenty-four hours the swab was re-wet

with the ice water from the glass containing the Aconite, every twenty minutes. The child began to recover, the convex appearance of the fontanelle began to subside and contrary to all expectation, the child recovered, and in our opinion no remedy can take the place of Aconite in the first or inflammatory stage of hydrocephalus. In several cases we have given Aconite in the first stage with satisfactory results. In the second stage we have given Arsenicum, Apis, Hyoscyamus and other remedies, with variable success. In some a beneficial and others without benefit. The arachnoid cavity when filled with fluid with few exceptions is the precursor of stupor, convulsions and death. Hydrometra is a rare form of dropsy, a dropsy of the womb. Having never seen a case we have no experience in the treatment. Hydrocele is regarded a surgical disease. It is in fact a dropsy of the scrotum of a compound character. It is either a collection of water in the cellular texture of the scrotum or in some of the coverings of the spermatic cord.

The accumulation of fluids is often so large as to be a source of great inconvenience. In some instances in very young persons, the ordinary remedies for other local dropsies have proved salutary in bringing about absorption and ultimately a cure. But in adults, it is seldom cured by remedies. An operation to draw off the water with an aspirator gives more speedy relief. The operation is not painful. A little ether spray brought to bear on the surface to operate on, will so freeze the integument as to render it insensible to the introduction of the needle, and then the tunica albuginea may readily be relieved of its burthen of water. That which sometimes occurs after scarlet fever has been cured by Sulphur and Pulsatilla. A boy eight years old, son of Prof. A. L. S. was cured of an enormous hydrocele believed to have been caused by a cold, by Helleborus and Dulcamara. Dulcamara was tried first and was followed by a favorable change. The tumor had somewhat lessened and then appeared to remain stationary, then Helleborus in the 3d, and afterward in the 30th dilution was administered and the lad recovered entirely from the affection. A boy nine years old similarly afflicted after scarlet fever was cured by first giving a dose of Sulphur, 6th dil. and following it with Helleborus, 6th dil.

The treatment of every dropsical cavity is based comparatively on few symptoms. There is in many cases no *pain* and yet great discomfiture.   If idiopathic the unmistakable pressure of the fluid indicates a vitiated constitution.   If only a symptom developed during the progress of some acute fever, or exanthematous disease, the cause of the affection must be taken into account and the remedies must be affiliated accordingly.

CHAPTER XX.

DISEASES OF THE RESPIRATORY ORGANS.

Under the head of Respiratory Organs are included the Schneiderean membrane, nasal cavities, the larnyx, the trachea, the bronchia and lungs. Besides there are accessory organs which may require attention.

The Nasal Cavities.

These externally are in sight and extend upwards and backwards until they reach the larnyx. The larnyx is bounded anatomically from above to below by the epiglottis and the inferior ligaments of the glottis, in which voice is produced, and the entire surface is lined by a mucous membrane, which is a prolongation of that of the pharynx. "On examining the interior of the larnyx two clefts are perceptible, one above the other. These are formed respectively by the superior and inferior ligaments of the glottis, and between them are the ventricles of the larnyx."

The inferior ligaments of the glottis meet at a point behind the thyroid cartilage," and this causes that prominence in the neck called Adam's apple (pomum Adami). They form a triangular cleft, the glottis or rima glottidis, the posterior extremities of which are attached to the arytenoid cartilage, the cleft being diminished or enlarged by the contraction or relaxation of the arytenoid muscles, which pass from one arytenoid cartilage to the other.

The thyro-arytenoid muscles form with the ligamentous structure and mucous membrane the gates or inferior ligaments. These muscles have usually been esteemed dilators of the glottis. "The intrinsic muscles of the larnyx receive nervous supply from the pneumogastric nerves."

Shortly after the pneumogastric leaves the cranium it gives off the *superior* laryngeal which is distributed to the muscles that close the glottis, and after it has entered the thorax it gives off a second, which ascends toward the larynx, and is hence called the recurrent laryngeal. It is distributed in part to the thyro-arytenoid muscles, no ramifications going to the muscles." (Magendie.)

Others maintain that these muscles receive a filament from each of the inferior laryngeals. This difference of sentiment envelops the precise functions of the different branches of the pneumogastric nerve in obscurity.

If the contractor muscles of the glottis receive the sole distribution of the superior laryngeal, and the dilator muscles the inferior laryngeal, it would seem apparent that the former would be concerned in the dilatation and the latter in the contraction of that aperture.

It has been shown by experiment that complete aphonia results when both the laryngeal nerves and the recurrent nerves are divided. Any injury to either of these important branches affects the voice, and this fact gives a satisfactory idea of their function.

The contractive muscles close the larynx when any irritating substance reaches it. It is evident that this action is excito-motary. We have an analagous manifestation in coughing and sneezing. The sensitive nerve conveys the impression to the nervous centre and the motor nerve excites the appropriate muscles. Mr. J. Reid maintains that the sensitive nerve is the superior laryngeal and the motor the inferior. From numerous experiments it seems to be quite evident that the inferior ligaments of the larynx are the grand organs through which the voice is produced, although the superior ligaments and the ventricles may be called into requisition for its modification and perfection.

It may be readily understood, therefore, why any morbid state modifies the condition of the lips of the glottis, as in inflammation, ulceration, œdema, which interferes with the actions of the intrinsic muscles so as to modify the character of the voice, or that may result in the total loss of voice, if the lesion is considerable.

The intensity of the voice depends upon the force with which the air is sent from the lungs, and this will vary according to the condition and the general powers of the body.

Continuous with the larynx is the trachea, which is also lined by a continuation of the same mucous membrane. It divides into two large tubes, the bronchi, one of which goes to each lung and then subdivides into numerous branches, which ramify and become imperceptible in the lung. All these branches are lined by a continuation of laryngeal mucous membrane, and it is maintained by some anatomists that the air cells of the lungs are but the blind extremities of countless numbers of bronchial tubes. It is not known whether the mucous membrane extends so far or not.

The trachea and large bronchial tubes are provided with cartilaginous rings; which extend two-thirds of the entire circuit of the tubes, and the remaining third where the cartilages are wanting is composed of muscular tissue which performs the office of regulating the calibre of the tube, as occasion may require; or so that the air may be forced through a narrower channel, and thus relieve the mucous membrane of adventitious matters. In the small bronchial vessels these muscular fibres appear to be wanting.

Their existence however, has been affirmed by some pathologists, in order to account for asthmatic phenomena.

In our examination of thoracic diseases, it is to be borne in mind that the lungs occupy a position at the sides of the chest, and that the heart has a central location, each of the air cells, or minute termination of the different bronchia, is associated with a radicle of the pulmonary artery, and of the pulmonary vein and in addition to these organic constituents, the lung has the bronchial artery for its nutrition with corresponding veins and lymphatics.

The nerves are from the pneumogastric and the ganglionic. All those elements are bound together by interlobular cellular tissue, so as to constitute the lungs as we observe them when cut into. Each lung has a proper fibrous capsule, and is covered by the serous membrane of the pleura in such manner that there are two pleura; each of which is confined to its own half of the thorax, lining the cavity and covering the lung.

Where the two pleura approximate each other behind the sternum is the mediastinum in which the heart is situated. As each pleura is reflected over the lung, and lines the parites of the thorax; the former is termed pleura-pulmonalis and pleura-costalis. The two pleura must be brought into contact when the lungs are distended with air.

The fluid secreted by the pleura, so lubricates them, as to

prevent friction when in health, but if through any cause this secretion becomes arrested and a morbid production presents the constant smoothly gliding over each other, the sound of friction becomes distinctly audible.

At every inspiration even in ordinary breathing when the ribs are raised by the appropriate muscles, the pleura-costalis is of course raised at the same time and consequently when the pleura is inflamed a sharp pain is experienced at each inspiration.

The pleura-costalis and the pleura-pulmonalis, frequently and very often too, unite under such circumstances, and this is commonly the case in phthisis pulmonalis so that the affected side does not rise in inspiration like the other, and the same result occurs, if one lung is obstructed so that it cannot receive its proper quantity of air.

When the costal pleura on both sides are much inflamed, there would be so much pain that respiration would be seriously affected, and dependent almost wholly upon the facility with which the diaphragm is depressed to void the pain consequent upon the elevation of the ribs. For the like reason relief is obtained by lacing a bandage tightly around the chest.

On the other hand cases of hepatitis, the breathing is almost entirely costal and the diaphragm if inflamed is the seat of great pain.

The muscles concerned in inspiration are relaxed during expiration, and in full expiration many muscles that draw down the ribs are thrown into action, simply because the vital activity of the lungs demand it.

The quantity of air inspired depends upon the capacity of the lungs, and the muscular strength of the individual. It might seem important to test the capacity of the lungs in different stages of disease which involves their texture, to enable us to infer the probable extent of hepatization or the obstruction of the air cells.

The practical application of a respirometer is surrounded with difficulties and always distressing to the individual and as the system of the patient suffers from gradual loss of strength as disease progresses, it is not probable that the test of pulmonary capacity will or can be made available. He should give much attention to the number of respirations in the different individuals. The average is to be eighteen in adults, but this necessarily varies. The young respire more frequently, and the aged respire less frequently than those in robust health at the middle period of life. Women of the same age and temperament breathe a greater number of times than men. The female child breathes more rapidly than the adult female, and adult male breathes less frequently than the female. It must be borne in mind that in adult age, emotions, exercise, and excitements of any kind may accelerate the respirations, so as to exceed the average number per minute. We have thus far exemplified the mechanical phenomena of respiration, and now let us turn our attention to the chemical phenomena of respiration.

It is necessary that a *quantum sufficit* of pure air should be received into the lungs, in order to promote and sustain pure health; and that this air should contain the chemical equivalents, viz., one part of oxygen to four parts of nitrogen.

The contact of the atmosphere with venous blood as it permeates the veins of the lungs is essential to hæmatosis, or the conversion of venous into arterial blood.

This chemical change is necessary to prolong life; or otherwise there would be a stasis of blood which would take place in the lungs as in asphyxia, and death would follow. But when the oxygen contained in atmospheric air is imparted at each respiration, hæmatosis or arterialization takes place, and then through the pulmonary veins it is returned to the heart, to be distributed to supply the means of repairing the waste in various parts of the body and at the same time the blood loses its venous properties and assumes the arterial.

Sir Astley Cooper maintains that this change of the venous into arterial blood is to be attributed to the influence of the pneumogastric nerves over the various respiratory phenomena, mechanical as well as chemical, and their diversion results in dyspnœa and death.

When the phrenic nerves are tied the most distressing asthma occurs; the breathing goes on by means of the intercostal muscles, the chest is elevated by them to the utmost, and in respiration the chest is singularly drawn in.

Sir Charles Bell asserts the pneumogastric and phrenic nerves form a part of the nervous respiratory system. But this is disputed by other physiologists, who maintain that there is no special column of the medulla spinalis set apart to control the respiratory movements, either voluntarily or involuntarily. We therefore gain nothing practical from these unsettled conclusions. We will therefore proceed to note from that which is apparent.

Physical Examination of the Chest.

It is only within the last half century that physical examinations have been regarded indispensible as a means of ascertaining health or disease of the contents of the thorax. By the physical signs of the healthy or diseased condition of the heart and lungs, as well as that of the pleura, we mean the evidences that are afforded the senses, uninfluenced by the vital properties of their contents, as distinguished by symptoms, which are the evidences afforded by the living contents in action. The viscera of the chest are surrounded by a bony framework " which prevents information from being obtained, in the case of the deeper seated structures, by any of the senses." Those diseases of the viscera were comparatively obscure until *Aurenbrugger* conceived the plan of percussion, that the sense of hearing might be made instrumental in detecting the pathological condition of the thoracic viscera by sounds. *Laenec* afterwards invented the stethoscope that he might detect the various conditions by the sense of hearing through the aid of this instrument.

Previous to this, diseases of the respiratory system were but poorly understood. *Marshall Hall* says the diseases of the respiratory system could scarcely be said to be understood until the era at which *Laenec's* incomparable work appeared.

The combinations of auscultation and percussion constituted the basis of *the diagnosis*, and the pathology is scarcely less indebted to that extraordinary man.

1. What is Percussion.

It was introduced by *Aurenbrugger*, of Vienna, in the year 1761. But it remained almost neglected for nearly a half century when a translation of this pioneer's work attracted the attention of the profession to this method.

The object of percussion, as a means of diagnosis, is to appreciate the sounds rendered by various parts of the chest when struck, both in the healthy and diseased condition. As the lungs always contain a large quantity of residuary air, and the parietes are possessed of a certain degree of elastic tension, if they are struck or pressed a hollow and somewhat tympanitic sound or resonance is elicited, the intensity of which is diminished by whatever interferes with the elasticity of the parietes or by any adipose or other soft deposition, if in considerable quantities, in the integument.

From this description it might seem to be evident that the resonance of the chest will be greater over those parts in which there is nothing but lung tissue and where the parietes are the thinnest and their tension the greatest; and on the other hand, if any disease has solidified the lung so that it does not receive the air, or any effusion has taken place in the chest, the resonance, instead of being hollow as in health, becomes dull; and again, if the amount of air be augmented, as in pulmonary emphysema, the natural resonance may be largely increased.

The following tables from *Laenec* and Williams, will exhibit the sounds rendered by the various regions in health; where any solid viscus interferes, the sound of course will be dull.

The sounds elicited from internal organs in the various regions of the chest are as follows:

1. The sound from the subclavian organs elicited by percussion in the situation of the clavicle, beneath which is the apex of the lungs *is very clear towards the sternum, clear in the middle. Dull close to the humerus.*

2. The sound from the infra-clavicular region which is situated between the clavicles and fourth ribs beneath which are the superior lobes of the lungs, large bronchi near the sternum is *very clear.*

3. The sound from the mammary region situated between the fourth and the eighth ribs beneath which are the middle lobes of the lungs, large bronchia in the upper part near the sternum. The heart generally covered by the lungs *is very clear;* in women a clear sound only by mediate percussion.

4. The sound from the infra-mammary region which is situated between the eighth ribs and the margin of the cartilages of the false ribs and, beneath which the liver on the right, the stomach on the left, covered only by the thin margin of the anterior inferior lobes of the lungs on the upper part, *is dull on the right side, irregularly dull on the left* or *unnaturally resonant.*

5. Superior sternal region embraces the upper part of the

sternum; beneath are the large bronchia, the sound on percussion is *very clear*.

6. The middle sternal region embraces the middle part of the sternum, beneath are the margins of the middle lobes of the lungs. *The sound is very clear*.

7. The inferior sternal region embraces the lower part of the sternum and ensiform cartilage, the sound is *clear in the upper part, less so in fat persons; below at times more dull at others tympanitic*.

8. Axillary embraces the axilla above the fourth ribs, beneath are the upper parts of the lateral lobes. *The sound is very clear*.

9. Lateral region embraces the space between the fourth and eighth ribs at the sides, beneath are the lateral lobes of the lungs; *the sounds are very clear*.

10. The inferior lateral region embraces the space below the eighth ribs, at the sides, beneath are the margins of the lateral lobes of the lungs, the liver on the right side, the stomach and spleen on the left; sound same as infra-mammary.

11. The acromial region is the space between the clavicles and upper margin of the capsulæ, beneath are the upper lobes of the lung and large bronchia; on percussion, when direct the sound is dull, by mediate percussion a somewhat of a clear sound, especially near the clavicles.

12. Scapular region embraces the scapulæ and muscular ridge below them, beneath are the middle posterior lobes of the lungs. Mediate percussion elicits the pectoral resonance.

13. The inter-scapular region embraces the space between the inner margins of the scapulæ, beneath are the roots of and inner parts of the posterior lobes of the lungs. The sound on percussion is *tolerably clear* when elicited through a pleximeter, or when the arms are around and the head bowed forward. The spinous processes of the vertebræ sound well.

14. The infra-scapular region embraces from the inferior angle of the scapulæ, beneath are the base of the lungs; the liver encroaches on the right side and the stomach on the left side, the sound is clear in the upper portion by striking on the angle ribs or by moderate percussion. The sound below is often dull on the right and unnaturally resonant on the left side.

Immediate percussion is by striking upon any of the above

regions with the tips of the fingers and also mediate percussion
is to elicit the sound through a medium called a pleximeter.
The fingers of the left hand with their inner surfaces towards the
chest are the best pleximeter, they must be laid flat, transversely
over the part to be percussed, and then struck with the tips of
the fingers of the right hand, or with the stethoscope. The shirt
may be drawn tightly over the part to be percussed or where
delicacy will permit may be made over the exposed surface. The
sounds rendered will be more distinct if the patient hold his
mouth open whilst the chest is struck.

In all cases percussion must be practiced over the corresponding
parts of each side and the result be compared. It may be effected
either when the individual is in the horizontal or erect posture.
In the latter case if the object be to examine the anterior part of
the chest it should be thrown forward by causing the patient to sit
erect with the head raised and the arms carried backward. To
examine the posterior part the head must be bent forwards, the
spine slightly inclined forwards and the arms crossed.

Auscultation.

Percussion is in reality a form of auscultation; the latter term
is commonly restricted to the audible evidences afforded by listening, either with the ear applied to the chest or through an instrument called the stethoscope, in the former the auscultation is said
to be *immediate* and the latter mediate.

Laenec was the inventor of the stethoscope, though for convenience we have various forms of construction of this instrument, there has been no variation of the principle from that of
the original inventor. It is an accoustic instrument consisting of
a cylinder with a tube running through, funnel shaped at one end,
that the sonorous vibrations that fall within it, may afterwards
reflect as in the case of the common ear trumpet be concentrated.

Every auscultator should exercise care in selecting a stethoscope adapted to his ear. Those which consist of the funnel part
only are the least satisfactory, because of the confusion of sounds
resembling, in some measure, those that are heard when a hollow
shell is applied to the ear. It is always requisite that the instrument should have, in addition to the funnel-shaped portion, space
enough for one or two inches of cylinder that the concentration
of vibration may be less imperfect.

The double cylindrical stethoscope, with an adaptation tube for both ears, made of elastic material, is now much used and very much preferred.

Every auscultator should practice percussion and auscultation on healthy subjects, after making himself familiar with each and every region of the chest, until he thoroughly understands the normal sounds, and then he will be able to detect those which denote disease.

Children are excellent subjects to practice upon, because some of the sounds are better developed than in adults, and it is requisite that both mediate and immediate auscultation should be practiced.

When any part of the chest opposite the lungs is auscultated a murmur is heard which we denominate the respiratory murmur, or murmurs of pulmonary expansion; as *Andral* would say the murmur of the cells. During inspiration the murmur is more distinct. The reason for this is believed to be the gradual expansion and contraction of the air vesicles and the friction of air against their walls. The vesicular murmur is louder during infancy and childhood, and is therefore termed *puerile.* There is a manifest difference in the respiratory murmur of various individuals of the same sex, and this murmur was different in every part of the chest. Many are subject to feeble respiration who have no lesion of the lungs, while others have it very loud and puerile. (Such are the views of Laennec.)

The sound is heard most distinctly in those regions where the lungs are situated, contiguous to the walls of the chest (*i. e.* in the axilla). When the murmur is not heard distinctly on one side and distinctly on the other, it is an evidence of disease.

It is important to bear in mind that a difference of opinion exists as to the inspiratory murmur of the two sides under the clavicle, which is the most common seat of tubercle. Dr. Girard, of Philadelphia, maintains that the bronchial respiration is decidedly more distinct in the right lung than the left, especially at the summit.

He accounts for it by the greater diameter and straight course of the tubes at the summit of the right lung, that are not lengthened and curved as on the left side by the pressure of the aorta.

Fournet differs from Dr. Girard in opinion. He maintains

that in persons of healthy lungs the sounds of inspiration and expiration are absolutely identical in all corresponding parts.

The exceptions were, when some doubt existed of the entire healthy condition of the lungs. He further entertains the opinion that from the physical condition of the two lungs there is no reason why there should be a difference in their respiratory sounds. Others, again, differ from *Fournet*. From much practical observation we have come to the conclusion that there is no difference in a large proportion of healthy subjects in the intensity of the murmur in either lung, but that at times there is a difference; the respiratory murmur being greater on the right side, and at others on the left.

We find that respiration is more "blowing," or the French would term it *soufflante*, when we listen over the inter-scapular region. This is owing to the large calibre of the bronchia at the root of the lungs. The trachea, owing to its size, affords an excellent type of this souffle or "blowing" sound. When this sound is heard over the parts mentioned, it indicates their healthy condition; but if the respiratory murmur is not heard and the souffle is distinct, it is an indication of disease and denotes that the respiration takes place through the trachea and bronchia, frequently termed respiration because the sound is formed altogether in the tubes.

If any portion of the lungs is impervious to air, the respiration must be effected by the remaining portion. In such cases inspiration and expiration occur through the tubes with great force and noise.

Andral terms this respiration supplementary. When the ear is placed at the lower region of the chest in the front and behind a gurgling noise is sometimes heard.

This must not be mistaken for that which is occasioned by muco-purulent matter in the cavity. It is produced unquestionably by the movement of the contents of the stomach or intestines.

We have already mentioned the friction of the pleura-costalis and pulmonalis.

There is no distinct sound produced by this friction except in cases of disease.

If the bronchial tubes be entirely free from disease, the sound will be of the character we have already described; but if they become inflamed or obstructed by mucus, pus, or blood, there will be various sounds, bronchial rales or rattles will be heard; which will be more particularly noticed in considering individual disease.

We have thus far considered the auscultation of healthy respiration. The voice also affords physical signs of great moment. We will describe those only heard in health, because they form the basis of our diagnosis in disease.

"When the voice is produced in the inferior ligaments of the larynx the sonorous vibrations not only pass out by the vocal tube but they proceed downwards along the trachea and resonance is distinctly heard when the ear or stethoscope is placed to the chest."

When the stethoscope is placed over the larynx or trachea, when the individual is speaking, it appears to the auscultator that the voice passes immediately to his ear, and is louder than that which passes to the other ear. This phenomena is termed the laryngeal or tracheal voice and indicates health.

Nevertheless we meet with something similar in disease, when an empty cavity exists in the lungs. The voice seems also to pass immediately through the stethoscope to the ear of the auscultator.

This constitutes the cavernous voice or pectoriloquy. "When the stethoscope is laying over the sternum and subjacent trachea or between the spine and scapulæ in the middle of the back over the subjacent large bronchial tubes the voice is heard to resound very strongly; but it does not pass up to the ear in adults like the tracheal or laryngeal voice."

In children this bronchial resonance is hardly distinguished from the voice from the larynx.

It is easily inferred that a dilatation of the bronchial tubes will greatly develop these sounds.

The resonance of the voice can be felt by placing the hand on the chest, the resonance is not heard from the minute ramifications of the bronchial tubes.

The vesicular texture is a bad conductor of sound and consequently presents the resonance of the voice in the bronchia from being transmitted to the parietes of the chest, excepting, when bronchia of a certain size pass close to the surface.

But if the vesicular structure becomes consolidated from any cause, as by the formation of tubercles, then the broncophony or bronchial resonance becomes very distinct and aids materially in our diagnosis.

When a modification of the transmission of the vocal resonance to the ear of the auscultator by the existence of fluid in the chest it may be regarded a physical sign of disease; as is presumed to be the case with egophony to be hereafter mentioned.

If the tips of the fingers be placed over the part of lung where consolidation exists the thrill may be distinctly felt at times running up the arm, when the patient speaks; while in portions of the lung that are free from disease no such sensation is experienced, or at least it is very different from the gentle vibration felt in the opposite lung if in a healthy condition; all these phenomena are better appreciated in their persons. In those chests which are well covered with muscles and fat and whose voices are deep bass the natural resonance of the voice is obscure and of limited extent. A proposition has recently been made to unite auscultation with percussion, *i. e.*, to listen with a common stethoscope or with one modified for the purpose while the part is struck in the ordinary method. Dr. A. Clark, of New York, has assigned some value to this combination of auscultation and percussion, but Fournet affirms this mode to be deceptive; the perceived sound bearing no precise relation to the condensation or rarefaction of the subjacent parts.

Among the physical signs we may include inspection, succussion, palpation, etc., of the chest.

Inspection of the chest, the raising of the ribs, the extent of costal respiration, etc., by succussion and palpation to detect fluctuation; by mensuration of the chest to discover the difference of capacity, between the side of the chest, which contains a lung whose function is impaired by disease; and one in consequence of the diseased condition of its fellow is perhaps executing more duty. All these methods may be referred to when necessary.

We have detailed quite minutely the means for physical exploration of the chest. It affords valuable evidence in regard to the nature and amount of structural disease; still all physical signs can only be regarded as valuable adjuncts, but cannot be implicitly trusted. In some cases organic affections of the chest afford the same physical signs; but the difference is indicated by the general symptoms.

It requires much patience and practice to acquire a useful

knowledge of auscultation and percussion, but there are some, though very few, who ridicule the whole doctrine of physical signs as useless.

But we can assert in truth that no one who has practiced physical examinations who does not regard them as a valuable means in diagnosis; it being easiei to decry its usefulness than to acquire the knowledge necessary for making physical examinations available.

The stethoscope enables us to distinguish between diseases whose general symptoms are alike. It enables us to pronounce on the existence of tuberculosis and also whether the tubercles have gone on to softening, when otherwise we might cherish a doubt, and thus enable us to encourage or discourage according to the evidence afforded. In the former case, we have relied on the stethoscope for determining the condition that might subject our patient to the necessity of finding a more genial climate, and in this case to support the drooping spirits with well founded hopes of benefit from the change, as well as to prevent all the inconvenience, misery and privations which might attend a hopeless expedition. In all probability too much attention has been directed to the exclusive study of physical signs of thoracic disease, inasmuch as these signs are dependent upon careful observation. In fact, it might be expected that unnecessary refinement would be introduced in the detail of the sign elicited.

So many and so varied have been many of the subdivisions seemingly minute and useless, that even those who place great confidence in auscultation are disgusted on account of this exaggeration. Trousseau says: "I have much greater pleasure in meeting with a man who will teach me the best method of mixing a poultice, than with the man who professes to instruct me in the difference between the rale sonore soufflante and the rale sonore, or how to distinguish the rale sibilant from the soufflant rale, or the latter from the turturrin rale or this again from the roucoulant rale, or the caverneux from the covernuleux rale, and all such petty distinctions." Raceboski says: "the greatest error that has been committed in regard to auscultation is having attached too conclusive importance to it, and having esteemed it as it were a science of sounds, each of which must indicate a different morbid condition."

This much is certain, and we are desirous of insisting on it particularly, there is no rale which has a very determinate and invariable. value, and that any one rale being given it is important to tell from it alone the name of the disease to which it belongs.

I defy any one whatever to distinguish in all cases, with his eyes shut and without interrogating the patient, the majority of cases of incipient tubercular pneumonia in the first stage, œdema of the lungs, hæmoptysis, or even pulmonary emphysema. This sibilant ronchus, or the base string ronchus, does not indicate the existence of simple bronchitis more than of pulmonary emphysema or tubercles, for they may both be heard equally well in the three cases.

The bronchial souffle no more proves hepatization of the pulmonary parenchyma than it proves the existence of pleuritics. The ronchi, even, which seem to belong more especially to a particular affection, have not such a determinate value as to enable us to pronounce positively the nature of the disease when they are present.

The gurgling, which is in some measure regarded as a pathognomonic to tuberculous cavities, may really be the result of pulmonary abscesses or the effect of the dilatation of the bronchia, and the metallic tinkling itself may either be the result of pleurisy with effusion of a pulmono-pleural fistula or of a simple pulmonary excavation. It is to be regretted that many practitioners are accustomed to observe or listen more than to reflect.

Stokes remarked that the art of reasoning justly upon the physical signs rather than enquiring into their physical character themselves, to which attention ought to be directed, and on which most observers fail, is indispensable. It cannot be too often repeated, added Dr. Stokes, "that physical signs only reveal mechanical conditions which may proceed from the most different causes, and that the latter are to be determined by a process of reasoning on their connection and succession; on their relation to time and their association to symptoms." It is in this that the medical mind is seen; without this power, I have no hesitation in saying, that it would be to wholly neglect the physical signs and to trust in practice to symptoms alone.

We are inclined to favor a medium course; as symptoms denote the struggle which nature makes to rid the air passages of certain obstructions, we can only determine their location by auscultation and percussion. It therefore appears evident that symptoms in connection with what the stethoscope and pleximeter are made to reveal, will conjointly appeal to the reflection of the practitioner, who may devise thereby some measures of relief.

We therefore recommend the study of physical signs in connection with symptoms as the course altogether preferable to pursue.

Catarrh.

Catarrh is the common affection arising from cold which produces an inflammatory condition of the mucous membrane lining the nasal cavities.

This membrane known as the schneiderian is preternaturally exposed to the vicissitudes of the weather and is dry, yet though when it is dry, when inflamed it is difficult to breathe through it because the nostrils are obstructed, not by the accumulated mucus, but by the mere swelling of the membrane.

The sense of smell becomes perverted or lost. The parts are evidently red, tender and irritable. The contact of atmospheric air a little less pure or a little colder than usual provokes sneezing.

Sometimes this affection extends into the frontal sinuses and headache participates and the lachrymal glands are so affected as to produce a copious flow of tears, at the same time there is frequently a chilliness and shivering.

There is slight fever and in the latter part of the day and in the evening a slight acceleration of the pulse is noticeable; after the usual dryness a thin serous fluid of acrid properties is secreted; for the membrane reddens and frets the alæ nasi, and upper lip over which this fluid flows.

This thin serous fluid gradually becomes opaque and yellow; at length the secretion resumes its natural quality and is reduced to its normal quantity again.

The swelling of the membrane disappears entirely. This is the natural history of the cold in the head, when it first makes its appearance, and is confined to the nasal ducts causing a swollen condition of the schneiderean membrane; and an obstruction of the lachrymal ducts and the reaction from this state is called coryza.

TREATMENT.—From the dryness of the nostrils and swelling

of the membrane, causing an obstruction, give Aconite 3x and repeat the doses every two hours until the dryness disappears.

Arsenicum.—When a fluent coryza sets in of an acrid or burning character, producing excoriation of the orifices of the nostrils and upper lip give Arsenicum 3x trituration, two grains every three hours until the acridity and flow disappear.

Mercurius 3x trit. is another remedy for fluent coryza when the discharge is of a less acrid character. When the discharge begins to thicken and gradually assume a yellow appearance, attended with some headache and slight depression of spirits Pulsatilla may be given every two hours until relieved.

Hephar sulph.—When the discharge gradually hardens and becomes opaque attended with some soreness of the nostrils, Hepar sulph. 3x every three hours in two grain doses I have found decidedly effectual.

Nux vomica 3x or Sambucus 3x are valuable remedies, a globule at a dose will soon remove obstructions of the nose of new born infants.

For febrile catarrh the remedies are *Aconite, Nux vom., Gelsemium, Veratrum viride.*

The modern Allopathic treatment for nasal catarrh is Sulphate of Quinine in three grain doses four times a day; certain kinds of snuff that were formerly recommended are now entirely discarded as being more hurtful than beneficial.

Dr. Watson says, you may stop a cold by twenty drops of Laudanum. Another prescription is to take a beaker of hot wine negus, with a tablespoonful of syrup of poppies on going to bed. This mode of treating catarrh is very objectionable, subjecting the patient to a liability to a return of the trouble in consequence of these palliative measures rendering him more impressive to the action of cold.

Chronic Catarrh.

Acute catarrh, which results from a cold and characterized by the usual symptoms, by being neglected may assume the chronic form.

TREATMENT.—One of the best remedies for treating chronic catarrh is *Sulphur*, given in pellets saturated with a tincture, four pills at a time night and morning. If severe headache attends the catarrh, or there is an obstruction in one nostril, Mercurius and Belladonna may be administered in the third attenuation, the former in trituration two grains every six hours, and the latter may be given in pills every two hours until the head is relieved.

Pulsatilla is the remedy when the patient is depressed and suffers most during damp, hot weather, and when the slightest exposure aggravates the difficulty and the patient suffers from depression of spirits.

Arum triphyllum 3x is indicated when the discharge from the nose is hot and acrid, and also when the secretion of the lachrymal ducts is also hot, and when there are little sores or vesicles about the base of the nose, and sometimes in the angle of the mouth; saturated pellets may be given, three at a dose and repeated once in three hours until relief is obtained.

Catarrh is very often met with and consists in a chronic inflammation of the mucous membrane of the air passages. The schneiderian membrane becomes chronically affected and the mucous secretion obstructs the nasal cavities; and when attended with any degree of fever, there is usually a dull, oppressive headache.

There is also an inclination to drowsiness when seated by a hot stove or in any warm room.

The slightest cold aggravates and provokes sneezing. From which it will be perceived that in the chronic form of this disease there may be a succession of acute attacks.

The mucous membrane, ever sensitive and soluble, no sooner suffers from one attack than another is liable to succeed.

If the mischief was confined to the schneiderian membrane the sufferings from the disease might be palliated, so as to secure a tolerable degree of comfort for the patient; but so long as this inflammation lasts without positive relief from remedies it is liable to provoke acute inflammation of the mucous membrane of the bronchial tubes, the suffering thus entailed is very often the sequel of chronic inflammation of the mucous lining of the nasal cavities.

Morbid growths will sometimes show themselves as a product of this chronic difficulty.

Nasal polypi are frequently met with and require attention and even removal by the aid of a suitable instrument in order to afford any relief to the patient.

Sometimes ulceration will result from chronic inflammation affecting the vomer and other tissues involved in the structure of the nasal cavities; and finally it may be said that chronic inflammation of the mucous tissue of the nose may pave the way for chronic bronchitis and bronchial consumption; and this fact is sufficient to stimulate exertion to arrest the difficulty before it descends to the bronchial tubes and results in similar mischief.

In addition to the remedies mentioned in the beginning of this article, I will suggest the use of Tartar emetic, when there is a sensation of constriction in the nasal ducts rendering it difficult for the air to pass in or out of the nostrils.

Silicea, the sixth attenuation is indicated when there is a discharge of pus from the nose indicative of a fistula.

To remove obstructions of hardened mucus from the cavities *Mercurius solubilis* and *Hepar sulphur* in all probability will have the desired effect. They may be administered in two grain doses of the 3x trituration alternately night and morning.

Epistaxis or Nose Bleed.

This symptom is so common that very little attention is paid to it by persons in general as it may occur from trivial causes.

It is regarded as a harmless hæmorrhage. Sometimes it is a remedy, sometimes a warning, sometimes really in itself a disease.

"The readiness with which the mucous lining of the nasal cavity pours forth blood is familiar to every school boy who often wipes a bloody nose."

Any strong bodily effort or a slight blow, a fit of sneezing, brisk exercise or summer heat is sufficient in many boys to make the nose bleed, and this facility for nose bleed often furnished an index to something abnormal in the circulation; and especially indicative of hyperæmia of the cerebral center. The import of this symptom, however, is not always the same, but we may regard it in the light of an epitome of the various forms of hæmorrhage by exhalation.

It is idiopathic in childhood, dependent upon active congestion. In youth it is nature's method of depleting a plethoric subject. In old age it is probably the result of passive or mechanical congestion and probably venous.

In some persons it is habitual and of periodical occurence and its suspension becomes a token of disease or of danger.

In young women it may be vicarious, in amenorrhœa, and

finally it may proceed from disease, in the nares themselves, or it may form a part of an extended hæmorrhagic disorder.

It is not necessary to go further into the phenomena of epistaxis. The main phenomena are obvious both to the patient and his associates.

The blood usually flows in drops, but they may follow each other so rapidly as to give the appearance of a stream. A moderate nose bleed is often a source of relief to the head, and the patient feels refreshed. A profuse bleeding from the nose may exhaust the system and cause faintness, debility and even death.

TREATMENT.—Nose bleed is generally arrested by the application of cold water to the forehead, back of the neck and to the bridge of the nose.

Nurses apply some cold metallic substance to the backs of children to check the flow of blood.

In cases of profuse epistaxis, blood letting from the arm was formerly the Allopathic resort.

The Homœopathic remedies *Aconite, Pulsatilla, Nux vom., Crocus sativa;* of debilitated persons, *China,* from cold *Pulsatilla,* if caused from tendency of blood to the head, *Belladonna,* if in typhoid fever *Rhus tox., Arsenicum,* if in children affected with worms, *Cina* or *Mercurius;* for females who menstruate scantily *Pulsatilla, Secale* and *Sepia;* if when the menses are too profuse *Calcarea, Crocus* and *Sabina;* for nose bleed in consequence of being stimulated by spirits, *Nux vom.* Belladonna, Bryonia; for debilitated persons in consequence of loss of blood and other losses, *China, Carb. veg.,* Ferrum; if caused by a blow, contusion, or by bodily exertions, *Arnica, Rhus tox., Calcarea,* for the disposition to nose bleed give *Calcarea, Carb. veg., Sepia.*

Diseases of the Larynx and Trachea.

Inflammation of the epiglottis. Midway between inflammation of the pharynx and larynx, we have that of the epiglottis. It will be recollected that the office of this organ is to perform a service in deglutition and also in respiration; consequently both functions are implicated in the disorder.

The epiglottis is not so important an organ as was formerly supposed.

The universal belief prevailed at one time, that the epiglottis was the sole barrier against the intrusion of substances into the larynx. This however, is affected by the motions of the larnyx by which it is drawn upward during deglutition and of the muscles whose office it is to close the glottis.

It would seem, therefore, if the muscles whose office it is to close the glottis so that if the laryngeal and recurrent nerves be divided in an animal and the epiglottis is left in a state of integrity the act of swallowing becomes extremely difficult; the principal cause which prevents the introduction being removed by this suction. Several physiologists, viz: Magendie, Trousseau, have related instances of persons entirely devoid of an epiglottis who were able to swallow without difficulty.

The instances are rare in which inflammation of the epiglottis occurs without indications of contiguous parts being implicated.

On this account epiglottidis has been described under laryngitis, and pharyngitis.

A recent writer has collected several examples of this character; when inflamed the epiglottis exhibits a red color, enlarged on drawing the tongue forward, inerect as it were, or covered with false membrane; and to the touch it has been swollen hard and prominent.

In every case of inflammation swallowing has been effected with great difficulty; which appears to be of a double character, partaking both of the pharyngeal and laryngeal.

The former is mechanical in its character and mainly attributable to the narrowness of the passage for the food into the pharynx; at others owing to the excessive sensibility of the epiglottis and to the kind of struggle caused by the pain during the contraction of the pharynx; the laryngeal dysphagia depends upon a small portion of liquid passing into the larynx during the act of swallowing and occasioning a convulsive cough for its expulsion.

When uncomplicated with active inflammation and great swelling of the tonsils, this difficulty of swallowing indicates inflammation of the epiglottis, taken alone it merely indicates the existence of inflammation of the superior portion of the larynx involving the epiglottis.

Sometimes there is a sensation as if some extraneous body were in the fauces with pain at the superior part in the front of the neck above the larynx, the moving of the tongue produces pain especially in protruding it and as the root of the epiglottis is studded with glands the inflammatory irritation stimulates them to an increased secretion of the mucus which is detached with difficulty and this occasions constant efforts which greatly harass the patient; sometimes producing paroxysms of fainting and sleeplessness. Cause, mainly exposure to cold or from mechanical irritation.

TREATMENT.—The Allopathic treatment consists in the application of a solution of nitrate of silver in the proportion 3 grains to one ounce of distilled water, applied by placing on the finger some ·soft covering, or a pledget of lint sewed upon it, which dipped in the solution can have a ready application to the inflamed epiglottis.

The tenacious mucus which collects about the top of the larynx in this and in other diseases may often be removed by the same agency.

HOMŒOPATHIC TREATMENT.—*Aconite.*—If there is any febrile symptom or a full bounding pulse this remedy in the third or sixth attenuation may be given in powder or pellets dry on the tongue. *Argentum* we have used in the third trituration, two grains morning and evening with good effect. Belladonna, in all cases where there is difficulty in swallowing, which seems to arise from a congested condition of the epiglottis; we have found Belladonna an invaluable remedy and it may be administered in the third or sixth decimal attenuation in dilution or in pellets every two hours.

Mercurius solubilis may be given in inflammation of the glottis involving also the pharynx when the deglutition is very difficult and when there is but little fever of a general character.

Phosphorus, we have found this remedy to answer the best purpose when the epiglottis has a dry appearance, and when there is great difficulty in deglutition.

Sulphur is a good remedy when the trouble seems persistent and does not readily yield to other remedies.

Inflammation of the Larynx.

The older writers mention of this disease in the nosology of Good, that the term laryngitis is not met with. It was evidently not studied as a distinct disease but was included with cynanche trachealis; cynanche stridula, or croup and some other affections of the larynx and trachea; yet although inflammation of the lining membrane of the larynx, the trachea and the bronchia may greatly resemble each other; there is a propriety in making a distinction which seems to be well founded.

Andrel makes another distinction; *first*, laryngitis with simple redness of the mucous membrane, and *second*, tumefaction of the membranes, *third*, with copious secretion of mucus, *fourth*, with copious secretion of pus, *fifth*, with production of false membrane, and *sixth*, œdematous laryngitis.

There are these objections however, to Andral's classification. No great advantage arises from a distinct consideration of the three first varieties. Fourth is the chronic form of the laryngitis and therefore will be treated under that head.

The fifth requires a distinct consideration under the head of croup. Nevertheless there is propriety in considering croup a form of laryngitis sometimes productive of false membrane. I have found in my practice many cases of croup which seem to partake of this character; another distinguished pathologist divides laryngitis in two varieties; one involves simply the mucous tissue and the other the sub-mucous tissue.

But this division is no better than the still more one of the acute, chronic, and œdematous laryngitis.

Acute laryngitis has proved a fatal disease in many instances in which it has been known to occur. To insure success in the treatment the patient must be seen early and the nature of the malady must be clearly seen and the source of peril thoroughly understood.

Then in most cases the sufferer may be relieved both of the disease and the danger that hangs over him. It is of the greatest importance, therefore, that we should be able to recognize laryngitis when we meet with it, and that we institute a judicious and effective treatment.

What are characteristic signs of laryngitis? In what does it consist? It simply means an inflammation of the parts that compose the larynx, especially of the mucous membrane which covers the laryngeal cartilages and the epiglottis. Sometimes the inflammation is limited to the larynx; at others it extends to the posterior fauces and contiguous parts.

DIAGNOSIS.—The patient complains of sore throat; you will commonly see some redness of the velum, uvula and tonsils.

There is a degree of restlessness and anxiety manifested by the patient in a greater degree than the inflammation.

The dangerous symptom which occurs early in the disease and ought to excite alarm, is difficulty of swallowing, for which no adequate cause can be discovered.

And to this is added difficulty of breathing, for which we can discover no adequate cause in the thorax. There are peculiar characteristics for the respiration. " It is attended with a throttling noise. The act of inspiration is protracted and wheezing, as though the air was drawn in through a dry, narrow reed.

The patient in complaining of the seat of distress usually points his finger to the *Pomum Adami.*

If he coughs, he coughs with a peculiar hard, or hoarse husky sound. He either speaks quite hoarsely or speaks in a loud whisper, all power of audible voice in the larynx is lost and he speaks by means of his lips and tongue, only in a rough whisper.

The cartilages of the larynx are tender to the touch, and when they are pressed externally they become painful. The face is flushed, the pulse is full and bounding, the skin hot and dry, the eyes protrude, he is distressingly unquiet and impatient for relief. He signifies his wish for air, begs for broad ventilation from the windows and open doors. All this avails but little if he finds no relief. He soon strangles and perishes.

The pathology of this malignant disease can be briefly stated; the membrane covering the interior surface of the larynx suffers inflammation.

The effect of inflammation in the mucous membrane is in the onset to produce thickness and dryness; and the membrane becomes turgid and swollen.

The subsequent effect is the effusion of serous fluid in the subjacent areolar tissue.

The rima-glottidis is narrowed by the swelling or thickening of the mucous membrane; and whenever the membrane is lifted and protruded by infiltration of the tissue, the rima-glottidis is still further contracted in breadth. It is nearly closed up and prevents the air from passing inward in sufficient quantity to sustain the invigoration of the blood. A small portion only of this fluid returns to the lungs, from the right ventricle of the heart, undergoes by aid of the air its accustomed resurrection to life.

Now the distressed patient exhibits a bluish discoloration of the skin; becomes drowsy and delirious and gradually dies of asphyxia. If the rima-glottidis becomes quite closed the life suddenly departs and puts an end to his suffering.

We may say here that the danger of an inflammation depends upon the part implicated. It will be seen that this is eminently so with laryngitis.

The inflammation in some instances is limited to less than a square inch of membrane.

The same area of the same membrane inflamed in the same manner and degree would present but little danger; but inflammation of the larynx becomes perilous, because creative of obstructions to free respiration of the atmosphere and the replenishing of the system with arterial blood.

The larynx is designed for vocalization and by its nervo-muscular structure is able to accomodate itself to any sound high or low in pitch, or any modification demanded by rhetoric. It also forms a portion of the channel through which air is conveyed to the lungs.

The faculty of speech may be entirely impeded without endangering the life. The function of respiration which is an organic function, under the influence of the will, will not dare to be suspended, even for a few minutes, and even a serious impediment to respiration inflicts a brief abridgement of life.

Sometimes laryngitis is accompanied by difficulty of swallowing, yet this trouble is not always present. Cases have been described where it did not occur at all. If the inflammation is confined entirely to the laryngeal membrane, the pharynx may not be implicated and the organs of deglutition not interfered with.

In very severe cases dyspnœa occurs at short intervals with spasmodic force and the danger of suffocation is apparent, with great distress and restlessness.

The eyes appear to be starting from the sockets followed by evident sinking of the vital powers and death and all the melancholy accompaniments of tubercular phthisis. There has accordingly been a species of this disease spoken of as laryngeal consumption; but in most if not in all cases this laryngeal affection is only a part of the complaint under which the patient labors, and what I have farther to observe respecting it, may be postponed until we take up the subject of tubercular consumption.

Again the membrane lining the cartilages of the larynx is not unfrequently thickened and ulcerated in secondary syphilis giving rise to a hoarse croaking voice, and a noisy and painful breathing. In case of chronic thickening of the same parts from chronic inflammation, you may do great good by the administration of *Mercurius vivus* in the first trituration. This in two grain doses may be repeated every two hours for two days; and if the gums should appear red and swollen discontinue the medicine.

We have seen many instances of this uneasiness about the throat, the noisy respiration. In all cases of disease of the respiratory organs, the symptoms are liable to spasmodic exacerbations and a fatal result occasionally arises from this cause as well as from the obstruction produced by inflammation.

There are various causes why hæmatosis is imperfectly excreted but this prevents its excretion except very sparingly and insufficient to support life.

When the laryngitis is slight, general inconvenience may not be great but when very severe, the great disorder of innervation may eclipse the local mischief. There is generally a congestion of the capillary vessels of the pharynx as an inspection of the throat will prove. The duration of the disease when it proves fatal, varies according to the constitution of the patient, the extent of the lesion and the effect of remedies.

The duration is three or four days and yet it has proved fatal in from twelve to twenty-four hours. General Washington, the first president of the United States, died of this disease. Preston Brooks, of South Carolina, fell but too early a victim to the disorder, and we have read of eminent physicians within the last half century together with many members of the clerical profession who became victims of the disease. As before remarked there was no accurate description of this disease until within the last fifty years. It is probable that much of the fearful fatality attendant on what was termed throat distemper was due to this disease.

CAUSES.—Exposure to cold as in every other case of internal inflammation has been assigned as a cause. Exanthematous diseases may be reckoned among the causes of acute laryngitis which may occur in all, from that of the newly born infants to adult age.

It is, however, extremely rare in childhood, whilst inflammation of the larynx and trachea with production of false membrane is exceeding common in childhood and rare in adult age.

There are but few cases on record of deaths having been produced by acute laryngitis in persons under twenty years of age. We have no exact data in regard to the influence of age as predisposing to this disease. Of twenty-eight cases, taken indiscriminately from various works; twenty-two in males and six in females. This may be owing to the former being more liable to irregular exposure, and to the more powerful exertions of the vocal organs.

This has been assigned as the cause of acute laryngitis as well as the chronic form.

ALLOPATHIC TREATMENT.—Dr. Watson says that in some cases copious bleeding has apparently saved the patient. The application of leeches is also a favorite resort; but says the same author, for bleeding to be of any service, we must not let the opportunity pass for prompt bleeding. There are two or three cases on record where repeated bleedings have been followed by recovery. Gen'l Washington was bled and died. Dr. Francis, of New York, recovered, but to be serviceable or safe, bleeding must be performed early. The main treatment therefore suggested is either local or general blood letting. Counter irritation is sometimes resorted to. The effect of the blister in producing serous effusion often extends beyond the skin, and it is possible that the œdema of the glottis might be produced or augmented in consequence of these topical remedies. The application of leeches over or near the laryngeal cartilages is thought to be of less utility than by the abstraction of blood by cupping from the back of the neck; and if we wish to apply a blister we must do so at the superior part of the sternum rather than to the front of the throat. Medicines are believed to be of but little advantage in any stage of the disease.

HOMŒOPATHIC TREATMENT.— The early administration of well chosen Homœopathic remedies, has apparently been of greater service, and has proved to be the source of more frequent relief than either blood letting or other depleting measures.

Aconite.—In the earliest stage of the disease, and the manifestation of the first febrile symptoms, this remedy in the first dilution may be given every fifteen minutes until the febrile symptoms pass off.

Belladonna, first dilution may be administered after Aconite and repeated every hour in drop doses.

Argentum, in the sixth attenuation may follow Belladonna in drop doses every two hours.

Argentum ni'ricum may be given the same way.

Bryonia, when this formidable disease occurs in damp weather and the patient complains of feeling worse from the slightest motion.

Ignatia may be administered when a cold is the cause, and the patient is suffering from grief.

Kali bichromicum at the first symptoms of hoarseness, or anything like croupal breathing may be given in the sixth dilution dropped in water every half hour.

Lachesis, 30th attenuation, says Dr. Herring and some others will exert a powerful influence over the disease.

Mercurius vivus, in the third trituration may be administered in a dose of 2 grains every hour when inflammation extends to the pharynx and renders deglutition difficult, and also when the throat is red and inflamed.

Sulphur and Hepar sulphur, are remedies that may be consulted, and we doubt not their utility in conducting off the disease after it has passed its severest stage.

Accessory means.—As acute laryngitis is one of the most dangerous diseases that assails the respiratory system, its early manifestations must be met promptly by every available means to arrest its progress.

A gargle made of chloride of potassium, two drachms to a tumbler of water; tincture of hydrastis may be added to the water in the proportion of twenty drops for half a tumbler.

Emollient poultices are sometimes resorted to, but great caution must be exercised both in changing and removing them. Compresses of warm water may be thrown around the neck with dry covering over them.

Chronic Laryngitis.

Besides the affection we have just now described, or referred to, the larynx is liable to chronic disease, to chronic inflammation, chronic thickening of the membrane, slow ulceration, necrosis of the cartilages; chronic inflammation and ulceration of these parts are very common in consumptive patients.

It is attended first with hoarseness, then with aphonia, a barking or stridulous cough, rough or whispering voice, all cease directly after employing Mercurius vivus in the third attenuation.

It is not always certain what may be the course of this chronic thickening; for there are other causes besides that of syphilis, from which the difficulty can originate; but one thing is certain, Mercurius vivus has a specific action on the affected part and in all probability will cure the affection.

·A lady aged twenty-five years, of a bilious temperament, who had been married six years, began to experience an uncomfortable sensation in the throat, accompanied by hoarseness which was indicated by a noisy, rough and difficult respiration. It was not known whether the cause of the difficulty was syphilis or otherwise; she nevertheless lost the trouble after taking five or six doses of Mercurius.

The complaint returned again in about six months, with nearly the same symptoms and was again relieved permanently by the same remedy. Another female patient who was long under Allopathic treatment, with similar symptoms without having been benefitted, was permanently relieved by the same preparation.

There are some reasons why these chronic affections of the larynx may have insidiously developed from the syphilitic diathesis. It is said that a little practice will enable a person to pass his finger into the patient's throat and to familiarize his sense of touch with the ordinary condition of the upper part of the respiratory apparatus, so as to be able to detect swelling, or irregularity or thickness of the glottis. A great advantage is said to have been obtained by applying remedies directly to the affected part.

Nitrate of *Silver* has been advantageously used in solution, applied by the probang to the diseased or thickened part of the affected organ.

A lad of eleven years who was unable to speak only in a whisper, and who complained of difficult breathing and cough; he drew in his breath with a loud wheeze, his cough had a whistling sound, as through a narrow tube and very troublesome at night, the expectoration of mucus not being great in quantity. He suffered this way all winter, having had whooping cough in the preceding autumn. He had cups applied to the throat;

little can be heard in the chest on account of the loud wheezing eclipsing all other sounds.

In about two weeks, having taken *Mercurius* persistently without improvement, on further examination it was discovered that the trouble arose from mechanical irritation and had progressed so far that remedial measures were unavailing.

It has been a difficult question to decide, whether in case of the tumefaction becoming so great in the larynx it is not warrantable to relieve the patient's breathing by tracheotomy. There are on record many cases where obstructions to respiration which seem to be located in the upper part of the trachea and larynx have prevented the lungs from receiving the *quantum sufficit* of pure air to provide for the arterialization of the blood; and therefore surgery has been called into requisition in the performance of tracheotomy, so that the aperture might be sufficient to keep the system replenished by the imbibition of pure air into the lungs. Is this warrantable? when it becomes evident that the air passages, by reason of obstruction in the larynx are incapable of admitting a sufficient quantity of air the operation should be commended.

We learn from various sources that this operation has been successfully performed in a number of instances; and where there is no other way for the lungs to inspire from the atmosphere than through an aperture made in the trachea, no one can dispute the utility of the operation.

TREATMENT.—In Allopathic practice the treatment is by topical applications, or counter-irritants applied to the region of the disease. In short the treatment is surgical, there being no medical treatment at all reliable.

HOMŒOPATHIC TREATMENT.—Chronic laryngitis, when the face is flushed and there is acceleration of the pulse and a hot skin with some thirst, give *Aconite* every hour until the fever is subdued. Give *Belladonna* after *Aconite* when there is soreness of the throat which interferes with articulation and deglutition.

Hepar sulphur is indicated for hoarseness and hoarse cough.

Phosphorus, for cough with rawness and hoarseness, and expectoration of tough mucus.

Spongia is indicated for pain in the larynx on touching it and turning the head; for difficult respiration, as if the chest were closed with a plug; preventing the passage of the air, for stridulous breathing, barking cough from efforts of inspiration.

Causticum, for chronic hoarseness and loss of voice, as from weakness of the laryngeal muscles.

Kali bichromicum, for chronic laryngitis with ulceration, expectoration of thick yellow mucus and hoarse croupy cough, aggravated when undressing; somewhat relieved after getting warm in bed.

For chronic affections of the larynx supervening upon syphilis, I have found no remedy so effective as *Mercurius solubilis* in the first, second or third trituration. I have also found *Nitric acid* a valuable remedy for syphilitic ulceration; for ordinary ulceration, *Calcarea* is entitled to the highest consideration.

For what is called the clergyman's sore throat or teacher's sore throat, as well as for those who use the voice continually; *Calcarea*, *Argentum metallicum*, *Lachesis* as well as *Carbo vegetabilis* may be consulted.

ACCESSORY TREATMENT.—Patients suffering from considerable accumulation of mucus in the larynx and throat may be greatly relieved by a copious draught of warm water. Patients suffering from chronic laryngitis must avoid extremes of temperature, especially a draught of cold air, or sitting in a cold room.

They must be warmly clad in the day time and they must be careful to have sufficient covering during the night. As the patient's appetite varies, it is proper for him to partake of any nutritious aliment which he may prefer, provided it is non-medicinal and free from irritating properties.

Œdematous Inflammation of the Glottis.

A distinction has been made between laryngitis and œdema, which is a just and real distinction.

Laryngeal inflammation and especially laryngeal œdema, not unfrequently occurs, and is suddenly fatal in the course of other diseases. I have observed that in severe tonsillitis the inflammation frequently extends to the larynx. We have seen two or three cases of erysipelas, attended as it almost always is, with sore throat, wherein death took place suddenly and unexpectedly; and where the epiglottis and the edges of the fissure of the glottis were found to be œdematous.

The inflammation of the throat had extended to the areolar

tissue beneath the mucous membrane of those parts and had led to the serous effusion there.

In small-pox, and measles, and scarlet fever, attended with sore throat, the very same thing is apt to occur. I have known a mercurial sore throat in a broken down constitution, to result in an inflammatory œdema. The laryngeal affection in these cases is consecutive and secondary and in all of them the great remedy is the formation of a sufficient aperture beneath the obstructed glottis.

In all of them also the essential symptoms warranting and demanding the operation of tracheotomy are the same. "Œdema of the loose areolar tissue subjacent to the mucous membrane of the glottis is indeed one common consequence of inflammation of that membrane. But it may occur independently of inflammation. The lips of the glottis become tumid and dropsical in consequence of a low inflammatory action in the throat, but sometimes also from the obstruction of the veins leading from that part."

The main practical difference between mere œdema glottidis and acute laryngitis is this: In the former there is no fever or inflammation; and the operation of tracheotomy becomes the sole resource to which in the extremity of danger we can look for help. Mere œdema glottidis is seldom attended with difficult deglutition; but not so in laryngitis.

If the epiglottis be involved in the œdematous swelling, and unable to shut over the glottis, the act of swallowing will be followed by a strangling cough, and increased difficulty of breathing.

The larynx is sometimes subject to ulcerations and necrosis of the cartilages. The inflammation that produces this slow ulceration is first attended with hoarseness, then with aphonia and a stridulous cough. But in most if not all cases of ulceration of the larynx, the patient labors under other difficulties, which we shall attend to when we treat of tubercular phthisis. Secondary syphilis sometimes finds its way to the larynx and produces thickening of the membrane which lines the laryngeal cartilages and this gives rise to a hoarse croaking voice and noisy and painful breathing; and sometimes again and again the uneasiness about the throat, the loud respiration, the whispering voice, with all its roughness, will cease immediately under the influence of *Mercury*. We therefore look upon *Mercury* either in the form of a trituration or a lardaceous preparation to apply externally a *grand specific* for syphilitic affections of the larynx; although it may seem that a repetition of this fact is quite unnecessary; yet the practical importance of it to the medical profession warrants this "line upon line."

The lining membrane of the larynx is liable to excrescences, in the form of warty growths which impede the entrance and exit of air, to and from the lungs. There is an incident on record of a boy who speaks in a whisper and complains of difficult breathing and a cough. Every inspiration he makes is attended with a loud wheeze, or cough, with a sort of a whistling sound as if made through a narrow tube, and most frequently at night. There is considerable expectoration of mucus yet limited in quantity. He has been ill all winter having had whooping cough in autumn.

The case finally terminated fatally; and when his body was examined, there was found at the very top of the larynx and vocal cords a warty growth closing the rima glottidis almost entirely. These warty excrescences sometimes occur and close up the aperture in the larynx and are certain to result in death.

The question arises, if some artificial means of introducing air into the lungs cannot be recommended. Ought not tracheotomy be performed in such cases? and ought not a tube be inserted through the opening into the trachea, through which the function of respiration can be easily and surely aided? It is true that tracheotomy is hazardous, and a greater proportion of those operated on are apt to die, nevertheless as all are sure to meet death without the operation and a fair percentage are benefited by it, we must say in all candor there is a warrant for the operation. In the case of a young man aged fifteen, son of a popular clergyman, laryngitis had progressed sufficiently to produce a tumefaction which apparently interrupted respiration. In view of the certainty of death occurring speedily, as a dernier resort tracheotomy was performed and the patient recovered.

CHAPTER XXI.

CROUP, CYNANCHE TRACHEALIS.

This disease is a violent inflammation affecting the mucous membrane, which lines that portion of the air passage, which lies between the laryngeal cartilages and the bifurcation of the trachea, the primary bronchia. It is in other words, an inflammation of the trachea or wind pipe; for this is the seat of the disease; but the inflammation sometimes implicates the larynx above and encroaches on the bronchia and their ramifications.

Dr. Condie maintains that croup commences in the larynx, that the mucous membrane in this cavity inflames first, and then extends into the trachea. The disease is therefore, strictly speaking, a laryngeal tracheitis. He also asserts that the mucous membrane of the larger bronchia may first inflame and afterwards it may extend to the trachea; from my own personal observation I am persuaded that croup is very rarely restricted to the trachea. I do not recollect but few cases, where either the larynx or bronchia and perhaps both were not implicated to a greater or less extent. Some writers maintain that the milder forms of this disease consist in an *inflammation* confined exclusively to the trachea, that when the mucous lining of the larynx partakes of the inflammation it becomes a suffocating croup and more severe.

In fatal cases of membraneous croup, it has been ascertained that the chief inflammation was in the mucous lining of the larynx; and yet this may be true only in a limited sense. We have encountered many formidable cases of croup, where the trachea only seemed to be the seat of inflammation.

During a violent and dangerous attack of croup where the inflammation of the mucous membrane caused a rapid exudation and formation of pseudo-membrane, we have found the action greater about the larynx, glottis and upper portion of the trachea, while at other times the bronchia are attacked and the disease is more protracted but not the less fatal.

Cullen, who first described the disease made no distinction between cynanche laryngea and cynanche trachealis, yet the boundaries between the two are unmistakably fixed.

Their anatomical situation is different, and they differ in malignity, though both are serious diseases. Croup usually occurs in childhood, but inflammation of the larynx is a disease which commonly affects adults. Croup is usually sudden and more serious, because it comes on without warning, and but little can be done to prevent its course.

Laryngitis gives sufficient warning of its approach to admit of topical or mechanical means of relief, as well as with well chosen remedies.

We have said that croup was peculiarly a disease of childhood. It occurs, if at all, between the periods of weaning and puberty. But few cases occur in children under a year old; a greater number, it is said, suffer from the disease in the second year than any other. In all probability this is owing to a change of diet consequent on weaning.

From the second year onwards the number of children affected with croup gradually decreases. An experienced writer says only one case in ninety occurred among children in his practice after the child was ten years old. But the disease does occasionally occur after the age of puberty. We are inclined to the opinion, however, that these, if carefully examined, would prove to be cases of laryngitis.

Croup is frequently preceded by what is commonly called a cold, which slightly affects the mucous membrane of the air passages.

The child at first sneezes, coughs and is hoarse. This last symptom sounds the note of alarm. Dr. Cheyne says hoarseness never arises from a common cold in a child only when it indicates the approach of croup.

It seldom attends common catarrh, and therefore when it occurs at a season or in a district where croup among children is common, the nurse or mother should take heed and provide protective measures. The medical attendant should be prompt with curative and prophylactic remedies. Much depends upon the early treatment of the disorder.

In addition to these symptoms the child is feverish and fretful, wakeful and restless. In a few days, if not arrested, the symptoms peculiar to croup begin to show themselves; such as difficult respiration, harsh inspiration, attended by a noise much like what is heard in whooping cough, rough voice, loud metallic ring to the cough, and considerable fever.

These are the symptoms which characterize croup.

The sonorous inspiration is almost enough of itself to identify the disease. The cough sounds peculiar and much as if the victim coughed through a tin trumpet.

The croupy cough is seldom mistaken after having once been heard. There is not any difficulty in swallowing, the face is flushed, the skin hot, the pulse is full and bounding, and there is considerable thirst. All these symptoms taken collectively enable us to judge of a case of croup. There is no disease that so resembles croup as laryngitis; and yet, except in case of thickening of mucous membrane of the larynx, or some syphilitic sore affecting the larynx, we find no cough that is liable to be mistaken for that of croup. At the commencement the fever generally runs high, and this is quite important in diagnosing a case of croup; as the obstruction of the air passage increases, the blood fails of receiving invigoration from the oxygen of the air, and then of course the skin becomes dusky, bluish, the pulse feeble and irregular, and the extremities cold, and as the disease progresses the cough changes its tone, and ceases to be loud and clanging and the voice sinks into a whisper, the pupils dilate, the respiration becomes more feeble and difficult, a cold sweat covers the surface and a hard, dense membrane forms in the trachea.

Life is destroyed in pure circumscribed tracheitis, by the accumulation in the windpipe of a concrete membrane like substance which often attends the disease, and gives to it the name of membraneous croup. In cases of recovery this membrane becomes dislodged, and thrown off in the form of a tube, or a cast of the trachea.

In severe cases this exudation is not confined to the windpipe, it extends downward to the bronchia and often enters its ramifications into the lungs.

The false membrane has been known to extend from the tip of the epiglottis to the large bronchia, sometimes this adventitious exudation extends even to the termination of the bronchia. On the other hand there are cases in which the adventitious membrane does not form at all, the inner surface of the trachea is seen to be merely reddened and tumid and covered with viscid mucus, or perhaps with a small exudation of concrete albumen here or there.

"The difficulty of breathing and the characteristic sounds that accompany it, depend in part, it is believed, upon spasmodic contractions of the small muscles of the larynx." For remarkable aggravation of the dyspnœa, or difficulty of breathing, are apt to occur and to subside again; and these aggravations may be brought on by deglutition and other sudden causes. I have observed in many cases of croup the spasmodic constriction of the glottis, but may here remark that doubts arise about its having anything to do with the difficult breathing; such doubts to say the least are in all respects reasonable, for the glottis can be closed by an effort of the will so as to prevent the passage of air to and from the lungs; a contrary opinion is entertained, that this is merely affected by the action of the little muscles that bring together the arytenoid cartilages and that these muscles like other muscles concerned in respiration, act independently of the will, and therefore through the reflex function of the spinal cord.

This independent and spasmodic action is apparently a providential provision for admitting in the healthy state the vivifying air; and for barring the entrance against hurtful gases, and against solids and liquids which would be injurious to the respiratory system.

We know that if a drop of water, or a crumb of bread, or a whiff of carbonic acid gas, gets past the epiglottis and into the larynx, spasmodic action of the little muscles in question occurs immediately.

These intruders so effectually elude the sight, that they cannot be voluntarily resisted, but these little muscles act as an unsleeping sentinel to guard the passage. We may, therefore, conclude that the audible respiration as well as the difficult respiration of croup are partly caused by spasm.

Dr. Condie maintains that all the diagnostic signs of croup may be suddenly produced by gastric irritation, caused by indigestible food, and will be as suddenly removed the moment the cause of gastric irritation is expelled. A medical gentleman in Philadelphia gives the case of his own child, who invariably exhibited the symptoms of croup after fish, and was relieved by an emetic immediately.

The reason why children when suffering from membraneous

20

croup throw back the head, is in all probability the presence of
the tubular membrane in the trachea; in that position the
cylinder of the membrane is kept open, whereas if the head were
bent forward, the membrane would be bent upon itself, and the
aperture through it would be obstructed.

It has been maintained that this concrete exudation, under
certain conditions, may exhibit the phenomena of adhesive inflammation. Similar films are formed or are thrown off the mucous
surfaces of the intestines and uterus. "Whether they are identical with the layers of coagulable lymph, poured forth in inflammation of the serous and areolar tissues, may be made a question."
We think most certainly there are some points of distinction
between them. "The concrete membrane of croup is more brittle, less fibrous, more decidedly albuminous than the false membrane that covers the inflamed pleura, pericardium, or peritoneum; a still more remarkable difference is this, that it is not
plastic in the sense in which that term was formerly explained,
it never becomes organized, never connects itself to the surface
by blood vessels from which it precedes. On the contrary it is
partially detached, and by degrees if the patient lives long enough,
it is completely separated from the subjacent parts." It has been
extensively observed that tracheal inflammation is limited to the
early period of life. Some have started one hypothesis and some
another to account for this fact, Dr. Stokes thinks the great production of white tissue in children accounts for the frequency of
croup with them. Dr. Williams starts the reasonable supposition
"that the inflammation involves the subcutaneous areolar tissue
which is abundant in youth, and that the natural product of the
phlegmonous inflammation transudes readily through the thin,
simple and delicate mucous membrane proper to that age."

Both the formation and renewal of the adventitious membrane sometimes appear to be quite rapid; a fact illustrative of
this is related by an *English writer* who upon the very brink of
suffocation performed tracheotomy upon a child and instant relief
was afforded the little sufferer, and she fell into a sweet sleep of
six hours, and breathed with perfect ease. In the meantime the
pseudo-membrane reproduced itself, and when the surgeon
returned to witness his triumph he found the child dead; an
autopsy revealed the fact, that the trachea was filled with false

membrane which had formed within six hours after the first tube had been removed.

Croup is not regarded as a contagious disease, although like tonsillitis, and for the same reasons, it is found in several members of the household at the same time or follows in rapid succession.

We knew a family of six children, the oldest ten years old, and the youngest seven months; the third child, a little boy, took the croup and suddenly died, and in quick succession the oldest and next to the youngest contracted the same disease, and in spite of the most strenuous exertions to relieve them, they died also; and yet the other three living in the same house and surrounded apparently by the same influences did not take the disease. I have sometimes noticed that tonsillitis will assail one or two or three of a family about the same time, and the remainder will escape. Dr. Gregory had two children seized with croup on the same night. Both had been exposed to a cold wind while walking on the seashore the previous evening. This accords with the theory that croup is almost always nocturnal in its attacks, and in some districts and near large bodies of water it seems to be endemic. Attacks are more frequent in the winter and spring near the seashore, where chilling winds and storms are the most prevalent, and it has been remarked that children sleeping in newly-washed rooms are liable to sudden attacks of the disease. From the fact that children who suffer from one attack are predisposed to succeeding ones, relapses frequently occur even after an apparent recovery, and these relapses are viewed as perilous, and aside from this liability to a recurrence the little patients are often affected with cough and hoarseness and even aphonia, for a long time, and while these symptoms remain the croup is easily brought back again.

The prognosis of croup is always uncertain. Formerly a very large proportion of cases terminated fatally. But since the disease is better understood the mortality is not so great. When the disease progresses rapidly and the child's lips become blue, the skin cold, the pulse feeble and intermittent, and a drowsiness and coma supervenes, we may conclude that life will soon become extinct. The mortality may be greatly decreased by attention to the early symptoms and by an immediate resort to vigorous remedial agents.

TREATMENT.—In Allopathic practice the three principal remedies consist of blood-letting, tartarized antimony and calomel.

Bleeding in the onset is unhesitatingly employed when the child is plethoric and strong; after the first depletion, either by cups or leeches, or when practical by bleeding from the arm, an emetic of tartarized antimony sufficient to produce copious vomiting is recommended, and this is followed by a brisk cathartic, when the tartar emetic acts severely upon the bowels it is often combined with laudanum or syrup of poppies according to the age of the patient.

HOMŒOPATHIC TREATMENT.—I have rarely lost a case of croup when early called to administer for the child's relief. Bleeding is objected to because of its depression of the vital forces and injury which in this respect must follow. *Tartar emetic* in doses to produce vomiting is also liable to a similar objection; it taxes the stomach and prostrates the patient without removing the cause, and cathartics do more harm than good by still further reducing the strength of the patient and more completely depriving the system of the power of vital resistance to the advancement of the disease.

We object to blisters, hive syrup, and all depressing agents, such as plasters of Scotch snuff and other relaxing resorts.

In the first or febrile stage, when the pulse is full, I have found *Aconite* in drop doses of the tincture, every twenty or thirty minutes, to mitigate the symptoms at once. After *Aconite*, if the croup symptoms remain with great difficulty in breathing and danger of suffocation, I have given the 1st dilution of *Spongia* in drop doses every fifteen minutes; ten drops are to be dissolved in ten teaspoonfuls of water, and a teaspoonful of it is to be administered every fifteen minutes until the respiration is relieved, and the apparent danger of suffocation is past and only a hoarseness remains.

I have found Hepar sulphur, third trituration in two grain doses and repeated every hour, to complete the cure. In the majority of cases the above three remedies will arrest and cure the disease in the catarrhal stage, but when the inflammation of the larynx and tracheal membrane is so great as to cause a pseudo-membraneous exudation, it becomes more formidable; in this case the danger increases as this adventitious membrane collects in the windpipe.

In such cases *Aconite*, so long as the fever is active, followed by Spongia and Hepar may mitigate if not cure. These remedies may be followed by *Iodium* if the dyspnœa continues and the disease appears to be persistent. I have known *Iodium* to be followed by a discharge of the adventitious membrane and to apparently steel the system against its reproduction. In the case of membraneous croup in a little boy four years ol l, after many reme lies had been given and no relief obtained, I was called in consultation with the attending physician; after examining the case I suggested *Bromium*, 2nd dilution, drop doses each in a teaspoonful of water every thirty minutes; after the second dose a violent struggle for breath, a cough which seemed like a fatal effort ensued, after which the adventitious membrane was expelled, and the respiration began to improve immediately and the child recovered.

We have also witnessed a recovery from this distressing disease, after all hope had been abandoned by the Allopathic medical attendant; by oft repeated doses of the 3x trituration of *Tartar emetic*.

In a severe case of asthmatic croup which persisted for several days Ipecac 3x dilution given frequently in drop doses soon brought about convalescence.

Kali bichromicum cured an apparently malignant membraneous croup, the 3x dilution, ten drops mixed with half a goblet of water was administered iu tea-spoonful doses every thirty minutes internally, while some of the crude drug was thrown into boiling water for the purpose of impregnating the air which surrounded the little sufferer with its fumes, after a few hours the child breathed easier and coughed up pieces of membrane, a gradual improvement followed until recovery was complete. The late Prof. W. E. Payne, M. D., had more than ordinary success with this remedy in membraneous croup. Aconite croup, according to Prof. Payne's observations is characterized by "invasion in the evening, after first sleep, preceded by restlessness, accelerated pulse and dryness of the skin. The patient usually rouses from sleep, with restless, impatient movements, tosses from side to side; cannot be calmed, and on attempting to swallow cries, as if from soreness and pain in the throat, followed immediately by a shrill, barking cough. The cough is frequent, *following every expiratory effort, but absent during inspiration.*

This seems to result from a tickling sensation. excited by rush of air through the over-sensitive and irritated larynx from the lungs; the sibilant or sawing respiratory sound is also heard *only during the expiratory act,* and not during the inspiration as in some other forms of croup. The cough is more or less paroxysmal, but the stridulous breathing continues until after midnight, when both gradually remit and toward morning nearly or wholly disappear; but often to return on the following night.

Some five years ago our attention was first attracted to the above peculiar concurrence of the stridulous respiratory sound, and barking cough in the case of a boy about four years old. The disease resisted all our efforts for four days, no remedy touched it; but we gave *Aconite* when the whole trouble vanished as if by enchantment.

In order to distinguish between *Aconite* and *Spongia* croup we will give the characteristic symptoms of the latter remedy.

Spongia croup.—" Hollow cough with expectoration and pain in the chest and trachea," roughness in the throat (night with weeping expression), breathing aggravated as from a plug in the throat, slow or quick panting larynx; painful as if from pressure, worse when touched, scratching, burning, or constrictive sensation in the larynx and trachea, stinging in the throat and sensation in the outer parts of the neck as if something were pressing out, morning and evening, painful tensions on the left side of and near the *Pomum Adami;* when turning the head to the right side, the eyes are sunken, the urine deposits a thick, grayish white sediment, general morning sweat, pulse quick and hard, drowsiness, lassitude of the whole body, out of humor, everything puts him out of humor, even talking and answering questions. Dr. Payne says: "it seems that *Spongia* covers nearly the same symptoms as *Aconite* with this difference and condition.

In Spongia croup the stridulous respiratory sound is always during *inspiration* and the cough less constant and excited only by the inspiratory act, and the cough and sibilant respiratory sound are not so constantly concurrent as in *Aconite croup.*

There is also in *Spongia croup* fluent coryza and sometimes sneezing with saliva dribbling from the mouth, which we do not see in *Aconite croup;* neither of these remedies have any Homœopathic relation to *membraneous croup*, either in their symptomatic or pathologic bearing, and in such cases, the time expended in their use, in our judgment, is so much time lost. Our experience is in confirmation of the above. Teste says that this remedy is only applicable in the second stage of croup.

Hepar croup, violent fits of coughing as if he would suffocate or vomit, deep distress on account of the tightness of breathing, husky, accompanied with painful soreness of the chest at every time of cough which is violent, the air rushing violently against the larynx, occasioning a pain in that part; sensation of scraping, scratching, with mucous expectoration, the cough being caused by tittilation in the throat, or by a scraping in the trachea, and increased unto vomiting by a deep inspiration, weakness of the organs of speech and chest, short breathing, pressure in the throat, occasioning a constrictive feeling as if he should be suffocated; urine pale, clear while being emitted, afterwards becoming turbid, thick, depositing a white sediment, or flocculent, turbid while being emitted, or dark yellow, burning during emission; great unconquerable drowsiness; profuse sweat day and night, viscid profuse night sweat, sweat before midnight, and apprehensive and inclined to weep.

Bromine croup.—Formations of pseudo-membrane in the larynx and trachea, spasm in the larynx occasioning suffocating cough with croup sound, hoarse, wheezing, fatiguing cough, not permitting one to utter a word; sneezing, with violent suffocating fits, expiration characterized by mucous rattling, wheezing, alternately slow and suffocative, and hurried and superficial breathing, painful, oppressed; gasping for air; heat in the face, increased secretion of urine, pulse rather hard, slow at first, afterwards accelerated.

Caustic ammonia croup.— Deep. weak voice, fatiguing, interrupted speech; increased secretion of mucus in the bronchia, violent cough with copious expectoration of mucus, especially after drinking, difficult rattling, labored breathing, stertorous breathing, suffocative fits, spasm of the chest.

Bichromate of potash croup.—Symptoms approach gradually and insidiously, at first slight difficulty of breathing when the mouth is closed, slight elevation of the temperature, pulse irregular, and intermittent; or frequent and small; as the disease progresses, the difficulty of breathing increases; the sound of the air as it passes through the trachea is shrill, whistling, as if it passes through a metallic tube, voice hoarse, cough not frequent, but hoarse, dry, barking and metallic, deglutition difficult, not painful, tonsils and larynx swollen red and covered with an appearance of false membrane; after a time breathing affected in part by the action of the abdominal muscles, and those of the neck and shoulder blades, head inclined backwards, breath offensive, finally, diminished temperature of the skin, prostration and stupor.

The medicines here described as to their pathogenetic symptoms, are those which are most completely specific against croup.

It is true that *Aconite, Iodine, Belladonna, Nux vom., Hyoscyamus, Sambucus, Tartar emetic, Phosphorus*, etc., cover in their pathogenesis many of the symptoms of non-membraneous croup; but they cannot be regarded positive and reliable remedies for fully developed cases.

We have in ordinary cases of croup followed successfully Dr. Bæhr's method of treating croup, that is, we give Aconite if the disease commences with fever, drop doses, every fifteen minutes; in the first, second or third dilution—then after a rest of one or two hours, we give *Spongia*, second or third dilution in drop doses every half hour, according to the severity of the case; we then follow with *Phosphorus, Hepar sul.* or Tartar emetic according to the symptoms, and as we before remarked our success has been satisfactory.

Tartar emetic croup.—Voice weak, burning under the sternum, cough and sneezing, mucous rale in the bronchia with effusion. Eating excites cough and vomiting of food and glairy mucus, short hoarse cough caused by tickling in the middle of the larynx; heat and sweat on the forehead when coughing which is very fatiguing. Tartar emetic is not only useful in the early stages of croup, but it is also useful when there are signs indicative of partial paralysis of the pneumogastric nerve, viz., face livid and cold, cold sweat on the forehead, or body, respiration short, hoarse and exceedingly difficult; head thrown back, pulse small and quick, or feeble and slow, difficulty in swallowing and disposition to sleep. This remedy should be given in the 2d trituration two grains every twenty minutes until relief is obtained. Tartar emetic must be given at short intervals and according to our observation, it succeeds best in low dilution.

The worst symptoms of catarrhal croup diminish rapidly under its effects when given every fifteen or twenty minutes, the victim falling into a gentle sleep, without vomiting or purging or profuse sweat. The cough soon becomes loose and the expectoration free.

Note.—Dr. Bœninghausen's treatment of croup is thus given: five powders numbered from one to five. Thus No. 1 and 2, *Aconite* 200, 3 and 5 Hepar 200, No. 4 Spongia 200. He says the symptoms of croup nearly always disappear after the first powder if no other remedies have been given. One hour should always pass between 1 and 2. If there should be improvement after No. 1, the second powder should only be given after twelve or eighteen hours. No. 1 and 2 remove the inflammatory symptoms, and No. 3 removes the cough.

Dr. Dansford relies upon *Aconite, Hyoscyamus* and Belladonna, for the cure of spasmodic croup.

Dr. Ludlam confirms this view, and cites from his practice many cases where the above treatment was speedily useful.

Prof. Hoyne finds high potencies of *Aconite, Spongia* and *Hepar sul.* more decidedly effective in croup than low ones, but it requires great care to affiliate the remedies correctly, and in the treatment of such cases only as afford a plain indication for their use.

Prof. Hoyne is a careful observer and reliable authority. He maintains further, and we think very plausibly, that the high and even the highest potencies of all the croupal remedies will act more speedily and satisfactory if selected according to the indications which the symptoms afford rather than as general remedies for croup.

Dr. Marcy says: "In addition to high febrile excitement, we must alternate with *Aconite*, the proper local specific, in accordance with the croupy symptoms, as Acon. and Spongia or *Aconite* and *Hepar* or *Aconite* and *Tartar emetic*, etc., he also recommends the use of the probang with a weak solution of Nitrate of Silver applied directly to the affected membrane; he further maintains that this treatment is strictly Homœopathic and curative in all stages of the disease when internal remedies may prove unavailing.

Dr. Hering recommends a low potency of *Tartar emetic* in catarrhal croup. *Hahnemann* after a practice of *twenty years* decided that the 30 centesimal dilutions were efficient.

Bœninghausen after eighteen years experience with the 200 was never inclined to use lower potencies, because he found them more efficient.

Prof. Carroll Dunham endorsed the views of Bœninghausen and carried them out in his practice.

With becoming liberality we must admit facts and thereupon the best possible testimony goes to prove that the administration of remedies in order to be curative must be upon the Homœopathic principle and that from the lowest to the highest potency, success will attend such administration.

Cold water compresses about the throat, says Dr. Holcombe, are with him a *sine qua non* and so successful has he been with them that he would not dare to undertake the treatment of a serious case of croup without them. We regard Dr. Holcombe high authority because in a large practice of many years he has never lost a case of croup. As an accessory means of curing croup, my experience accords with his.

Dr. Tate includes among the croup remedies *Ipecacuanha*, and we think very justly, but the indications for its use are the agreement between the symptoms of the disease and the pathogenesis of the remedy, as for ourselves we have cured asthmatic croup with it when all other remedies seemed to fail.

1. Diphtheria arises from a specific invisible cause, which in order to produce the legitimate pathological points, must first be introduced into the blood.

2. The means for the introduction of this virus into the blood are two in number, viz., through the respiration and by inoculation.

3. We cannot conceive of an epidemic cause which fails to occasion more or less contamination of the atmosphere. Local circumstances may concentrate such a taint and thus render susceptible persons in a community more liable to contract the disease from breathing this atmosphere.

4. In exceptional cases the diphtheria may spread in this manner by a thorough poisoning of the air which is breathed, but as a rule it is much more feebly contagious than either of the eruptive fevers. There is no evidence that it is ever conveyed by *fomites*.

5. The only known method of successful inoculation is that a portion of the vitiated secretions from either the mucous membranes or the skin of a diphtheritic subject be applied to an absorbent surface.

6. But these methods of communicating the disease will fail unless the individual constitution and local habits and surroundings of the subject afford a congenial soil, in which the specific cause may develop its specific effects.

"All of these symptoms and sequellæ point to the constitutional character of diphtheria. There is no question but that it is a systemic and not merely a local disorder which owes its essential character to the presence of a species of parasitic growth whether it be algous or fungous. It is zymotic in its origin, its characteristics and its sequellæ. It is a disease *per se* and not alone a dyscrasia. Like the typhoid fever, it has its general and special lesions, the one systematic and the other local."

Certain English physicians maintain that the specific cause of diphtheria is a depressing poison which acts primarily on the nervous system as the sudden sinking and death of patients without apparent cause would indicate. Sometimes patients not considered dangerously ill drop off suddenly, at other times a longer duration of the disease ends in some particular or peculiar form of paralysis, occurring some weeks after the first attack of the disease. "This paralysis is not due to mere poverty of the blood or the *spanæmia* induced by the preceding disease, but rather to the presence in the system throughout all the stages of the disease of a specific poison whose special affinity is for the nervous tissue, its action is shown in the first instance by a general vital depression and subsequently by a more or less complete suspension of the function of particular nerves or system of nerves and loss of power of the limbs.

After reviewing the published opinions on diphtheria and from facts which have come under our own observation, we cannot avoid the conclusion that a peculiar morbific influence which so far affects all the inhabitants of large tracts of country at a time, so as to modify more or less all common forms of disease, is the origin of diphtheritic development.

Predisposing causes inherent in the constitution, such as a scrofulous diathesis or psora or glandular swellings, are apt to invite the diphtheritic miasm as an exciting cause, sudden change of temperature, exposure to cold or derangement of the digestive apparatus, all serve to render the system impressible.

That we may better understand the nature and scope of the disease, let us examine closely *the symptoms.*

In some localities the patient is suddenly seized with violent vomiting of a thin yellowish white matter of an offensive odor; then purging of matters of similar appearance and smell. This vomiting and purging lasts for a longer or shorter period, and is followed by great prostration and stupor. This is followed by sopor more or less profound from which it is difficult to arouse the patient. The skin is hot, pulse 100 in adults, in children 140 or 160, tongue bright red, great thirst, the patient drinks with avidity and immediately vomits. The purging mentioned above is not common to all localities.

There is a characteristic odor of the breath, peculiarly offensive, which frequently gives the first conclusive evidence of the impending danger; even if the symptoms have revealed nothing alarming. The infection of the breath is undoubtedly from the specific zymotic poison operating in the secretions of the parts implicated as well as upon the blood. In the early stages the patient feels no soreness of the throat, although on critical examination, the tonsils, soft palate, and back of the pharynx, are found to be of a bright red and of a smooth shining appearance. The small vessels as in ordinary sore throat do not appear to be congested, but smooth and shiny as if covered with varnish; a tenacious film of white fluid is seen at this stage hanging from the *velum palati* which bursts before the expired breath, and sends its film down over the mouth and the *depressor linguæ*. This film or curtain is reproduced at once, and is again burst, and in a moment a similar curtain is formed.

In from sixteen to twenty hours the condition of the system undergoes a change. The stupor disappears and delirium takes its place; there is hectic fever, quick pulse, rapid respiration, shrill and thick voice; a short and dry cough; indications of approaching croup; puffiness of the neck; tongue coated with white fur in spots, which in a very short period conglomerates and forms one thick plastic deposit, which in time is liable to cover the whole palate to the teeth presenting the appearance as if the whole mouth was painted white. The powers of life begin to fail rapidly; the delirium subsides and distressing sensations of choking and suffocation come on; the sufferer tries to tear open his mouth; tears at his neck with his nails, although deglutition seems unimpaired he gradually swallows whatever fluid is offered him.

The extremities exhibit signs of purpura; diarrhœic discharges occur constantly from the bowels.

There is muttering delirium and finally a long tetanic convulsion which usually ends in death.

It is seldom that we find many cases of true diphtheria in any locality yet invaded by the disease. The exudation resembles wash-leather, and there is a fetid discharge from the nostrils, ulceration from the tongue, gums and fauces, a seeming loss of vitality or deficiency thereof from the beginning of the disease. In the severe cases apthous ulcers are found on the tongue, palate and tonsils, and in most cases a small rapid pulse and moisture on the surface and great weakness.

When the disease is more intense white elevated spots are found on the tonsils, uvula arches of the palate or posterior wall of the pharynx appearing like a tumefied and hardened mucous membrane covered with white patches varying in size from that of the smallest fish scale to that of a piece of white kid sufficient in size to cover the posterior surface of the buccal cavity and throat. A deep red border surrounds these patches and when removed it leaves a raw, rough, and often bleeding surface.

These patches frequently form and spread rapidly; under successful treatment they loosen, break and are thrown off with sanious and bloody discharge; the breath is very offensive, the pulse small and rapid with profuse perspiration and finally with extreme debility.

From an article in the *North American Journal of Homœopathy*, February, 1862, in sixteen cases, of whom four died, there occurred in addition to the above symptoms "constant cough provoked by swallowing, and worse from crying, hoarseness and rasping respiration, such as characterized membraneous croup." In some cases the peculiar membrane was visible covering the epiglottis. In three cases the membrane came away in fragments leaving a rough and bleeding surface. In but one case it formed a second time on the same spot. "One patch thrown off and preserved in alcohol, is nearly an inch square, and of the thickness of the heaviest kid, of spongy texture and yellowish white color; the under surface is rough with elevations and depressions corresponding with the granulations of the tonsil from whence it came; upon close examination it appears like the mucous membrane thickened by an interstitial deposit of a white cheesy substance.

It must have left the surface of the tonsils whence it came completely minus the mucous membrane."

DIAGNOSIS.—The differential characteristics between diphtheria and croup may be contrasted as follows:

DIPHTHERIA.

In diphtheria there is an exudation of an albuminous or coagulable effusion on the surfaces of the fauces and air passages, and most always commences on the tonsils and pharynx, extending along the nares velum pendulum palati, and sometimes downward to the larynx. It seldom passes beyond. It may descend into the larynx and trachea and produce all the symptoms of true croup.

Sometimes this false membrane may manifest itself upon other parts of the body denuded of the outer skin.

It has been known to cover the conjunctiva of one eye and the surface upon the arm.

Diphtheria usually selects feeble subjects who are surrounded by unfavorable conditions. Inflammation

CROUP.

Genuine croup has its seat in the trachea and lower portion of the larynx.

It commences there and seldom, if ever, implicates the larynx or any part of the fauces.

There is no vomiting or diarrhœa.

Croup is essentially a sthenic disease. It is highly inflammatory in its nature; generally traceable to exposure to cold and damp air. It is seldom epidemic and never contagious. The symptomatic fever is inflammatory throughout its course. It has been caused by some known exposure, as sudden suppression of perspiration, wet feet or a current of cold damp air. Exposure to cold, bleak winds and chilling blasts, and large bodies of water have a tendency to check perspiration and

DIPHTHERIA.

In diphtheria, from the first, assumes a gangrenous or putrid character and the fever attendant on this disease is distinctly typhoid. Under this fever, which results in the loss of the vital power and exhaustion, diphtheria is essentially a zymotic disease.

The specific poison is a toxical agent which acts on and depresses the nervous system.

CROUP.

produce chilliness of the surface, the perspiration being driven inwards towards the mucous membrane.

Period of Life.

DIPHTHERIA.

Diphtheria is common to all ages, considered to be the most fatal during childhood and adolescence.

CROUP.

Croup is confined to the period of infancy and childhood.

The victims are found all the way from the period of weaning to that of puberty.

Character of the Effusion.

DIPHTHERIA.

In the light cases of diphtheria there is no effusion and when there is, its features are not uniform or permanent. In some instances the matter effused consists of a lymph-like albuminous deposit, and is the product of an active inflammation of the fauces as in cynanche pharyngea and tonsillaris. In other cases it is soft, shreddy, in patches on one or both tonsils; the palate or fauces resembling sloughy mucous membrane. It is accompanied by all the symptoms of typhus fever as in cynanche maligna and in some of the worst forms of scarlatina and measles.

CROUP.

"The false membrane in laryngeal croup is strong, dense fibrinous, often organized and it often exhibits a well marked vascular derangement."

Principal Symptoms.

DIPHTHERIA.

We never observe the short sibilation of croup when the disease is confined to the upper part of the larynx.

We do not see the spasm with fits of suffocation, but a kind of a mucous rattling in the course of forty-eight hours with marks of a slow and progressive asphyxia during which discharge the nose becomes putrid.

In no locality have we yet found

CROUP.

In croup there is a hard hoarse cough which is afterward stifled. Spasms of the larynx are followed at least by asphasia and suffocation. The agitation and extreme agony which distinguish the last stage of croup, contrast strongly with the livid palor of the surface, the delirium, profound depression, somnolent tranquility and adynamia which belong to this stage of diphtheria. The dyspnœa is paroxysmal,

21

DIPHTHERIA.	CROUP.
all cases presenting the peculiar diphtheritic exudation though we may distinctly recognize all the other distinctive features of the epidemic. We find the same erysipelatous patches of inflamed surface on the tonsils, the same swelling of the glands of the parotid and sub-maxillary region, the same disposition to a low state of the system. We find these states in the same localities and in the same families in which the more strongly marked cases of *true diphtheria* are seen. Diphtheria can be communicated by inoculation from the thin film of the poisonous exudation.	invariably worse at night, in the intervals the breathing is almost natural. The patient alternates between suffocation and repose. There is no eruption, no acrid coryza, no especial liability to hæmorrhages from the mucous membrane, no alimentary disorder, no albuminuria. The glands of the neck are not swollen; there is no after tendency to paralytic prostration. Croup can not be communicated by inoculation.

Distinction between Diphtheria and Scarlatina.

Many people and some physicians maintain that diphtheria is but a masked scarlatina, because they have some features in common. Thus in both are enlargement and inflammation of the tonsils and glands of the neck, ulceration and rash upon the skin which does not appear in all cases.

Similar premonitory symptoms, general depravation of the blood, shown by a tendency to gangrene; albuminuria is common to both. In reply to those who maintain the identity of scarlatina and diphtheria, and that the latter is scarlatina slightly modified by some epidemic influence; we will cite the fact that diphtheria has prevailed as an epidemic in many localities where scarlatina was not only absent, but had not been heard of for years.

That there is much confusion in the minds of physicians, in regard to the diagnosis between this disease and some others is evident by the fact that consulting physicians very often disagree about the name of a disease which is before them.

It would seem from the history of the disease together with its progress for the last few years that its existence would be coupled in some measure with scarlet fever. It was observed in New York city in 1860 that when diphtheria prevailed extensively there was more scarlet fever than was ever known before in that city.

In 1858 the two diseases prevailed together quite extensively in England, and physicians frequently confounded the two diseases.

DIPHTHERIA.	SCARLATINA.
Diphtheria comes on insidiously with slight heat and subsides early.	The invasion is sudden and violent; the skin is hot and the fever high.

Liability to a Second Attack.

Persons who have had diphtheria once are very liable to a second attack. Dr. Dake mentions nine cases, each of whom had a second attack of the disease several weeks after apparent recovery.

In scarlet fever the patient recovering therefrom is not generally liable to a second attack, and having had diphtheria does not protect him from scarlatina.

Eruption.

DIPHTHERIA.	SCARLET FEVER.
In diphtheria the eruption, if there is any, appears and disappears suddenly, and is more like measles than scarlet fever, and is not followed by desquamation.	The eruption in scarlet fever is a prominent feature of the disease. The rash does not come out suddenly but gradually ; and after remaining upon the surface for a day or two, or even longer, it terminates in desquamation.

The Angina.

DIPHTHERIA.	SCARLATINA.
Commences by patches on the tonsils, and spreads sometimes so as to invade the respiratory passages. There is no false membrane formed in many cases, because death occurs before the time for the formation of this false membrane is reached. In slight cases there is none that attracts attention.	The inflammation of the throat tends to localize itself in the whole cavity of the fauces and posterior nares, and tends rather to invade the oesophagus than the larynx.

Dropsical Affections.

We have never known dropsy to occur as a sequel of diphtheria.	The albumen is chiefly eliminated by the kidneys.

Modes of Termination in Death.

DIPHTHERIA.	SCARLATINA.
Death takes place from this disease in consequence of the extreme prostration, and the symptoms by which it is preceded are those which result from the action of a malignant septic poison. The poison in cases of slow recovery still manifests its power in general vital depression, more particularly in the form of paralysis.	The immediate cause of death from scarlatina is suffocation, cerebral congestion, or effusion or dropsy. In all these affections there is a high degree of septicæmia ; but it does not show its effect in general or partial paralysis which often follows diphtheria.

Diphtheria and Scarlatina Anginosa.

This is known by the name of ulcerated sore throat of the older writers. The coating of the tonsils, etc., consists of an erysipelatous redness, which is soon superseded by patches of a gray, tenacious, firm, transparent membrane.

The tonsils and contiguous tissue are covered with a thick, heavy, pultaceous exudation of dull, whitish or dirty looking color.

Diphtheria and Syphilitic Ulcer on the Tonsil.

The diseased surface is not depressed; the membrane can be separated from the tonsils.

In this last affection the surface is depressed, except in secondary syphilis, and the false membrane is adherent.

Relations between Diphtheria and Erysipelas.

The points of coincidence in these diseases are as follows: They are both dependent on causes little understood and they occur in subjects predisposed by previous disease to fall under the influence of any epidemic that may be prevalent.

Persons of scrofulous diathesis are liable to be attacked by both of these diseases. Damp weather and damp districts are most favorable for the spread of both of these diseases, and the same remedies are called into requisition in the treatment of both; when one has recovered from an attack of diphtheria he is a good subject for the other, and the reverse is true. An attack of phlegmonous erysipelas prepares the system for an attack of diphtheria if the poison is in the atmosphere or the disease is prevailing epidemically.

One celebrated physician says he saw several cases in which erysipelas spread over their faces after the peculiar false membrane of diphtheria had disappeared.

In these cases it would seem manifest that erysipelas is liable to affect the skin; and diphtheria spends its force on the mucous membrane.

The *distinction* between erysipelas and diphtheria is sufficiently obvious to any observer. It is well, however, to study critically into the nature of pseudo-membranes.

What is a false membrane; what is understood by the term? A French writer says, "A false membrane is a morbid product which is most frequently deposited upon a tegumentary surface— either of mucous or serous membrane, sometimes adventitiously, and which is formed or exuded by that part of the body which it invests."

It has been recognized by the most extensive practitioners that diphtheritic poison, when introduced into the system has an affinity both for the nervous centers and the mucous membranes which line the internal cavities.

We have observed in many instances the tendency of diphtheria to invade the respiratory passages, the nasal fossæ, the larynx and the trachea. An apthous eruption it is believed occupies a portion of the alimentary tract, the stomach and the œsophagus, but never extends to the mucous surfaces of the larynx or bronchia.

The pathology of diphtheria is calculated to throw some light on the morbid tendencies, and to suggest important practical hints. A writer on the *Medical Times and Gazette* says, "that a parasitic fungus was always present on the affected part in those cases which came under his own observation."

From this fact he was led to believe at first that this fungous growth constituted the chief characteristic; but on taking an opportunity to examine the films which occasionally form in the mouths of those sick with various diseases and submitting them to the test of a microscope, that they all indicated the presence of fungous growths that could not be distinguished from those of diphtheria.

The diphtheritic deposits, according to Laboulbene, are plastic products which are morbid and are deposited upon a tegumentary surface, the skin or mucous membranes, by exudation upon those parts which they are to invest and are not persistent.

The same author says that we mark the existence of plastic products of a grayish or yellowish hue and which appear to be located upon the thickened mucous membrane.

At different periods of their formation these pseudo-membranes are opaque, somewhat delicate and thicker towards the center; others are grayish or yellowish. The first,—the more delicate, are easily detached, the adhesion and tenacity of the latter being well marked, they adhere to the mucous membrane.

This plastic product forms more or less extended, and not little islands which tend to coalesce. Sometimes the plastic exudation covers the entire tonsil and also the uvula. Sometimes also it forms a lardaceous coating located at the base of the pharynx. The subjacent membrane which is reddened, is bloody in little patches, but the surface is not ulcerated; the mucous membrane which surrounds the cast is tumefied. The submaxillary glands are congested, painful and the neck swollen.

If we examine at a more advanced stage of the disease we discover the false membrane in a state of putrid solution. These membranes detach themselves in threads which are mingled with the saliva, or which are attached to the posterior part of the mouth by some points upon their surface.

Where the plastic product is not adherent below, the diphtheritic false membrane has been reproduced, it resembles an ulcer in appearance, which has thrown off threads of decayed mucous membrane.

The lesion of the superior alimentary and respiratory passages are not more important to include in the natural history of diphtheria than many diseases of innervation. We cannot witness the immediate and sudden prostration which bears no proportion to the duration or severity of the disease, the excess of heat and other disorders, calorification, the rapid pulse, the dilated pupil, etc., without coming to the conclusion that there is a profound disturbance in the functions of the nervous centers of animal and organic life. I have observed an uncertainty of gait, as well as stiffness and lameness in the muscles of the neck; incontinence of urine and involuntary stool, which leave no doubt of these centers being poisoned.

PROGNOSIS.—Children under eight years of age are less likely to recover from a severe attack of diphtheria than older persons. I have observed in some cases that children predisposed to croup are difficult to cure, because of the imminent danger of the diphtheritic exudation in the larynx. The disease in adults is not so hazardous to life. Dr. Willard, of Albany, lost but three out of 188 cases in adults. When we hear the peculiar noise caused by the glottis involved in the disease, it forebodes an unfavorable prognosis.

When the child throws his head back to an angle of about 45° it indicates an instinctive position taken by the child to facilitate respiration.

When we see this instinctive effort, it argues that the exudation of adventitious matter in the cavity of the larynx is closing up the aperture and rendering it difficult for the inspiratory movement to supply the lungs with a *quantum sufficit* of fresh air.

Under such circumstances the blood fails of receiving the requisite amount of oxygen to promote the arterial circulation, and this fact forebodes an unfavorable prognosis. When children under eight years old become suddenly prostrated in its early stage, and sight becomes affected and a low delirium sets in recoveries are very rare.

Those subject to glandular enlargements are liable to be swept away by this disease.

The incipient stage of diphtheria, if met with well-chosen remedies may be cured and under Homœopathic treatment the prognosis may be more favorable.

TREATMENT OF DIPHTHERIA.—Under Allopathic treatment a very large percentage of the victims die of the disease. A persistent use of the proper Homœopathic remedies will cure a great majority of the cases of this malady. In our treatment of some hundreds of cases including many of a malignant type our losses have not exceeded two per cent. We make this statement in order to show the importance of being exceedingly critical in selecting the specific remedies at our command. *Kali bichromicum* and *Mercurius hydriodicum* in the first trituration are salutary remedies. They should be employed as follows: *Kali bichromicum* of the first trit. dissolved in water in sufficient quantity to tinge the liquid with a yellow color should be given in teaspoonful doses every hour. If the deposits do not disappear under the use of this remedy change to the *Mercurius hydriodicum* and give a small powder, dry on the tongue and repeat every hour. If the deposits have not disappeared entirely *Biniodide of Mercury* may be substituted for the Hydriodate.

Aconite and Belladonna may be employed as adjuvant remedies in case there are indications for their use. Attention should be paid to the demands of the system for an appropriate diet.

Meat broths, wine whey, milk punch and the like should be given judiciously from the commencement of the disease, in order to preserve the strength and counteract the typhoid tendency. In case there is a sense of threatened suffocation, the vapor of ammonia water may be inhaled to aid in detaching the albuminous depositions. Ammonia is an excellent solvent of albumen and will often conduce materially to the comfort and safety of the patient. *Ammonia* may be used as an internal remedy when there are strongly marked symptoms of a typhoid character; and when there are indications of decomposition of the blood. It must be employed, however, after the remedies named above.

So important a disease as diphtheria and one which manifests itself in various localities, should not be passed over without a full presentation of the views of physicians. The treatment of diphtheria is necessarily based upon correct principles of pathology.

Quite a number of remedies in the hands of different practitioners have been employed in the constitutional treatment of this disease.

Aconite.—In the forming stage of the disease is one of the first remedies to be employed; it may be given in the lower dilutions in water, five drops in a cup of water may be administered in teaspoonful doses every hour or two according to the condition of the patient.

Belladonna may follow *Aconite* when there is a bright scarlet redness extending over the mucous membrane, the tonsils somewhat swollen, and the posterior portion of the fauces presents a diffused inflammation. Ten drops of the third decimal dilution may be put in a glass of water and a teaspoonful may be given every hour during the stage of inflammation.

Colchicum prepared as above has been found efficacious for the swollen and engorged tonsils when attended with headache and fever.

Rhus tox. when the inflammation of the fauces presents a dark red appearance or when there are dark crimson patches scattered over the inflamed surface. The *Iodide* of *Mercury* has been extensively prescribed in certain forms of diphtheria when the deposit is located upon the mouth, tonsils, uvula, velum, palati and pharynx. I have witnessed the good effects of this remedy in those cases characterized by a tough viscid secretion of the mucus follicles and particularly in those cases where the deposit was loosely adherent and limited in extent, and also in some cases where the false membrane is not completed, but falls off spontaneously. In the admirable work of Prof. R. Ludlam on Diphtheria, this remedy is commended for those cases which are marked by derangement of the alimentary system and also when there is the least appearance of membraneous deposit or swelling of the glands of the neck. He recommends the persistent administration of the Merc. protoiodide 3x trituration every two hours until these symptoms disappear. Dr. Paine says he gave it in the first trituration and the effect in arresting and detaching the false membrane was in many cases most gratifying.

Biniodide of Mercury is commended by Dr. Marcy as having a specific action in the disease when there is high fever with inclination to sleep by day, fever increasing towards evening and delirium, rapid pulse; when aroused complains of difficult deglutition. A *few doses of Aconite and then* a few doses of Belladonna 3d were given first and then the remedy above named has afforded satisfactory results. Some cases of diphtheria have been reported cured when there was great prostration, high fever and inclination to sleep; difficult breathing with considerable stridula and when the head was thrown back; by BELLADONNA and Mercurius solubilis given in alternation every hour; in addition to the *Protoiodide of Mercury* taken internally, the *Muriate tincture of Iron* has been recommended as a local application and this treatment in some cases proved successful.

Kali bichromicum.—This remedy has received great credit for having produced wonderfully successful results when the diphtheritic effusion is on the superior portion of the pharynx, nares, larynx, trachea and bronchial tubes, even down to their ultimate ramifications, the deposit being of a firm texture and of pearly appearance, elastic, fibrinous, securely attached to the subjacent integument. Cases in which a transfer of the local disorder to the larynx or trachea is threatened. There is soreness of the larynx when pressed from before backwards. Aphonia, croupy inspiration or croup, desire of the patient to lie with the head thrown far backwards, in order to throw open the glottis, tonsils enveloped by a thick and well organized deposit, incessant cough, tendency to ulceration and deposit upon remote surfaces, as the uterine and respiratory epithelial surfaces. When putrid symptoms begin to be manifested the remedy should be superseded by some of the *arsenical preparations* or *Nitric acid* or *Carbo vegetabilis.*

Kali bichromicum should be administered in the third decimal trituration, and about two grains should be given every hour, two

hours, or three hours, according to the condition and strength of
the patient.

Dr. J. S. P. Soule feared the use of this remedy in a low
potency, because of the aggravations he had known it to produce. When given every hour he said his patients invariably
grew worse. Cough was almost constant, except in the night
when asleep. It ran up from a slight hacking to suffocation,
which was only prevented by the inhalation of the remedy, whenever the cough became dry and the respiration whistling, and the
suffocation seemed to be imminent. Inhalations were employed
with prompt palliative relief, of course temporary; but it was a
respite. It did not fail in a single instance of relieving the
breathing and loosening the cough, and the ejection of membrane
or large portions of stringy mucous.

The method was simple—about two or three grains of the
Kali bichromicum put in a small tin tea-pot and a half cup of
boiling water poured on it, the vapor passing from the spout was
inhaled. *Aconite* and this remedy appeared to yield satisfactory
results, so much so that in all subsequent cases this treatment was
relied upon, and the Doctor says he had no reason to repent of
this resort.

Kali hydroiodicum.—Dr. Robinson, of Auburn, N. Y., calls
the attention of the profession to this remedy, because he has
tried it, and has never found any remedy attended with such happy results. Used in the same way as the *Kali bichromicum.*

Tartar emetic.—No one can doubt the utility of this remedy
who has given it a fair trial. Laboulbene has shown that this
drug is capable of producing the false membrane in the cavity of
the mouth, especially on the tongue.

They are described as "having the form of irregularly formed
patches, whitish, or grayish in color, somewhat thickened, of a
marked consistence, and firmly adherent.

"In the œsophagus they are small, delicate, pale and easily detached from the subjacent tissue. Beneath the false membrane
the surface of the tongue is excoriated, echymosed, wrinkled, and
forms an elevated margin around the plastic deposit, which is red
and somewhat distended. The œsophageal mucous membrane is
ulcerated; the borders of the ulceration are not elevated, but en-
closed by a red circle, the base being softened and grayish, and at
some points echymosed."

Dr. Ludlam recommends this remedy for sudden swelling of the cervical glands and tonsils in scrofulous children, who are predisposed to catarrhal or asthmatic affections, occlusion of the larynx or lower respiratory passages, by excess of mucus of a feebly organized plasma, with cough, dyspepsia, difficulty of breathing, gasping, which compels the patient to sit upright, or to seek the open air, retching or vomiting of tenacious mucus, without any considerable thirst. Small circular patches, like small-pox pustules, on and upon the mouth and tongue; hepatization of the lungs impending or progressing by closure of the pulmonary air vessels by solidification of effused serum. Our own observation confirms the statement of Prof. Ludlam, who seems to have observed critically the remedial power of this drug.

Arsenicum.—We have found this remedy to act well when the breath is fetid and the nostrils discharge a viscid, foul secretion, and great and increasing prostration.

Arsenicum iodatus seems equally efficient, if not more so in removing putrid offensiveness of the breath in the latter stage of the disease.

Bryonia, Capsicum, Baryta carb., Nitric acid, Lachesis, Cantharis and other remedies have severally a place to fulfil in the hands of the skillful practitioner in the treatment of this formidable disease, and we have only to study their range of action and to correctly affiliate them to conditions for which they are indicated.

CHAPTER XXIII.

SPASM OF THE GLOTTIS.

This disease is of rare occurrence; it was known, however, to the older writers. Dr. J. Clare gave a description of it under the name of "a peculiar species of convulsions of infant children." The disease has been described by modern schoolmen under the name *Asthma* Thymicum.

DIAGNOSIS.—There is no probability of mistaking spasm of the glottis by one who has encountered a case.

It is so alarming in its character, that it immediately excites the attention of parents. It consists essentially in a diminution of the aperture of the glottis so that respiration is occasionally interrupted for a moment, and after violent efforts the child ultimately succeeds in drawing its breath, with a sound approximate to that of croup or whooping cough, occasioned by the very narrow chink through which the air passes. After a time the attack ceases and the child remains in ordinary health, but sooner or later the disease returns, at first the child waking out of sleep in one of them, but subsequently this may occur in his wakeful moments.

The intervals between the paroxysms are at first considerable, but they become less and less until the child has them frequently, so that it scarcely recovers from one before it is assailed by another. During the paroxysm the face often becomes swollen and livid, and the veins filled with black blood.

At various intervals, from a few seconds up to a minute, or at times nearly two minutes, air is at length admitted through the glottis, passing through the contracted rima glottidis, and giving occasion to the peculiar crowing sound. To these symptoms not unfrequently succeeds a fit of coughing or crying which terminates the scene, or if the glottis be not even partially open the child will die in two or three minutes at the utmost. Pallid and lifeless it will die of asphyxia and fall exhausted on the nurse's arm, and it is then the child is generally said to have died in a fit.

I have met with but two cases in my practice of more than thirty-five years, and I noticed in one case the noise of breathing was such as an increased secretion of mucus in the air passages would produce.

The symptom is seldom absent and communicates to the affection the appearance of catarrh and especially of the *catarrhus suffocatio*, by which name it has been known by some. There occurs during the disease a slight swelling of the hands, feet and the fingers and toes become rigid and the thumb is frequently drawn into the palm of the clenched hand; it is not, however, the flexor muscles that are alone affected; the spasm has been observed in the extensors, producing a permanent spreading and extension of the fingers, which by some is regarded as a favorable indication that the nervous system is less seriously affected than when the opposite condition was manifest. These symptoms are sometimes accompanied by general or partial convulsions, though not always. Several authorities have written sentiments in confirmation of this view of the disease.

PROGNOSIS.—From the description we have given it would seem that nothing very flattering to the hopes of the parents could be said by the physician and though by many it is looked upon as a disease of the most serious nature, it has been maintained that it is rarely fatal by NORTH, while others think it will yield to proper remedies. Several children of the same family on attaining a certain age have died of this trouble, and I have never received information of a case of permanent recovery. It is certainly an alarming affection and quite surely will prove fatal.

CAUSES.—In the cases which came under my personal observation, one was congenital, and the other was supposed to result from injury inflicted by the carelessness of a midwife at the time of the child's birth.

From what we have previously written it may be inferred that a predisposition to this affection is laid in the organization, —a circumstance confirmed by many observers.

If not congenital it may be said to be constitutional and liable to occur before the period of the first dentition. Some think damp houses or damp seasons may provoke an affection of this kind, but almost all writers agree that it occurs generally in children of a constitutional taint. Among the exciting causes, must be considered fright, or any influence that over-excites the nervous centers or any part of the nervous system. The bare removal of a child into new surroundings will sometimes provoke a paroxysm.

TREATMENT.—Allopathic—Soda to correct the acidity of the stomach, and Iodine against the scrofulous diathesis, or *Iodide of potassium* for the same purpose. The Allopathic treatment varies to suit the different pathological views; some recommend active cathartics, some, counter-irritation applied to the throat, and others recommend an embrocation composed of soap liniment and other ingredients, and others simply a regulation of the diet, and free exposure to pure air.

HOMŒOPATHIC TREATMENT.—For children, *Aconite* when the spasm comes on, followed with *Belladonna*, *Cuprum*, *Gelsemium* and *Sulphur*. Accessory means consist in keeping the child warm, and applying warm water with a sponge to the throat.

Spasm of the Glottis in Adults.

Spasm of the glottis occurring in adults owing to pressure on the larynx and trachea, or on their nerves, has been separated from the spasm of the glottis in children; although the symptoms, causes, etc., are much the same. In adults, however, the affection is secondary, whilst in the child this is doubted by some and affirmed by others.

CAUSES.—Irritation of the trachea or œsophagus in the vicinity of the larynx, bronchocele, aneurism, etc., all of which must be ascertained by careful examination.

PROGNOSIS.—When the affection is persistent the great object is to obviate the suffocation, by obviating all the circumstances that may provoke the paroxysm.

This is difficult, and therefore the prognosis must be unfavorable, and yet it is incumbent on the medical attendant to enjoin freedom from mental and corporeal agitation.

Perfect quiet, an inclination of the body forward so as to favor the respiratory effort and warm bath during the continuance of the paroxysm.

ALLOPATHIC TREATMENT consists of opiates in connection with the warm bath.

In hysterical females, a spasmodic affection of the laryngeal muscles is by no means uncommon, giving rise to what is termed hysterical croup. The paroxysm consists of a long, protracted, loud and convulsive cough, followed at times by a crowing inspiration and by dyspnœa so great as to threaten suffocation. This state may continue for two or three hours, or until the patient faints or a decided hysterical attack supervenes. The Allopathic treatment is that recommended for hysteria; during the attack dashes of cold water over the face and neck, or a douche from the spout of a coffee pot. Spirit of ammonia applied to the nostrils, and when the patient is able to swallow, *Sulphuric ether* and assafœtida pills may be administered freely.

HOMŒOPATHIC TREATMENT.—Between the paroxysms requires *Ignatia, Platina, Cimicifuga* and *Aurum* of the 3x in half-hour doses of the remedy selected. For the fit *Camphor* and *Moschus*. The Camphor when there is a general coldness of the surface. The Moschus is to be administered in case of a fit, every thirty minutes. Ignatia if there is weeping, or great sensitiveness and inability to sleep. Other remedies may be consulted and prescribed according to the symptoms. *Assafœtida, Belladonna, Pulsatilla, Staphisagria, Valerian, Hyoscyamus* are remedies to select from according to symptoms. This practice has a decided preference over the Allopathic, inasmuch as the natural struggle to rid the system of the disease is materially aided.

Morbid Productions in the Larynx and Trachea.

The cartilaginous structure of the larnyx and trachea are liable to hypertrophy, and when the mischief proceeds so far as to occasion narrowness of the larynx, signs of suffocation ensue. No serious inconvenience results when the hypertrophy or the different cartilages are moderately increased above the normal size. There will, however, be a sense of constriction in the larynx in a greater or less degree, which if neglected may progressively increase and interfere with respiration. Unless some means are brought to bear to arrest the overgrowth, there will be an increasing dyspnœa and signs of suffocation. The cause of this increasing dyspnœa, if not known during life, becomes apparent on dissection if the enlargement is accompanied by tenderness on pressure. An iodine ointment has been prescribed for application to the affected part and rubbed in night and morning. Leeches have also been recommended.

But this treatment is less certain of affording relief than carefully selected Homœopathic remedies. Argentum nitricum in the 3x or 6th centesimal trituration if given in daily doses may arrest and remedy the difficulty. Also *Aurum muriaticum* if the hypertrophy has supervened on syphilis. Ossification of the cartilages in old people frequently occurs, but with little inconvenience, unless hypertrophy at the same time causes the difficulty described above. It is only when the cartilages are entirely ossified that a fatal result is likely, and this rarely happens.

Total dysphagia must take place if it ever occurs, and death is inevitable. It is said that no danger can result from ossification of the cartilages of the trachea, notwithstanding it is a morbid change. In consumptive individuals tubercles are sometimes met with in the mucous membrane. If they primarily occur in the larynx, they may undergo softening and give rise to all the phenomena of chronic laryngitis and require a similar medical treatment. Polypoid tumors may form in the larnygeal and tracheal mucous membranes, similar to those on other mucous surfaces. As there are no positive signs of their presence, no Allopathic treatment is recommended. But if suspected, Calcarea carbonica may be given in the 30th attenuation. We can have no positive knowledge of their presence except by dissection after death, and this has been the case with other morbid formations, either calculous concretions or hydatids, which never come to light except by dissection.

Foreign Bodies in the Larynx and Trachea.

The effect of foreign substances passing into the larynx of adults is sufficiently known. But in children there is not the same facility. In case of some foreign bodies being impacted in some portion of the air passages they have often been mistaken for spasm of the glottis or croup. If it be known that some solid substance has passed into the larynx of a child, the earliest resort to means to get rid of the trouble is desirable.

The most simple resort is mustard water, make the child drink it freely until it vomits, if this fail give hive syrup for the same purpose. The act of vomiting may relieve the wind pipe of the foreign body. If these means should fail of giving relief, more trouble may ensue. If all these measures fail, tracheotomy is recommended. The earlier the resort the less dangerous for the child.

CHAPTER XXIV.

DISEASES OF THE BRONCHIA AND LUNGS.

Inflammation of the bronchial tubes like other inflammatory diseases admits of two divisions, acute and chronic; the former may be subdivided into the ordinary acute and the epidemic form.

Acute bronchitis in the ordinary form has usually been regarded in the light of a catarrh, which consists of an acute inflammation of the mucous membrane of the bronchial tubes. It is properly a pulmonary catarrh, as that which affects the lining membrane of the nares is termed a nasal catarrh. A defluxion of mucus from any of the open cavities is very properly termed a catarrh which must be distinguished by a term indicating its locality.

Pulmonary catarrh therefore is confined to the mucous membrane which lines the bronchial tubes and is synonymous with bronchitis. The milder forms of bronchitis, constituting what is usually termed catarrh of the chest, are quite familiar, and no one passes through life without having experienced to some extent the nature of them. They are readily managed and commonly need no medical attention.

The symptoms which attend the ordinary form of acute bronchitis, are those of a common cold, as inflammatory irritation of the lining membrane of the nose is indicated by sneezing. So is that of the bronchial tubes by cough, both being due to the reflex action of the nerves. The same reflex action gives occasion to a convulsive respiratory effort on the part of certain muscles, to drive the air swiftly through the air passages and thus to sweep away from the mucous membrane any source of irritation that may exist there.

Cough, consequently, in these affections is a mere symptom although formerly it was regarded as a *disease* by itself.

When the cough first begins, it is dry, because the first effect of inflammation of mucous surfaces is to diminish or arrest the discharge from them; but this stage soon passes away and the mucous follicles secrete more profusely and much larger quantities than in health, and a fluid of unnatural character; the pathological state again resembling the cold in the head, in which the nasal mucous membrane is first dry and devoid of mucous secretion, but is soon subject to a reaction and secretes profusely. It is this condition which we term a "common catarrh" and is usually accompanied by a moderately hurried respiration and slight febrile heat.

When the inflammation is more deeply seated in the bronchial tubes a pain is experienced in the chest with a sense of heat under the sternum, frequent cough, at first dry, difficulty of breathing, rapid pulse, more or less headache, especially when coughing or after the paroxysm of coughing.

If the inflammation is great and the face is red and tumefied, there is generally a corresponding amount of fever, loss of appetite and thirst; the tongue has usually a white coating upon it, and the mouth a clammy taste.

The paroxysm of coughing sometimes provokes vomiting, and for the most part there is an aggravation of all the symptoms towards evening. Occasionally, too, the bronchitis is attended by phlegmasia of other mucous tissues and a protracted febrile indisposition to which the name "catarrhal fever" has been given, although the term is nearly another name for acute bronchitis.

In severe cases the cough is violent and occurs in violent paroxysms producing severe pain and a sense of laceration which is often referred to the lower portion of the sternum. The pain shoots with violence from the ensiform cartilage to the back, and owing to the exertion of coughing the various muscles of the chest and abdomen are painful on pressure.

About the third day, the cough, which up to this period has been exceedingly dry, becomes more moist, a thin, frothy secretion is expectorated, sometimes with comparative ease, and at other times with more or less difficulty. The sputa gradually increases in quantity, and becomes more consistent, viscid and ropy and at length thicker, more opaque and less in quantity.

Toward the termination of the disease it becomes white, yellow, or more frequently of a gosling green color, and if expectorated in water it is suspended at or near the surface.

Pus is occasionally united with the mucus of bronchitis, especially in cases of measles; we have treated cases of this kind and were surprised at the quantity of pus secreted by the bronchial mucous membrane. There was apparently no cavity, and yet at times the expectoration seemed to be streaked with blood, and sometimes, though rarely, tinged with bile.

We have seen distinct membraneous formation thrown off by the cough having the shape of the bronchial tubes. This pseudo-membraneous secretion requires violent efforts at coughing to expectorate it, and yet there is not that danger of fatal suffocation, as in cynanche trachealis.

Not much can be elicited by physical examination, the signs are mostly negative. Percussion reveals a clear sound over every part of the chest, indicating that there is nothing like a morbid deposit in the tubes.

Auscultation indicates a sibilant or whistling, dry ronchus or *rale* exhibiting a contraction of the tubes by reason of the thickening of the mucous membrane. At a later period when there is an increase of the mucous secretion, the mucous *rale* is heard.

There may be such an accumulation of mucus as will obstruct the ramifications of the bronchia and temporarily obscure the respiratory sound which is usually heard when the ear is placed over any region of the thorax. The duration of the disease is from one to two weeks. The mild cases commonly classed under the head of catarrh generally terminate favorably.

The same may be said of the majority of cases of the severer form, but occasionally, owing to the extension of the inflammation, to the small bronchial subdivisions and to its narrowing the tubes and filling them with mucus, death takes place from asphyxia. The disease may likewise pass into the chronic form, or may become complicated with pneumonia; and there would seem to be no doubt that tubercles may form and pass through their various stages; so that death may result from phthisis.

It is proper to remark that simple bronchitis almost invariably commences in the lower and posterior portion of the lungs, usually attacking both sides and advancing from upwards, whilst the opposite is the case in phthisis.

The causes are the same as those of inflammatory affections of the respiratory apparatus in general. The inhalations of any irritating vapors or gases may induce it; the inhalation of extraneous bodies contained in the atmosphere, as the dust from gun-cotton, steel-grinding, etc. It forms a part as it were of eruptive fevers, measles, variola, varicella, whooping cough, scarlet fever and other diseases.

TREATMENT.—It is usual with Allopathic practitioners to make a cough mixture of ʒi ss. of mucilage of gum arabic, ʒi of the syrup of poppies and ʒiij of water.   Dose, a tablespoonful when the cough is troublesome; or ʒi of mixture of almonds and ʒi of Sulph. of morphine.   Dose, a tablespoonful when the cough is troublesome.   Bathing the feet in warm salt and water or mustard water is recommended as accessory means; warm wine whey as a stimulating diaphoretic, or perhaps a mixture of syrup of squills and sweet spirits of nitre to promote *diuresis* is regarded a useful adjuvant.   But we regard this treatment as attended with some danger in inflammatory affections of this kind.

HOMŒOPATHIC TREATMENT discards these means as well as bloodletting, antimonials, expectorants, blisters, as being decidedly injurious.   In the first stage we have given Aconite to reduce the fever and the attendant symptoms.   This remedy always acts favorably in removing irritable fever and in producing regularity of the circulation, and in many mild cases is the only remedy required.

In those cases attended with pain in the chest and a sensation of heat under the sternum, and particularly when the cough produces pain in the head and is aggravated by motion, we have obtained satisfactory results from Bryonia.

Belladonna is indicated when the patient complains of chilliness, dryness of the throat and dry cough, and great soreness beneath the sternum with continuous pain in the head or sensation of rawness caused by capillary congestion.

In the second stage when the mucous membrane yields a copious secretion and still the pain and soreness remains, when the cough is constant and much mucus is expectorated we have found Phosphorus decidedly beneficial.

When the bronchial vessels fill rapidly with mucus, and but little pain and soreness is felt in the chest, we have found Tartar emetic capable of affording prompt relief.

We have also found Gelsemium, Causticum, and Hyoscyamus, among the useful remedies when indicated.   Hyoscyamus in troublesome night cough and in the advanced stage; when the sputa becomes thick, we have found Hepar sulph. and Pulsatilla useful. Mercurius is useful when the expectoration is thick or plastic.

Diet as in all inflammatory affections should be light, barley water and flax seed tea may be used as emulcent drinks. Toast and black tea if the patient has any appetite.

Epidemic Acute Bronchitis or Influenza.

This peculiar affection has prevailed epidemically throughout whole regions of country and has received a nomenclature corresponding to each place, each region or country. In Germany it has been called Spansiher Ziep, Pips. This was an epidemic which prevailed in 1580. The same disease became *Shafhusten*, a fashionable disease in the 16th and 17th centuries and it is now called *influenz*. In France it has been called Grippe. Other terms in different countries are used to signify the same bronchial disturbance. In England and America the term influenza prevails, though some writers retain that of epidemic catarrh. The disease has prevailed epidemically in this country at four different times, at least, since 1833, and what is regarded as remarkable, a very large proportion of the population in all the chief cities was attacked about the same time.

Symptoms of the approach of the disease are very much like an ordinary cold, with sneezing, sniveling and profuse coryza. The stage of invasion is marked by chilliness, and general aching in every part of the body, followed by fever, thirst, quick pulse and inflammation of the nasal and bronchial mucous membranes, and accumulation in the air passages amounting almost to suffocation.

In some cases of children and aged persons, especially in those inclined to pulmonary catarrh, it has proved fatal; but generally the disease runs its course rapidly and terminates in health.

CAUSES.—It is as difficult to define the precise cause of this epidemic as that of other epidemic diseases. It has spread in all countries with equal severity and without regard to seasons, and so far as can be observed, independent of all conditions of the atmosphere. It has therefore been conjectured that certain influences arising from the soil or from variations in physical conditions operating on the surface of the earth have led the way, but this is very unsatisfactory. Sometimes the disease is character-

ized by considerable irritation of the mucous membrane lining
the air passages and sometimes by actual inflammation of them,
and also to implicate the lungs in the extended inflammation, and
thus it would seem that the air taken into the lungs had been
contaminated by some irritating substance and readily detected.

We have observed that the nervous system is liable to suffer
to a greater or less extent from this disorder, that digestion and
the circulation are also impaired, and on the totality of these derangements a low nervous fever has supervened that has accompanied the disease throughout its whole course, provoking an
irritation of the pulmonary mucous membrane.

This again might seem to indicate the presence of malarial
influences depressing to the nervous system.

TREATMENT.—This disease has such a diversity of symptoms.
In Allopathy no fixed rules are laid down. Blakiston recommends
blood-letting at first. Graves endorses this treatment. Dr.
Wood says that in simple uncomplicated cases very little treatment is required, except the keeping of the patient in bed with
prudent nursing, as in ordinary acute catarrh. Leeches have been
recommended by some applied over the sternum, and cupping by
others. Andral recommends an emetic composed of fifteen or
twenty grains of *Ipecac*, or two grains of *Tartar emetic*. When
the mouth is clammy or bitter, the tongue coated and loss of
appetite, and a sense of weight in the epigastrium, Cartwright
recommends antimonials, to keep the patient nauseated to prevent pneumonia or pleurisy. Counter irritation with blisters
over the chest, and opium to mitigate the severity of the cough,
is recommended by some; others recommend a Lobelia emetic to
conduct off the disease at once. Graves says foment the neck
and chest with very hot water, and Blakiston adds to the hot
water stimulants and tonics. But nothing can be said in favor
of the above modes of treatment, because they are liable to do
more injury than good.

HOMŒOPATHIC TREATMENT.—Aconite in the febrile stage, is a
most valuable remedy. We have seen the effects of the early administration of it in aborting the disease. We gave the 30th
attenuation to a patient who complained of pain in the head,
dryness of the nose and mouth, frequent sneezing, pain in the
back and loins, and at a time when thousands were suffering from
influenza, and repeated the dose once in two hours for a day, and

the patient recovered so rapidly that we had no need of other remedies.

Arsenicum is indicated when there is not much fever, heat or thirst; but great restlessness of the patient at night, drinks often but little at a time, very weak, simultaneous chilliness and slight fever, discharge of acrid and corrosive mucus from the nose, which has a violent burning and excessive soreness of the *nares* with fugitive pains in the loins and extremities. We have been successful in curing when we have employed this remedy in the lower attenuations; but of late we have preferred the high and highest attenuations with satisfactory results.

Nux vomica. — Alternate chills and fever in the evening, when there is much discharge of mucus during the day, and the pituitary surface becomes dry at night, without much thirst, lightness of the chest, constipation, and great heat in the head and face. We have given this remedy in various attenuations with beneficial results, but we prefer the high in mucous fevers of this epidemic type.

Mercurius.—When there is constant sneezing, soreness of the nose, with constant watery discharge, offensive smell, profuse perspiration at night, worse in the morning, can't bear cold air, and particularly when many persons are affected at the same time.

Hepar sulph.—In persons who have taken much Calomel, and who become assailed by epidemic influenza, with fever and pains in the limbs, aggravated by cold air, and motion causes a headache.

Lachesis.—When the influenza is characterized by severe catarrhal symptoms and running of watery fluid from the nose, which at the same time is swollen and very sore, we have many times employed the three last named remedies in various attenuations, in the treatment of influenza, and when correctly affiliated we have without exception cured our patients. But latterly we are induced to give the high potencies credit for the greater promptness in affording relief.

Euphrasia and Alium cepa have been satisfactorily employed by us in that stage of influenza characterized by a white mucous discharge from the nose, with watery eyes, sore and running.

Pulsatilla when there is loss of appetite and smell, and the discharge from the nose is thick yellow mucus; sometimes greenish and offensive.

Ipecacuanha, Arsenicum, Bryonia for asthmatic breathing in influenza. The above remedies in medium potencies, if well affiliated, will satisfy the patient and reward the practitioner.

Chronic Bronchitis.

Chronic bronchitis is a catarrhal affection which is very common in the temperate regions of the globe, especially observable in the fall, winter and spring when its worst features are often exhibited.

It is only in the present century that its pathology has been comprehended. In 1808 Badham wrote an interesting treatise on Bronchitis, and Hastings wrote on the chronic forms of the disease, and from that time to the present, inflammatory affections of the mucous membrane lining the bronchial tubes have received considerable attention from pathologists.

The mucous lining of the trachea itself may be affected with chronic inflammation independent of the laryngeal and bronchial mucous membrane. It is liable to extend, however, so as to implicate either the laryngeal membrane or that of the bronchia. In case the trachea alone is affected, it is denoted by a slight *cough* at first, but subsequently it becomes violent with mucous expectoration, at times streaked with blood, and occasionally purulent. The pain is sometimes severe and is felt from the base of the cricoid cartilage to behind the last portion of sternum. When the tracheal mucous membrane is ulcerated and swollen, a whistling sound is heard during respiration, from which it is sometimes suspected that the trachea is obstructed by a tumor.

Dyspnœa sometimes accompanies this condition of the mucous membrane. The voice is rough, but not extinguished unless the inferior ligaments of the larynx are also inflamed.

The general symptoms are the same as in chronic laryngitis and phthisis trachealis may be the result.

Chronic bronchitis may or may not be the termination of the acute. It exists in some instances when there has been no acute form of the disease to initiate it. The symptoms are not always uniform. In all cases there is cough; this, however, varies in character and intensity. The bronchial cough is more marked, perhaps, than other affections of the respiratory organs. There is also great variation in the appearance of the matters expectorated. They are often clear and transparent and at other times very frothy, and again they are viscid, adhesive and contain small white lumps which attach themselves to the vessel.

These lumps have been mistaken for tuberculous matter and indicative of phthisis.

But this is doubtful as may be proved by placing them on a piece of paper and exposing them to heat; if they are merely sebaceous matter from the mucous follicles of the fauces and larynx they will leave greasy stains on the paper, while tubercular matter from the lungs will not.

In other cases the sputa will be greenish-yellow puriform mucus, commonly devoid of odor; but at other times they are disagreeably fetid; under the proper kind of treatment many cases have recovered. We once treated a lady for chronic bronchitis where the room was filled with the almost insupportable odor of the sputa, which she was constantly expectorating; she recovered entirely from the disease under the influence of *Muriatic acid* and Carbo veg.

There is a great variation of quantity of matter expectorated. Sometimes with little effort the quantity is sufficient to exhaust the patient, while in others the cough is severe and exhausting, while the expectoration is trifling; when the former is the case it has been termed *humid* and in the latter, *dry* catarrh. We have now under treatment a gentleman about fifty years of age, who has suffered every fall, winter, and spring with chronic catarrh for the last fifteen years; his cough is exceedingly distressing and exhausting, but his expectoration very trifling, and at times he suffers from paroxysms of retching and struggling to throw off the smallest quantity of this mucus, which seems to irritate the air passages. The only respite from this retching and coughing is from the internal use of Ipecac and Tartar emetic.

In the less severe cases the respiration is not much affected; but in those more affected the breathing is sometimes oppressed and not unfrequently wheezing and asthmatic, which comes on in paroxysms.

In a majority of cases there is but little pain unless the paroxysms of coughing are frequent and severe. The general symptoms are not usually very marked or disturbed.

There is seldom any fever as a rule. Though in some cases a subacute inflammation and fever may attend cough. The fever is usually of the hectic type and seriously affects the nutritive sys-

·tem as is evident from the gradual emaciation that attends it. It comes on daily in the afternoon and evening, with circum· scribed redness of the cheeks, quick and irritable pulse, under which the patient sinks away.

The symptoms of the severer forms of chronic bronchitis approximate very nearly to those of *phthisis pulmonalis*. In-milder cases persons may be affected for years with chronic cough and expectoration without the general health being materially, impaired at all.

Generally the disease mitigates as the warm weather of the spring comes on, and almost disappears or is decidedly improved during the summer. It returns again in the fall and winter. This may be repeated uniformly for a series of years and gives occasion to the name, winter cough.

It has been observed, however, that victims of chronic bron-chitis gradually wear out and die, and therefore the disease has been appropriately named "lingering consumption."

It is not at all unlikely that death may occur in old people especially, owing to the copious secretion of mucus in the smaller bronchial vessels, interfering with hæmatosis, so that the nutrition of the nerve is in this way modified by the deprivation of duly oxydized blood, the system in the other parts suffers and the patient succumbs.

In some instances chronic bronchitis may be affiliated with some affection of the lungs and pleura or some chronic affections of the heart, which must be duly noted in order to form a sound· prognosis and to establish proper indications for treatment.

The physical signs of chronic bronchitis are like those of the acute, purely negative. The normal resonance of the chest may exist throughout. Nearly all the phenomena observed in acute bronchitis are found in the chronic form. The bronchial rales are heard as in the acute form of the disease, and these scarcely ever obscure the vesicular murmur, and this is the same in the chronic form of the disease.

Sibilant rales of different character, which in certain cases have been compared to the clicking of a valve or to the pronuncia-tion of the word TIC, gurglings like those of phthisis are heard where dilatations of the bronchial tubes exist, and also cavernous respiration, pectoriloquy and other distinct sounds. The diagnosis of chronic bronchitis is generally very easy, but difficulties hard to encounter may occur. Then in incipient phthisis, before the lung has become much engorged, and tubercles are not present in sufficient numbers to give a dull sound, there might be a difficulty in deciding whether the trouble is bronchial or tubercular. By careful observation, or it may be said by critical observation, it is possible to avoid this dilemma. The general symptoms, it is true, are somewhat alike; but the mucous rhonchi or rales will be found to occupy quite different situations in the two diseases.

In phthisis the rales are heard at the summit of the lungs, while in chronic bronchitis the rales are heard over the various regions of the chest and they vary in their character at different periods.

The dilatation of the bronchia which may give rise to obscurity in the diagnosis is rarely accompanied by induration of the lung in a sufficient degree to diminish the sound of percussion as in phthisis around the tubercular cavities; and moreover, the dilatation is not always found at the apices of the lungs, but in most cases it is observed in the middle portion where it may exist for some time without apparent change or augmentation.

CAUSES.—Although chronic bronchitis is frequently the sequel of the acute form, it, as before remarked, may occur as a primary disease.

In advanced age, and particularly in subjects worn out by excesses, it is not uncommon. It sometimes occurs after whooping cough in children, and in some cases it is associated by some organic lesion of the heart, or tuberculosis. The same irritating substances floating in the air which give rise to acute bronchitis may also occasion the chronic form.

The repercussion of measles or other eruptions or the suppression of some habitual flux, such as hæmorrhoids, may be reckoned among the causes which occasion this disease.

TREATMENT. — In Allopathic practice the treatment is regulated by circumstances; when there is much febrile excitement an antiphlogistic treatment is recommended and especially if the bronchial inflammation is attended with pain and soreness of the chest; counter-irritants are applied to the chest; such as ointment of tartarized antimony, croton oil and intermittent blistering; while tartar emetic is administered internally as an alterative. Stokes recommends a liniment composed of turpentine and acetic acid, so as to keep up an erythema upon the surface. Emetics are also recommended as an occasional resort. Groves recommends a mixture, tartar emetic and ipecac, for evacuating the bronchial tubes, and Dover's powders to allay the cough; and with these agents an indefinite number of expectorants and balsams to palliate the sufferings of the patient; all of which it must be confessed only detract from the vital condition of the system, and seldom afford permanent relief.

HOMŒOPATHIC TREATMENT.—The object of this treatment is to strengthen and uphold the struggle of nature to regain her normal condition when depressed. This cannot be done by any system of depletion and therefore it must be apparent that this (the Homœopathic treatment) is by far preferable in all bronchial inflammmations.

Aconite.—In those cases of chronic bronchitis characterized by acute paroxysms of fever, rapid and full pulse, hot skin, dry cough, thirst, and a dull pain in the head. When these attacks occur Aconite may be given either in solution or pellets until the fever subsides. The doses may be repeated every hour.

Belladonna may be given in the same way as Aconite when there is oppression and weight in the chest, chilliness, short and anxious, and even rapid respiration, a shaking, spasmodic cough, pain in the head, over the eyes and shooting through the temples.

Bryonia is useful in those attacks which have the following symptoms: Headache aggravated by movement, pressure in the eyes, dryness in the throat, respiration difficult, short and anxious, pressure on the chest as if from a weight; stinging in the chest, cough with stinging in the chest, and with severe aching pains in the head. This remedy as well as Belladonna may be administered in pellets or solution every hour until there is a subsidence of the symptoms; and we will remark that there exists a great similarity between acute bronchitis and the acute attacks of chronic bronchitis.

Patients may entirely recover from the former; but in the latter patients may be suffering steadily with chronic bronchitis; when from a trifling exposure to a bleak wind *all* the symptoms of acute bronchitis may supervene suddenly; and during a long siege of chronic bronchitis, the patient may suffer from a series of these acute attacks. It will therefore appear sufficiently plain why the same remedies prescribed in acute bronchitis, are called into requisition in these seasons of acute suffering attendant on the chronic forms of the disease.

Tartar emetic is indicated when there are severe paroxysms of coughing and obstruction to the respiration amounting almost to suffocation, when there is a wheezing respiration, a mucous *ronchia*, a shortness of the breath, and anxious oppression of the chest, great anxiety and agitation, palpitation of the heart, pains in the back and loins, pressure in the eyes, pains in the head and throat.

During the progress of acute and chronic bronchial affections, severe paroxysms of coughing, with rattling of mucus in the bronchia, difficult respiration, cough aggravated by eating, speaking, inhaling cold air, or lying down. Repeated doses of this remedy rarely fail of affording relief.

Rhus toxicodendron is indicated when worse in the evening, at night and when at rest, mitigation of symptoms on rising and walking about, when external cold aggravates and frictions and warm applications alleviate them. Gentle exertions may relieve while violent exercise may aggravate them.

We have known violent and convulsive paroxysms of coughing with considerable oppression and mucous rattling by day and greatly aggravated towards night, to be relieved by Rhus, and when there was a return in subsequent seasons of cold weather, the same remedy always relieved.

It is said on good authority that when fatiguing paroxysms come on worse in the evening, about 8 o'clock that a medium potency of Rhus, caused at first aggravation, but afterwards there was great improvement the same night.

Nux vom. is regarded an analogue of Bryonia and its use is indicated by similar symptoms, viz., symptoms aggravated by motion, in the open air and after eating, worse early in the afternoon.

Phosphorus is indicated when there is complete loss of voice, and when there is more or less pain in the larynx, constriction of the chest, cough with frothy or rust colored sputa. Dread of coughing.

Causticum after Phosphorus in case of loss of voice, a hoarseness and roughness of the throat in the morning, constant tickling in the throat causing a short hacking cough. Pain over the hip when coughing and involuntary urination.

Hepar sulphur is also indicated when there is rattling of mucus in the trachea or dry hoarse cough and roughness in the throat. Rattling, choking cough worse after midnight. Hoarse anxious wheezing respiration with danger of suffocation when lying down. This remedy is particularly applicable to bronchial irritation from exposure to cold west winds, 3x or 6x trituration every two hours, or three times a day.

Mercurius solubilis when the whole mucous membrane lining the bronchial tubes is affected, hoarseness and sore throat, violent racking cough at night, as if it would burst the head and chest.

Pulsatilla.—We have seen the salutary effects of this remedy in a loose cough, with copious secretion of yellowish or greenish mucus, and also for a troublesome dry cough at night, with scraping and dryness of the throat, chilliness even in a warm room. Hot, dry skin with little or no thirst; suitable for persons of a mild temperament, or sensitive disposition. In severe cases we have given the third decimal dilution every hour.

Sanguinaria canadensis.—This remedy has a wide range of action and occupies a prominent place among remedies for various diseases. In chronic bronchitis attended with dryness of the throat and a sensation of swelling in the larynx. Severe cough with circumscribed redness of the cheeks and pain in the cheeks.

Fluent coryza and a watery diarrhœa, burning in the hands and feet at night; it is an excellent remedy in chronic bronchitis, to remove the peculiar irritation of the pre-tubercular state. This remedy when indicated may be given either low or high in dilution; we have seen the 30th dilution in drop doses administered every hour produce a satisfactory result, and we have seen severe coughs yield readily to the 3x trituration in two grain doses every two hours.

Sulphur in chronic bronchitis is an indispensable remedy in many cases. It is indicated by hoarseness and loss of voice, and for the sensation as of something creeping in the larynx and particularly for a loose cough with expectoration of thick mucus and soreness in the chest; stitches in the chest extending to the back; pain in the left side. Frequent weak and faint spells; constant rattling in the chest. This remedy is the most useful in long standing cases when the cough and expectoration is gradually wearing upon the system. It has been observed that lean people who bend forward when they walk, are the subjects most likely to derive benefit from this remedy. A single dose of this remedy once in twenty-four hours is sufficient.

Chronic bronchitis, as before stated, exhibits its worst features in cold weather. During the summer it may entirely disappear.

This fact suggests that change from a cold to a warm climate may prove beneficial. If a limited season of warm weather effects so favorable a change, what will a change to some genial, warm climate like that of St. Croix or St. Thomas in the West Indies, where cold weather never chills, or the heat of the weather never oppresses. Diet, when a paroxysm of fever in chronic bronchitis destroys the appetite, it is not for the interest of the patient to compel himself or to be compelled to take solid food in such quantities as might weaken the system by overtaxing the stomach. It is decidedly better to give such patients gruel, toast-water, broth, with rice-water and beef tea, and when the fever disappears and the appetite returns, a more generous diet is always allowed. Much of the time during the progress of the disease the patient may have a good appetite and should be allowed his preference for any kind of non-medicinal food, and if he chance to find an article which disagrees with his stomach let his physician or his own good judgment admonish him not to indulge in a repetition.

Summer Bronchitis or Hay Fever.

This singular variety of chronic bronchitis is frequently met with in this country and Europe.

It has received various names indicative of the season and the cause of its occurrence.

With us it is commonly called *hay fever* or hay asthma, because it usually occurs about the termination of the hay harvest.

The most common symptoms are itching of the eyelids, and at times of the inner canthi of the eyes, with irregular attacks of violent sneezing, sense of weight on inspiration; and at times considerable difficulty in breathing, and copious discharge of mucus, thin and watery, and often acrid, from the nasal cavities; sense of smell and taste very often impaired during the attack. There is also redness of the eyes, and sometimes sense of weight in the forehead.

A gentleman, of Bristol, England, in reading a description

of this kind of catarrh, writes that with little exception, he has suffered with the disease every June for seventeen years; he further writes as follows, being a physician: The attack generally begins with me in the latter part of May, with great itching of the eyelids, particularly at the inner canthi; from which I regularly during the month extract some cilia which grow very near the corner and increase the irritation.

My most troublesome symptom is sneezing. It is of a violent kind and often continues eight or ten times. The defluction from the nostrils is most copious at these periods of the day; while in the intervals I have no catarrhal symptoms.

Expectoration of clear mucus is also considerable. My sneezing attacks are sure to come on while I am visiting my patients—to my great annoyance.

This comfortless state generally continues five or six weeks, but is never sufficient to interrupt my employment, or render any confinement necessary; though I am always free from it while in the house.

How far grass or hay has anything to do with this affection I cannot satisfactorily determine. There are certainly several hay-fields within a quarter of a mile from my house. The air seems to make me worse and an open window is my abhorrence, while I am thus indisposed.

Last week I spent an hour or two in a friend's hay-field with a party of ladies, but the syllabub or the ladies' pastoral sports had no amusement for me and I was glad to get to a corner of the field where my streaming eyes and nostrils and noisy sternutations might escape both remark and commiseration.

Certainly during that afternoon in the hay-field was the worst attack I ever had; but whether it was the air which was cooler than usual, or the hay I could not tell; I must, however, confess that my *fancy* on the subject has always leaned more to the effect of some subtle particles of an irritating nature; than to the ordinary causes of catarrhal affections.

My lungs are rather asthmatic, formerly I had a good deal of asthma; I have never found time to try any remedies.

Another gentleman, not a physician, who has long been a sufferer from this disagreeable affection, says his first attack was from undergoing an operation for the removal of hæmorrhoidal tumors; which he had suffered from since his boyhood; and they were wont to *bleed freely*. This operation arrested the discharge. The attacks usually occurred after the middle of July; always very suddenly without any apparent predisposing cause. He suffered worse when he ate fruit, such as peaches in particular.

Having great heat in his nose, he says he resolved to restrict himself to a cooling diet, eating fruit freely and drinking ice water; he never had the disease as bad or so long, or sneezed so much as when upon this diet. He had two general sneezing attacks each day until the middle of October. A daily discharge of limpid fluid from the nostrils, heat in his head; and he complained of being unable to collect his ideas, so as to write anything but stupid articles, because of the confusion of his head, at times he had fever, and at times he had not; the feet hurt when at rest. He says he has tried countless remedies, regular and irregular, and nothing has cured. He thinks *Prussic acid* with black drops three times a day has sometimes palliated the disease and rendered the suffering more tolerable.

He says his doctor called his disease a peculiar form of gout, that cannot be cured and that the dribbling from the nose is ceaseless for five or six weeks, because the head required it, or otherwise the *gout* might fall in the eyes, at any rate he found it a mighty trial of faith, patience, good nature, etc.

It is obvious from the foregoing details that the disease does not belong to *Asthma*, as now defined, neither nervous or spasmodic; but that it is an inflammatory irritation of the mucous membrane of the eyes, more than of the whole respiratory apparatus and that the asthmatic dyspnœa is attributable to this, and this fact renders it proper to classify the disease with chronic bronchitis. We have known of many cases of this distressing trouble, and have prescribed Mt. Washington for the weakness and Mt. Desert for the rock to be taken *ad libitum*, though not always salutary, as remedial measures.

Before we proceed to detail the treatment which this formidable disease requires, we will consider what pathologists say about the *causes* of this unique affection.

Some attribute it to motes in the atmosphere escaping from decaying vegetation, some to the fine and almost unobservable irritating spores that escape from grass in its flowering season. Some to the same invisible agents which float in the air from the flowers of other plants, and notably from the *rag weed*, a species

28

of *Ambrosia* which grows wild in waste places in cities. Some to fresh-cut grass, and some to well-cured hay. But most of these causes seemed to be well supported. Those who make hay seldom suffer, and the disease is on the whole rare; not a very large proportion of the inhabitants ever suffer a six-weeks' siege with it, and we must therefore look for another specific cause. It is probable that some congenital idiosyncrasy exists as a predisponent in those who are its victims, or that some incidental changes, which other forms of disease may have produced in the physical system, have rendered it impressible to exciting causes either from hay or flowers, and caused this annoying trouble. What is called a rose cold belongs to the genus " hay fever," and there are many persons who can never smell a rose without suffering immediately from an attack of asthma.

It seems to be a disease which affects only about one in a hundred, and is an annual visitor. I once knew a lady who suffered annually from an attack commencing on the 20th of August and lasting about six weeks. The first invasion of the disease in her case was soon after her first child was born, and she suffered annually after this for many years. She finally had a respite from the disease after passing through a second period of gestation and parturition, fourteen years after the first attack.

TREATMENT.— It would seem from the confession of Allopathic physicians that but little advantage had been derived by them from medical treatment. Dr. Oliver Wendel Holmes prescribed "gravel ten feet deep as the only positive cure." Dr. Philip Sing, physician of Philadelphia, said he had utterly failed in every case which came under his care.

Others have maintained that *it ought not to be cured*, that the catarrh was nature's prophylactic against the gout. But it hardly seems probable that nature could be so Allopathic in her prophylactic measures. It is affirmed also that cold shower baths are the best prophylactic to employ before the period of expected recurrence, accompanied by the internal use of the Sulphate of Quinine and Sulphate of Iron, as follows: Give a pill three times a day, made of three grains of Sulphate of Quinia and one grain of the Sulphate of Iron.

Several cases are cited where this was an effectual protection, for persons who previously had been severely afflicted, and especially when they were exposed to the same influences as before, and have brought upon themselves all the agonies of spasmodic asthma.

It has been advised to visit the seashore, but in some instances this has proved injurious by causing a development of the plague before the time of its expected visit. The chlorides of lime and soda have, it is asserted, been successively used by Dr. Elliotson in aborting the disease.

A gentleman sprinkled a solution of the chloride of soda all around his room or bedchamber, and he did so with perfect success.

HOMŒOPATHIC TREATMENT.—But little can be said affirmatively concerning the successful treatment of hay fever with Homœopathic remedies. It has baffled the skill of the best practitioners, and yet there have been many cases of the kind cured. It has been my fortune to have many ladies and gentlemen to treat with the best skill I could bring to bear. Some cases have apparently yielded to remedies, but by far the greater number have run on for weeks in spite of all efforts to relieve them. The following remedies have often palliated, and in rare instances cures have been made:

Aconite, Arsenicum, Arum triphyllum, Allium cepa, Bryonia, Euphrasia, Ferrum, Hepar, Ipecac, Mercurius sol., Nux vom., Pulsatilla and Sulphur. We have prescribed these remedies, and all with some satisfaction.

Aconite, when there is some sense of fullness of the head and heat in the nasal cavities, with frequent paroxysms of sneezing, will remove the febrile symptoms, and for a time mitigate the catarrhal symptoms.

Arsenicum when there is a burning sensation in the eyes and nasal cavities, and also when the thin limpid fluid discharged from the nostrils causes a smarting and soreness of the nose, and also when there is much sneezing and asthma, will palliate all these symptoms and greatly relieve the distress.

Arum triphyllum when there is much itching of the eyelid and the inner canthi of the eyes, and inclination to sneeze several times in succession, smarting of the upper lip, by a discharge of acrid fluid from the nose, and paroxysms of asthma. Eyes inflamed, nose very sore. Arum trif. has been given with great benefit. It has sometimes aborted the disease. We had two patients during the last summer who have not failed for many pre-

ceding years of an attack of hay-fever about the middle of June
that would last until September. We gave each of them, when
they first began to complain of itching and smarting of the eyes,
the Arum trif. in the 30th potency, in pellets; we prescribed
four pellets every three hours. One of these gentleman was
cured of these premonitory symptoms, and was able to attend to
business daily through the remainder of the summer, without
being interrupted by an attack of this annoying trouble. The
other gentleman was not so fortunate; his attack gradually grew
worse, and much to his annoyance, because his business required
his presence. Finding that Arum trif. did not serve him as well
as I wished I gave him Mercurius sol. three times a day, from
which he derived benefit. All his symptoms became mitigated,
and he remained in this partially cured condition for ten days.
I then gave Hepar sulph. and this worked well; he gradually
became better, and at the end of four weeks he was gratified to
find himself well.

A gentleman subject to annual attacks of that disease came
to us in June and said he felt the premonitory symptoms of his
annual trouble. His eyes and nose were slightly implicated; I
gave the 3x of Allium cepa, and it took effect very soon and he
was better for several days, faintly hoping that the remedy would
cure him.

In a week he returned much discouraged and said his nose
was in a sad condition, discharging but little, but he could scarcely
breathe through the nostrils because the schneiderian membrane
was so swollen. I gave him Silicea 30th; did not repeat the
dose. The next day he was decidedly relieved of the symptoms;
gave placebo. He still remained somewhat relieved, but not
cured. In two weeks Mercurius sol. was given and whether it had
any curative effect we cannot say, but he gradually recovered
from an attack which lasted four and a half weeks.

With Sulphur as well as Silicea, we have often witnessed
good palliative effects and when patients have been much depressed. Pulsatilla has worked well. I could occupy considerable space in detailing cases where I could but believe the duration of the case was abridged and the suffering greatly palliated.
I will close this article by asserting that summer bronchitis, hay
asthma, or by what other named, or by what other name it may
be called, is in all probability a curable disease and the more we

study into its nature, and the more closely we can affiliate remedies Homœopathically, the better will be our success. As for example: S. B.—Esq., a merchant annually subject to this disease, commencing in July and terminating about the first of the following October; when he first felt his last attack coming on he came to us for a prescription. The lids of his eyes looked red and his nose was affected with a tickling in the nostrils. Hepar, the 6x was given, and the next day he was better of these symptoms, but complained of obstruction of the nasal ducts and heat and soreness of the nose and eyes, with frequent inclination to sneeze. Mercurius 3x trituration was given and in forty-eight hours these symptoms were removed, and although relieved of the itching of the eyes and nose, and the burning and obstruction, together with the sneezing, he was suffering from another feature of the disease which was spasmodic asthma, for which Ipecac was prescribed with but little advantage. After, Ipecac, Hyoscyamus, and for twenty-four or forty-eight hours there was considerable improvement. The treatment was followed up to meet the variations from day to day, until the disease passed off and the gentleman himself admitted that his suffering was very greatly abridged in duration from what it had been in former years.

During the continuance of this disease the patient may or may not have his usual appetite for food. Avoiding condiments generally except salt, he may select his diet as his appetite may dictate while under treatment.

Since writing the above I have been informed that Prof. E. M. Hale has succeeded in aborting several cases of hay fever with Sabadilla.

Whooping Cough, Tussis Convulsiva.

This disease may be conveniently divided into three stages: 1st, the catarrhal, which resembles the ordinary bronchitis. There is more or less indisposition, chilliness, depression, suffusion of the face and eyes, increased secretion of tears, sneezing and discharge from the nose, along with a dry, fatiguing cough, which comes at short intervals or fits.

During that stage there is more or less fever which is more apparent during the night. The duration of this stage varies; in some instances it lasts but a few days and others several weeks. 2nd, we have the nervous, convulsive or spasmodic stage, which marks the peculiarity of the disease. The cough is now so extremely violent, convulsive and distressing that the patient feeling its approach runs and lays hold of any support he can reach until the paroxysm is over, and after a short period of rest another paroxysm ensues, and these are usually of more frequent occurrence at night than by day. The cough consists of a rapid number of unequal expirations which seem to follow so quickly that inspiration is impracticable. The return of blood is interfered with thereby and the face becomes swollen and livid. The eyes are copiously suffused with tears, the veins of the neck are prominent, a profuse perspiration breaks out and suffocation seems to threaten. But in a short time small and imperfect inspirations are effected and then a long and distressing inspiration attended by a peculiar noise which has been termed a whoop from which the disease takes its name. The cough sometimes ceases after this peculiar inspiration, but other paroxysms with similar peculiarities may succeed until a viscid, ropy, colorless secretion is with difficulty expelled, sometimes attended with vomiting. It is supposed that the sonorous inspiration is owing to the entrance of the air into the trachea through the glottis, the opening of which is spasmodically closed in part or contracted; a severe pain is sometimes felt in the forehead which requires attention. Some, indeed, have regarded this symptom as indicative of the encephalic origin of the cough. The duration of the paroxysms are from one to four or five minutes and this recurrence varies in like manner from every five or ten minutes, but others are not more than six or eight times in twenty-four hours. When the paroxysms are not very long or fatiguing or very frequently repeated, the child resumes its play immediately afterwards, but when they return with great violence and difficulty of breathing, pain in the chest and general indisposition remain. Fright, crying or any sudden mental emotion or rapid running may bring on a paroxysm of coughing. Stimulants of any kind promote the frequency of the coughing paroxysms. Sometimes blood will flow freely from the nose, mouth and ears during a fit of coughing.

We have seen in one or two cases a violent determination of blood to the head, in one of those fits causing the child to faint and appear prostrate as in epileptiform difficulties.

In excessively severe fits of coughing the bowels and bladder may be subject to involuntary evacuation.

Hernia is sometimes the result, and also prolapsus ani, from severe straining, and protracted paroxysms of coughing.

Between the fits there is but little if any indisposition, unless some complication is present that keeps the system depressed. The duration of whooping cough varies, sometimes the first and second stages will pass away in from two to four weeks. The third stage is that of the decline of the cough. This is indicated by the decline of the spasmodic phenomena, less frequent and less severe.

Every day the intervals between the paroxysms lengthen and the fits of coughing become shorter and shorter.

The peculiar whoop becomes less and less, and ultimately disappears altogether. The fluid expectorated becomes opaque and thicker, of a greenish hue generally, though sometimes puriform, although the cough is reduced to the level of an ordinary catarrh, and gradually ceases, especially if the case runs its course in the spring or autumn; but if in the autumn and winter it may be more protracted.

The entire duration of the three stages of the disease varies from six weeks to three months. If frequent colds are contracted during the existence of the disease, the sequel may prove to be serious. We have known several cases to terminate fatally when a sequel of bronchial catarrh has been entailed. Whooping cough has also been complicated with pneumonia, and at times with tubercles, which are developed and formed as a sequel.

CAUSES.—But little is known of the causes of whooping cough. It is one of the diseases which invariably assumes the epidemic form. It rarely occurs as a sporadic disease, and persons once afflicted with it rarely have a recurrence. Seldom does it occur twice in the same person, yet some do have it several times, and some it is asserted are liable to take it every time it prevails epidemically. When whooping cough prevails extensively the mortality is considerable. It is often the agent of stirring up latent dyscrasies, which united with it soon wear out the system. Whether whooping cough is contagious or not is yet a mooted question. Some maintain that it is propagated by direct contagion, and cite many facts in favor of this theory; others again contend that epidemic influences, confined to restrictod districts, are the overpowering agents in generating the disease.

Those who regard the disease contagious fix upon a period at which it becomes so, and when it ceases to be so. From our own observation, we are inclined to the opinion that it is contagious, and may be communicated at any period until the whooping ceases.

TREATMENT.—The Allopathic treatment is merely palliative, for the opinion is cherished that the disease must run its course, and cannot be aborted or abridged, nevertheless a treatment is laid down for the three stages of the disease as follows: First stage, expectorants. Second stage, anti-spasmodics and laxatives. Third stage, gentle means are commended.

HOMŒOPATHIC TREATMENT consists of affiliating well chosen Homœopathic remedies, and this for the protection of patients, and for preserving their constitution and aiding nature in her struggles seems altogether the best. No drugs at all depressing to the nervous system can be useful or curative, and therefore in each stage of the disease such remedies are to be employed as the symptoms may indicate. It must be admitted that each stage is characterized by a distinct class of symptoms.

First or primary stage, *Aconite* when the cough is dry, hard, or wheezing with burning pains or tickling in the trachea, more severe at night, skin hot and dry, high colored urine with general feverishness, repeat the doses every hour until the skin becomes moist.

Belladonna.—Persistent cough which is sudden and violent, with sore throat and headache, worse at night; nose bleed or effusion of blood in and around the eyes. Dose, repeat every hour.

Secondary stage. Drosera is indicated for the convalescent stage when the following symptoms are manifest: whooping with frequent and severe paroxysms of hoarse loud cough and at times hæmorrhage from the nose, eyes, mouth and ears. There may be little or no fever, except perspiration, vomiting of food, water or slimy mucus. Hahnemann speaks of this remedy as curative or at least efficient in the treatment of epidemic whooping cough, except in scrofulous children, who may first require antipsoric remedies, such as *Calcarea carbonica*, *Carbolic acid*, and *Sulphur*. A dose of either may be given first and then a dose of the *Drosera* after every fit of coughing.

Ipecacuanha is indicated when in the convulsive stage, every paroxysm of coughing brings on vomiting of mucus and food, and ends in asthmatic breathing; watery or bloody discharge from the nose and eyes, violent cough which threatens suffocation. Often useful at commencement of second stage.

Corallium rubrum.—Teste mentions this remedy as occupying the first place among the remedies for the spasmodic symptoms and whoop of the second stage. It is a remedy much esteemed when the symptoms are violent, and when the fits are attended with a flow of blood from the ears, nose, and mouth, with violent retching and vomiting.

Cuprum met.—For the violent forms of whooping cough, causing convulsions; the body becomes rigid, the cough suffocating, and the breath nearly suspended during the paroxysms which occur frequently and generally attended with vomiting; great prostration and slow respiration; two grains of the 3x trituration may be given after each paroxysm.

Kali bichromicum is indicated when there is much cough, glairy phlegm, which adheres to the throat and frequently causes vomiting. This remedy has been commended for night perspiration in this disease. 3x trit., 2 grs. after each fit.

Hyoscyamus when the paroxysms are frequent, but not so violent, and when they are much worse at night; and not attended with fever, and also when the expectoration is mucus of a thick greenish color; and also when the cough produces sparks, scintillations or spots before the eyes. This remedy may be given in the 1st dilution, ten drops in a half tumbler of water; a dessert spoonful after each paroxysm until they begin to mitigate in frequency and severity, and the patient can rest quietly at night.

Alumina.—Dr. C. Hering regards this remedy exceedingly valuable in the treatment of the catarrhal stage of whooping cough, when the bowels are constipated. Dose, of the 30x dilution, four or five times a day.

Arnica montana when the cough has produced muscular soreness of the throat and chest, and also when the patient dreads the approach of the paroxysm on account of its provoking a painful soreness of the chest. Arnica should be administered after each fit of coughing, ten drops in half a tumbler of water, dessert spoonful for a dose.

Bryonia is indicated when there is rheumatic soreness of the chest, and considerable heat in the air passages which renders it distressing to cough.

Bromide of Ammonia is highly regarded as a specific remedy for whooping cough in England. We have no provings of the drug except of an incidental character. The same remark will apply to *Bicromide of Mercury* and the Bromides generally.

Cina.—In whooping cough when the child is troubled with worms, the signs of which are itching of the anus, and picking of the nose, fretfulness, and variable appetite.

Nitrate of Amyl is said by Dr. Ruddock to be capable of arresting the paroxysms by inhalation.

Tartar emetic has had a beneficial effect in cases of fully developed whooping cough when there has been much vomiting after the paroxysm.

Sulphur when the whooping ceases; which is the *third stage*. This stage requires careful treatment that *débris* of the disease may be carried off effectually.

Hepar sulphur is also indicated in this stage, particularly when the phlegm is tenacious, and persistently adheres to the parietes of the air passages.

DIET should be light, digestible, and nutritious, and if either children or adults have any appetite for food they should be allowed it in moderate quantities.

More than the stomach will kindly receive will provoke paroxysms of coughing. Toast water, flax seed tea, barley gruel, or oat meal water are severally grateful to patients and are often all that the system requires.

Whooping cough is a painful disease to witness; and when mothers see the distress and suffering attendant on each paroxysm they are often led to inquire if there is no immediate relief. It would gratify any physician to answer in the affirmative. But all he can do is to point to the *accessory measures* for protection and relief.

Infants should be immediately taken up and cared for; for when a fit occurs they should be held and supported in the best and most favorable posture.

Friction with goose oil, or olive oil, or soap liniment is soothing and the impression prevails that much relief is obtained from this resort.

Vaccination with non-humanized matter is on good authority an excellent palliative. A child who has not been vaccinated, should receive this attention as soon as the first whoop is heard.

During the latter part of the past winter and commencement of spring, our attention has been directed to the peculiarities of this disease. In many instances it has apparently made its appearance as the sequel of exposure to wet and damp weather. After the feet have been wet, the child begins to cough as from an ordinary cold, and suffers more or less from chilliness, depression, suffusion of the face and eyes, increased secretion of tears, discharge from the nose, paroxysms of a dry fatiguing cough, attended with more or less fever, and worse during the night. Finding but little success in the treatment of a cough of this kind when the above symptoms were present, I have in most cases observed that after one or two weeks the cough would assume a nervous or spasmodic character, and would come on in violent paroxysms, and very soon would ensue the distressing characteristics of whooping cough. From the beginning to the end, remedies seemed to be of little avail in mitigating the violence of the cough, and yet they proved exceedingly efficient in removing concomitant ailments. In what is usually termed the catarrhal stage, or the stage of invasion, I have found several remedies which apparently relieved the patient of much suffering. Under their influence, I have seen the undue excitement of the lachrymal gland pass away. I have seen asthmatic breathing removed, and the soreness of the chest of which many victims complain, and also the fever entirely dissipated.

On the 5th of February, I was called into a family of six children, the oldest of which had seen but ten summers, and the youngest but a year old. Now, just previous to this, there had been some wet weather and rain, and the house had become damp. The older children played out on the sidewalks and in the yard, and even the youngest had been more or less influenced by the damp atmosphere. The temperature of the weather changed suddenly, and there was a variation of 23° in the thermometer between night and morning, and this group of children from the oldest to the youngest began to cough, and their eyes became suffused with tears, and,from the running at their noses and febrile symptoms we commenced treating them with *Aconite*, 3d dilution, in water. At first this treatment did well, as it subdued the febrile excitement and gave promise of speedy recovery. After an elapse of twenty-four hours, they still continued to cough. Gave *Belladonna*, 3d dilution, in water, dose every two hours for the next twenty-four hours, and still each continued to cough, complaining of much soreness of the chest and more or less headache at each paroxysm of coughing. Gave *Bryonia*, 3d, in water—a few drops in half a goblet—and a teaspoonful every two hours. This removed the soreness of the chest and headache, but still the cough became more violent and manifested itself in paroxysms at short intervals. But little expectoration attended the cough, and, during the intervals between the paroxysms, the children seemed quite relieved. Various remedies were given with the hope of mitigating the cough, with little effect, and, after ten days it became apparent that each was affected with whooping cough; and now we had a fine opportunity to select from the group of whooping cough remedies. We gave *Nux vomica* when the cough was dry, racking and worse after midnight, and in the morning, with vomiting, anxiety and suffocation, with bleeding at the nose and mouth. We also gave *Pulsatilla* for similar symptoms; but witnessed only a slight amelioration. Our plan was to dissolve a few globules of the 3d attenuation in a tumbler of water, and give a dessert-spoonful after each paroxysm, until we could note some change. Sometimes we found the effect favorable and the distress less, but subsequent trials proved that we had made but little headway in arresting the difficulty. At times when the cough was attended with great anxiety and suffocation, and when the face was of a bluish hue and at each paroxysm there was vomiting of mucus, *Ipecac*, given as above, evidently mitigated all these symptoms. When the cough was preceded with crying as if some sore trouble was dreaded, *Arnica*, in the same form, gave decided relief. But I found no remedy that seemed capable of entirely arresting the cough in the catarrhal stage. The nearest that any remedy approached this desirable result, was attained through the use of *Corallium rubrum*, 3d centesimal trituration, a two-grain powder twice a day. After the children had been coughing three weeks or more, this remedy was given as above, and there immediately followed a mitigation of the severity of the symptoms, the number of paroxysms began to lessen, and each returning one became lighter, and three weeks later the cough had disappeared entirely. But one peculiarity was noticeable in these children: they lost flesh, looked pale and sickly even after the cough had left them.

The etiology of whooping cough has been a mooted question among pathologists, and the causes that induce the disease have been difficult to define. It has been maintained that it originates from malaria, from the fact that it prevails in the heat of summer as well as in mid-winter, in the spring, or in the autumn; that it often prevails in frigid, temperate and tropical climates.

From our observation, an epidemic whooping cough may arise from exposure to damp and cold, and then spread from one to another, and from family to family, through some generating influence entirely disconnected from the primary cause. Bennett relates a formidable case that supervened upon wet feet, from which a contagion emanated and spread through a whole community, and that the average duration from the beginning to the ending of the disease, provided it progressed uncomplicated with other difficulties, is about eighteen weeks. It has, according to the observation of most writers, three distinct stages, each of which manifest the same degree of stubbornness, and rarely yields to any kind of treatment; and yet it is maintained that remedial treatment is constantly necessary in order to prevent local inflammations in the respiratory system. The first stage is termed catarrhal, and is attended with symptoms resembling an ordinary cold, and may be complicated with acute bronchitis, or pneumonia. This stage, then, requires special attention. If there is fever, *Aconite* will prove useful; if capillary congestion, *Belladonna;* and these remedies, if they do not remove the cough, may ward off an attack of pneumonia. We have seen the good effects of *Pulsatilla* in the catarrhal stage in removing inflammation from the mucous lining of the nasal ducts.

In the second stage, usually termed the nervous, spasmodic or convulsive, which is known by the characteristic symptoms of the disease, the violence of the cough may be mitigated by remedies. When the paroxysms come on more frequently at night and during the night, *Hyoscyamus*, 3d dilution, will often produce a perceptible amelioration; and in those cases where the victims are forewarned of the approaching paroxysm by a soreness and distress that causes them to cry out, *Arnica*, 3d dilution, has afforded considerable relief. Those cases of whooping cough attended with vomiting, and when the victim feels better during motion, *Drosera* is indicated. When they turn blue in the face as if suffocating, or when the paroxysms are preceded by weeping, *Cuprum* is indicated, and also *Arnica*.

Veratum album is indicated in cases of great exhaustion when children fail to recover strength after a paroxysm of coughing, and are inclined to lean their heads against something for support, and when they have fever with cold perspiration, especially on the forehead, intense thirst, small quick pulse, and emission of urine while coughing; and also when the cough ceases on lying down, and recurs when rising from bed.   A few drops of the 3d dilution, in water, and a dessert-spoonful three times a day for several days, has had favorable results. *Coccus cacti* given in the same way, has had a good effect when a ropy mucus is coughed up at each paroxysm. *Hyoscyamus*, when the cough is dry and occurs most frequently at night. *Conium* for scrofulous children when the attacks are violent and the face flushed, and the expectoration is bloody.

For the third stage of whooping cough, I have found *Sulphur* and *Hepar sulph. calc.* about the only remedies that availed any thing in promoting convalescence.

Hæmorrhage into the Bronchia—Hæmoptysis.

The expectoration of blood is always an alarming symptom; although not a common occurence. When the hæmorrhage into the broncial tubes takes place it is often the commencement of the existence of pulmonary tubercles; and yet when it is a single exhalation of blood from the bronchial mucous membrane it is of comparatively little danger.

When the patient is conscious of spitting blood he is alarmed, whether the blood comes from the bronchial tubes or the throat, unduly supplied from the posterior nares; this latter cause of spitting blood is quite common and really deserves no more consideration than common epistaxis. Hæmoptysis from the bronchial arteries is a rare occurrence; and yet from the mere spitting of blood from the posterior fauces, has been confounded with it; the impression is created that instances of real bronchial hæmorrhage are not rare.

It is not very difficult to discriminate between those of little danger from such cases as come under the head of *real hæmoptysis*. When practitioners boast of their great success in the treatment of hæmoptysis, and the great number of cases they have treated, it would undoubtedly appear from a close examination that by far the greater number of the reported cases would be classed among the examples of venous hæmorrhages; and only to a small extent from the pharynx.

DIAGNOSIS.—Hæmoptysis when it occurs is usually preceded by indisposition to a greater or less extent, and especially by a sense of weight, heat or an uneasy sensation about the chest, with oppression of the respiration and cough.

These signs indicate hyperæmia or congestion of the lungs and a sweetish taste of blood in the mouth.

In addition to these local symptoms the extremities and surface of the body are usually cool, rigors or chills are experienced down the back. The face is sometimes pale, at other times flushed; an accelerated action of the heart and a quick, vibratory, hard pulse; with these a distressing ebullition is felt in the chest, and this is a certain indication that there is an effusion of blood into the bronchi. The respiration becomes labored, and a sense of tickling and pricking is referred to the bifurcation of the trachea. The expectoration of mucus streaked with blood or of pure blood in greater or less quantity now follows. The blood is found on examination to be of a vermilion color, or florid and frothy if recently effused, otherwise it may be dark or black. When the effusion of blood into the bronchial divisions is about ceasing, portions of blood may remain in the tubes for hours and then when expectorated they may be of a dark color. We have many times seen extraordinary quantities of blood discharged from the rupture of some large vessel, and from or in consequence of the same the patients have sunk away and died immediately. Occurrences of this kind, however, are few compared with the great number of cases of hæmoptysis which may occur from constitutional debility.

These severe hæmorrhages are often the result of mechanical injuries or strains. The quantity of blood expectorated varies; sometimes it is mouthful after mouthful, almost amounting to vomiting and then there is usually a cessation and the patient feels relieved. The expectoration resembles red currant jelly, but at times it is not so much colored. Hæmorrhage after hæmorrhage is liable to occur, each of the same character. The quantity lost is at times astonishing, but more especially when it is vicarious as in suppressed catamenia; under such an influence the hæmoptysis may be a monthly occurrence.

Cough usually continues after a copious discharge of blood, with a slight quantity of dark liquid or coagulated blood which gradually ceases.

Percussion of the chest does not elicit any abnormal sound, and the reason is obvious. The blood is expectorated as fast as it transudes into the tubes and for this reason auscultation elicits no sound except the mucous rale.

The diagnosis between hæmoptysis and hæmatemesis may occasionally be difficult, and also between the former and epistaxis. The latter occurring from the posterior nares into the pharynx, may be expectorated along with the mucus of those parts. The color of the blood is nevertheless quite different. That which comes from the nares is not florid or frothy; while that which comes from the bronchia *is*. The blood which actually comes from the stomach may be distinguished in like manner from that evacuated in hæmoptysis as well as by other signs. In hæmatemesis there is a sense of weight in the stomach and a nausea; in hæmoptysis, there is cough and dyspnœa, and moreover blood that is vomited may be mixed with the contents of the stomach.

"The blood of hæmoptysis may proceed from the rupture of an aneurism of the aorta, but in such a case there is not much time for doubt, as the case speedily terminates fatally."

As hæmoptysis is rarely a primary disease, but usually symptomatic of some internal lesion, it becomes important to determine the nature and extent of such lesions, and ascertain if possible whether it is an actual tubercular dyscrasia. If this be so the prognosis will not differ from that of *phthisis pulmonalis*, and the existence of tuberculosis must be determined by the signs and symptoms which we shall describe hereafter.

Hæmoptysis may be the foundation of tuberculous deposits, even though nothing of the kind exists when it occurs if a predisposition of the kind exists in the subject. Andral affirms "that he has found less than one-fifth of those who have labored under hæmoptysis exhibit tubercles on dissection." There are many who have manifested a proclivity to this affection early in life and yet have physically risen above it and have attained a ripe age. It is quite certain however, that tuberculosis either precedes or follows this alarming difficulty.

CAUSES.—In order to fully comprehend the circumstances under which hæmoptysis is the result, we must take a critical view of the predisposing, as well as the exciting causes.

The *predisposing causes* are numerous; first phthisical habit, second, faulty organization, third debility, fourth, a strumous diathesis, fifth, hereditary taint and any organization in which the vessels are loosely protected by the parts in which they creep. Extreme youth or advanced age, these are severally predisposing causes and there are many others.

The *exciting causes* are also numerous, any change of atmospheric pressure may excite hæmoptysis. Exposure to cold winds or to extreme heat, over exertion, fatigue, etc. It is affirmed that women are more liable to this affection than men, and this we may infer from the effects of interrupted catamenia; vicarious hæmoptysis is commonly from this source.

It has also been affirmed that the spitting of blood is of more frequent occurrence in the spring and autumn when the days are warm and the nights are cool, or at least that there is quite a contrast between the cool of the morning and evening and the midday warmth. Andral also affirms that nearly every attack takes place either in the morning or evening. Any violent exertion that throws the blood towards the face or head or that creates considerable vascular action will often bring on an attack.

It has occurred with great severity immediately after sexual intercourse. It is recorded as having taken place during the act.

In the advanced stage of pulmonary consumption, hæmoptysis may be a symptom of abscess in the lungs.

It is averred that certain vapors from acids or dust from the type foundry or from that which ascends from pulverizing of certain drugs, as in that of Ipecacuanha, may provoke an attack and lastly on the authority of a distinguished pathologist a prolonged mercurial treatment has provoked an attack and the same author warns his professional brethren against the persistent use of Iodine; on the same account we are inclined to doubt the correctness of the observation.

TREATMENT.—Allopathic.—Derivative treatment in moderately severe cases, such as limited bleedings from the arm or a brisk cathartic with a low diet, absolute rest of body and mind; in cases less severe where mucus streaked with blood is constantly coughed up. Balsam of Fir has been recommended and occasionally a powder of Calomel, Jalap and Ginger. For immediate use when the attack is sudden, salt and water is recommended in a saturated solution in doses of a wine glass full repeated frequently

24

until the bleeding ceases, and then Balsam Tolu and Opium or Balsams and syrups with occasional cathartics are prescribed.

HOMŒOPATHIC TREATMENT consists in the affiliation of remedies in accordance with the symptoms: as a condition for successful treatment, rest and quiet are enjoined with a light diet of non-medicinal nutritive food. It is not inconsistent with the treatment to recommend a swallow of water saturated with salt, every half hour, when the attack is sudden and no physician at hand.

Aconite when the attack is preceded by fullness or congestion of the chest or burning pain, palpitation of the heart, anguish and restlessness, great fear and nervous excitability.

Arnica if caused by a fall or blow upon the chest or on the back, or expectoration of dark and coagulated blood. Tickling under the sternum, and when coughing produces a sore pain as if bruised in the chest, or when he feels a general soreness after the injury.

Belladonna when there is severe congestion of the chest and head with rigors passing down the spine, constant tickling in the larynx with cough and expectoration of bloody mucus, stitch-like pains in the chest, worse when in motion, very susceptible to cold, pain in the forehead and eyes.

China is an excellent remedy after great losses of blood or fluids, ringing in the ears and fainting fits, and when the patient is worse every other day. This remedy is called for when there is great debility from night sweats.

Hamamelis virginica is indicated for profuse hæmorrhage of venous blood coming into the mouth without any effort, like a warm current from out of the chest, mild, calm and at times taste of sulphur in the mouth.

Hyoscyamus when the hæmorrhage is preceded by a dry cough especially at night, obliging the patient to sit up; frequent starting from sleep with wildness of expression and red face, and when everything looks large this remedy does wonders.

Pulsatilla when hæmoptysis results from suppressed catamenia, and in obstinate cases where the blood discharged is black and coagulated. Well suited to persons of a mild disposition.

Ipecacuanha when hæmoptysis is so profuse that the patient spits mouthful after mouthful of blood, until he is affected with nausea. Ipecac is the remedy to procure speedy relief.

Phosphorus when there is much mucus tinged with blood and a cough which produces soreness with dryness of throat and mouth, or when the system is run down from emaciation; feels better after sleeping.

Rhus tox.—Suitable for dry cough which seems as if it would tear something out of the chest. Discharge of light red blood, tickling under the sternum which excites the cough. It is suitable for hæmoptysis caused by straining or lifting or reaching with the arms. There are many other remedies which may be called into requisition in the treatment of this disease as Bryonia, Crocus, Ferrum, Millefolium, Nitric acid.

We have obtained the greatest benefit from employing the above remedies in the 6th, 12th and 30th potencies. We have generally begun with the 6th—a few drops in a glass of water, and repeat in teaspoonful doses every hour, two hours, or three hours as the case may demand. We shall have reason to detail the benefits of Homœopathic treatment in this affection when we treat of pulmonary hæmorrhage.

Accessory treatment.—When lying on the back excites bleeding, the patient should lie with his head and shoulders elevated, inclining to either the right or left side.

Hæmorrhage into the Lungs.

This affection has been considered under the head of hæmoptysis, but pathologically there is a marked difference between an exhalation of blood from the bronchial mucous surface, and an effusion of blood into the pulmonary parenchyma, and the relation which they sustain to each other renders it advisable to consider hæmorrhage from the lungs next in order after hæmorrhage of the bronchia.

The disease which we are now considering is only a pulmonary apoplexy, and not an uncommon affection.

Rostan affirms that the affection is both common and yet rare; we have witnessed a sudden death from this kind of apoplexy, and we have read of other instances of instantaneous death by asphyxia. But usually the existence of the trouble is duly announced by a train of symptoms.

DIAGNOSIS.—The disease comes on suddenly and is marked by great difficulty of breathing; amounting at times to a threatening of suffocation.

The hurried and unequal movements of the chest exhibiting the greatest irregularity with great anxiety, are characteristic symptoms. The characteristic physical signs are absence of the respiratory murmur over that portion of the chest beneath which the hæmorrhage has occurred; and a crepitant rhonchus around the effused part; this accords with the observation of Laennec, but Andral says these signs would not appear constant, and in many it would seem percussion and auscultation have afforded no information. The expectoration of a black fluid devoid of fetor and resembling a solution of liquorice juice, has been esteemed a more positive sign of the collection of blood which has undergone some change prior to its expulsion. Laenuec says that where the blood is at the same time poured out into the air vesicles, the quantity expectorated may be enormous, as much as ten pounds have been lost in forty-eight hours.

The causes of hæmorrhage into the lungs are obviously the effects of heart disease; or pulmonary consumption. A case of an individual came under our immediate observation, a merchant aged fifty years who had suffered some from asthma and palpitation, but not sufficient to require his absence from his business.

He went on an errand after church on Sunday to one of the hotels; on taking a seat he began to breathe with great difficulty and his respiration rapidly grew more and more labored, for the next ten minutes when he expired. It was decided by the coroner that he died of pulmonary apoplexy, caused by the rupture of an aneurism, which an autopsy revealed.

Another case is related of a young man of consumptive tendency travelling for his health, who suddenly became a victim to pulmonary apoplexy from the softening of a tubercle and a hæmorrhage into the lungs.

TREATMENT.—The common Allopathic treatment for every kind of apoplexy is to bleed copiously, and not to be prevented from this course by apparent debility or feebleness of pulse. Dr. McIntosh remarks, however, that "the plan of bleeding in every case of bloody discharge from the lungs is very bad, because it is bleeding for a name without pathological consideration." When blood is flowing freely from ruptured tubercles, bleeding freely from the arm is recommended for the purpose of producing syncope in order to arrest the flow, or change the current of the blood toward the artificial outlet.

HOMŒOPATHIC TREATMENT.—For cases in which only a portion of the lung is filled with blood and the exit into the bronchial tubes is not rapid, Ipecacuanha 3x dilution may be given every hour, and Hamamelis in 3d dilution may be given in like manner.

Causticum, Belladonna, Pulsatilla, and Phosphorus may be consulted. So far as our own observation goes, no treatment can accomplish much. For when a blood vessel is ruptured and there is a hæmorrhage into the pulmonic tissue, there is but little hope for the patient, other than a brief and partial palliation of his sufferings, and yet the benefit of Homœopathic treatment in this fatal disease has been witnessed in producing a degree of absorption of the clot in the lungs; and to exert a styptic influence in arresting the flow or expectoration of blood and consequently of prolonging life. The worst cases of hæmoptysis have been mitigated with well chosen remedies, and hæmorrhage into the lungs which finds its exit through bronchial expectoration may also reap a corresponding benefit.

Pneumonia—Inflammation of the Lungs.

By the term "pneumonia" is understood inflammation of the lungs. Some writers have included in this, inflammation of the bronchial vesicles or air cells, or the inter-vesicular tissues, or of both combined. If we, however, regard the vesicles or air cells, to consist of terminal extremities of the bronchial tubes, it is difficult to separate pneumonia from bronchitis, which as we have seen is an inflammation of the cells and minute tubes. But some writers believe that it differs from bronchitis in the ordinary acceptation of the term, merely in the occurrence of parenchymatous inflammation, such as solidification, suppuration, or abscess phenomena, not proceeding from any inherent difference in the disease, but a result of anatomical structure. Inflammation of the lungs admits of the divisions which may be termed acute, chronic and typhoid.

Acute inflammation of the lungs has been described as *vesicular* inflammation of the lungs or lobular or *double* according to the part of the lungs affected. Vesicular pneumonia is that in which the vesicles alone are supposed to be implicated. *Lobular pneumonia* is applied to the disease when all the vesicles of a lobe are implicated. Lobular pneumonia when all the lobes of a lung

are concerned, and double pneumonia when both lungs participate in the inflammation; and it is termed pleuro-pneumonia
when both the lungs and pleura are implicated at the same time.

Lobular pneumonia occurs more frequently in the inferior
than in the superior lobes. This is confirmed by Andral and
others. It has been claimed that the right lung was more liable
to participate in the inflammation than the left and especially so
in children under six years of age.

A much larger proportion of children suffer from double
pneumonia than adults, and the progress of the disease differs in
some respects from the same in adults.

From the extreme delicacy of the texture implicated, hepatization in some part of the lung is more liable to occur with
children than with adults.

DIAGNOSIS.—Pneumonia begins with febrile excitement,
cough, viscid, bloody, or purulent expectoration. The cough is
dry and fails to disclose the degree of inflammation; shortness of
breath and breathing with difficulty are symptoms which may
accompany other affections, and yet taken with physical signs are
sufficiently positive indications of acute inflammation of the lungs
with other symptoms; much pain is experienced in the chest or
in that portion where the inflammation exists, sometimes in the
right lung and sometimes in the left. Pain in the external part
of the chest in connection with other symptoms is regarded a
sure indication of inflammation of the lungs. The presence of
this pungent heat over the surface of the chest in nineteen cases
out of twenty is quite a certain diagnostic sign.

When we take into consideration the characteristic symptoms
in the order of their development, there seems to be but little
difficulty in referring them to the lungs.

At the commencement of the inflammation, there are general
febrile symptoms, a dry cough sets in. If some degree of bronchial irritation has preceded the attack, the first expectoration
may be mucus; about the second or third day, however, the matter of expectoration becomes characteristic; consisting of mucus
intimately mixed with blood; yet this appearance is by no means
constant.

Andral says the disease may occur without any characteristic
expectoration, and when the bloody and viscid sputa are present

their appearance may vary from yellow or rusty to florid red in the same day.

After awhile in the progress of the disease, the sputa increases in density, and becomes viscid, transparent and so tenacious as to adhere to the sides of the vessel; and it may remain in this condition until the disease is about to terminate, when it varies according to the nature of the termination.

If the inflammation of the lungs terminates in resolution, the sputa loses its red color, and great viscidity, but these will return in case of any reccurence of the inflammation; or on the other hand if there is any serious aggravation of the disease, the sputa becomes less, and even very small in quantity; difficult to expectorate and sometimes utterly suppressed. This suppression may be real, or the sputa owing to its viscidity, and the depressed condition of the patient may accumulate in the bronchial tubes and induce death by asphyxia.

The rusty sputa is found in cases of pneumonia which occur in persons of a robust habit, and is regarded valuable as a diagnostic sign. But in a great variety of cases of feeble persons and children as a sequel of fever, Dr. Stokes says "it is esteemed of little value." It is probable that many cases of pneumonia begin and run their course and terminate either favorably or unfavorably, when that which is expectorated varies but little from that which is bronchial. It is also noticed that when pneumonia occurs in the course of another disease the absence of the characteristic expectoration is also seen.

When pneumonia terminates in suppuration the expectoration is either purulent or in the form of a fluid which is muco-purulent, or of a purplish red color; having the consistence of gum water, and similar in appearance to prune juice. This latter form of expectoration occurs when the pneumonia is of a low grade, and in broken down or greatly impaired constitutions, and the former in consequence of acute pneumonia in healthy persons.

Dyspnœa sometimes occurs in pneumonia but not so often as in bronchitis or pleuritis. We cannot estimate, however, the extent of the obstruction by the amount of difficulty in breathing, in some attacks of pneumonia there is great oppression of the chest accompanied with anxiety, lividity of the face and a sense of suffocation.

These cases frequently have a fatal termination. On the other hand the breathing is singularly easy, especially after the employment of certain remedies even though a considerable portion of the lung is hepatized. The pain in pneumonia is believed to result from pleuritis, which generally accompanies this disease and involves parts of the chest, especially at the commencement the pain is most severe. The cough augments it as does inspiration, change of posture, percussion and lying on the left side.

With regard to the complication of pleuritis and pneumonia in children there have been various opinions. Dr. Gerhard, of Philadelphia, thinks such complications rare, others think it a frequent occurrence.

Andral says when there is no pleuritis present, that a kind of weight and sensation of heat is experienced in the chest. The idea has prevailed that pneumonia patients always lie on the affected side, but this is erroneous says Andral, the decubitus is generally on the back.

The most distinguished pathologists recognize three stages of pneumonia.

First, the stage of engorgement of the lung with blood, and a crepitating ronchus is heard.

Second, solidification takes place with its physical signs. Third, interstitial suppuration occurs, or rather the condition which precedes an abscess supervenes.

Other eminent pathologists maintain that in the first stage the lung is dryer than natural with intense arterial injection; no effusion of blood in the cells. Second, the cells are engorged with blood; no change of structure. Third, solidity and softening. Fourth, interstitial suppuration. Fifth, abscess.

In the *first stage* the chief derangement is local puerility of respiration, which may be esteemed diagnostic if it occurs along with fever and excitement of the respiratory system, and especially if percussion elicits a clear sound which indicates that no permanent alteration of structure has yet occurred.

It is not unusual for the sound on percussion to become obscured until the second or third day and sometimes later. In the second stage of Stokes and the first of Laennec, the crepitation is heard along with a gradually diminishing respiratory murmur.

This crepitating rhonchus has been compared to the sound

produced by rubbing a lock of hair close to the ear, "as a physical sign," says Dr. Stokes, "it points out a secretion or effusion into the vesicles, but to determine that it is pneumonia, the increasing dullness and gradual obliteration of the respiratory murmur must be combined with comparative dullness of sound on percussion."

" In the third stage of Stokes, the second of Laennec, there is solidity with softening; the cells are obliterated while the large tubes remain pervious; there is, therefore dullness of sound with bronchial or tubal respiration and a loud resonance of the voice. These are signs which indicate solidification."

Andral maintains that solidification may occur without the usual preceding signs, the lung passing in a few hours from an apparent state of health, according to every physical sign to solidification; when this, according to indications takes place suddenly, without preceding crepitating rhonchus, it has been regarded as pathognomonic of pleurisy with effusion, but the physical signs are equally indicative of the condition just described.

"When pneumonia is on the eve of terminating by resolution and to pass from the *third* stage to the second, the crepitating rhonchus returns; this has been termed the returning crepitating rale; tubal expectoration diminishes; the broncophony gradually disappears; the crepitating rhonchus fades away, little by little until finally the sound of normal respiration is heard. Different physical signs may be elicited in many parts of the lungs indicating that they are in different stages of inflammation, and at times after other signs have ceased, a crepitant rhonchus may remain.'

This is an important circumstance and should keep the physician on his guard against a relapse, or some other trouble from insidious inflammation.

Laennec was of the opinion that as solidification of the lung passes off the fact is always announced by a return of crepitating rhonchus, but Stokes entertained a different opinion. The signs of the fourth and fifth stages of pneumonia, according to Stokes are the following:

If there be tubal respiration with a sharp and peculiar mucopurulent rhonchus, these signs taken along with the previous history of the disease and the existing symptoms, will lead to the conclusion that there is interstitial suppuration.

"The signs of pneumonic abscess do not differ from those of

tuberculous cavities, the former are generally at the inferior portion or about the root of the lung, and are not so slow in their
formation as tubercular abscesses." (Stokes.)

But little can be learned by percussion or auscultation when
the pneumonia is deep seated towards the base, center or root of
the lungs. In like manner when some isolated lobule is inflamed,
the physical signs may yield no information as to the existing
affection.

In pleuro-pneumonia where both the lungs or pleura are inflamed, the solid fluid or æriform secretions may modify the signs
of pneumonia; notwithstanding the frequency of adhesions, the
sound of friction is rarely observed in pneumonia. When air is
secreted into the pleura, it is indicated by the sudden appearance
of tympanitic resonance over the affected portion of the lungs.
"This sound may be distinguished from the cracking sound of
caverns and differs from the clear sound rendered by percussing the
lower portion of the lungs over the stomach distended with air.
(Stokes.)

The bellows sound of the heart, as well as the throbbing of a
large portion of the chest, which have been observed in pneumonia are synchronous with the systole of the heart during the
early stage of the disease. It has been surmised that the bellows
sound is owing to inflammation either of the pericardium or endocardium accompanying the pneumonia, and that the throbbing is
attributable to the semi-fluid condition of the lungs, the pulsation
of the heart being propagated through these organs and occasioning phenomena analogous to those of aneurism. (Stokes.)"

The duration of pneumonia averages from twelve to twenty
days. Often it continues only two, three or four days; at other
times it may go on thirty or forty days. It is always a serious
disease. It may pass into the chronic form or lay the foundation
of tubercular or pulmonary consumption.

Pneumonia is not the same in all cases or in all persons. In
some, intense pneumonia may exist without giving rise to dyspnœa or cough or the characteristic sputa and it would appear
that auscultation may afford no sign, yet this form of the disease
has been termed *latent pneumonia* by Andral. It is rarely primary, and generally occurs in the course of other diseases. We
have already attested to the differences which are manifest in
pneumonia in children. With them there is less power of resis-

tance, and the disease often terminates fatally before it reaches the third stage, the appearance in dissection being much like that of engorgement of the lungs.

In old persons more rapid prostration is produced than in those of robust manhood, and hence the term pleuro-pneumonia; nothing has been applied to pneumonia in them as well as to chronic bronchitis, which latter affection is indeed very apt to be complicated with pneumonia, sometimes causing intense difficulty in breathing.

That there is a practical difficulty in diagnosing the symptoms of pneumonia when it occurs in the course of serous fevers, pleurisies, pericarditis, arachnoid inflammations, gastro-enteric inflammation, pulmonary tubercles, etc.

The peculiar influences which modify this disease so as to constitute the *bilious* and *typhoid* forms of pneumonia, we shall have occasion to advert to hereafter.

CAUSES.—Pneumonia occurs in all countries and in all climes; although like other inflammatory diseases, it occurs with greater severity in changeable climates, than in less so, as in Australia, Colorado, and the Californias. It is not so common in warm and equable climates, in temperate regions; some parts of the country are more affected by the disease than others.

In our own country, the United States, the disease is quite common. According to statistics that have been taken, it would seem it occurs much more frequently, even here, in some places than in others. Dr. Emmerson, of Philadelphia, confirms this fact by the following statistics. They give the average mortality from consumption and acute diseases of the lungs in those places. The annual average of general mortality to the population of New York is one to 39.36; in Boston, one to 44.93; Philadelphia, one to 47.80; and in Baltimore, one to 39.17. From consumption alone the average mortality compared to the general is 5.23; in Boston, 5.54; in Philadelphia, 6.38; Baltimore, 6.21. Average of consumption and acute diseases of the lungs, one in 4.07 in New York; in Boston, 4.47; in Philadelphia, 4.90; and in Baltimore, 5.33. It must be obvious that in cold and variable climates, in which humidity and frost are ever disturbing the evenness of the temperature, and where the country is open to cold winds, from the ocean, the surroundings are worse for those liable to affection of the pulmonary organs. In like manner, pneumonia is more likely to occur in cold and moist seasons.

It has been extensively observed by different surgeons on the medical staff of the army, that at posts on the coast of New England, 233 out of every thousand became affected during the year with catarrhal diseases; while there were but 143 out of one thousand on the coast of Florida.

It is said that in French hospitals three times as many cases of pneumonia have been observed the last six months of the year as in the previous half year.

It has already been stated that pneumonia is liable to occur in the course of other diseases. It would seem that chronic inflammation of any organ has a tendency to predispose to inflammation of the lungs; so that it would seem that a patient may suffer for a long time with some chronic inflammation, and finally die of an acute attack of pneumonia. A predisposition to the disease may be produced by injuries, or surgical operations, or by repeated attacks of any painful disease. Dr. Pleasants includes among the predisponents, toothache the painfulness of which unsettles the nervous system and affects the respiratory organs.

In a statement of forty-one deaths which occurred in the *University Hospital, London*, it appears that twenty-three of the cases were either in the second or third stages of pneumonia. On this account it has been suggested to defer operations during very severe weather and when pneumonia prevails epidemically.

Pneumonia occurs in all ages. It has been found in the still-born and consequently is an intra-uterine disease. It attacks men and women alike, although it is averred that men are more liable to the disease than women. This is accounted for because of their greater exposure to exciting causes. In order to adapt a therapeutics in pneumonia, our attention is chiefly directed to ante-mortem phenomena; we might write many pages giving a description of post-mortem appearances, from which we might derive some information of the termination of the disease in death. We might acquire a knowledge of the solidification of the lungs, and the air vesicles rendered impervious to the air. But such information affords but a slight aid to therapeutics.

TREATMENT.—An early resort to the lancet has been universally commended by the Allopathic profession. Of late, however, the views of leading men are quite at variance on the subject. The late Prof. Geo. B. Wood recommends thorough depletion, but Dr. Todd, of London, says bleeding should never be tolerated, because it multiplies the chances for a fatal termination of the disease. This is said in reference to the first stage of the disease as recognized by Laennec.

Bouillaud recommends extensive cupping over the chest and the abstraction thereby of large quantities of blood. This treatment he claimed was attended with marked success.

In seventeen cases of double pneumonia, eleven recovered under this treatment, while but two cases out of fifty-five terminated fatally where only one lung was involved. He further claimed that the average duration of the disease under this treatment was from nine to thirteen days, while fifty cases treated by Louis less actively, averaged fifteen days.

In more modern times nearly all practitioners are agreed that such copious and repeated abstractions of blood are neither necessary or advisable. Next to blood-letting the tartrate of Antimony and Potassa, given in large doses has been commended.

The tartrate of Antimony and Potassa is administered as follows: Tart. Ant. et. Potassi grs. iij, Aqua cinnamomum ℥ ij Acet. opii grs. vij. M. Dose, half an ounce every two hours. Another revellent when this is inadmissable and after blood-letting, is four grains of Calomel, twelve grains of conserve of roses, mixed into a pill mass divided into four pills, one to be given every six hours. To this treatment may be added blisters and leeches and mercurial ointment applied externally, both as a dressing for the surface denuded of the skin by blisters, and as a clinical administration of the Mercury. During the whole course of the disease mucilaginous or gummy drinks are allowed, as gum water, barley water, flax-seed tea, etc. Brisk cathartics and alteratives enter largely into the treatment of the different stages of the disease.

If the cough is troublesome expectorants are freely recommended. The air of the sick room they recommend to be kept at a comfortable temperature, especially at night, and mental and corporeal quietude are strongly enjoined; when this subsides, milk, farinaceous preparations, as arrow-root, sago, etc., are allowed with great circumspection. It is true that variations from this treatment of pneumonia may be found with different practitioners.

HOMŒOPATHIC TREATMENT.—The advent of Homœopathy created a marked change in the treatment of pneumonia. The disease under any circumstance is serious; and Homœopathic treatment has had a grand success in lessening the severity and abridging the duration of the disease, as well as the diminution of its fatality. In an experience of over forty-five years we have treated a large number of cases of pneumonia and with a comparative success which no other treatment has excelled; our treatment after satisfying ourselves of the nature of the disease, has been to place the patient in the most comfortable situation for treatment in the beginning. I will illustrate the treatment by a citation of cases and the treatment employed.

CASE I. A boy, aged 12 years, who had been attending school. From a warm school-room he returned to his home in a cold rain storm from which he became chilled; he soon began to experience a sense of oppression in the chest, a dry hacking cough, a dull, deep-seated pain or tightness in the chest, rapid and difficult respiration; attending the cough was a viscid tenacious expectoration of a greenish or pale color, sometimes tinged with blood; great heat of the skin, headache, thirst, full pulse, somewhat accelerated, general restlessness; urine red, scanty and hot. From these symptoms we recognized the first stage of pneumonia, although it was but the third day after leaving the school-room. Our first prescription, March 5th, was Aconite, third decimal dilution, ten drops in half a glass of water, a teaspoonful to be given every hour. In 24 hours we found the inflammatory symptoms had subsided—the pulse was not so hard, the urine was not so hot or highly colored. But the constriction of the chest was the same, and the headache was worse, and March 6th we gave him Belladonna, prepared and administered in the same way as the Aconite. March 7th, twenty-four hours after, the headache was relieved and the constriction of the chest was somewhat relieved. But the boy complained of stitches in the side and difficult and anxious respiration, and a troublesome cough; which made the headache return at every effort. We prescribed Bryonia in the third dilution, in the same manner as the Aconite. March 8th, 24 hours, we found our patient unmistakably better, and convalescent, and yet the cheeks were flushed, and the soreness of the chest remained, the thirst had disappeared, and the tongue was moist, and the temperature which was 103, was reduced to the normal standard.

We continued the Bryonia March 9th, patient still improving. March 10th all the disturbing symptoms were gone, and the appetite returning.   The duration of this attack was   nine days.

CASE II.   Was that of a young lady, aged 22 years, who fell into my hands when in the second stage; with the following symptoms (how the first stage was treated we could not learn): Her breath was labored, her cough almost constant, cheeks flushed; very pale around the eyes and mouth; palpitation and inclination to syncope, pulse irregular. Percussion over the right lung elicited a dull sound, no respiratory murmur, no crepitus rhonchus could be heard.   The left lung was free, the respiratory murmur distinctly heard.   There could be no doubt but that the right lung was extremely hepatized.   The difficult and anxious respiration of the left, and the cough with the muco-purulent expectoration was evidence of the severity of the disease, as well as the coolness and moisture of the skin, tongue red at the margin and covered with a dry dark fur.   The bowels were constipated.

After examining critically the pathogenesis of several remedies, we decided to give Tartar emetic, 3d attenuation.   This remedy was administered in the two grain doses every two hours. The patient had then been quite ill for six days.   We gave the first dose of Tartar emetic on the eve of the sixth day; the next morning she complained of great debility; had not rested during the night.   She had drank a little arrow root gruel during the night; at about day break she had a copious movement of the bowels.   We regarded this favorable, and directed the medicine to be given at intervals of two hours.   The next morning her cough was less painful and her respiration somewhat improved. The percussion over the affected portion of the lungs still elicited a dull sound and no respiratory sound could be detected in the right lung.   As some of the prominent symptoms had yielded, we continued the Tartar emetic in the 6th, dose and repetition the same.   In twenty-four hours more we perceived that absorption was taking place and that the engorgement was fast disappearing. But the heart's action was not improved, and we prescribed *Veratrum viride* 3x.   Twenty-four hours after we found a general improvement.   The coating had disappeared from the tongue and the patient had taken a little nourishment.

From this time convalescence was gradual until all the functions became established.   The duration of the entire attack was seventeen days.

No inflammatory symptoms were manifest afterwards: the expectoration gradually became normal and in time there was a full return of strength.

CASE III.   We were called on the 5th of November to a mother and daughter whom I found suffering from the pains and aches usually attendant on the first stage of pneumonia.   The mother aged forty-two, a stout fleshy woman, complained of headache which was constantly aggravated by a hard and somewhat frequent cough, dull pain in the chest. The clinical thermometer indicated 102°, pulse 114 and a sense of constriction which interfered with easy respiration.

She had considerable heat over the chest and her skin was hot and dry. She expectorated a viscid mucus, very tenacious. She had but little thirst and her heart was quite active and her pulse somewhat accelerated and full, 114 a minute; urine highly colored, and a brick dust sediment. We gave Bryonia 3x, ten drops in half a tumbler of water, a teaspoonful every hour. Nov. 6th we noted but little change, but feeling sure that Bryonia was a well chosen remedy we continued it. Nov. 7th we noted relief of the head and found that her cough did not provoke the pain in the head that she had experienced the past few days. But her other symptoms were no better, her cough was quite as frequent and the expectoration was darker and streaked with blood, the lungs were both implicated and engorged, but no physical sign of hepatization. - Nov. 8th, the expectoration was of a rusty color, the soreness of chest great. The difficulty of breathing greatly increased.

Phosphorus, 6x ten drops in half a tumbler of water and a teaspoonful every hour was prescribed. Nov. 9th, found the soreness of the chest better, the cough less severe and expectoration of mucus of a yellowish or greenish color; we also found the skin moist, and a natural secretion on the edge of the tongue.

The action of the heart was moderated, the pulse nearly normal, the urine of a more healthy color. Nov. 10th, Phosphorus 30x was continued. Nov. 11th, still further improvement, the cough and soreness of the chest in a less severe form remained, the bronchial tubes seemed filled with mucus, and so profuse was the secretion that she was almost suffocated; yet she felt no pain. Nov. 12th, no fever or inflammation manifest. In this case a troublesome but painless cough was entailed which was kept up by constant tittilation in the respiratory passages. It will be seen that this case ran about nine days, after which the entailed cough gradually passed off, but not wholly until spring when warm weather set in.

CASE IV. The daughter, aged 23, on Nov. 5th was coughing continually, and with painful soreness of the lungs, considerable thirst, hurried respiration; the pulse was full and quick and in brief cessations from coughing she felt a dull, heavy pain in the chest. This case was less severe than that of the mother, but an unmistakable case of double pneumonia. Seeing that her skin was hot and her breath feverish, Aconite 3x as before prescribed was given every hour. Nov. 6th her skin was not so hot and her cough less painful. Nov. 7th, Aconite continued; respiratory murmur perfect in both lungs, but her head had commenced aching and coughing aggravated the pain. Nov. 8th we gave Bryonia 3x prepared as before, and administered every two hours. Nov. 9th there was a change in the disease; the head ceased to ache, but the expectoration continued with much blood and the patient suffered from several paroxysms of dyspnœa, was very feeble and could not move without experiencing an aggravation of her suffering. Pulsatilla was substituted for the Bryonia and on Nov. 10, Pulsatilla continued. Nov. 11 she was decidedly better, but still she had some fever, and the cough was troublesome and she raised considerable mucus, sometimes yellowish, greenish or streaked with blood. Nov. 12th all the characteristics of pneumonia had disappeared and that a little time would be the best remedy to complete the cure. Duration of the disease seven days.

In looking over Jousset's Clinical Lecture on pneumonia translated by Prof. R. Ludlam, I have concluded to give it entire and no apology is needed, for it will be seen at once that both the lecture and the notes are a choice specimen of clinical literature and so practical that no one can fail of being profited who reads it.

The summary of the lecture is as follows: " Of pneumonia *case* rapid termination of the disease; lack of deferescence; importance and difficulty of diagnosis, of individualizing and of curing by name or title. Arsenicum and Tartar emetic case of pneumonia with absence of the usual signs. No deferesence. Critical days. Necessity of examining all febrile patients by auscultation. The expectant system and the errors and fallacy of its statistics. The boasted success of Dr. Hughes Basset. Puerperal pneumonia case."

" *Pneumonia cured on the ninth day. Gentlemen:*—In a former lecture we have already spoken of pneumonia and its clinical treatment by Bryonia and Phosphorus. *Apropos* of two cases.

CASE LXVIII. Mr. Charles B.—, aged 45, was admitted on the 31st day of January and discharged the 26th day of February. (Men's ward No. 2.) The antecedents of the patient have been bad and his general condition on being admitted into the hospital was very unfortunate. He tells us that for ten years past he has taken cold in winter and summer and that generally he coughed for several months together. Ten days ago he was forced to take his bed. Although he is not sensibly emaciated, and has never raised any blood, yet he looks like one with phthisis. From the beginning of winter his health had been very good and he had not the least signs of trouble when four days ago he was suddenly seized with severe chills. The next day he had some cough and a violent dyspnœa which has not left him since that time.

"The observable symptoms do not accord in their gravity with those revealed by auscultation; he appears to be seriously ill. There is a profound adynamia and the face is red and swollen; the breathing is difficult, and fever intense.

"On the evening of his admission the temperature was 108.1° and the pulse 124. The cough is frequent and the expectoration difficult; the sputa are not characteristic, but white, purulent, slightly aerated and somewhat tenacious. There is a complete loss of appetite, with a foul tongue.

"Percussion shows a slight dullness over the middle lobe of the right lung; and auscultation detects some loud and sibilant rales on both sides of the chest, but more especially upon the right one.

"Feb. 1st, fifth day, morning temperature 101.1°, pulse 96; evening temperature 102.5°, pulse 96. Bryonia and Ipecac, 12th dil.

"Feb. 2d, sixth day, morning temperature 101.3°, pulse 104; evening temperature 102.1°, pulse 108. The patient had been very restless during the night. The dyspnœa was as bad as at the beginning, and the debility still more pronounced. The expectoration is a little more copious, and the sputa more sticky. This morning auscultation reveals a tubercular souffle at the summit of the right lung. Tart. emetic trit. He was also ordered two large spoonsful of brandy.

"Feb. 3d, seventh day, morning temperature 102.5°, pulse 108; evening temperature 103.1°, pulse 108. To-day the general condition of the patient is very bad; the temperature is very high and he complains of a constant oppression in the right lung. Besides the blowing sounds there are crepitant rales. Tartar emetic, 1st trit., during the day and Arsenicum, 3x trit., at night.

"Feb. 4th, eighth day, morning temperature 101.6°, pulse 100; evening temperature 101.8°, pulse 96. The general condition of the patient is not improved; but the temperature has fallen nearly one degree, and auscultation reveals instead of the souffle a mixture of the mucous and crepitant rales. The sputa are bloody and viscus. Arsenicum, 3x trit., alone.

"Feb. 5th, ninth day, morning temperature 99.9°, pulse 60; evening temperature 98.9°, pulse 64. As the thermic curve shows that the temperature has fallen to the physiological point, the general condition of the patient is much better than it was yesterday. Now, the sputa are quite characteristic, they adhere to the bottom of the vessel, and have the color of barley sugar. There are sub-crepitant rales in the right lung. Arsenicum, 3x trit.

Feb. 6th, tenth day, the temperature remained 98.5° both morning and evening. The dyspnœa of which he complained has ceased. We still hear some moist rales in the lung, but we also perceive a slight souffle of expectoration at its apex. Arsenicum, 3x trit.

"Feb. 7th, eleventh day. The patient is going on well, he was allowed to eat some porridge and to drink a little wine and water. There is a very copious diarrhœa. The same treatment.

"Feb. 8th, twelfth day. The appetite is returning very decidedly and expectoration is becoming less and less copious. Continue the Arsenicum, 3x trit., and give him an egg.

"Feb. 9th, thirteenth day. The respiration in diseased lung is normal again. The mucous rales have entirely disappeared.

"Feb. 11th, fifteenth day. The patient still continues to have a mucous expectoration. The cough, however, is infrequent. Tartar emetic, 1x trit.

"Feb. 14th, eighteenth day. The cough and expectoration less than before; the digestion is very well performed. The same remedy was continued for two more days, and the patient effectually cured.

Now here is a case of pneumonia occurring in a man who was worn out and ill, which terminated on the ninth day and the convalescence from which was complete after eight days.

Seventeen days' have therefore sufficed for the disease and for the convalescence. When these patients were subjected to treatment by bleeding *coup sur coup* by blisters and by large doses of Tartar emetic such rapid results were unknown.

It is worthy of remark that in this case properly speaking there was no defervesence, since it required seventy-two hours for the temperature to return to its normal state. In fact on the seventh day the temperature was 102.3° in the morning and 103.1° in the evening, *ril est* it varied only one-sixteenth of a degree during the day; on the ninth day it fell one degree and it was not until the tenth day that it reached the normal point, 98.5°

It is worthy of note that the ninth day which in pneumonia is the most pronounced of all the critical days, marked the term of the morbid evolution.

The diagnosis was beset by a difficulty which is not often encountered in such diseases as have their proper physical signs; for although auscultation was practiced every morning and evening, yet it did not give the characteristic signs of pulmonary hepatization until the sixth day of the disease.

Until that time we had only heard the rales proper to bronchitis, and therefore diagnosticated the case as one of grave bronchitis. What was the cause of this anomaly; undoubtedly it was the adynamic state of the patient and the feebleness of the respiratory movements.

"This crepitancy or physical diagnosis is quite as possible in pulmonary disease or elsewhere and under different conditions the case corresponds with the detection of uterine deviations. One physician examines a case and fails to find any displacement. The next day another physician may be equally positive of the existance of prolapsus or of some version or flexion of the organ. Both were right, both were wrong; if either had insisted that a mistake had been made in the diagnosis; when the change of condition of diseased or abnormal states had developed what were not recognizable at first and under different circumstances. A little common sense would often keep physicians out of a snarl in these matters and more careful observation will make us all more charitable."

When our patient had reached the sixth day, the diagnosis suddenly illuminated the whole pathological picture, and with a positive proof of the lesion, the therapeutics ceased to be doubtful and uncertain. The treatment was immediately changed to the two remedies which are suited to a dangerous form of pneumonia, viz., Tartar emetic and Arsenicum. When the fever was intense, 103.5°, the prostration very profound and the nightly agitation had afforded the principal indication for Arsenicum, it was given alone and it established convalescence.

We also prescribed a small quantity of brandy and we believe that a moderate use of alcohol has not been without its influence in the happy issue of this case.

It is especially in the pneumonia of old people, *senile* pneumonia, in some forms of typhoid pneumonia and in the disease occurring in patients with a broken down constitution and unpromising antecedents as in Case LVIII, that alcohol in some form is of excellent service. We could cite a number of cases from our own experience in which if judiciously used, certainly was the means of saving life.

This example also shows you, gentlemen, that it is not necessary to restrict or limit the treatment which we apply to all diseases of the same kind. We must study earnestly the indications which are furnished by the symptoms of the individual case. This is what I call individualizing, in the medical sense of the word.

You should in fact guard yourselves against two errors, one of which consists in founding the indications upon certain symptoms that are proper to the sick person and in taking no account of the diagnosis; the other in making, as it is sometimes styled, a cure of the disease; or by the use of a treatment which is arranged beforehand for all the diseases of the same name or kind, without reference to the particular indications in each case. After the first of these methods one might prescribe Chamomilla, for example, in tuberculosis, meningitis, croup or the colic, *if the child is only quiet when* it is carried in the arms. In the latter case one should not obstinately treat such pneumonia as we have just detailed by Bryonia and Phosphorus, else the patient will be apt to die.

Spinal Schlerosis with Inter-Current Pneumonia.

Here is a second case of pneumonia which bears some resemblance to the preceding one.

CASE LXIX. Mr. George P.—, aged 86 years, admitted on the 3d of February, 1876. (Men's ward, No. 6.) The patient, who was attacked some days after his entrance into the hospital with pneumonia, asked to be treated also for a spinal affection from which he had suffered for about two years. He was a janitor and had lodged in a damp room, but he had never been very ill, and declared most positively that he had not been of dissipated habits.

The disease set in abruptly, with such weakness of the limbs that it was impossible for him to walk, except for a very short time without great fatigue.

He had had bruised pains in both legs but had never experienced the sharp, terrible pains that are usual in locomotor ataxia. From the beginning of his disease there was a continual oppression with occasional fits of violent suffocation. He had also had vertigo for some time. Now we find him with the following symptoms:

The general condition is pretty good. There is, however, a slight emaciation of the lower extremities. When his eyes are open he walks with comparative ease and the legs have not the irregular, jerking movements that occur in locomotor ataxia, but when his eyes are bandaged he walks with the greatest difficulty and threatens to fall at any moment There is an habitual constipation, difficulty in passing urine and he cannot empty the bladder entirely.

The cutaneous sensibility is preserved, and so is also the muscular sensibility; for some time, however, his vision has been a little weak. He was given Phosphorus, 12x dil. This remedy was continued, but without improvement, until Feb. 10th. The night before he took a little walk in the court, and afterwards complained of a violent headache and a great oppression. He also had fever, the temperature being 101.3° and the pulse 100.

Feb. 10th, second day. The patient complains severely, but is not so oppressed as during the night; and does not cough. Morning temperature 101.1°, pulse 120; evening temperature 101.3°, pulse 120. Aconite, 6x dil.

Feb. 11th, third day, morning temperature 101.8°, pulse 108. He is not doing so well. He does not cough, and there is no sign of an acute affection of the lungs.

Feb. 12th, fourth day, morning temperature 104°, pulse 120; evening temperature 104, pulse 112. The fever is intense; the patient had some bleeding at the nose during yesterday, and this was followed by a pretty frequent cough. Auscultation of the back part of the thorax gives a negative result. Aconite 6x dil.

Feb. 13th, fifth day, morning temperature 103.25°, pulse 112; evening temperature 103.6°, pulse 124. He continues to cough but raises nothing; the headache of which he complained at first is better; at our morning visit there was an adherent, yellowish, sticky sputa which clung to the bottom of the vessel, and which was a little streaked with blood; auscultation of the thorax both anteriorly and posteriorly, revealed intense souffle which was located in front and in the upper portion of the right lung, there was no rales. Bryonia, 3x dil.

Feb. 15th, seventh day, morning temperature 102.5°, pulse 116; evening temperature 103.25°, pulse 120. This morning the general condition of the patient was very bad; the souffle extends both to the front and behind; there is complete prostration, and the tracheal rale can be heard at a distance. Tartar emetic, 1x trit., for the day, and Arsenicum, 3x for the night.

Feb. 16th, eighth day, morning temperature 101.6°, pulse 100; evening temperature 100.4°, pulse 100. There is a decided improvement in the patient's condition; the dyspnœa is less marked and the facial expression is better. During yesterday he had a slight epistaxis; to-day auscultation discloses blowing and crepi‑tant rales. The same prescription.

Feb. 17th, mouth dry. The fever is completely broken. The evening temperature was 96.6°, the respiratory souffle has disappeared, Arsenicum 3x trit.

Feb. 19th. He still coughs a little, and complains of a slight pain in the right side. There are some mucous rales in the chest. Bryonia 3x dil.

Feb. 22d. He coughs but very rarely, the pain in the side has left, his strength returns very slowly. Phosphorus 6x dil.

Feb. 25th. Last evening he had a slight oppression with a pretty sharp pain in the epigastric region; Nux vom. 3x trit.

Feb. 28th. Respiration in the right lung is normal, but he still coughs a little; the digestion is better but not perfect. The same remedy continued. The patient had no more symptoms, but continued to improve during the month of March.

In this case the diagnosis has been very difficult on account of absence of the usual signs of pneumonia; neither cough, expectoration or pain were present; perhaps we were wrong not to have practiced auscultation more thoroughly. The seat of hepatization above in front of the chest is so rare that we have spoken of it. It certainly helped to prolong the error in diagnosis. The disclosures of the thermometer were those proper to pneumonia. There was a rapid rise in temperature without oscillation to 104°.

We should at least feel as kindly toward the failures of a physicial diagnosis as we do toward the failure of our remedies when we do not obtain the desired result from their employment. If we depend upon them to the exclusion of others, the signs revealed by auscultation and percussion are no more reliable than the general symptoms.

The author's point is well taken but he might have added, there are two forms of pneumonia in which one would almost entirely be misled if they should rely to any considerable extent upon this mode of examination, more especially in the early stages of the disease. These two kinds of pneumonia are that of infancy or of early childhood and that which occurs in the puerperal state.

In *infantile* pneumonia a careful physical examination of the child's chest, more especially the front part of the thorax, is often impossible (anæsthesia would keep the youngster quiet and overcome his opposition) add to this fact, in the lobular form of pneumonia the lesion may be so limited to the interior of the organ and so covered by the healthy tissue, as to be beyond the reach of the ear, and of the pleximeter; in such a case we cannot therefore depend upon physical signs exclusively any more than we can upon the subjective sensations of the patient when the little one is not old enough or wise enough to tell us the sensations he feels.

We shall add a clinical talk upon puerperal pneumonia at the close of this lecture.

In this case there was no proper defervescence. On the seventh day the temperature was 103.75°; on the eighth day 104° and on the ninth day 99.6°. There was, therefore, a regular though rapid decrease of the temperature. "Besides the last peculiarity there was the termination on a critical day,—the ninth day of the disease, and the rapidity of the convalescence, which was complete after two days."

"The *prostration* and *oppression* complained of were the symtoms which led to the choice of *Tartar emetic* and *Arsenicum*." We will omit the remainder of this clinical lecture as it relates to the expectant method, and its fallacies and the treatment of *pneumonia* by venesection and other methods, showing the comparative disadvantages of the various theories compared with the Homœopathic treatment.

In addition to the clinical experience which we have given above we will cite one or two cases illustrative of our treatment of typhoid pneumonia:

Case I. George M.—, aged 37 years, was seized by what he termed a bad cold, January 3d. For two or three days he neglected himself, thinking that his head would cease aching when his cold passed off.

January 6th was called to see the patient and noted the following symptoms, viz.: Severe pain in the head over the eyes, deep-seated pain in the right lung, tongue heavily coated, breathing labored, skin moderately hot, pulse 108, temperature 100°, complained much of pain when moved. Bryonia, 3x dil., dose every hour.

January 7th. No improvement, pain in both lungs, pain in the head as if it would fly to pieces every time the patient coughed, pulse not very full, but 120 a minute, temperature 101°, Bryonia continued.

Jan. 8th. The head had ceased its violent aching and the patient seemed dull and reticent, the pain in both lungs was increased, pulse 120, temperature 101½°.

Jan. 9th. Found the patient comatose, with countenance sunken and pale, cough quite frequent, which was attended with a moan of distress. Pulse more feeble, appeared very much prostrated, no inclination to take food. Temperature the same —101½°. Rhus tox. 3x dil. every hour.

Jan. 10th. Found the patient weaker, and comatose; cough very worrying, expectoration of a ropy, tenacious mucus, streaked lightly with blood. Phos., 6x dil., every hour. Temperature and pulse nearly the same.

Jan. 11th. Found the patient somewhat aroused, but inclined to dose, speaks very hesitatingly, complains of pain, labored breathing, seems confused, much sordes has collected on his teeth, breath exceedingly foul and short. Auscultation reveals a dull sound over the region of the right lung, and yet a slight murmur and mucous rale could be heard; continued *Phos.* and

Rhus tox. the former by day and the latter by night; directed the mouth washed with tepid milk and water, and to rinse his mouth with pure water, after the sordes had become softened.

Jan 12th. Patient has been very restless during the night; there was coldness upon the surface affecting the lower extremities; this coldness was followed by a febrile reaction and much thirst, pulse 120 and quite feeble. Temperature 102°. Gave Arsenicum, 3x trituration, two grains every hour.

Jan. 13th. The patient had been sick nine days and we were anxiously looking for a change. The fever had passed off, the pulse had a little more volume; the patient had drank a little gruel. The surface was warm, the pain less; but the cough more frequent and also the expectoration of dark colored mucus, bowels still constipated, and urine still depositing a brick dust sediment. Arsenicum continued.

Jan. 14th. Patient appears better; pulse 120, temperature 100°,cough loose, expectoration less tenacious, slight improvement of the pain in the chest, and the breathing was better and no dyspnœa. Patient was much prostrated and Arsenicum still continued.

Jan. 15th. Patient better, pulse 112, temperature 99°; patient had taken some nourishment in the form of gruel; slight appearance of saliva upon the margin of the tongue, cough loose but troublesome, more consistency to the expectoration, much mucus expectorated, and at times almost suffocated. Tartar emetic, 3x.

Jan. 16th. Convalescence not satisfactory, but evident slight mitigation of symptoms from yesterday. Tartar emetic continued.

Jan. 17th. Less fever, pulse stronger, appetite returning, unable to sit up and coughing quite overcomes the patient.

Jan. 18th. Had a good night, slept considerable; awoke feeling refreshed, no perceptible fever, no thirst, tongue clean, natural movement of the bowels, calls for something substantial in the way of food. Still very weak. China, 3x dil.

Jan. 20th. Cheerful and recuperating as fast as possible. This patient was several weeks regaining his strength, but ultimately fully recovered.

CASE II. March 15th. A child four years old began with a short, dry and hacking cough, very soon a high fever sprang up, pulse 130 a minute, temperature 103°. Gave Aconite, 3x.

March 16th. She still coughed incessantly, very little expectoration of viscid mucus; complained of much pain in the head, fever was intense, in the afternoon she began to be dull and inclined to sleep. Belladonna, 3x.

March 17th. Deep coma, breathing very labored, heart's action strong, pulse 136, temperature 103°. Takes no notice; moans when she coughs. Bry. 3x dil., every hour.

March 18th. No better, case looks unfavorable. Gave Gelsemium.

March 19th. About the same; pulse and temperature the same. No marked change of symptoms, except that the cough was less frequent, and the expectoration increasing. Rhus rad.

March 20th. Pulse the same, temperature the same, less stupor, cough more violent, expectoration tinged with blood. Fever not so high.

March 21st. Skin moist, warm perspiration, coma passed off, cough continued with great violence, rusty sputa. Gave Phosphorus, 3x dil., every hour; had her chest bathed with goose oil and a flannel over the chest. I could perceive no signs of the solidification of the lung or lungs although her breathing was difficult. But the course of the disease was rapid. Phos. continued.

March 22d. All the symptoms more favorable except the cough, directed demulcent drinks to be given, such as rock candy and water, flax seed or barley tea, and gave Phos. 3x.

March 23rd. The fever had subsided and the child called for food; her cough had become less painful, pulse 116, temperature 98° or normal.

March 24th. Heart palpitated from weakness, cough still considerable. Gave Pulsatilla 3x dil. every hour.

March 25th. Rapidly recovering, and in a reasonable time she was well.

CASE III. We had another child violently attacked quite similar to the one just detailed. Veratrum vir. broke it up entirely on the sixth or seventh day and the child grew better every day until her strength was fully regained.

The symptoms of pneumonia, and bronchitis or whooping cough are covered by Tartar emetic, Aconite, Mercurius, Phosphorus, Bryonia, Pulsatilla, Nux vom., Hyoscyamus and Ipecac.

Pneumonia of acute character, occurring in old people or feeble persons, showing a low grade of inflammation, will require Phosphorus, Lachesis, Sambucus, Lycopodium, and Arnica.

When pulmonary inflammation arises from mechanical injuries, Arnica 3x dil. every hour.

Chronic pneumonia is undoubtedly a rare disease, that is, simple chronic pneumonia as an original affection. But the scrofulous or tuberculous inflammation of the lungs, which is chronic in its character and accompanies the softening of tubercles is extremely frequent. We doubt the propriety of calling this kind of inflammation chronic pneumonia at all.

The general symptoms have a great similiarity to those of phthisis pulmonalis, and sometimes night sweats. Therefore in opposition to the views of some of the older writers, we shall think it manifestly proper to class this affection with that of pulmonary consumption and shall include ·its description and treatment next under this head, which will be deferred until we treat specifically of phthisis *pulmonalis*.

Typhoid Inflammation of the Lungs—Typhoid Pneumonia.

We shall include under this head, inflammation of the lungs, more or less latent, and accompanied by great prostration, and that may be attributable to the low state of the constitution, the complication with other diseases, or because the pulmonary affection results in a great measure from a general morbid condition.

This form of pneunonia is met with everywhere. It prevails in some localities more than in others, and unless the symptoms of prostration are very great, it is commonly called bilious pneumonia.

It has been seen as a complication of gastro-enteritis, of true typhus, of delirium tremens, of phlebitis, of malignant erysipelas, and sometimes proves to be the fundamental disease.

SYMPTOMS.—Typhoid pneumonia is often eclipsed by the disease with which it may be complicated.

Thus, a common gastric fever may appear to be the most prominent, and seem in reality to be the disease; but a close observation may reveal dyspnœa, and cough.

It is extremely insidious in its progress, and is not suspected, and the dyspnœa may suddenly become aggravated; the motion of the chest may manifest great irregularity and in as brief space of time, the disease may terminate in death from engorgement of the lungs.

It sometimes occurs that the only method of determining whether inflammation of the lungs exists at all, is by physical signs, these alone reveal the true nature of the disease. A trifling cough with or without expectoration, slight dyspnœa and hurry of breathing may occur; yet the patient may not complain of the chest; although extensive and fatal disease may be present.

It is asserted by Stokes, that in this disease, the stethescope will over and over again detect inflammation of the lung when there has been no preceding cough, pain, dyspnœa, or expectoration.

The same author also asserts that in this form of pneumonia, engorgement of the lungs and solidfication often take place most rapidly, but, although this is the fact, the progress of resolution is generally exceedingly slow.

Chronic hepatization with or without hectic fever, or a lurking congestion, may continue for weeks; and although under appropriate management, the disease may be ultimately relieved, or removed, atrophy of the lung with or without ulcerative disease is often established.

In certain cases months may elapse before the respiratory murmur is heard, and in many instances it is never re-established. On the other hand, typhoid pneumonia has been known to cease in a single day, on the supervention of an attack of gastritis or enteritis.

"Typhoid pneumonia may terminate in rapid and fatal hepatization—in gangrenous abscess, or it may induce chronic solidification or induration of the lung which may end in the tubercular condition."

TREATMENT.— In Allopathic practice bloodletting is commended in the early stage of the disease, and only in robust individuals where the bilious or gastric symptoms are more marked than the typhoid, or when contra-indicated the joint deflectory and revellent actions of cupping may be employed with advantage. In the earlier stages of the disease, the employment of mercury is recommended, until the system has been brought slightly under its influence; likewise under that of counter irritation. The patient should be warmly clothed in flannel next to the skin, and the extremities should be kept warm. In cases where gastric or bilious complication is considerable, and especially where gastro-enteritis is threatened leeches are applied over the stomach and a warm bread and milk poultice over the leech bites.   Great caution is exercised in the administration of cathartics, and instead emollient or anodyne injections are prescribed.

The debility that attends the lowest forms and stages of the disease, suggests the use of mild tonic stimulants such as wine whey; cold infusions of bark with acids, or any of the vegetable tonics.

The decoction of Senna or with carbonate of Ammonia is prescribed when the patient becomes hectic, with copious expectoration.

The diet is restricted to mild farinaceous articles such as arrow-root, sago, or tapioca, and as soon as the patient is able, a change of air is recommended.

HOMŒOPATHIC TREATMENT.—In the earliest stage after the nature of the disease has been fully comprehended and if the patient is in a well ventilated apartment which is essential to the success of good medical treatment, and for a patient of nervo-bilious temperament with moderately full pulse, and active fever, tongue heavily coated, breath hot—*Aconite* 3x dil. may be given and repeated every hour at first, if the cough is frequent, and a yellowish dark colored mucus is expectorated, and the patient complains of great thirst and difficult breathing, and there is a sallow complexion, or a bitter taste in the mouth. *Mercurius sol.* 3x trit. may be given in two grain doses every hour or two hours until there is a change.

Arsenicum alb. in the 3x trit. may be given in the same way; when there is great heaving of the chest or difficult respiration, coldness of the face, and cold hands and feet, with great prostration, cough and dark colored expectoration, patient craves cold air, and cold drinks, moans and tosses about in bed; and frequently sinks into a kind of stupor and particularly when the gastric symptoms are very marked.

Bryonia alb. when the patient is disposed to lie quietly, and cries out with pain when moved, and when there is considerable heat in the chest, and when the cough is attended by pain in the head; and the expectoration is of a reddish or rusty appearance, and also when there is considerable gastric irritability and the fever is moderate.

Carbo vegetabilis.—We have found this remedy useful in advanced stages; when there is great prostration of the vital forces: sensation of great weakness in the chest, coughs by spells, with brownish expectoration, paleness of the face and coldness of the extremities, weak pulse and hardness of the secretions.

Lycopodium.—In cases of a tuberculous tendency we have found *Lycopodium* 3x trit. especially useful, when there is circumscribed redness of the cheeks, and copious expectoration of mucus mixed with pus; and a fan-like motion of the nostrils, and sand-like sediment in the urine; we have also found this remedy useful in promoting absorption, when portions of the lung are hepatized, and also when complicated with affections of the heart.

Rhus tox.—When typhoid symptoms are present, and the patient lies in a half stupor and partially delirious. Terrible cough as if something would be torn out of the chest, and the expectoration is of a brick dust or bloody appearance, and the patient is disposed to get relief by frequent moving about in bed, and is very restless at night.

Sulphur.—Is particularly indicated in protracted cases, when the physical signs of hepatization are unmistakable, and when the patient has frequent faint spells, and flashes of heat. In a case of extensive hepatization of the inferior lobe of the right lung, Sulphur, the 30x dil., proved useful in promoting absorption and when the patient suffered from suffocation, and required a bountiful supply of fresh air in the room he complained of heat in the top of his head.

Tartar emetic is a valuable remedy in bilious pneumonia, when the gastric symptoms are so prominent that they obscure the condition of the lung; which is disclosed only by percussion, and when large quantities of mucus and bloody matter are found in the expectoration, and the patient frequently exhibits signs of suffocation. This remedy by its prompt action has undoubtedly saved many from a premature grave. To the above I will add the following memorable case. I was called in May to take charge of the case of Mr. L. G., aged 50, who was of a strongly marked bilious temperament, and of a debilitated constitution, whom I found on the 23rd suffering from a moderately severe gastric fever, and frequent retching and vomiting; he was very much prostrated, temperature 102° and pulse weak and 120 a minute, he craved cold drinks a little at a time and frequently; prescribed Arsenicum, 3x trit., every two hours.

May 24th. Temperature 103°. Found the disease had changed to a gastro-enteritis and that the breathing was labored and difficult, the face pale and cold, thirst intense, abdomen distended, the patient complaining of much pain around the umbilicus. There was no cough or apparent pain in the chest, pulse very rapid, and the gastric irritability so great that even the most simple efforts to satiate the thirst would excite retching; prescribed Ipecac, 6x dil., to be given every hour.

At 9 P. M. found the patient suffering from severe dyspnœa, occasional cough, with dark, bloody expectoration, breathing short and labored, cold, clammy perspiration upon the surface, cold hands and feet, pale face and pinched expression of the countenance, temperature 104° and pulse very feeble and quick; found the gastric and gastro-enteritic symptoms had disappeared and on percussion found the entire right lung in a hepatized condition. Auscultation revealed the fact that no air was passing into the lung. Gave Tartar emetic 6x dil., ten drops in half a tumbler of water, a teaspoonful every thirty minutes; remained with the patient during the night; at 7 A. M. found the patient rapidly sinking. Case terminated fatally on May 27th.

In this case the gastric and gastro-enteritic symptoms completely masked the latent pneumonia until the disease had assumed a fatal type.

From the above case we infer the exceedingly dangerous character of bilious or typhoid pneumonia, when gastric symptoms are so prominent at first as to mask the real nature of the disease.

The diet in these cases must necessarily be confined to farinaceous gruels or in some cases to a mild stimulant, as wine whey.

Gangrene of the Lungs.

Gangrene of the *lung*, which almost always results from inflammation.

This particular feature of pneumonia is not frequent, yet we have seen two distinctly marked cases which terminated fatally. It occurred in broken-down constitutions. In cases of this kind the breath becomes fœtid, emaciation evident, expression of anxiety; nostrils dilate during inspiration; respiration 60 per minute; face flushed, expectoration dark colored and of the odor of gangrene, pulse 130 or 140, small and quick, marked œdema of both feet. In both of these cases life was apparently prolonged by judiciously selected Homœopathic remedies, among which are *Arsenicum* 3x, *Carbo veg.*, *Secale cornutum* and *Lachesis.*

According to Allopathic authorities this affection always proves fatal. Their chief remedies consist of cupping and the administration of chlorate of lime or soda and other anti-septics or disinfectants.

Œdema of the Lungs.

According to Laennec this affection is not uncommon, but exceedingly difficult to diagnosticate. It occurs as the *super acute* at a time when the patient is in perfect health, or in the course of acute disease. The first indications are symptoms of suffocation, which in the course of two, three or four hours end in death by asphyxia. The acute is, though, characterized by considerable dyspnœa at first, and goes on increasing from four to twelve days and ends in complete prostration and finally proves fatal. The *chronic form* of *œdema* is characterized by *dyspnœa*, which may be slight for months, while the patient is in a state of rest, but becomes seriously augmented by coughing and expectoration and during exercise. *Percussion* in all these cases elicits only an obscure sound and auscultation shows great feebleness of the vesicular murmur, and that it is accompanied by a *subcrepitant rhonchus* much less than in pneumonia in the first stage, and apparently with moisture and more prominent bubbles.

The causes of this malignant affection are not known. It may occur as a primary affection or be developed in the course of different diseases,—acute bronchitis, or pneumonia, or heart disease, or cerebral hæmorrhage or general dropsy.

TREATMENT.—In Allopathy no specific treatment is laid down, but in Homœopathy it is believed that *Apis mellifica, Helleborus nig., Arsenicum* and *Apocynum can.* may be suggested.

Emphysema of the Lungs.

"Two forms of emphysema of the lungs have been described, one of which is termed *vesicular* and the other *inter-lobular*." The former is confined to the air cells, and the latter to the cellular tissue which connects and separates the lobules of the lungs. Modern writers have said this disease is common, and that inter-lobular emphysema is more properly termed emphysema of the lungs; as the *vesicular* concerns the terminal extremities of the bronchial tubes. We will consider the diagnostic signs of each, although properly speaking they may not be separate and distinct diseases, but complications of other affections involving the pulmonary tissues.

The vesicular emphysema consists essentially in dilatation of the air cells of the lungs, which as a matter of course become increased in size, and an increase in the quantity of air, as well as the capacity of the chest itself.

SYMPTOMS.—Vesicular emphysema is unattended by fever; is of long duration, commencing frequently in early life; but seldom after one has passed the fiftieth year.

1. Slight dyspnœa which generally continues without aggravation, for a number of years when it dates from infancy, and afterwards becomes more and more marked, occurring in paroxysms during which the patient appears at times to be threatened with suffocation. The dyspnœa is often preceded by a cough and is generally accompanied at some period or other during its course by bronchitis, which when aggravated would seem to be one of the most common causes of paroxysms of dyspnœa. Some pathologists ascribe the dilatations of the air vesicles to bronchial inflammation, but according to the observation of others, the emphysema is rarely preceded by bronchitis. The form of the chest appears to undergo some alteration causing the patient to stoop habitually, and in some instances the dilatation of the lungs crowds the heart downward. Its impulses become manifested in the epigastric region. Such are some of the chief symptoms of vesicular emphysema.

The *causes* productive of vesicular emphysema as already stated, may be bronchitis or pneumonia and in some instances intense moral emotions. The intrinsic cause of the dilatation of the vesicles we are unable to appreciate. It has been ascribed to a want of elasticity of the lung. The muscles of inspiration are ever active to dilate the chest, and thence by virtue of atmospheric pressure the air cells and when not counteracted by the natural elasticity of the lungs, the air cells as well as the cavity of the chest become permanently dilated.

TREATMENT.—It is maintained in Allopathic practice that a restoration of the vesicular murmur may be effected by the same means employed to remove bronchial irritation. In Homœopathic practice, the characteristic symptoms of the affection, such as a sense of suffocation, dyspnœa, or sensation of distension and fulness of the chest would seem to indicate such remedies as *Arsenicum*, Tartar emetic and Aconite, in the 6th dilution, if the circulation, as indicated by the pulse is abnormally vigorous.

26

2—Inter-Lobular Emphysema.

This variety of emphysema results from the infiltration of air into the inter-lobular cellular tissue. Prof. Gross, of Philadelphia, says it is a common affection in the *West*, but from quite extensive observation, we are inclined to doubt the correctness of the assertion.

The diagnostic symptoms, which enable us to determine the presence of this disease are dyspnœa and difficult expiration, a sense of suffocation, and a feeling of obstruction in the bronchial tubes which renders it difficult to breathe out the air. This is attributed to a want of elasticity of the lung.

The causes of this affection are believed to be various. Mechanical injuries from violent efforts. Sometimes the disease occurs spontaneously, and sometimes from the effect of other severe diseases such as dysentery, bilious and typhoid fever and inflammation of the lungs and whooping cough. In cases which have terminated fatally, autopsy has revealed the fact that the cellular tissue between the lobules of the lungs was infiltrated with air.

In cases of whooping cough with children when they are inclined to *coma* consequent on convulsions, and their faces are swollen and puffed abnormally there is reason to apprehend the presence of emphysema.

TREATMENT.—When the circulation is vigorous, the dyspnœa is worse; and heart's action more forcible. The chief treatment in Allopathic practice is Tartar emetic; with the tincture of Digitalis to reduce the circulation and respiration to the normal standard and to regulate the bowels with mild cathartics.

HOMŒOPATHIC TREATMENT is in accordance with the manifest symptoms. *Arsenicum* for rapid and labored breathing, *Aconite* for accelerated circulation and Veratrum viride to reduce the heart's action and relieve the dyspnœa; Tartar emetic to remove the apparent suffocation from an undue accumulation of mucus, may be administered in the 3x decimal attenuation drop doses every hour or two grains of the trituration may be given every two hours. The diet should be farinaceous and entirely free from stimulants. It is important in all of these cases to avoid stimulation, as adverse to the needs of the patient.

Asthma.

In the preceding affections of the lugsn we have frequently used the term dyspnœa, to denote difficulty in breathing, as associated with certain pulmonary diseases. But in the consideration of the disease known as asthma, that peculiar affection is meant which is characterized by laborious breathing and is preceded by some premonitory signs of its approach. "For a week or two previous to an attack of asthma, the patient will often be troubled with sneezing every morning, itching in the inner canthi of the eyes, irritation of the throat with constant inclination to hem or hawk, lassitude, dull pains in the head and back and limbs, loss of appetite, dry hacking cough and great depression of spirits." The first invasion usually occurs during the night, with tightness and constriction about the chest, urgent and distressing symptoms such as dyspnœa, aggravated by the slightest motion, inspiration short and strong, while the expirations are long, labored and wheezing; great and rapid motions of the nostrils, livid and bloated countenance, indicative of much distress and anxiety; inclination to sit up, and a decided inability to lie upon the right side or back from the first invasion, and during the forming stage, respiration very difficult as if from want of air, yet a breath of air or the wind from a fan cannot be borne without difficulty, face pale, pain through the temples; cannot lie upon a feather bed. The dyspnœa worse at night and better during the day.

Dry cough at first in a majority of cases, followed in a few hours by a viscid expectoration; excitement brings on an attack, such as grief and fear, also certain odors, or the inhalation of irritating substances palpitation during the attack; and this may occur in the season of flowers; tongue foul, breath offensive, eructations, flatulency, urgent desire for cool, fresh air, the circulation sometimes rapid and at other times variable.

The causes which produce asthma, or cause the paroxysms are not always the same. The paroxysms may be caused by crying, laughing or any emotional excitement when the predisposition already exists, and under like circumstances a cold, damp wind, or sitting in a draft of air, or from indigestible food, or exposure to a chilly night air. It was observed by Hahnemann that "asthma almost always occurs in individuals who are the victims of chronic miasm." We have observed in several instances, that urticaria partially developed and then suppressed, was followed by an acute attack of asthma. We think it safe to assert that the greater proportion of true asthma is attributable to the suppression of some cutaneous eruption, or miasm, which from some exciting cause has been thrown upon some portion of the respiratory apparatus. We have observed, also, that when an attack of asthma is threatened that the employment of such remedies as have the effect to develop an eruption like nettle rash, will relieve the air passages. We have used Bryonia and Pulsatilla in cold, damp weather with excellent effect, and also Cuprum aceticum in dry weather or cold, with similar results.

Other influences which may be reckoned among the exciting causes are atmospheric changes, easterly winds, and electric conditions of the atmosphere. The inhalation of irritable substances, or dust of Ipecac, or the odors of certain plants, imponderable in their nature, often cause severe paroxysms. Anger, fear, or any source of irritation, such as spinal disease and intemperate habits or a sedentary life, etc.

Asthma, though a distressing disease, "never kills," is the expression of Dr. Salter, who, in his extensive observation, had never seen a case in which a paroxysm proved fatal.

When accompanied with organic disease of the heart, and more or less disease of the lungs, the patient gradually wears out and dies.

But in young subjects of sound chest when the attacks are short and the intervals between them long, no permanent shortness of breath, no cough or expectoration, and especially if the attack becomes milder and less frequent, and the exciting cause can be obviated, the prognosis is favorable.

If the patient is advanced in life and his lungs are not sound, and the attacks are frequent and severe, the breathing more or less impaired, never quite free, and when the cough and expectoration indicates that the disease is gaining ground, and remedies have a mere palliative effect, no favorable prognosis can be given.

TREATMENT.—In Allopathic practice, the common emetics such as Ipecac, Sulphate of Zinc and Tartrate of Antimony are chiefly relied upon, in connection with warm stimulating manipulation or pediluvium sinapisms applied to the wrists, and over the anterior or posterior part of the chest. Galvanism has been extensively employed with pronounced good effects.

HOMŒOPATHIC TREATMENT is mainly appropriate or well affiliated remedies.

Arsenicum alb, " is employed with advantage in bad cases occurring from suppressed eruptions or catarrh; also in persons of feeble or impaired constitutions whether from excesses, previous sickness or old age." The following symptoms indicate the special use of this remedy: Sense of extreme lassitude and debility; difficult stifling dyspnœa with attacks of suffocation; ▸spasmodic constriction of the larynx and chest; short respiration anxious and wheezing; irregular throbbings of the heart, sufferings aggravated by night by lying down, movement, eating, mental excitement, or exposure to cool fresh air; distension and cramp-like pains in the abdomen; frequent eructations, nausea, vomiting burning sensation in the stomach, fœtid breath, smarting or burning in the throat, burning and oppressive pains in the eyes, pale face, anxious and desponding. The remedy may be given and repeated according to the urgency of the symptoms in the 3x trit. or even in drop doses of the 6x dilution.

Bryonia is also applicable to cases of asthma arising from suppressed eruptions or partially developed nettle rash and also in catarrhal or pulmonary complications. The paroxysm generally occurs in the night, respiration difficult, short, sighing, impeded by stinging in the chest; cramp-like pains, aggravated by motion, apprehensive, tensive, or contractive, pain in the thorax, cramping, cutting, or shooting pain in the abdomen, bitter or sour eructations. Throbbing pain in the head, increased by exercise, a dose of the 3x or 6x attenuation may be given every half hour in urgent cases until better or worse symptoms occur.

Belladonna, according to Hartman, has been especially recommended in cases where there exists a tendency to spasms or any organic lesion. He asserts that it often proves radically curative, after the exhibition of some inter-current remedy, particularly in cases which have not become too chronic by repeated relapses, under which circumstances recurrence must be had to some of the anti-psoric remedies, as *Sulphur* or *Calcarea carb.* It is particularly indicated when the paroxysms come on in the night, in fits of short, difficult, irregular and suffocating respiration, accompanied by a dry cough, pressure on the chest, violent beating of the heart, vertigo or swimming in the head, pains in the small of the back and limbs, cramps in different parts of the body, anxiety, irritability and fretfulness. Dose of the 2x or 3x dilution every hour. In the flatulent asthma of children *Chomomilla* is an important remedy, and also that following a suppressed catarrh. It is likewise specific in those attacks caused by anger, or grief, fear, etc., in adults, distension or fulness of the stomach and bowels, pressure, anxiety, and fulness in the region of the heart, short wheezing respiration, great restlessness, dry irritable cough, bad taste.in the mouth, tainted breath. Dose and administration same as in *Belladonna*.

Bromine has been highly commended in some cases of asthma. Dr. Douglas cured a case of ten years standing in a girl 16 years old, who suffered in the meantime from dyspnœa which had remained after measles. So violent was the trouble that the girl was not able to walk or ascend the stairs. It disappeared after taking four or five doses of the 30x dil. of five pellets each. It is one of the few remedies which produce copious false membranes in the air passages.

Calcarea carb. has cured a case of dyspnœa, irregularity of circulation, blue discoloration of the skin in a young girl seven years of age, the 30x dil. in drop doses cured this case in six weeks.

Lobelia inflata has been highly recommended in large doses. Several cases of asthma of long standing have been cured by Lobelia infusion given in doses that would provoke vomiting and the reason must be that the above excessive and dangerous doses only cured because the remedy is capable of causing the disease.

Pulsatilla is indicated in asthma when it occurs in persons of mild temperament, light complexion, hair and eyes, and when it comes from *suppressed urticaria* or other rash, and also from cessation or other derangements of the catamenia, and inhalation of the vapor of sulphur. The symptomatic indications are short, suffocating, and extremely difficult respiration, as if from want of sufficient air or choked by some irritating substance, obliged to sit up, appears distressed and anxious.

For attack in warm and sultry, foggy weather, cramp-like and constrictive painful tension of the chest, and depression of spirits, short spasmodic cough, nausea, palpitation of the heart, fullness and distension of the stomach after eating. From the 3x to the 6x decimal dilution may be given every half hour or hour until relieved.

Ipecacuanha.—In asthma caused by retrocession of eruptions of milliaria urticaria, or by inhaling irritative odors. this remedy and Arsenicum are much relied on in asthma to relieve anxious and difficult respiration.

Much has been written concerning hygienic measures, either for the relief or prevention of paroxyms of *asthma* but it is difficult to establish general rules, every sufferer from the disease should breathe the air which he finds best adapted and most congenial to his case.

Sometimes long journeys and sea voyages and even the hardships of military life have wrought favorable changes in patients who had long suffered from the disorder.

Tubercles in the Lungs.

The presence of tubercle in the lungs gives rise to pulmonary consumption, yet they cannot be regarded as synonymous, inasmuch as tubercles may unquestionably exist there, and yet remain quiescent so that no symptoms of pulmonary consumption become manifest. But the latter cases are exceptions.

The word *phthisis* means, *to dry up*, *fade;* and consumption means, to emaciate or decline from any cause. Hence the older writers, as well as many of the modern authors, make mention of *laryngeal*, pulmonary, gastric, hepatic, and renal phthisis to denote the marasmus caused by diseases of the larynx, stomach, liver, etc. In the more modern periods the term phthisis has been applied to diseases of the lungs only.

By one distinguished writer on this subject it is asserted that as many species of phthisis are laid down as there are organic lesions which would in their development lead to wasting and death; hence he has enumerated the tubercular, granular, cancerous, melanotic, calculous and ulcerous.

Since the arrival or appearance of Laennec, writers on pathology have admitted but one species, under the head of tubercular, and that the existence of tubercles of the lungs constitute the proper character of phthisis.

Williams in his work on Consumption thinks it is well to include under this term all those forms of disease of the lungs; which arise from tubercular formations, or of depositions, and indurations, which are allied to them, in the substance of the lungs. In order therefore to give a correct view of this morbid condition it is proper to enquire specifically into the pathological character of tubercle.

Tubercle.

We now call attention to the nature of tubercle. Many have been the theories and speculations on this subject, and not more than one can be true, and this must not be founded on any conjecture or forced conclusion from facts that have been made to conform to certain pre-conceived notions.

The fruits of honest and independent inquiry freed from all selfish motives are what is needed, and these only can prove of practical utility in the study of therapeutics in connection with the disease, and considering the nature of pulmonary tuberculosis we must consider and determine upon the degree of truth found in various theories, honestly put forth and defended, from the best of motives and conviction of their truth, by so doing we may find well-settled principles and facts which may throw light upon the nature of the disease.

The first claim we shall notice is that tuberculosis is an inflammatory disease, and that its principal feature is arterial degeneracy.

Dr. Williams says in his Principles of Medicine that tubercular matter may be found within the blood vessels themselves, as he has repeatedly observed something presenting all the external appearance of yellow tubercle in the blood vessels of parts remote from the lungs, and that where fibrin may coagulate, its degraded form of tubercle may occur.

Rokitansky in his Manual of Pathology, maintains with considerable plausibility that tubercle is a fibrinous modification and that the tubercular crasis is but the arterial elaboration of fibrin which forms its cardinal feature. He also maintains that in consequence of the alteration of the nature of fibrin, tubercular matter is constitutionally deposited even when the blood is very deficient in that constituent; all the fibrin is thrown out in the form of tubercle. The rapid coagulation of tubercle—blastema, which must be effused in a fluid form, has a tendency, when coagulated, to soften. Its formation being favored by active arterialization and prevented by a venous condition, this author regards as highly indicative of a real affinity between tubercle and fibrin. From the fact that tubercles are often found in the lungs when no suspicion of their existence had been entertained when the patient was alive, and that the tissue around them is found to be perfectly healthy and presenting no sign of inflammation, we cannot subscribe to the theory that tubercles form centers of inflammatory action, and when inflammation exists we must conclude that it is a consequence rather than a cause of tubercles, which may form independently of inflammation, and be the cause, the same as other foreign bodies, of provoking inflammation. In this opinion Laennec concurs, as well as other authors who have examined the subject. It would seem, therefore, that tubercle is the result of defective nutrition, as Dr. Colten remarks that tuberculosis is a peculiar condition of the whole system in which instead of the healthy nutritive material required for the growth and reparation of the body, there is produced in the blood a morbid substance which sooner or later appears as tubercle, or tuberculous matter in the pulmonary structure. He regards this condition very nearly the same as that of scrofula.

The same author says that in consumption as in other diseases we are permitted to recognize the disease only by its effects. It is evident that there must be something which constitutes the malady, but it would be vain to search after it because it has no individuality; yet we are permitted to study its laws and in some measure control its actions. We are inclined to regard the generalization by Hahnemann under the generic name of psora as the probable source of tubercular deposits, and that individual characteristics may present themselves in different subjects. Dr. Epps is inclined to look upon tuberculosis as the result of a special cachexia of its own in different cases, and that the pretubercular stage also varies in different subjects. Imperfect nutrition, which is always attended by debility is the primary source of the vitiated condition of the blood when devoid of material necessary for sustaining the various tissues. When the blood is deficient of its elementary constituents it fails of producing the appropriate matter required by the tissues for their support, nevertheless the struggle of the defective fluid produces something which aggregates in the form of tubercle, which becomes deposited in various tissues. Dr. Pope concludes that malnutrition is undoubtedly one of the earliest features as well as one of the most fatal characteristics of tuberculosis, but like other authors he concludes that the primary cause of tubercle must be the predisposing cachexia before alluded to, and we are also inclined to the opinion that the predisposing cause of tubercles is a vitiated condition of the whole system, an inherited cachexia, or that which may be acquired by exposure to a class of influences which impoverish the vital condition of the blood.

If it be true that imperfect nutrition lays the foundation for the generation of tubercle, we must look first to the possibilities of invigorating this function.   The blood is the immediate source from which is derived the proximate principles which become allied to the various tissues and supports them by a perpetual contribution to their substance.   This can only take place when the blood is in a normal condition or when its essential constituents are present in exact and definite proportions.   When the blood is in this state it will yield just such material as can be utilized by the various structures.

But when the blood is deficient of one or more of its elementary constituents the product it yields not being convertable into any of the animal structures, becomes deposited in the form of tubercle which cannot be utilized in repairing worn out tissues. These tubercles are of different forms, the milliary not being larger than a mustard seed, while the aggregate tubercle may be of the size of a pea and even of larger dimensions, and being like foreign bodies they find a lodging place in various localities, and especially in the pulmonary structures, the effect of which is an interruption of nutrition and consequently results in an irr tating fever, wearing the flesh, and destructive to the adipose tissue.

In view of the fact that the lungs suffer from tubercle and consequent emaciation in a much greater degree than any of the other internal organs the term pulmonary consumption is not inappropriate.   We will therefore consider briefly the nature of pulmonary consumption.

Pulmonary Consumption.

In order to impart information concerning one of the most common diseases and one which is usually regarded fatal, it is my purpose to compile from the best authorities as well as from my own observation such facts and theories as may lay a foundation for a successful treatment.

But before we proceed allow me to give some historical data concerning the disease and its ravages and the possibility of guarding against it, of curing it when it is manifest, or at least of ameliorating it so as to prolong life.

With regard to the primary origin of the disease it may be claimed that its antiquity is not chronologically known, for in the earliest history of the human race after the fall, its inroads have been noticed. It is quite certain that consumption has been regarded as fearfully fatal from time immemorial. So great are the numbers that have fallen victims to its ravages that it is more dreaded than any other sickness that befalls mankind.

In view of the facts that the best skill has only been attended with a partial success and no attempt at concealment has been made, that with the aid of all the approved appliances, confirmed consumption must still be regarded a most destructive disease and one in which the hope of beneficial treatment lessens in a remarkable degree in every stage of its progress, let us minutely examine its characteristics with the hope of guarding against its primary development. Much undoubtedly can be accomplished acquiring a familiar knowledge of the natural history, its tendency, progress, and various phases of the disease, the class of subjects most liable to it, the earliest signs of its approach. It is therefore our manifest purpose to note these particulars.

First, consumption as the term signifies, implies a wasting of all the vital or functional powers, extreme emaciation, or consuming of the adipose tissues and flesh. The term is of late restricted to this peculiar wasting effect of tubercular matter in the lungs and the changes which it undergoes and which it works. But in these cases it will be an error to restrict the disease to the lungs, though a continuance of the lung trouble would in time destroy life; but its mortal tendency is very greatly accelerated in nearly all cases by parallel characteristics in other organs. The lung trouble is beginning to be regarded as only a fragment of a great constitutional disease which plays its most conspicuous part in the air vesicles of the lungs.

These complications of pulmonary phthisis which I shall note more fully hereafter are sufficient to establish the all important fact that *tuberculosis* is not exclusively a disease of the lungs. Like its kindred scrofulosis it may invade other organs. Dr. Watrous says it is a disease so closely linked with scrofulous diathesis that the formation of tubercles may occur in any locality where this diathesis is present.

Viewing pulmonary consumption and its kindred difficulties in the light of a constitutional disease from which the whole organism suffers, we are naturally led to inquire into all its characteristics and also into the constitutional peculiarities of its victims. It has been observed that consumption is peculiar to certain families, but in what way these unfortunate families become thus exposed is a question yet to be settled and though difficult we shall attempt to arrive at some satisfactory conclusion upon the subject. In a normal condition the human race would not suffer the pain of infirmities. It is therefore evident that there has been a departure from the original condition and it is probably within the province of science to restore the physical status of man to its normal or healthy state. It is not to be expected that this can be accomplished in a single generation with the present knowledge upon the subject and by the aid of modern appliances; the hereditary tendencies may be partially or wholly restrained. The healing art has for its object the restoration of the physical constitution as it originally was: a perfectly normal condition of the human organism, is absolute health. Were an infant without hereditary taint to be perfectly trained in accordance with the laws of its constitutional nature, and it pass through life, from one stage of development to another, from infancy to childhood, to youth, virility and old age, and even to the termination of its earthly existence in the sleep of death without disease or pain. But any violation of the laws of health brings disease. When the numerous violations of the laws are taken into account we need not wonder at the inroads that have been made upon healthy constitutions. When parents become the victims of constitutional disturbances from inattention to the laws of health, the effect is transmitted to the succeeding generation, which by additional violation will degrade still further the inherited constitution and so on; from generation to generation, until the physical degeneracy becomes complete, and now the whole system is filled, consequently, with predisponents that only await exciting causes for the development of diseases.

When the present state of the human family presents itself for the consideration it must be admitted that the physical infirmities of the preceding generations are apparent. A gradual

departure at first increasing from generations has resulted in a
multiplication of predisposing influences to disease of a constitutional character.   The question under consideration is "can these
influences be eradicated?"   What measure can be brought into
cordial co-operation with the remaining vis-medicatrix to effect a
gradual return to that sound condition of health which alone is
capable of waging a stern resistance to exciting causes of
disease?

It is well known that tuberculosis springs up in vitiated
constitutions and that it is a constitutional disorder which can be
transmitted from parents to their offspring and the only way to
rid the human race of this most formidable disease is to begin the
work of restraint in the present generation, that the next succeeding one may profit by the effect and the next still more and
so on until the warfare is accomplished.

We shall endeavor to explain as far as present knowledge
upon the subject will permit, all the stages of the disease in order
that we may be able to institute timely effort to prevent its
development.

It has been demonstrated that in certain stages *consumption is
curable*, that in other stages the disease can be restrained and that the
lives of individual cases may be prolonged, that obstacles to nutrition can be removed, and moreover that suffering and pain can
be greatly ameliorated.   But to accomplish this we must become familiar with the nature, history and progress of the disease,
the peculiarity of the subject as confirmed by observation, the
first indications, the characteristics of the various stages, the
kindred derangements. together with all the obvious phenomena
demanding the most skillful resources and appliances, which the
most modern science furnishes; complete or even partial success
in warding off or mitigating the painfulness of the disorder depends chiefly upon advising a treatment for each phase that presents itself.

1.   *The obvious peculiarities of those predisposed to the disease.*
—When we see a man or woman with a narrow contracted chest, a
little inclined to bend forward as if it were an effort to stand or
sit, and one who has black hair and pale countenance, one whose
digestion is easily disturbed, and who generally exhibits a melancholic expression of the countenance, we shall generally find that

his or her antecedents, as well as the general appearance would indicate one predisposed to consumption.

2. The first or earliest indication of the development of the disease will generally be that of ordinary fatigue, respiration as if tired, an apparent want of vim, a tendency to tire easily upon the slightest exertion. The appetite may be tolerably good but the food taken into the stomach does not digest vigorously, neither does it appear to nourish and keep up the flesh and strength, loss of weight, of warmth, and a proneness to chill quickly on the slightest exposure. The countenance is generally pale, and with all there is an apparent listlessness and inactivity, and the patient is not conscious of any actual disease. The careful physician will regard this preliminary stage as one of unusual importance, as demanding judicious hygienic measures to stimulate nutrition, by well chosen therapeutic agents. If a restraint is not here interposed the disease will progress.

3. A short, dry, hacking cough is usually the next stage, as if a slight cold had been contracted; very little, if any, expectoration attends the cough, and the patient is inclined to think it of little consequence. But if a careful, competent physician is consulted in this stage, he regards the cough, the dryness of the throat, the proneness to chilliness or fever, "as prophetic" of more serious disturbance, and here his skill is taxed to change the condition of the system, if possible, by hygienic and therapeutic measures.

4. If the cough is not quieted, and the nutritive function kept up, it will increase insensibly until signs of hæmoptysis become apparent, the patient begins to spit up a little blood, but as but little pain has been realized and only a sense of debility comes over him, the matter is viewed as trivial or temporary. But the physician regards the symptom as a formidable tax upon the vital condition of the respiratory system and where his skill is again called into requisition to devise measures to in some way strengthen the nutritive function, and by therapeutics of a styptic influence, to arrest the hæmorrhage and to guard against its recurrence.

5. Either before or at the time of the spitting of blood, which sometimes is slight and sometimes is very severe, the patient will generally have distinct marked chills, followed by fever, and for some time during each day the pulse will be weak and accelerated, the cheeks will be flushed, a circumscribed red-

ness will appear on the cheeks denoting a *hectic*. Here again the faithful physician finds an opportunity to restrict by his prescription the progress of the fever, to restore the appetite which has become impaired, that the patient's strength and flesh may be preserved and life prolonged.

6. If the arrest of the disease is not accomplished, the patient's strength begins to fail more rapidly and *night sweats* set in sometimes very profuse, at other times less so. These sweats are apt to occur at the limitation of every *hectic* paroxysm and rapidly detract from the strength of the patient, during each paroxysm of the *hectic*, the respiration becomes hurried and difficult, the cough and expectoration profuse. But little hope remains of doing anything further than to mitigate the suffering.

7. All the while the cough has been increasing in severity and the expectoration has greatly increased, at first it has been muco-purulent, then, although purulent, frequent paroxysms of suffocating cough and copious sputa will be productive of a humid asthma distressing to witness.

But as there are constitutional peculiarities in each and every subject, our treatment of this formidable disease will depend upon the correctness of noting first the cachexia, and then the symptoms which indicate the struggle that nature is making to rid the system of what is foreign to its purpose.

Physical constitutions are inherited, and if subject to any hereditary taint it becomes a predisponent of its corresponding disease, nor can it become so unless operated on by some voidable or unavoidable exciting cause. By early attention to diet, nutritive in its character, and such as is suited to the demands of the nutritive system, the inherited predisposition may be restrained and rendered less susceptible to the action of exciting causes. Nevertheless a vast majority of the cases of pulmonary consumption are victims of hereditary taint.

Our treatment therefore at first must be adapted to the pre-tubercular stage; it must be hygienic, and must relate to the quality and quantity of food and drink, fresh air, and exercise.

We have known persons of slender constitution, feeble nutrition, descendants of families known to have been visited by this disease, who have become robust and apparently vigorous by adapting an hygienic regimen for their constant observance.

When a man or woman with crow-black hair, slim, and in-

clined to throw the arms forward as if bending a little, though
otherwise in good health, it may be inferred that he is of the
consumptive tendency, and that his diet should be adapted to the
state and condition of his nutritive system; we would recommend
such persons to the habitual use of cooked salt codfish at least
once a day, as it furnishes food for the nerves, and thereby
strength to the digestive processes. We have known such persons having more or less inappetence to experience a favorable
change in this respect after a few meals of nicely prepared codfish
in milk. When the appetite is once established other articles
of diet may enter into the daily living. The greatest variety of
food free from any medicinal quality is allowable provided no injurious effect is felt from its use; regular times for eating and
drinking should be observed, while daily exercise in the open air
and gymnastic exercise for the arms will greatly promote digestion as well as equalize the circulation. The only way to prevent emaciation is to supply such nutritive material for the blood
as contains all the proximate principles; and a compensation for
waste is provided for. For as stated above, the blood must be in
a normal condition and constantly replenished, or it fails in its
efforts to supply the necessary elements of nutrition. The indications which the appetite affords will generally suffice for the
regulation of the choice of aliments.

With regard to beverages, it is in accordance with the laws
of the physical constitution that natural thirst should be satiated
with the pure " *Aqua Fontana* " water. But in a low vital condition and tardy digestion a little wine may be taken for the
stomach's sake. The persistent use of stronger stimulants will
sooner or later ripen into an exciting cause which may arouse the
latent tendency to tubercular deposits.

As for the therapeutic agents employed in the treatment of
the various stages of the disease, it may be remarked that none
except those which have been thoroughly proven upon persons in
health should be called into requisition, and these only when
their pathogenetic symptoms are similar to those presented by
the disease at the time of their administration. The consideration of this, the ultimate object towards which all the preceding
investigations tend, will be worked out in reference to the action
of medicine in connection with the various stages of the
phthisical disease.

TREATMENT.—The Allopathic treatment of pulmonary consumption is by no means uniform in any stage of the disease. In persons predisposed and feeble, tonics and stomachics are freely recommended with a view of promoting the activity of the nutritive function. But if in spite of these efforts the system becomes more feeble and emaciation becomes apparent the various preparations of cod-liver oil are called into requisition and sometimes with apparent good effect.

In case of failure of arresting the disease at this stage, by this remedy, and a cough sets in of a dry hacking nature, some expectorating preparation such as the syrup of Ipecac and squills, is given to loosen the cough, and to give some palliative relief to the patient; nearly the same treatment in the second stage except when febrile symptoms show themselves, small doses of quinine are given frequently, and this treatment is kept up to a greater or less extent in the succeeding stages of the disease, not with the expectation of curing the disease, but merely as palliative measures.

HOMŒOPATHIC TREATMENT though fraught with many difficulties, looks to a more desirable result, for beginning with the symptoms of the pre-tubercular stage and faithfully establishing the similitude between the pathogenetic effects of the chosen remedy and the phases of the disease, it is not improbable but that the struggle of nature may be so aided as to finally have a curative effect, but at the very point where the warfare commences the affiliation must be accurately made or little or no beneficial result can be hoped for. In order to make ourselves more clearly understood in this respect we will present the outlines of a few cases, and their treatment. Case 1st. In a subject, J. H——, aged 25 years, who is subject to frequent epistaxis or flowing from the nose of blackish blood, coming on suddenly during day or night, this would indicate the use of *Aconite*, as this symptom is prominent in its pathogenesis, because *Aconite* has the power of producing a similar vascular excitation.

Now, if in connection with the epistaxis the patient has a contracted chest and suffers from the bleeding of the nose at night, or early in the morning, we may infer that there is a cachexia which produces it and a critical examination will point to *Calcarea carbonica*.

In the case of the patient under consideration we find the

Calcarea cachexia intimated by the tall and slender frame, light hair, and blue eyes, fair complexion, very sensitive to cold, and inclined to eruption on the skin, and freckles, we therefore select for this case, *Calcarea* as the remedy, because we find it indicated by the nosebleed and other symptoms which we have noted.

By referring to Hahnemann's Chronic Diseases it will be found that nearly all the symptoms that are recorded in the pathogenesis, of the similitude of the symptoms of this disease, as found in this case, and the success which has attended the administration of this remedy in the higher attenuations has been quite satisfactory; when this remedy is prescribed in the pre-tubercular stage, when early symptoms, such as epistaxis and other peculiarities of the cachexia show themselves, it will be very likely to stay the disease from further progress, but if it has progressed further on, the same remedy if it accords with the symptoms may have a curative effect.

If called upon to treat a case of this kind when the pre-tubercular stage has passed, it will be necessary to make a critical record of all the symptoms in order to search for their similitude in the pathogenesis of some of the antipsorics, and the one approximating the nearest in point of resemblance will be found the most effectual in the treatment of this stage of the disease. There are in the human family a great variety of physical constitutions and habits of body, each of which may have its individual cachexia, which will correspond to its remedy, as the Causticum cachexia, Lycopodium cachexia, Cal. carb., Nitric acid, Baryta carb., and each and every other remedy that has been useful in treating tuberculosis. In the case above cited *Calcarea carbonica* had a satisfactory effect, all the symptoms present in the tubercular stage disappeared, the hectic fever ceased, and the patient has remained comparatively well for several years. In the first stage of phthisis we generally find emaciation and a dry cough, which is apt to be worse at night. This dry cough is sometimes attended with running at the nose and a mucous expectoration streaked with blood, with a sense of rawness and a wounded feeling in the chest. It will be seen that all these symptoms are found in the pathogenesis of *Calcarea carbonica*. In the second stage of phthisis the mucous expectoration often has a color and a sweet taste. This is also a symptom found in the pathogenesis of

Calcarea, and we may go on through the various stages of phthisis, and we may find that the cheeks are frequently red, and that there is a burning in the hands and feet, oppressed respiration, uneasy feeling, quick pulse, which varies but little either in the cold or hot stage of hectic, and also copious night-sweats. *Calcarea carbonica* is evidently the remedy to be consulted in phthisis.

We will briefly consider the action of *Lycopodium*, which in many respects is an analogue of *Calcarea* and therefore both are Homœopathic to the symptoms of the various stages of phthisis. When the bleeding occurs in the afternoon and not in the morning, Lycopodium is more especially indicated; in the second and third stages, when there is evidence of ulceration and the hair falls off easily, when there is considerable expectoration of sanious matter, and evening fever, and sweat towards morning, *Lycopodium* is Homœopathically indicated.

There are many points of resemblance between the Calcarea and Lycopodium cachexia, and also of the symptoms attendant in the different stages of phthisis. The distinction between the action of Calcarea and that of Lycopodium, is to be found in the fact that the Lycopodium manifests its action most frequently at night. We may add also that this remedy has a different action on the kidneys and urine.

In case of tedious constipation in phthisis, Lycopodium, by virtue of its primary action, would be indicated; it therefore becomes clear from these views that the remedy has a curative relationship to those cases of phthisis characterized by tedious constipation, hard stools, disease of the kidneys and great debility. The cachexia, for which Nitric acid is suitable, and the symptoms of phthisis which have not as yet been covered by the pathogenetical facts of Calcarea and Lycopodium, may point to Nitric acid to furnish a curative means, for the pathogenetic effects of this drug bear a similitude with many symptoms exhibited in some cases of phthisis, more directly than those of Calcarea and Lycopodium, and would be likely, therefore, to exert a more decided curative action.

Sulphur is a remedy which may be employed in the cure of consumption when its peculiar cachexia is present. Among the pathogenetic effects of this remedy the symptom of itching of the skin is prominent, and its power to eliminate upon the surface in the form of eruptions which itch, smart and burn, would indicate its value as a remedy for those forms of consumption which originate from suppressed scabies and other forms of psora. In the group of remedies which collectively furnish the curative means in the treatment of consumption, we also find *Sepia*, *Kali carb.* *Arsenicum*, *Cal. phos.*, *Sticta pulmonaria*, and many other remedies, which if carefully studied and correctly affiliated in accordance with their pathogenetic effects, and the symptoms of the disease, would furnish the practitioner with the therapeutic means of almost every form of treatment pointed out in Homœopathic science. We will now recapitulate: Homœopathic treatment, in the premonitory stage, for the nose-bleed, *Aconite* and *Calcarea* have a great correspondence. With the symptoms attendant upon nose-bleed in the primary stage, *Aconite* is useful for erethism which attends the age of puberty and gives rise to epistaxis at this period. It is also Homœopathic to that peculiar sense of fulness of the chest so common at the age of puberty, more especially so where the conditions of the lungs connected with tubercular disease are present, as all the phenomena of inflammation are found under the pathogenetic effects of Aconite,—and therefore this remedy would be Homœopathic to any local or general inflammatory action; as for instance very painful inflammation of the eyes and a sensation of the eye being much swollen; in inflammatory catarrh of the nose attended with bleeding from the nasal ducts, or where bleeding from the lungs is present in any individual having symptoms of inflammation; and this is why the persistent use of Aconite will cure such bleeding.

It is nevertheless in the action of Calcarea that the cure of the cachexia which causes the bleeding of the nose arises, therefore the indications for the employment of Calcarea are flowing from the nose of a blackish blood, a period of several days with some bleeding of the nose at night, and early in the morning. It is also useful for affections of the throat, rawness of the top of the throat, and painful deglutition; a piping in the superior portion of the trachea when lying down, a tickling irritation in the larynx producing cough; this symptom suggests also the use of Nitric acid. It has been observed that many persons of a phthisical cachexia are subject to freckle especially in young subjects when exposed to country air during warm weather. In those decidedly

phthisical the freckle is present whether in country or town, Calcarea is indicated when these pimples, or freckles, are numerous
and attended with itching. Calcarea is indicated when sweating
is produced by the slightest exercise and the patient is very sensitive to cold air; and the feet feel as if dead; or when he walks in
the open air he feels depressed in spirit and suffers from an oppressive headache, which is only relieved by lying down; even the
symptom of sneezing in a phthisical individual with a sensation
of a stoppage of the nose this remedy is indicated, or when there
is itching of the eyelids in the evening or early in the morning;
or falling off of the hair, or an eruption behind the ears, or when
there is a sense of fullness in the narrow chest as if puffed up
with blood, causing an anxiety in the chest with anxious breathing
and tremulous action of the heart, spitting of blood. Calcarea is
indicated in the first stage of phthisis, for dry cough on retiring
at night, and after midnight when the cough is attended with discharge of mucus from the nose and irritability of the lachrymal
glands; and when the cough ceases to be dry, and there is a discharge of mucus from time to time early in the morning and after
lying down at night and the expectoration is tenacious, tasteless,
and inodorous, and also when the expectoration of blood through
coughing and hawking, leaves a sense of rawness in the chest,
and in the more advanced stages when the expectoration is
streaked with blood, has color, taste, and smell, it is also indicated
in the second stage; when sweating commences on all parts of
the body and when the patient finds it difficult to keep awake,
and yet does not sleep soundly; and sweats much, early in the
morning, has dry throat without much thirst; the sweat is very
exhausting. Another characteristic symptom for which Calcarea
is indicated, relates to the sweats of the lower extremities, the legs
and feet; a great many other symptoms would indicate the use of
Calcarea, such as delirium and a variety of characteristic peculiarities of the phthisical disease. Lycopodium has the power of removing many diseased conditions believed to be premonitory
signs of the approach of consumption.

The peculiar cachexia for which this remedy is adapted may
be ascertained by studying carefully its pathogenesis and their
Homœopathic relationship to the symptoms present in consumption, but in order to arrest the progress of the disease it is necessary to employ Lycopodium as in the case of Calcarea as early in

the disease as it is possible to note the cachexia and symptoms which point to its Homœopathic applicability.

We may remember the same concerning Nitric acid, Causticum, Carbo animalis, Carbo vegetabilis, etc., the entire group of remedies which sustain any relation to the phthisical condition in order to utilize them as curative agents must be studied and affiliated in like manner.

With regard to diet, in the treatment of phthisis in the curative stages, it must be carefully selected to meet the demands of the system; salt fish which has undergone no fermentation, nicely separated from its bones, may be cooked and eaten with cream; when the patient is subject to much nervous excitability, well-fed beef and mutton may be supplied *ad libitum;* if indicated by the patient's appetite.   A farinaceous diet with eggs and milk, and cocoa with almost any other non-medicinal and nutritious material may enter into the regimen.

CHAPTER XXV.

DISEASES OF THE PLEURA.

The pleura is a serous membrane which lines the thorax, the pleura costalis and reflected over the lungs is termed the pleura-pulmonalis, it is subject to inflammation, the portion that covers the lungs is subject to modification in the phenomena presented by inflammation, differing somewhat from that which pertains to the portion which lines the parietes of the thorax, by reason of its contiguity with the viscus which it covers; the acute inflammation of the pleura is denoted by acute pain in the side or in some part of the thorax, cough, difficulty of breathing, fever, more or less dullness on percussion, with egophony, followed by enlargement of the effected side and avolition of all sound of respiration and voice; great variety however exists in the phenomena, which renders a further inquiry into the character of the symptoms and signs necessary.

One of the most constant symptoms of the disease is pain, yet in some cases, and particularly in that form termed latent pleurisy, no pain may be experienced, especially in weak and debilitated subjects; with such the inflammation may have existed for a long time accompanied by copious effusion in the cavity of the pleura as clearly ascertained by auscultation and percussion.

Generally pain is felt in the region of the nipple, on one side or the other, extremely acute and lancinating, and greatly aggravated by the slightest attempt at inspiration, the sensation of severe pain in the axilla, under the sternum or clavicle, or the region of the scapulæ, the margin of the false ribs, etc., may be experienced.

When the inflammation is seated in the pleura costalis it is increased by pressure on the intercostal spaces, and by percussion, inspiration, or coughing or motion of the body in general, compelling the patient to make short and repeated inspirations, with a dread of the slightest mechanical change induced by unavoidable movements.

In acute pleurisy the pain exists from the outset, but not

always fixed, and this is the reason why it is sometimes confounded with pleurodynia, or rheumatism; it becomes fixed, however, and constant and expressively severe, and then its severity gradually diminishes even to obscurity before the termination of the disease. When the pleura that covers the parietes of the thorax becomes inflamed and the intercostal spaces become so sensitive and sore as to interfere with the motion of the chest in respiration, the diaphragm is called into requisition to carry on this function; but when the lower portion of the pleura in contact with the diaphragm becomes the seat of the inflammation and renders this organ unable to assist in performing the function of respiration and the pleura-costalis and intercostal spaces are not implicated the function is then performed by the elevation and depression of the parietes of the thorax or ribs while the extreme pain is experienced at the margin of the false ribs.

When both pleuræ are implicated and their serous surfaces become so dry for want of lubrication as not to glide easily over each other a sound is produced resembling the creaking of leather; at other times the serous surfaces may become adherent from the inflammation and render respiration exceedingly painful, because the painless gliding of the surfaces when in health becomes obstructed by the adhesion.

When effusion of any kind takes place in the cavity of the pleura, the extent of the respiratory movements are necessarily diminished in the direct ratio with the quantity of fluid effused. The sound of respiration will likewise be diminished in the affected side, but more extensive than natural in the unaffected side.

When the patient articulates during the existence of effusion no vibration can be felt as in health; pleuritic effusion may be detected by passing the hand under each scapulæ, when this absence of vibration is apparent, especially when auscultation has revealed dullness of sound. There are many other indications of pleuritis and subsequent effusions or adhesions which might be enumerated and described, but the characteristic symptoms already given will assist in making an unmistakable diagnosis.

TREATMENT.—The Allopathic treatment is much the same as in pneumonia; blood letting is a general resort and this is repeated several times until the system becomes lowered and then topical depletion over affected region; this is followed by an emollient poultice and massive doses of mercury given until the mouth becomes affected, tartar emetic in sensible doses is administered for the purpose of producing an alterative effect upon the stomach and bowels.

It is maintained that the salivation should be kept up, and that the effusion is absorbed and that the cough should be constantly quieted by full doses of opiates. After the violent symptoms have subsided and effusion still remains, diuretics and active cathartics, sinapisms, blisters, and other counter irritants are called into requisition; the entire course of treatment is objectionable from the fact that those who submit to it are greatly reduced and have less power of recuperative action in the system.

HOMŒOPATHIC TREATMENT.—Aconite when the disease sets in with a chill and inflammatory fever, and is characterized by a dry hot skin, a full bounding pulse, agonized tossing about, violent thirst, shortness of breath, and great nervous excitability, this remedy is plainly indicated. It is also indicated for piercing and stitching pains in the chest interfering with respiration, with dry cough, inability to lie on the affected side.

When the patient experiences a sensation as if the ribs were broken or bruised, with stitching pains in the left side and a short, dry cough, Arnica is indicated; this remedy is also indicated for sore feeling as if from a bruise, shock, or other mechanical injury, when the cheeks are flushed and hot, and the patient finds his respiration greatly oppressed, and the pain augmented by the motion of respiration, or when his position is on the affected side.

Bryonia is indicated when the head aches as if it would split open, has nausea and faintness when trying to sit up, and thirst for copious draughts of water at long intervals, and also for constipation of hard, dry stools as if burnt, and also when the patient is easily fired up with anger, and is exceedingly irritable.

When the violent stitching pain does not yield to this remedy, Kali carbonicum may be substituted; especially when the darting, shooting or cutting pains are in the right side of the chest, and generally with violent palpitation of the heart. Kali carbonicum is a suitable remedy for a dry cough which becomes severe about three o'clock in the morning.

Mercurius solubilis is suitable for soreness and burning in the chest, stitching pains in the right side of the chest—through from the shoulder blade, cough worse at night and when lying on the left side, when the tongue is moist and the thirst is great, copious perspiration which affords no relief, an aggravation of all the symptoms at night. In cases of bilious pleurisy where there is great pain, restlessness and constipation, *Nux vomica* given in the evening may follow this remedy.

For **short, difficult respiration**, lancinating pains, or sharp pains when pressing upon the intercostal spaces, or sense of tightness across the chest with shaking cough, *Phosphorus* may be consulted, especially if there is sensation of weakness, and emptyness in the abdomen, cutting pains in the bowels, and not unfrequently with gastric derangement, long, narrow, hard stools difficult to expel.

Rhus tox. is called into use when pleurisy accompanies rheumatism, or is brought on by exposure to wet weather, or from straining, lifting, or overexertion of any kind. In cases where the febrile symptoms have subsided, and wandering pains still affect the chest, and there is shortness of breath with general debility, this remedy is indicated, and also when the patient suffers intolerably when at rest, obliging him to move continually to get a little relief.

When the disease is complicated with pneumonia, or does not yield to well-chosen remedies, Sulphur is indicated, particularly when there is some soreness remaining which becomes manifest when moving, and also for a short, dry cough with stitches in the chest extending through to the left shoulder blade when aggravated from the least motion, and also for flashes of heat over the chest and on top of the head, accompanied at times by fainting. In case of burning, dry, hot skin and covered with perspiration, with hurried and difficult respiration, *Tartar emetic* is indicated, and also when there is a loose cough and much apparent rattling of mucus without expectoration, with vertigo and drowsiness, and paralytic weakness of the lungs.

To promote absorption of the serous effusion, *Arsenicum* and *Phosphorus* may be consulted; for the hydro-thorax, which supervenes upon inflammation of the pleura, *Arsenicum, Apis mellifica, Apocynum cannabinum, Hellebore* and *Jalapa* form a group from which to choose according to their pathogenetic action.

Accessory means.—Light poultices of linseed meal, or compresses of very warm water may be applied to the region of the pain.

Chronic form of Pleurisy.

Weak and feeble persons after an acute attack of pleuritis may suffer from the chronic form; the symptoms of chronic pleuritis are not unlike those of the acute, only less severe. The sequel of chronic pleuritis is usually emphysema or chronic contraction; the symptoms and signs are chiefly those that denote copious effusion into the pleura of the affected side and they are the same in all forms of the disease; difficulty in breathing, tickling cough, and hectic fever, are the usual concomitants of the disease.

The fluid diffused may be absorbed in process of time, and the chest may return to its normal condition, and this, too, when the affected side, involving the intercostal spaces, has been much swollen; this is usually the most favorable termination.

TREATMENT.—Allopathic treatment consists of cathartics and the administration of half a grain of *Iodine*, twelve grains of common *salt*, and one pint of distilled water, for internal administration, while blisters may be used externally with prescription in promoting absorption.

HOMŒOPATHIC TREATMENT.—which has been found to be more effectual, consists entirely in the administration of attenuated Homœopathic remedies. *Iodium* the 6x, *Kali* hydriodicum 6x, Sulphur and other remedies.

Typhoid inflammation of the Pleura.

The remarks that were made on typhoid inflammation of the lungs, are not inappropriate to apply to typhoid pleurisy. The diagnosis and method of treatment are in all respects the same; bilious pleurisy usually occurs in broken down constitutions, and is frequently the sequel of some other morbid condition. It may be insidious, the signs are often latent; being indicated rather by the sinking of the powers of life, than by any new suffering as in typhoid pneumonia; it is slow of removal; it is frequently combined with gastro-enteric disease.

Bilious pleurisy is frequently a secondary disease in the course of typhus or spotted fever, in typhoid arthritis and diffuse inflam-

mation, in severe forms of erysipelas in phlebitis, and by many it
is conceived to be a consequence of purulent absorption.   Louis
thinks it does not occur frequently as a complication of typhus.
In many of these cases the cavity of the pleura is known to contain collections of purulent or sero-purulent matter, although during life the symptoms of pleurisy were either wanting or slightly
marked; at other times the invasion of the disease is accompanied
by severe pain.   In all these cases the physical signs denote effusion; the treatment of bilious pleurisy requires the same care and
caution detailed in that of typhoid pneumonia.

Pleurodynia.

This is a form of neuralgia which sometimes suddenly attacks
the side, giving rise to a stitch of a longer or shorter duration,
and seems to be seated in the intercostal muscles, rather than in
the pleura, it may be distinguished from acute pleuritis, by the
absence of fever, and the physical signs that indicate pleuritis;
there is also more or less soreness manifest on pressing the muscles of the chest.   The class of patients most frequently assailed
with pleurodynia, are the nervous and hysterical, which apparently
suffer intensely at times.

TREATMENT.—The Allopathic treatment for this peculiar suffering is by scarification, and cups, sinapisms, and hot applications,
and sometimes by bags of heated salt, or hot flannel, and volatile
liniments.   For internal administration, opium pills, or sulphate
of morphine are prescribed.

HOMŒOPATHIC TREATMENT, which is by far the most preferable, consists in the administration of carefully selected Homœopathic remedies, among which are *Bryonia*, *China*, *Calcarea carbonica*, *Gelsemium* and *Sulphur*, while us accessory means, flannels
wet with the extract of *Hamamelis virginica* may be applied externally.   When the disease is connected with hysteria, *Ignatia*,
Hyoscyamus, and *Pulsatilla* may be consulted in all such subjects.
A generous diet is to be commended.

Dropsy of the Pleura.

Like other serous cavities that of the pleura is liable to dropsical effusion; the disease is comparatively rare, yet sufficiently
frequent to merit attention, as in the case of pleurisy, the

fluid is contained in the cavity of the pleura, and is essentially an accumulation of the secretion which takes place from the pleura, and which in a healthy condition is intended for its lubrication, and like other dropsical accumulations it may occur from an exaggerated secretion of the exhalent vessels, beyond the normal power of the absorbent vessels; or the exhalent vessels may only pour out their normal quantity, while the absorbent vessels may take up too sparingly; in either case dropsical accumulation would inevitably take place in the pleural cavity; should there be any obstacle that prevents the proper return of blood to the center of circulation the result may be a passive hydrothorax.

The *symptoms* and physical signs which denote dropsy of the chest are not unlike those which become manifest during the effusion which takes place in pleuritis; it is therefore difficult to discriminate between a slight attack of acute pleuritis and an active dropsy of the chest.

There is however, an entire absence of febrile symptoms, though dyspnœa which is in proportion to the amount of fluid effused, difficulty of lying on the affected side, and in case of double hydrothorax, panting respiration, and difficulty of breathing except when in the sitting posture, energetic action of all the respiratory muscles and extreme anxiety of countenance and œdema of the lower extremities.

The physical signs are dullness of the affected side, egophony. If the fluid is small in quantity, another physical sign is the absence of the respiratory murmur in the part corresponding to the effusion.

With the substitute of tubal respiration when the accumulation is restricted to one side, there is an enlargement which corresponds to the amount of the effusion, this swollen condition is · sometimes associated with enlargement of the intercostal spaces. The causes are the same as those of general dropsy.

The disease may occur at any period of life, though most commonly at the age of forty or upwards, it must be borne in mind however, that it frequently occurs as a symptom of some abdominal or thoracic disease.

TREATMENT.—In the regular Allopathic practice *Digitalis* and *Opium* is made into a mixture with gum-arabic and water;

this is employed extensively in nearly all cases of dropsy of the chest.

HOMŒOPATHIC TREATMENT has proved far more effective and desirable in curing this disease; the remedies employed to restore equilibrium between the secretory and absorbent vessels are *Arsenicum, Apis mellifica, Apocynum can., Digitalis, Kali hydriodicum, Lachesis, Helleborus niger* and *Sulphur*.

Arsenicum in the third decimal trituration, if there is considerable prostration, thirst, and a burning sensation in the epigastric region, and a difficult respiration and palpitation of the heart.

Apis mellifica when the dropsical effusion is evinced by panting respiration and œdema of the lower extremities with scanty urination.

Apocynum when there is but little disturbance of the heart's action, but great pressure upon the lungs from the accumulation of water in the cavity of the pleura, and when there is a sense of suffocation, shortness of breath, with considerable enlargement of the affected side.

Kali hydriodicum is particularly indicated when the secretion of the urine is scanty, and the signs of accumulation are indicative of pressure upon the lungs to a degree that respiration becomes mechanically obstructed, and when, also, there are slight rheumatic pains darting through the chest, and in sympathy, apparently, with similar pains affecting the trunk and lower extremities.

Lachesis is particularly indicated for hydrothorax attendant upon *menopausis*, the critical age of women.

Helleborus niger is a suitable remedy for hydrothorax when it supervenes as a sequel to exanthematous diseases.

Sulphur is also a remedy that may be employed in the treatment of hydro-thorax with œdematous swelling of the lower extremities.

Dietetic regulations for dropsies in general.—The diet should consist of the lean as well as the fat *beef* and *mutton* cooked without vegetables. Very little water should be drank, and only a restricted amount of other fluids.

Air in the Pleura.

It is difficult to discriminate between the symptoms of pneumothorax and hydrothorax, for in many instances their symptoms are so analagous, and yet there is a difference; the patient complains of great difficulty of breathing, which is in the ratio with the quantity of air effused, and the rapidity with which the effusions occur; the affected side is rendered prominent in many instances, and there is an unusual clearness on percussion over the whole affected side, or if the patient be sitting up the resonance may be marked at the upper portion of the chest, while it may be dull beneath, denoting the presence of the liquid beneath.

This unusual sonorousness is accompanied with absence of the sound of respiration except near the root of the lung, where it is tubal; pneumothorax and hydrothorax may each exist at the same time, the lower portion of the pleural cavity may contain considerable fluid while the upper portion is filled with air.

The cause of air in the pleura may be a wound of the chest, or communication from the lungs with the cavity of the pleura; this communication may consist of a tubercular excavation with a fistulous opening into the pleura. Some authors say that when the effusion of air or of air and fluid is considerable there may be signs of displacement.

TREATMENT.—The prevailing treatment for years has been of a palliative character, and the impression is that the disease, being connected with tuberculosis, is incurable, but in rare cases it has terminated favorably by absorption.

A distinguished French author says, when the affection is uncomplicated it need not terminate unfavorably, and even the incurable cases may continue for years, or until some new morbid condition arises to aggravate the difficulty.

HOMŒOPATHIC TREATMENT has been found serviceable and not unfrequently curative.

Sulphur will sometimes hasten absorption.

Calcarea carbonica, when complicated tubercular degeneration, when the air in the pleura is supposed to receive through the fistulous opening of the cavity a continued supply.

Silicea is indicated and its effect will be to close up the fistulous opening and afford a better opportunity for the absorption; this remedy is also supposed to arrest tuberculosis.

A case of phthisis pulmonalis with perforation, the subject being a bricklayer, made several extraordinary rallies under the use of this remedy, and several times returned to his occupation, his life was apparently prolonged for nearly two years.

In the case of a gentleman, aged twenty-six years, of a consumptive tendency, was after a brief illness an unmistakable victim to this trouble.   It resulted, it was supposed, from some insidious communication between the bronchia and the pleura. Lycopodium was given to the patient first, and apparently with good effect; he was emaciated and rather inclined to dyspnœa. Lycopodium administered twice a day for several days was followed by a change in the lubricative system, his appetite became improved and he gained in flesh and strength and though he had previously been subject to hectic fever it totally subsided; and he took exercise every day, he could ride on horseback if not for the interference of the splashing of the chest, absorption gradually took place under the use of this remedy. A number of other cases are reported by different authors where Homœopathic treatment has been successfully employed.

Asphyxia.

By this term is understood a want of pulse, or an interruption of the circulation. In this sense it was formerly used, and the same meaning to a certain extent is preserved, but what is commonly understood by asphyxia, is suspended animation. Many distinguished authors of late, however, use the term to signify apparent death, or suspension. The diagnostic difference between syncope and asphyxia is this: asphyxia denotes apparent death from the suspension of respiration, and syncope is usually applied to death commencing in the heart. The epithet of asphyxia has been applied to the malignant type of cholera, when the patient appeared to be pulseless and in collapse.

CAUSES.—Anything that produces sudden prostration and sinking in the system, or that interferes with the æration of the blood, causes asphyxia. Pseudo-membraneous formations in the larynx, trachea, and bronchia, are frequently followed by asphyxia. Asphyxia may be considered under various heads: First, asphyxia from drowning; this varies according to the submersion being complete from the first, or as risen again and again to the surface. When a person falls into the water and remains beneath the surface, the first effort to inspire draws in the water until it reaches the glottis, causing the muscles which close it to contract spontaneously so that little or no water can pass or enter, and death takes place from strangulation, but little can be learned of the changes that take place in persons while drowning. Louis instituted several experiments with a view of testing the matter. On immersing animals in colored liquids he discovered these in the trachea, and sometimes in the ramifications of the bronchia. Others experimented in the same way with other fluids and with similar results, but even if small quantities of water enter the bronchial tubes, it may be supposed that the victims rose to the surface after falling into the water and made an attempt to breathe, and the inspired air mixing with the water and mucus would produce the froth or frothy mucus sometimes met with in recently drowned persons. Many have been the phenomena described by different authors pertaining to the imbibition or non-imbibition of water into the different cavities of the body during the process of drowning, but one thing is certain, death will result from asphyxia produced by submersion in the water unless perchance the persons are rescued before life is extinct, and the asphyxia can be overcome.

TREATMENT.—No time should be lost when a drowned man is taken from the water, his mouth and throat should be cleansed and then he should be turned on his face that the water may escape from his mouth and throat, and then artificial respiration should be attempted, rolling the victim over and over for a few minutes and then draw his tongue forward and keep it in this position; and sometimes by blowing into the patients mouth, at the same time manipulating the chest respiration may be established. The use of the flesh brush is also commended; due regard should be had to the patient's position, he should be placed on his back on an inclined plane and then his arms should be worked gently upwards and downwards in order to give a motion to the chest, in gently lifting the arms above so as to meet; the active inspiration may be stimulated and aeration of the blood may proceed and on turning the arms of the patient down expiration may be facilitated.

Inspiration may also be excited by tickling the nose with a

feather or some kinds of snuff; during these operations tepid or
warm water may be dashed upon the chest and face, which should
be briskly rubbed.

After respiration becomes established wrap the patient in a
dry blanket and briskly rub his limbs until the surface becomes
warm to the hand, when the power of swallowing has returned
the patient may take a little wine, warm tea, or coffee.

Second, asphyxia from hanging, requires first the removal of
the ligature about the neck and then nearly the same manipulations as in the case of drowning, and if no injury has occurred to
the spinal cord, circulation may become established and the respiratory function duly restored. Third, asphyxia from smother-
ing does not differ in its essential appearance from other varieties;
it is exceedingly rare to find an occurrence of the kind except in
the case of children, and even in them, it is an unusual occurrence·
It is possible for an adult in a state of intoxication to get into a
position that may obstruct the entrance of air into the air passages. In numerous instances through the carelessness of nurses,
or mothers, children have been smothered in bed; a young infant
pressed too closely against the side of its mother during her sleep
may result in death from asphyxia from the arrest of the respiration; and sometimes an anxious care of the mother in wrap-
ping her infant too closely in flannels has resulted unfavorably.
The treatment is precisely the same as has been laid down for the
other varieties. Fourth, asphyxia from tumors and other morbid
conditions.

Whatever obstructs the entrance of air into the lungs, gives
rise to asphyxia. In some exceedingly rare instances, quinsy sore
throat has so obstructed the entrance of air into the air passages
as to produce asphyxia. Laryngitis may close up the aperture of
the larynx, and other obstructions not necessary to enumerate
may have a similar result.

Asphyxia of new born Infants during Uterine Life.

It is well known that no more blood passes through the lungs
than is necessary for their nutrition, and that the blood of the
fœtus is sent back to the placenta, whence it passes back by the
umbilical vein. It is probable that the blood after being sent to
the placenta undergoes a change which better adapts it to the nutrition of the fœtus before it is returned by the umbilical vein.

From this fact it may seem that the placenta is a respiratory organ for the fœtus; and if this be so we can readily understand why the pressure of the child's head during parturition should obstruct the circulation by pressure upon the cord giving rise to asphyxia.

We can thus understand that if the cord comes down in such a manner as to be strongly compressed for some time before delivery, asphyxia may be produced.

TREATMENT.—When immediately after birth the child appears lifeless, and respiration has not been established, the earliest resort possible to excite respiration should not be neglected, manipulation of the chest, dashes of cold water upon the chest, and slapping it with the hand, exciting the nostrils by something volatile, will in the majority of cases excite the respiratory function and the child will begin to cry. If within the brief period of two minutes, there is no response to these measures, the accoucheur should place a quill or a small glass tube into the mouth of the infant into which he should blow his own breath, in order to inflate the infant's lungs; respiration by this means has frequently been established. In one instance a child suppose to be dead, began to cry six minutes after its birth. If any mucus is found in the child's throat sufficient to obstruct respiration it must be carefully removed by the fingers, some have recommended a warm bath; but so far as the author's observation has gone to prove, the bath weakens, though respiration may be excited by it. Another means of exciting respiration is by rubbing or friction. By employing these means the lives of many newborn infants may be saved; which in all probability would never breathe if carelessly neglected. It is evident therefore that the various forms of asphyxia must be treated with reference to the causes that produce them.

In very many cases the asphyxia of adults is liable to prove fatal. It is profitable to make use of all the means that have been suggested, as well as others that suggest themselves to restore animation.

Asphyxia from Anæsthesia.

This frequently results from the carelessness of the operator. Neither *Chloroform*, *Ether* or *Nitrate of Amyl* should be administered without facilities for free respiration in a good atmosphere.

From a failure to recognize the importance of this condition of the anæsthesia the muscles of the larynx may suddenly contract so as to obstruct respiration.

Spirits of Ammonia should be called into requisition and applied to the nostrils, while the tongue should be drawn forward and confined by a depressor in order to facilitate the entrance of fresh air.

In this way the asphyxia may be overcome, and the circulation and respiration may be re-established. Some practitioners resort to a saturated tincture of Camphor, a few drops of which is placed in the mouth, others again administer Ammonia in sufficient strength to antidote the effect of the anæsthetic.

The use of *Chloroform* and *Ether* as anæsthetic agents, subject to extremes may have a disastrous effect on certain persons; nevertheless the number of deaths resulting from the employment of these agents are exceedingly limited.

CHAPTER XXVI.

DISEASES OF THE CIRCULATION.

In morbid conditions of the blood common observation shows that the condition of the solids is materially influenced by that of the blood which bathes them and furnishes the pabulum for their support. On this account modern pathology is to look to the blood as the source of many diseases, which in former times were regarded as exclusively confined to the solids. Fullness of blood is a condition which enters into the conception of non-professional, as well as the professional, and that an opposite condition of poverty of blood, sometimes exists, there can be no question.

We cannot from common observation fully appreciate the effects of a moderate degree of plethora and anæmia. so well as when the fullness or deficiency is considerable. The blood is susceptible to some degree of modification caused by a change of element, or by agents which are sometimes administered for this purpose, such as the various preparations of *Iodine, Mercury*, etc., and likewise its character may become essentially changed. The effect of disease upon the blood has been observed by Andrew Magendie, and the still more modern writers. A part of the history of individual diseases consists of the effects which they produce in the blood, as it will farther appear when certain blood diseases are considered. When the blood is circulating through the vessels. it consists, apparently, of a fluid portion which is termed serum, and a solid portion under the name of fibrin. When the blood is drawn and left to stand in a vessel, the fluids and the solids separate, the serum rises to the top and the fibrin intermingles with the red corpuscles and sinks to the bottom, as will be made apparent by washing.

The specific gravity of the blood differs in different individuals, but it is difficult to account for this obvious fact. The mean specific gravity varies, 273, according to observations. It is therefore difficult to fix the standard. It is easy to conceive of a change in the specific gravity of the blood in case of copious losses, because the solid portions are not readily generated, while the diminution in the quantity of the circulating fluid increases absorption. The specific gravity of serum affords more precise information.

, The proper proportion of saline matters does not raise the specific gravity of serum above that of distilled water more than five parts in a thousand.

The excess beyond this is owing to the presence of albumen so that the specific gravity of serum pretty nearly indicates the quantity of albumen contained in it, and hence it becomes a useful guide in Bright's disease.

In certain cases of disease when albumen is carried rapidly out of the system, as in renal difficulties, dropsies, and profuse hæmorrhages; the specific gravity of the serum which in health averages 1027 has been observed as low as 1013, while in other conditions where both the water, and salts, are removed as in cholera, O'Shaughnessy found the specific gravity as high as 1041. There is a material variation also of the proportion of fibrin to the serum in different diseased conditions; the state of the vital fluid may be particularly described, under the head of such diseases, as the state of the blood has been specifically noticed.

Plethora or Fullness of Blood.

From observation it is manifest that too much blood is formed and the vascular system is more or less burdened on this account. There is at times a fullness of blood in the general system which the term polyæmia is used to signify; while a surcharge of the capillary system is termed hyperæmia.

A general fullness of blood is regarded by some as a predisponent of disease, and creates a tendency to local congestion.

One of the causes of plethora is believed to be a full habit of eating and drinking, and excess of nourishment. A want of mental and physical exercise.

TREATMENT.—In Allopathic practice for a fullness of the blood, depletion of some kind is constantly called into requisition; but this practice is very objectionable.

HOMŒOPATHIC TREATMENT for general plethora is mainly dietetic, consists in the regulation of the diet, by substituting vegetables for animal food, and a proper restriction as to quantity. For the removal of a general sense of fullness *Aconite* may be administered three or four times a day; for local congestions such as a rush of blood to the head or hyperæmia, Belladonna may take the place of Aconite.

For other derangements consequent upon plethora such as drowsiness, giddiness, headache, flushed face and bleeding at the nose, such remedies as have these marked symptoms in their pathogenesis may be administered.

Persons at all subject to plethora must avoid alcoholic stimulants, wine and beer.

Paucity of Blood.

By the term paucity of blood is understood both a deficiency of blood and that condition in which the watery portions largely predominate.

Hydroæmia, symptoms, paleness of the countenance and skin, and those portions of the mucous membrane which connect with the outer tegumentary tissue, sometimes, however, the vessels of the skin of the face are turgid with blood, and the cheeks become vividly red, as in hectic fever, which presents the appearance of a livid and circumscribed flush.

Chronic inflammation of the liver or spleen accompanied by general anæmia is often attended with this circumscribed flush of the cheeks.

A slow, feeble pulse, or a frequent, small and almost imperceptible pulse indicates paucity of the blood.

In nearly all anæmic subjects, there are disagreeable beatings in the chest, and of the neck and head, frequently attended with syncope.

The nervous system becomes very impressible under the influence of *anæmia*, and the most trivial excitement on this account may produce irregularities in the circulation; this is strikingly manifest in the headache, beating of the carotid and temporal arteries, which suddenly intervene, and the suffusion of face that quickly supervenes upon losses of blood, as in metrorrhagia; anæmia is also attended by a disturbance of the cerebral function, as vertigo, dimness of vision and noises in the ears; anæmia is also attended with more or less œdema of the lower extremities; the symptoms of anæmia are so plainly manifest in opposition to those of plethora that no further detail of them is necessary in diagnosticating the disease.

The causes of anæmia are, any circumstance that deprives the organism of the blood necessary for the nutrition of the tissues, as copious depletion or spontaneous loss of blood as in metrorrhagia, hæmoptysis and other hæmorrhages; next to the loss of blood, insufficient nourishment, absence from food, or any interruption of the nutritive function. Excessive fatigue, want of rest and imperfect ventilation, or confinement in apartments which exclude the light of the sun; and lastly we may include diarrhœa, cholera, dysentery and other morbid fluxes from the bowels, including hæmorrhoids.

Anæmia may be symptomatic of various diseased conditions of an organic character such as operate to impoverish the blood and produce paleness of the countenance; emotional excitement or an exceedingly irritable disposition which frequently becomes manifest in fits of ungovernable passion, may temporarilly at least induce anæmia; fevers also have a tendency to exhaust the richness of the blood, and may be included among the causes, the paleness of the countenance during a chill, as well as that of the entire body are not indicative of anæmia, there being a recession of the vital fluid from the surface to await a natural reaction.

TREATMENT.—In all cases where the function of nutrition will admit, the patient must be supplied with a nourishing diet and especially so if the anæmia has been caused by starvation. In as much as the stomach under such circumstances is exceedingly impressible, the caution and prudence of the practitioner must be exercised.   The patient must be placed in well ventilated apartments and be supplied with a "quantum sufficit" of fresh air and sunlight.

The various preparations of iron in massive doses are much relied upon by Allopathic practitioners, together with the different mineral and vegetable tonics including *Cinchona*. To allay the nervous excitement a prescription of hydrocyanic acid, four drops; mucilage of gum arabic, three drachms, and six ounces of camphor water; dose a wine glass every six hours; this treatment from observation has not been so successful as a judicious Homœopathic affiliation of remedies. For losses of blood by depletion, *China;* for hæmatemesis first give Ipecac and then follow with China, in habitually anæmic conditions indicated by extreme paleness, *Ferum metallicum*; for anæmia caused by metrorrhagia, *Crocus sativa,* or *Ipecac* may precede the use of *China;* after the use of *Trillium* and *Erigeron* to arrest metrorrhagia; if any anæmic condition remains, *China, Ferrum met, Cansativa, Natrum mur., Nux vom.,* etc. For the paleness and debility which sometimes precede menstrual derangements, the *Pyrophosphate* of *Iron* is required. For scrofulous anæmia or that which results from a protracted dyspepsia, or confinement in an impure atmosphere generally attended with loss of appetite, confusion, giddiness in the head, sleeplessness, noise in the ears, like the singing of a tea-kettle, *Cinnabar, Sulphur, Cal. carb., Arsenicum* and *Pyrophosphate of Iron.* Each Homœopathic remedy mentioned above should be given in drop doses of the 3d dilution and two grain doses of the 3d trituration, repeated every two hours.

In many cases of lymphatic anæmia treated Allopathically with Iron and without success the Homœopathic use of *Kali hydriodicum, Merc. hydriodicum, Ferrum iodutus* and *Sulphur,* 3x dil., has proved successful. Nevertheless the treatment of anæmia in all cases must be with reference to the cause, temperament and age of the patient guided by the peculiar symptoms in each individual case.

CHAPTER XXVII.

DISEASES OF THE CIRCULATORY ORGANS.

Diseases of this class may embrace those of the heart, arteries, veins and capillaries; first, disease of the heart and its membranes; taking it for granted that the anatomical position of its location, and the anatomical structure of the heart is well understood, we may proceed to note the obvious phenomena of its healthy action that we may note accurately the derangements or departures from this normal standard; first, sounds of the heart; when we place the ear to the præcordial region we hear first a dull or slightly protracted sound which corresponds to the arterial pulse, this is instantly succeeded by a sharp quick sound like that of the valve of a bellows or the lapping of a dog, it corresponds to a part of the interval of the arterial pulsations; these sounds are believed to result from the dilatation and contraction of the ventricles, the impulse of the heart seems to be a back stroke felt at the end of each pulsation and is attributable to the refilling of the ventricle; the regular or normal action of the heart is readily ascertained by the pressure and regularity of these sounds. The substance of the heart is essentially muscular, it is invested by a membrane of a fibro-serous character lubricated by a serous secretion, this membrane is termed the pericardium, which forms a closed sac and contains the liquor-pericardiæ. The endocardium is the serous lining which differs on the two sides of the heart, that of the right heart being very distensible, resisting and not very liable while that of the left side is scarcely extensible, remarkably brittle, and the most liable to ossification; these membranes are liable to attacks of inflammation of both the acute and chronic form.

Inflammation of the pericardium, acute pericarditis, may be readily recognized by the following symptoms: an acute, pungent or lacerating pain in the region of the heart under the sternum, extending towards the epigastrium, and sometimes between the shoulders; a sense of more or less oppression, rapid breathing; sometimes in the progress of the disease the respiration

442

is panting, palpitation irregular, jerking or intermittent pulse, a dull sound over the region of the heart; at times it sounds as if two dry surfaces were rubbed together or of the creaking of new leather when there is an entire absence of any sign of pneumonia or pleuritis; for the most part there is an inability to lie on the left side, the diagnosis of pericarditis is rendered somewhat difficult because certain of the symptoms are common to different cardiac diseases, inflammation of the pericardium not unfrequently is denoted by a very dull pain and so slight as to require careful percussion to detect it. It may also be detected by pressure upward on the epigastrium and also by pressure on the left hypochondrium in the vicinity of the disease.

When the disease is complicated with violent pneumonia or articular rheumatism the pain which accompanies these diseases often makes the pain in the pericardium; when positive pain is not experienced, a disagreeable sense of constriction and weight in the chest, which induces the patient to lie on the back is felt; in some cases these feelings are aggravated by lying on the left side. In the advanced stage of the disease the patient prefers the sitting posture, slightly inclining his body forward or to the left side; the dull sound over the cardiac region is only present when effusion has taken place in the pericardium, the period of effusion may be determined when the impulse of the heart is so feeble as not to be readily felt by the hand.

The first effect of inflammation is to diminish the serous secretion, the second is a reaction and serous effusion; during the first effects of inflammation it is observed to produce a sound of friction, and the second or that of effusion of the cavity, may very considerably obscure the sounds of the heart and cause them to appear at a distance; this secretion occurs early in the disease and is sometimes very profuse but susceptible of being absorbed when the disease terminates in health; pericarditis was once regarded as a fatal disease, but in modern times a different estimation has been placed upon the affection; it may terminate fatally in a few days, or at longer periods when preceded by signs of cerebral disturbance.

CAUSES.—From a chill or exposure to a cold damp atmosphere; it may be produced by violent exertion, excessive grief, or any intense emotional excitement, it frequently occurs in connection with inflammatory rheumatism, and has been regarded at least a concomitant if not a part of this painful disease; it is sometimes complicated with endocarditis and the latter as well as the former may become chronic.

TREATMENT.—Like all internal inflammations, and particularly those of serous membranes, the treatment must be active; in Allopathy blood-letting was practiced freely, followed by small doses of *Tartrate* of *antimonia* and *potassia*, the latter is employed as contra-stimulant or nauseant, tincture of digitalis is sometimes added to the tartar emetic in the proportion of forty drops to two grains put in four ounces of water, one-fourth of which to be given every three hours; this treatment is liable to many objections, in the first place it detracts from the strength of the patient, without a successful antagonism with the disease.

HOMŒOPATHIC TREATMENT.—*Aconite* in rheumatic cases for inflammation of the pericardium is indicated when there is a double friction sound and a laboring pressure of the heart upwards, before there is effusion of serum into the cardiac cavity.

Aconite, from the 3x to 30x, is also indicated in pericarditis when there is pain in the region of the heart extending over the whole sternum, tightness of the chest and inability to take a long breath, or to cough, and when there is a restless condition of the patient, and an anxious expression of the countenance.

The pain and uneasiness of pericarditis, the consequence of rheumatism, is more marked and severe than when the disease is from another cause; pericarditis not consequent upon rheumatism and characterized by little pain, palor, an occasional distress of countenance, and willingness of the patient to lie on the left side and the pain if any about the heart shoots upwards to the shoulders and the pulse is full and strong, Aconite is still the remedy. If the patient is unwilling to lie upon the left side and suffers an increase of pain from pressure or motion, *Bryonia*. When the pulse is full and bounding and there is shortness of breath, or suffocative constriction of the chest, Spigelia is indicated; we have also found this remedy of great service in obviating an irritable condition of the nerves of the heart, and also for dyspnœa. *Arsenicum, Cactus* and *Veratrum* are also to be consulted in reference to these symptoms, each in 3x dil. When accompanied by violent palpitation of the heart which is visible and easily heard, *Digitalis*, drop doses of 2x dil.; these remedies with their analogues are indicated early in the disease. When effusion has taken place *Arsenicum, Apis mel., Digitalis, Hellebore, Spigelia, Apocynum can.*, and Croton tig. may severally be consulted and prescribed in accordance with the symptoms in drop doses of the 6x dil.

Dropsy of the Pericardium.

Dropsy of the pericardium; independent of the serous effusion into the pericardium there is a dropsy, or accumulation of water into this cavity. The symptoms and signs referred to under acute inflammation of the pericardium, as indicative of effusion, are the same as present themselves in hydro-pericarditis. It has been affirmed that patients suffering from dropsy of the pericardium cannot lie in a horizontal position. The patient is easily fatigued, and is often affected with laborious and rapid breathing, with frequent inclination to sigh, with sudden starting during sleep, anxious and depressed expression of countenance; the patient has a sense of fullness in the chest, and puffiness of the face and extremities, a limited secretion of highly colored urine and irregular pulsations of the heart.

TREATMENT.—Hydrothorax and hydro-pericarditis are so intimately connected that the one cannot exist without the other; the treatment, therefore, includes the same surgical and therapeutic agents. Paracentesis in some instances has apparently been successful in prolonging life, but this is at best a palliative measure; a better result has been obtained from the Homœopathic treatment of this affection. The disease not being idiopathic, but generally the sequel of some acute inflammation, must be treated in accordance with the symptoms, and under the table of the pathogenetic effects of *Apis mel., Arsenicum, Apocynum, Digitalis* and *Helleborus niger*, may be found all the characteristic symptons of this disease. In some cases cures have been effected, but the prognosis in general is by no means favorable. In pericarditis, where there is much palpitation and a whirling motion of the heart *Asclepias tuberosa* and *Cactus grand*, 3x dil., we have given with satisfactory results. The region of the heart during treatment should be covered with warm compresses, and gentle friction over the cardiac region is also to be recommended.

Endocarditis.

By this term is understood inflammation of the fibro-serous-membrane, which lines the interior of the heart, the causes, symptoms, and constitutional conditions are the same; in both pericarditis and endocarditis the latter is often latent and the friction sounds of the former are often difficult to determine the presence of the cognate disease, the friction sounds are restricted to the cardiac region in pericarditis; the valve murmurs are heard beyond this region. The mitral as well as the valves of the aorta are generally affected, though sometimes the mitral alone is implicated. In children subject to acute rheumatism, the mitral valve is liable to partake of the difficulty, and in adults or aged persons disease of the aortic valve predominates; it is more frequently fatal in children and young persons. A systolic mitral murmur audibly entending an inch and a half beyond the nipple is most probably due to mitral regurgitation; you can only distinguish the existence of an aortic murmur in the neck just before the sternum over the innominate artery. If after listening to the first sound, the second follows clearly and distinctly after, there is probably no affection of the aortic valves, even if there be a loud systolic murmur; if however, the second sound is inaudible, indistinct or prolonged, or be replaced by an astolic murmur, the lining membrane of the heart is undoubtedly inflamed, a careful examination should be instituted of the muscular and functional state of the heart in order to ascertain if its force and vigor are above or below that which is normal; or if it be liable to excitement from slight causes, irregularity of the rythm, feeble pulse and an evident want of blood in the arteries, we are led to suspect an implication of the tissues of the heart.

PROGNOSIS.—The heart is liable to become hypertrophied or enlarged from endocarditis if the valves thicken or shrink or adhere at their margins, and the lesions remain persistent; when the dilatations of the cavity of the heart exceed the hypertrophy the danger is increased; in as much as the muscular tissue of the heart becomes soft and flabby, as the blood becomes impoverished, and the tone of the system is lowered.

Endocarditis is rarely fatal; though the valvular disease which ensues gradually becomes so; the unfavorable signs include a feeble pulse, imperfect filling of the arteries, rigors, swelling and pain of the spleen, albuminuria, hemiplegia, and softening of the tissues of the heart.

TREATMENT.—The treatment of endocarditis varies in some degree from that of pericarditis, as the symptoms are different and point to a different class of therapeutic agents, among the remedies found serviceable in cases of acute rheumatism, we may select *Spigelia, Aconite, Veratrum viride, Bryonia*, Digitalis and *Rhus radicans*, each in 3x dil.

Aconite has a powerful effect in acute rheumatic cases implicating the mitral valve. *Cactus grandiflorus*, 3x dil., may be employed in accordance with the symptoms; which are fluttering of the chest, dyspnœa and labored breathing; in all cases of acute rheumatism ending in endocarditis, the patient should be kept free from excitement, and restricted to a diet and regimen that comports with the condition of the patient.

Hypertrophy or Enlargement of the Heart.

An abnormal enlargement or growth of the muscular tissue of the heart, and an increase of its size and weight is termed hypertrophy; the most simple form of enlargement of the heart consists in the thickening of the walls without interfering with the capacity of its cavities, or in other words the simple enlargement of the muscular structure of the heart. The thickening of the walls with dilatation of the cavities is termed eccentric hypertrophy; whereas the thickening of the walls with diminution of the cavities is termed concentric hypertrophy; a thickening or growth of the walls of the heart without effecting a change in the cavities is very uncommon. Eccentric hypertrophy which affects an abnormal dilatation of the cavities is the most common.

CAUSES.—When the heart is compelled into excessive work as in the effort to overcome obstruction to its action, it contributes to its enlargement; excessive emotional excitement is also an obvious cause. We once knew a gentleman who was accused of crime and sentenced to a long term of imprisonment whose anxiety and grief on account of his separation from his family, compelled his heart into such excessive action that it acquired an enormous size; this hypertrophy of the organ proved fatal; an autopsy revealed the fact of enormous muscular growth, and diminution of the cavities; the heart weighed three pounds and fourteen ounces. Excessive physical exertion and general plethora may also be included among the causes of hypertrophy of the heart, as the right arm of the blacksmith acquires vigor and enlargement of its muscles by their constant exercise; so the heart compelled into double or triple service undergoes a similar change.

SYMPTOMS.—The symptoms of hypertrophy are excessive beating, and palpitation; imperfect action of the valves, and especially if they are diseased is an unmistakable symptom; a strong impulsive movement of the heart, dullness of sound in the cardiac region, and evident bulging or swelling of the left side, that can be felt by the hand, irregularity of rythm, shortness of breath, distress and anguish, deranged digestion and frequently a tickling cough, bronchial irritation, and other symptoms that interfere with respiration.

TREATMENT.—*Aconite* for acute palpitation; *Cactus grand.* for hypertrophy with valvular disease and dropsy of the pericardium. Digitalis for strong beating of the heart with contracting pains under the sternum and a feeling of oppression, it is a most efficient remedy in restoring regularity of the heart's action. Arsenicum for anæmic persons with dilatation of the right heart and a tendency to dropsy. Ferrum pyro-phos. in case of constitutional debility. In all cases patients suffering from hypertrophy must avoid violent exertion of every kind, such as ascending steps, climbing hills and long walks, mental excitement, and anxiety. As a rule rest of body and mind is indispensable.

Angina Pectoris.

Sudden severe paroxysms of pain or spasms of an enfeebled and diseased heart, with intense anxiety, a burning sensation and constriction; this disease occurs more frequently in aged persons.

SYMPTOMS, are intense pain centering in the heart and extending through the anterior portion of the chest up the shoulder and down the arm. The patient has fear and anxiety and fear of instant death; he suffers from faintness and dyspnœa, an agonizing palpitation and weakness. If walking he is sometimes compelled to stop and seize upon some object for support in which position he becomes pale and the surface of the body is covered with a cold, clammy perspiration. The paroxysms come on suddenly with variable duration; some longer and some shorter.

There is a liability of their recurrence with greater severity until they prove fatal. The cause of angina pectoris is primarily disease of the heart or obstruction of the coronary arteries in consequence of which the muscular fibres of the heart become impaired; with these predisposing influences, muscular exertion, flatulent distension of the abdomen or intense mental excitement may provoke these paroxysms.

TREATMENT.—The Allopathic treatment consists chiefly of counter irritants, leeching and a mild mercurial course and other palliative measures.

HOMŒOPATHIC TREATMENT. — The Homœopathic remedies called into requisition are *Arsenicum*, *Digitalis* and *Veratrum viride*, for the diseased condition of the heart; the selected remedy administered should correspond pathogenetically to the symptoms of the disease, for the paroxysms and during their existence we have used *Aconite, Bell., Cactus g.* and Spigelia, each in the 6x dil. In very recent cases attended with great anxiety and throbbing, *Aconite*, and particularly in plethoric persons, Aconite is evidently the remedy, but in persons advanced in life when attacked frequently and suddenly *Digitalis*, 3x dil., is indicated. In cases of slow intermittent pulse, with cold feet and hands, and a cold perspiration, *Veratrum alb.*, 3x dil.; when the patient has a pale and haggard face, feeble and irregular pulse, *Arsenicum*, 30x trit., is the remedy, especially when there is extreme dyspnœa, increased by the slightest movement. *Cactus grand.* is indicated when there is a feeling as if the heart were clasped and compressed as with an iron hand, and particularly if the patient has had rheumatism. A critical study of the cause of angina pectoris or rather the paroxysms might result in the selection of many other remedies; when the paroxysm comes on from grief, Ignatia may be consulted, when from indigestion and distension of the abdomen, *Nux vom.* and *Pulsatilla*, 3x dil. Inhalents such as *Chloric Ether* and *Nitrate* of *Amyl* have been found useful and palliative.

The accessory treatment should be gentle stimulants, warm fomentations over the region of the heart, and flannels wrung out of quite hot water applied to the extremities.

In verification of the correctness of the above treatment, the following case is cited: Hon. K. H. was suddenly seized with Angina Pectoris, and suffered intensely for twelve hours or dur-

ing an entire night. Several well-known remedies were tried
without effect. At last he complained of chilliness. Hot applications were made to the region of the pain and a dose of the
3x dil. of *Bell.* gave speedy relief.

Fainting Fits, Swooning or Syncope.

By the term syncope is understood loss of animation, volition and muscular power; when one faints there is a complete or
partial loss of consciousness, owing to nervous depression; the
causes of fainting fits or syncope are apparently inherent in the
constitution, prominent among which is debility from constitutional causes, or loss of animal fluids, hysterical diathesis, stirred
up by sudden joy, grief, fright or the sight of blood, a wound, or
from unpleasant sights of any kind.

TREATMENT.—The treatment of syncope is mostly by olfactories, Camphor, Musk, Carbonate of Ammonia, and even Aconite
may be applied to the patient's nose, and as soon as the patient
can swallow, Pulsatilla, 3x dil., or Cimicifuga, 3x; at the same
time loosen the patients' clothing, expose them to the cool air,
and wet the face frequently with cold water. The horizontal
posture is best for the patient during the fit and should not be
interfered with. For the constitutional debility, *China, Arsenicum,
Canchalagua,* and *Jodium.* When the fainting fit is caused by
affections of the heart, either functional or otherwise, the remedies are *Veratrum viride, Digitalis,* and *Nux moschata.* For hysteric fainting, cold douches, or wet a soft towel, and dash it without being wrung on the face; repeat until reaction occurs. When
a patient is conscious of this proclivity to fainting fits, all exciting
causes must be avoided; all trivial circumstances which cause
fainting must be duly noted in order to correct the tendency.

Palpitation and irregularity of the action of the heart; when
the body is in normal health, the beat of the heart is scarcely perceptible, its perfect action therefore is indicated by a want of
consciousness of its pulsations; its movements are so quiet, and its
dilatation and contractions occur with such perfect accuracy, that
nothing interrupts the flow of blood, and the power of the heart
to drive it. Palpitation is a departure from this standard, and an
indication of a want of balance in the circulatory power of the
heart; it is not an evidence of excessive power, it is an overtax
upon its muscular power and therefore the demand upon it is ex-

cessive, it is laboriousness that is indicated by palpitation. When the palpitations of the heart are increased in force or in frequency this sensation occurs. Palpitation in organic diseases of the heart comes on slowly and without observation, whereas palpitation from functional disturbance generally comes on suddenly, in the former the distress and palpitation are constant, in the latter only at times. In organic affections of the heart there is lividity of the lips and cheeks, also œdema of the lower limbs. Moreover, very little acceleration of the pulse in organic affections, whereas in functional the heart's action is greatly quickened, then again in organic difficulties *instead* of palpitation, the patient complains occasionally of severe pain extending from the shoulder to the arm, in functional difficulties the palpitation is observable and much complained of by the patient, who has pain in the left side also, and lastly organic, or palpitation resulting from organic disturbance, is more common in males than in females. Functional troubles more frequently excite palpitation in females than in males. The causes of palpitation may be indigestion, and from this source alone palpitation may become so violent as to cause the greatest alarm on the part of the patient; a nervous temperament, or hysteria, and a full habit, and diseased heart are predisposing influences. The exciting causes are excessive joy and grief or sudden emotion of any kind, protracted running, and profuse menstrual discharge, or any circumstance disadvantageous to the heart may cause palpitation.

TREATMENT.—The Allopathic treatment consists of the administration of certain sedatives calculated to lessen the heart's action.

HOMŒOPATHIC TREATMENT of palpitation from emotional causes may be analyzed as follows: *Aconite*, for that which arises from excitement, *Chamomilla*, and *Nux vomica*, for that which results from passion, *Coffea*, that which occurs from joy, and wakefulness. For palpitation caused by grief, *Ignatia, Opium; or Veratrum viride* for that caused by fright, or fear. When over exertion causes palpitation, *Arnica*, or *Hypericum*. When it occurs from congestion *Belladonna*, or *Gelsemium*. When it occurs from indigestion, *Nux vomica, Pulsatilla*, and *Lycopodium* exercise a quieting effect; palpitation caused by nervous irritability is readily subdued by *Moschus, Bryonia, Hypericum, Spigelia, Cactus*, and *Valerian;* in treating the trouble the remedy must be

selected in accordance with the indications, and the totality of the
symptoms; for violent cases with irregular pulse, inability to exercise, etc., *Digitalis* has frequently afforded relief. To insure
success from the use of therapeutic agents the patient must avoid
exciting scenes, and stimulants of every kind, strong coffee, prep-
aratidns of Morphine. Pure air, cold water used internally and
externally, moderate exercise in the open air, digestible food, and
a contented and tranquil disposition are also valuable considerations.

Intermittent Pulse.

Sometimes there is a loss of the normal beats of the pulse of
one in every three, four, seven, or eight pulsations at the wrist;
the cause of this may be debility or some interference of the action
of the ventricles of the heart; the pulsations which succeed the
intermission are generally heavier and fuller, showing that the
ventricle is contracting on an extra volume of blood after a mom-
entary intermission. The cause of intermission is accredited to
deficiency of nervous force, and an overwrought brain; in a feeble
and anæmic patient we find the condition which is frequently the
source from whence this difficulty arises; sometimes grief from the
loss of friends; or the shock of failure in business, disappointments,
or any other *cause* that may result in an exhaustion of the nervous
force, may be associated with an intermittent pulse.

TREATMENT.—The treatment is mainly hygienic. Change is
recommended, sufficient rest, and sleep, and the avoidance of
fatiguing exercise, or over mental exertion. If recuperation does
not readily follow, resort may be had to the following therapeutic agents: *Digitalis*, *Spigelia* and other quieting remedies; *Ignatia* when the system has been exhausted by protracted grief;
Gelsemium when neuralgic pains accompany an anæmic condition,
A generous diet and active exercise in the open air are accessory
measures for the invigoration of the nervous system.

Aneurism.

An aneurism is a tumor caused by the dilatation of an artery.
It sometimes occurs at the junction of one artery with another,
and is invariably filled with blood. In an early stage pulsation
is distinctly manifest in the tumor with more than ordinary violence; in an advanced stage the blood is coagulated and deposits
itself in numerous thin layers.

Aneurism may be idiopathic or not referable to any definable cause, or it may be traumatic, caused by injury to an artery. The disease is of more frequent occurrence in men than in women, and is often fatal. There are several varieties. The *fusiform*, or spindle-shaped, sometimes called true aneurism, consists of an abnormal dilatation of an artery. The *sacculated*, this is a partial dilatation of all the coats of an artery. The diffused is simply an escape of blood from a rupture in contiguous tissues. This variety has sometimes been accompanied by all the symptoms of a shock, and when chronic it has been mistaken for a purulent sac, but if opened it is at the imminent risk of the patient's life.

The causes of aneurism are usually mechanical, and may arise from a wound, blow, a strain, violent muscular exertion, or any kind of injury. From the fact that men are subject to aneurism more than women, the cause in all probability will be found in great muscular exertion, as in gymnastics; the predisposing cause is unquestionably a weak or flabby condition of the coats of the arteries. These predisponents of the trouble, are excessive doses of mercury, syphilis, gout, rheumatism, and phthisis pulmonalis, hypertrophy of the heart, and lastly excessive use of alcoholic stimulants.

The diagnosis is sometimes attended with difficulties, such as have misled the most eminent surgeons. One of the characteristic signs is a lancinating intermittent pain with a continuous aching.

When the tumor is situated near the course of a large arterial trunk and has a distinct pulsation it is probably an aneurism.

TREATMENT.—In Allopathic treatment a resort to saline purgative and other antiphlogistic treatment, to quiet the circulation together with large doses of *Digitalis*, are the principal measures called into requisition.

HOMŒOPATHIC TREATMENT.—*Aconite*, gives relief from pain, and reduces the force and frequency of the pulse. *Kali hydriodicum*, and *Nitric acid*, are suitable for patients weakened by syphilis and mercurialization.

There is no remedy that can take the place of *Arnica* in traumatic aneurism, and the same may be said of *Phosphorus* in the idiopathic form. *Veratrum viride*, in recent cases is a valuable remedy for the arterial excitement, and in the deposit of fibrin; ten drops of the third dilution in a half glass of water may be given in dessert spoonful doses every three hours until the pulse is reduced to fifty or sixty a minute.

Avoid stimulants, except in the primary stage, for which experience has sanctioned their use. They are now considered valuable adjuncts in the treatment of internal aneurism. The most favorable position must be secured for the patient, and the apartments should be well ventilated and away from noise, he should be allowed but three meals a day, taken at regular intervals and if his appetite requires, as much as three ounces of broiled steak, two ounces of white bread and butter, and a teacupful of cocoa may be allowed for breakfast; about the same quantity of boiled meat with potatoes and bread, with a goblet of water for dinner, two ounces of bread and butter, and a cup of milk or tea for supper; his daily allowance should not exceed ten ounces of solid food, and ten ounces of fluid proportioned as above.

The restriction of the diet is for the purpose of moderating the circulation and to lessen the quantity of blood, so as to favor the coagulation of fibrin within the sac. A recumbent posture is enjoined in all cases of aneurism. It has been ascertained that recumbency reduces the force and frequency of the aneurismal pulse. This posture, therefore, is of itself an indispensable accompaniment of other remedial measures, and without which patients are seldom affected.

CHAPTER XXVIII.

PHLEBITIS.—INFLAMMATION OF THE VEINS.

The tissue of a vein, like other tissue, is subject to inflammation and the consequent changes in its texture, and a local coagulation of blood with a tendency to embolism. There are two varieties, adhesive and suppurative, the former arises from exposure to dampness and cold, and frequently affects one of the large veins of the lower extremities, and commonly in connection with varicose conditions it is quite painful but not particularly dangerous. The latter as suppurative inflammation is more dangerous than the adhesive, being caused by wounds or abscesses, it is sometimes associated with pyæmia, and by the severity of symptoms may indicate extreme danger, as leading to a fatal termination.

The Phlegmasia Dolens or Milk Leg.

This is an inflammation of the veins peculiar to nursing women. The symptoms of this disease correspond so nearly to those of phlebitis that the same therapeutic agents are involved in the treatment. The symptoms which indicate the presence of phlebitis are as follows: There is a reddish purple appearance of the superficial veins which are hard, swollen, and nodulated, darting pains through the limb when moving; and there is stiffness with more or less swelling of the part. In acute phlebitis the patient is subject to rigors, with depression of spirits, anxious countenance, weak and rapid pulse, brownish coating upon the tongue, a dry and a cadaverous appearance of the skin, attended with great prostration, and sometimes with bilious vomiting and a low muttering delirium. In extreme cases there may be excessive pain in the joints and purulent formations in various parts of the body.

TREATMENT.—At one time general bleeding as well as topical depletion was a general resort in Allopathy which now is universally condemned, and alterative doses of *Tartarized antimony* are advised as a contra stimulant to obviate depletion with the lancet. Next in importance *Digitalis, Calomel*, and other alterative agents are recommended.   This treatment throughout is objectionable, because it is an additional tax upon the vital forces of the organism.

HOMŒOPATHIC TREATMENT is not liable to the same objection and yet the most critical care is required in the selection of remedies.   The symptoms of every case must be critically and carefully recorded and the remedies must be selected in accordance with the symptoms.   In acute phlebitis the therapeutic indications point strongly or decidedly to *Aconite*, or *Pulsatilla;* when there are typhoid symptoms, *Arsenicum, Carbo vegetabilis, Hyoscyamus* and *Muriatic acid.*   In the chronic form of the disease, *Arnica, Hamamelis, Pulsatilla, Lycopodium, Nux vomica,* and *Zinc.*   In those cases where there is a secretion of pus, *Hepar sulphur, Mercurius corrosivus, Silicea* and *Sulphur.*   When the fever is moderate or has been subdued by *Aconite, Pulsatilla* will act efficiently upon the veins.   It is particularly applicable in those female cases subject to menstrual irregularities and leucorrhœa. The 3x attenuation of all these remedies is employed.

When persons are afflicted with varicose veins, have a flushed face, headache, throbbing in the temples, and brilliant staring eyes, *Belladonna* 3x dil. is indicated.   When there are varicose veins of the lower extremities which have a dark red appearance, *Belladonna* 3x is also the remedy.   The key note for the administration of *Arsenicum* in these cases is the extreme prostration.   *Carbo vegetabilis,* in those cases complicated with cyanosis.   *Silicea* and *Hepar,* for actual or threatened suppuration.

Æsculus hippocastanum 3x trit. is regarded an excellent remedy for hæmorrhoids; *Hamamelis* is a grand remedy for a general and healthy condition of the veins.   The accessory means to be employed in the treatment of varicose veins is the external application of the fluid extract of Hamamelis, warm fomentations in case the congested veins are painful, and also in case of painful congestion elsewhere.

Varicose Veins.

Varicose veins may be known by their enlargement or dilatation, tortuous, knotted, and divided into separate pouches of a dull leaden or purplish color, with considerable discoloration of the parts, and a swollen condition of the limb.

In case a great many small cutaneous veins are alone affected they present the appearance of a net-work. When standing or walking the enlarged veins become swollen and painful and
on assuming a recumbent posture the swelling diminishes, the
pain subsides; the causes of this varicose enlargement of the veins
may be by strains or over-exertion, which causes an afflux of blood
into them and causes their distension; occupations which favor the
gravitation of blood to the lower extremities.

Obstacles to the return of the venous blood, such as ligatures,
garters, or stays, and the gravid uterus, or impacted fæces, by
pressing upon one of the large venous trunks, occasion a varicose
condition that extends to all its branches. In some instances this
venous trouble arises from an hereditary predisposition and also
from an altered condition of the blood, or from the want of activity
in the circulation which leads to an enfeebled and relaxed condition of the walls of the veins.

The following disturbances may arise from varicose veins:
cold feet, severe, aching pain, fatigue and sense of weight after a
protracted walk, or from being too long in a standing posture;
then again a severe and dangerous hæmorrhage may occur upon
the bursting of a vein. The imperfect circulation, together with
the obstruction of the absorbent, and the defection of cutaneous
nutrition may cause ulceration on the lower portion of the outside of the leg. Varicose veins being intimately associated with
constitutional debility, incapacitate one for hard or long-continued work.

TREATMENT.—For the simplest form, see treatment for phlegmasia dolens; when associated with other disorders, such as constipation, and hæmorrhoids, *Sulphur* 3x and *Nux vomica* 3x may be
consulted. *Arsenicum* 3x is the remedy for varicose ulcers of the
leg attended with great debility and burning pains; for varicose
inflammation and fever, *Aconite* 3x, *Belladonna* 3x, and Hamamelis virg. The *Hamamelis* may be used in the form of a lotion
—one drachm of the strong tincture to half a pint of water, to
begin with. The strength of the lotion may be increased by one
part tincture to five parts of water, while the internal administration is indispensable.

The surgical means for destroying these veins, as recommended by Prof. Wm. Todd Helmuth, is by the application of an
escharotic paste composed of equal parts of caustic potash and

lime made into a paste with alcohol. This paste should be washed off in two or three minutes with vinegar and water, and the eschar allowed to separate; the hæmorrhage which ensues is easily controlled by an application of the styptic colloid. Those who have witnessed this treatment are favorably impressed with its superiority over other resorts for obliterating varicosis. The position of the patient, while subject to therapeutic treatment, must be such as to secure rest, with the limb in a horizontal posture to favor the return of blood toward the heart, and thus relieve the extended veins of the column of blood. Moderate compression by nicely fitted bandages or laced stockings, so as to afford that support to the blood which the valves can no longer give; they are essential in preventing increased distention. The pressure should be gentle and uniform, and should be applied early in the morning before the patient puts his feet on the floor, and they need not be removed until he retires at night. When only small portions of the vein are enlarged, a gentle pressure may be brought to bear by use of a strapping plaster, but even in these slight cases, long exercise or standing should be abstained from, and even after moderate exercise the limb should be raised and placed in a horizontal posture. The leg should be thoroughly washed and rubbed dry every morning.

Varicose Ulcers.

Varicose ulcers may be treated in precisely the same manner as other ulcerations. *Arsenicum*, and *Belladonna*, when they present the appearance of congestive inflammation, *Pulsatilla*, and *Macrotin*, when the ulcers are not painful or when they occur in persons of lymphatic temperaments.

Goitre or Bronchocele.

Goitre is an enlargement of the thyroid gland, it is peculiar to certain mountainous districts as in Switzerland, but not limited to any particular locality. The swelling is frequently termed the Derbyshire neck; the swelling is neither painful or dangerous, nevertheless it is regarded as a source of deformity especially when it acquires a significant size and presses heavily upon the trachea and œsophagus, interfering in some degree with deglutition and respiration; women are more frequently the victims of goitre than men. It is said that in thirty cases twenty-nine of them will be found in women. The right lobe is usually more swollen than the left, it is found more frequently in mountainous districts where the soil is chalky and it is often associated with cretinism.

The cause of this dyscrasia is believed to be the habitual use of water from magnesium limestone rocks, or water which contains the soluble salts of lime; where there is a ridge of magnesium limestone the inhabitants roundabout are liable to this affection, such is the case in many parts of England and Switzerland. The proof of this has been apparent in the fact that some who have refrained from drinking the water in these districts are known to not suffer from this disease.

Inasmuch as cretinism is frequently associated with and accompanies this deformity it is proper to consider it in connection therewith. It is true that all the goitres, are not cretins, and yet all the cretins are victims of goitre. Cretinism prevails in the region of the Alps, Pyrenees, and Himalaya mountains.

TREATMENT.—As goitre is usually the effect of some tangible cause, and intimately related to other derangements, the treatment must be in reference to these. For those living in valleys, *Spongia* is recommended, and also this remedy is better suited for children and young persons, and especially girls approaching puberty. *Iodine*, externally applied, is better for hard goitre. For bilious temperaments, in case no other symptoms are present,—in cases of long standing, *Mercurius iodatus* 3x is an effective remedy, especially when the swelling has progressed in spite of other remedial measures. In scrofulous persons *Calcarea carbonica*, 3x and even *Arsenicum* 3x are valuable remedies. Other remedies, such as *Kali hydriodicum*, *Bromine*, *Sulphur* and other antipsorics may be consulted. The external as well as the internal use of any of these remedies is to be recommended.

Goitre is difficult to remove, and therefore to favor this desirable result the patient must be careful to subsist on digestible elements, and such as will nourish the system properly. In uterine derangements there is a tendency to turgesence of the thyroid gland associated with anæmia, palpitation, and protrusion of the eyeballs. The cause of this difficulty is nervous exhaustion, such as in some cases may be brought on by metorrhagia or leucorrhœa in females, and by hæmorrhoids in males.

The symptoms of this variety of goitre are the following: a pinched expression of the countenance, brown, dull and soiled appearance of the skin, expression of distress, nervous agitation, and sometimes hysteria, a wild look of the eyes, and a protrusion of the eyeballs, swollen eyelids and a profuse shedding of tears, sensation like that of sand in the eyes, albuminuria, flashes of heat, palpitation, rapid pulse, copious perspiration, bowels constipated and an abnormal appetite.

TREATMENT.—The treatment of this peculiar malady requires strict attention to diet, and the selection of remedies in accordance with the prominent symptoms. *China* 2x is suitable for the prostration caused by the loss of animal fluids. When there is anæmia, *Ferrum* 3x trit. is the remedy; when connected with the symptoms which show that the heart is implicated, *Macrotin* 3x trit. or *Pulsatilla* 3x dil.; when accompanied by gastric disturbances and irritability, *Nux vomica* 3x.

CHAPTER XXIX.

DISEASES OF THE ARTERIES.

Anatomically, there are three coats traceable and separate from each other in the arteries, the outermost coat is cellular in its character, the next coat is fibrous and eminently elastic, if not contractible, the inner coat is of a serous character, and secretes a thin fluid which lubricates and prevents friction. The arteries are subject to acute and chronic inflammation and various other kinds of degeneracy, all of which would indicate the employment of therapeutic measures in accordance with the symptoms.

Inflammation of the Arteries.

Inflammation of the arteries may be circumscribed, or diffused, the former may occur from a bruise or a wound inflicted by some jagged or serrated instrument, inflammation of this kind will yield readily to the application of cold compresses, wet with water which contains about one-twentieth of the officinal tincture of *Arnica montana* to allay the traumatic fever, ten drops of this tincture may be mixed in a goblet of water and the mixture may be given in teaspoonful doses at intervals of two hours until the fever is subdued.

The arteries are by no means sensitive in a healthy state, but when inflamed to any extent, there is the presence of pain of so severe a character as to resemble neuralgia. The pain usually follows the course of the arteries implicated, the pulsations at the seat of inflammation become extremely energetic and are regarded an unmistakable diagnostic sign of the trouble, pressure upon the seat of inflammation increases the pain. These are the principal features of arterial inflammation.

When the inflammation is developed spontaneously it is from the operation of internal causes such as constitutional rheumatism, gout and erysipelas and the effects of other septic influences.

Toxical doses of *Mercury* and *Secale cornutum*. The result of arterial inflammation is frequently loss of elasticity to the vessel affected, softening of the coats to a degree that the rupture of them may occur from the slightest effort. Antiphlogistic treatment such as blood letting and saline purgatives were formerly regarded indispensable but since the advent of Homœopathy the therapeutic action of Aconite either in a higher or lower attenuation will take the place of these agents.

When gouty swellings are attended with much pain or when in other localities than the joints, myalgia may be present, *Aconite* either in a high or low attenuation will allay the inflammation and relieve the pain. *Bryonia* may follow *Aconite* when the patient suffers greatly on being moved. *Pulsatilla* may be given after *Aconite* in warm sultry weather in plethoric persons.

Nux vom., after *Aconite* will prove useful. The general rule with reference to dietetic measures in inflammatory diseases must be observed in the treatment of this disorder.

Ossification of the Arteries.

This difficulty is believed to be the sequel of *Gouty* or rheumatic affections and usually occurs at a late period in life. Syphilitic subjects whose systems have become mercurialized are more liable to this affection ordinarily than gouty or rheumatic persons.

There is no treatment yet discovered that will either prevent or cure this malady.

SYMPTOMS.—There are no symptoms which indicate ossification of the internal arteries, or deep seated in its earliest stage but where it has made much progress especially if the arteries are near the surface as in case of the radial artery at the wrist, there is a feeling of an indurated cord with abnormal or indistinct pulsations.

The indications, however, of ossification at the wrist are also significant of the same trouble elsewhere in the circulatory system, and most commonly about the heart, or in the heart; as may be determined by the abnormal sounds elicited by the stethoscope, when an artery becomes ossified it is easily ruptured, and is liable to become obliterated; by reason of ossification of any of the arteries or branches the circulation must necessarily be retarded, inasmuch as the elastic and contractile power of the parieties of the vessel is destroyed as a consequence of this lesion, aneurism, hyperæmia and hæmorrhages may result.

CAUSES.—As before stated ossification of the arteries is very common in old age. It may, however, occur in all ages, as the sequel of syphilis, mercurialization, rheumatism or gout.

TREATMENT.—In Allopathic practice no therapeutic agents are employed; and in Homœopathic treatment, the beneficial effect of remedies is extremely doubtful. *Arsenicum, Calcarea carbonica, Mezereum, Sepia* and *Sulphur* may be consulted.

Atheroma.

Atheroma is a morbid accumulation within some of the arteries, supposed by some authors to be intimately related to fatty degeneration of the heart. *The treatment*, if any, in order to be useful must be of a prophylactic character. The accumulation of fatty matters can be prevented by strong doses of Kali hydriodicum, 1x trit., 3 gr. doses every third hour through the day.

Embolism.

Embolism is an obstruction in the arterial circulation, from clots of blood and fibrine which may result from endocarditis, exceedingly dangerous and fatal. Aconite may act well as a palliative.

Thrombosis.

Thrombosis is an obstruction in the large veins by clots of venous blood, that bridge over the caliber of the veins and sometimes these thromboi form abcesses or open the way to septicæmia. *Iodo-phenique* has been used as a protective agent when signs of septicæmia become manifest.

CHAPTER XXX.

DISEASES OF THE CAPILLARY VESSELS.

The capillary system of vessels, holding any intermediate position between the arteries and veins is most important in its physiological and pathological relations, it is between the part of the artery, no longer visible, and the earliest perceptible radicle of the corresponding vein, that the change from arterial into venous blood occurs.

This change marks the nutritive action, and has been exerted upon the blood, and discloses the important agency of the capillary vessels.

The capillary system is a wonderful provision in the animal economy for the purpose of conveying from the arteries the elements of nutrition.

In conveying the elements of nutrition through this intermediate system it is easy to comprehend how obstructions may arise and become the source of many inflammatory difficulties. It has been a question with physiologists whether there is any action of the capillaries distinct from that of the heart.

While we shall not attempt to settle this question, the phenomena of inflammation are apparently sufficient evidences of the independent action of those vessels.

The blood is the pabulum of all nutrition and therefore a nutritive irritation may exist which demands a greater supply from this source. there is no spontaneous morbid condition of any tissue in which they are not the parts implicated. It is therefore requisite that the function of the capillary system in supporting nutrition as well as its susceptibility to injuries from obstruction should be carefully understood.

Hyperæmia.

This term has been introduced into modern medicine to signify an accumulation of blood in the capillary vessels in contra distinction from the term polyæmia, which signifies general plethora; the term has been used by some writers to signify inflammation, but the sense in which we use it merely signifies an increased quantity or congestion of blood in the capillary vessels.

Hyperæmia undoubtedly arises in an affected part when the arteries convey too much blood to the capillaries, or when the veins which constitute the returning channels become obstructed in a way that promotes accumulation in the capillary vessels.

Andral's division of hyperæmia into four distinct varieties, affords a general idea of the varied pathological conditions under which this affection apparently occurs may be stated as follows: that which is produced by irritation, is termed active, that which results from defective tonicity of the capillary vessels, is termed passive, that which arises from an obstruction in the venous circulation, is termed mechanical, that which occurs after death, is termed cadaveric.

Under this head of active and passive hyperæmia is included sthenic and asthenic, or active and passive inflammation.

In all cases of increased secretion from an organ, or of increased nutrition in any part of the economy, the vessels concerned receive an abnormal quantity of blood and thus become subject to hyperæmia or congestion. This, to a certain extent, may be healthy, but when it exceeds the limits prescribed by health, local disturbance of function is liable to occur. Passive hyperæmia may take place with but slight interference with a healthy action, as in case of venous obstruction retarding the return of blood to the artery. The extensive anastomosis of the vessels are, to a great extent, the safeguard against passive hyperæmia.

SYMPTOMS.—The symptoms of hyperæmia, or obvious indications, are redness of various shades, and more or less pain, according to the location, and greater or less activity of the congestion. We have an example illustrative of these various appearances, in the inflammation of the fauces. According to its character, in very active inflammation, the parts are a vivid red; when it partakes of the passive form, they are dusky, and vessels of a larger size containing black blood, may be seen distributed over the mucous membrane. That which applies to inflammation of these parts has a similar application to the stage of hyperæmia which precedes the inflammation. There is also more or less tumefaction with the redness owing to the capillary engorgement. In all cases of hyperæmia there is, necessarily, a degree of tumefaction, owing to the increased quantity of blood in the capillaries. This tumefaction is not perceived when it occurs in the internal organs, as it does not come within the range of observation. It may be inferred, however, from the following symptoms, to wit: chilliness, languor, depression of spirits, lassitude, weakness of the muscles, coldness of the extremities, with occasional paroxysms of the heart and arteries. These symptoms, however, may occur from other functional difficulties, and none of them can be regarded as distinctive evidence of internal hyperæmia.

The best pathologists believe that the sequel of hyperæmia is inflammation; it is easy to see that distension of the capillary vessels cannot continue in any organ without impairing its function and in some cases without its destruction for a time, or permanently abolishing it, as in apoplexy, induced by hyperæmia of the encephalic vessels. Epilepsy and mania and other kindred affections are viewed as resulting affections. The causes of hyperæmia of a predisposing character of the head or when moving the head causes a sensation of pain and paleness and throbbing in the temples *Bryonia* is indicated.

Pulsatilla is indicated for hyperæmia in women, subject to painful menstruation and heaviness and pain in the head.

Sulphur is particularly indicated in sudden encephalitis which may result from protracted hyperæmia, and threaten softening of the brain. The accessory treatment consists of a well regulated diet, regularity at meals and the avoidance of all kinds of excitement, the application of warm water to the affected parts during the action of therapeutic agents.

Inflammation.

It has already been remarked that hyperæmia is the initiate of inflammation. The former is usually the precursor of the latter, yet it is well known that hyperæmia may exist and pass away without the supervention of inflammation; when there is such an accumulation of blood in the capillaries as to distend them; in consequence of this over-distension a morbid process is set up which is denominated inflammation; when this over-accumulation of blood coagulates and forms an obstruction of the capillaries, changes occur in the vessels themselves and also in the cellular tissue, and the over-distended capillaries, which immediately communicating with the vessels induce in them an increased action and effusion of fluid; and when the inflammation is seated in the parts of great importance in the organism its impress upon the constitution is a general febrile reaction of greater or less severity. This is the best definition we can offer for the pathological condition termed inflammation, and this is far from being satisfactory. Magendie once remarked that a whole book might be made up of the idea represented by the word inflammation.

DIAGNOSIS.—When the inflammation is external or in any of the outlets with.n the range of vision it presents in the earliest stage certain phenomena or local signs or symptoms for it being synonymous with disease; when any irritating agent is applied to a part, the flow of blood through it appears to be accelerated, the arteries convey the blood more freely than in a healthy condition and the fluid is seen to flow irregularly and often in retrograde direction; and in a direction contrary to that previously taken.

If the part be examined by the microscope immediately after the irritation has commenced and the extreme vessels appear distended and in a state of hyperæmia, the flow of blood is evidently retarded, and soon after effusion of the serous portion of the blood takes place into the cellular tissue and if the inflammation continues the liquor sanguinious after a little time exudes, and finally morbid secretions may take place under the new affinities, therefore it is manifestly proper to ascribe inflammation to increased action, or to an increase in the contractility of the extreme vessels, and then again the absence of tonicity in those vessels from the first renders them passively subject to congestion and inflammation, and yet again one of the earliest phenomena is a turgidity or active expansion of the extreme vessels which corresponds to the diastole of the heart.   In case of internal inflammation we have then to perform our diagnosis from the general symptoms in association with a disordered function of the affected organ.

There are four signs that m iy be predicted of localized inflammation; pain, swelling, redness and heat; it is quite unnecessary to dwell upon the modus operandi, through which these are induced.

The pain is evidently the result of distension of a nervous filament produced by the new pathological condition of the vessels and surrounding tissues. When the vitality of the vessels undergoes a modification, the pain in the inflamed parts is of a pulsatory character. The heat is owing to the increased velocity, and greater quantity of blood passing through the permeable vessels. The swelling is attributed to the dilatation of these vessels and to the effusion of them into the cellular tissue; the redness is caused by the accumulation of red globules in the vessels.

Diseases of the Glandiform Ganglions.

The term glandiform ganglions has been given to certain organs which resemble the glands in many respects but differ from them in others. These organs include the thyroid and thymus glands, spleen, supra-renal capsules and the lymphatic glands.

It has been generally considered by eminent physiologists that these glands are immediately connected with the circulation of the blood and lymph and for this reason it is proper to consider their diseases in relation to the circulatory organs. These glandiform bodies differ from the glands in having no excretory ducts. They are all situated in the course of the lymphatics or venous circulation and may be viewed as purificatory organs in the venous circulation; that they have an important office to fulfil in the venous circulation in diverting under peculiar circumstances the blood from the portal system when seemingly overloaded.

Whereas the glands proper are so formed and placed at the confines of the arterial circulation and are so evidently concerned in the preparation or depuration of the blood, that it may serve its office in the animal economy, it will be seen that the glands which have excretory ducts are associated with those which have not, in forming a grand system of purificatory organs for absorbing every thing from the blood that cannot be utilized, in compensation of losses and the up-building of the tissues.

CHAPTER XXXI.

DISEASES OF THE SPLEEN.

The office of the spleen is undoubtedly essential in the depuration of the blood. It is situated to the left of the stomach in the left hypochondrium.

There are many phenomena which lead to the belief that this organ with the pancreas and liver is concerned in the preparation of the blood for its arterial journey for assimilation and nutrition.

In proportion to our knowledge of the function of this organ when in health, we can note the aggravation and changes produced by disease.

When the left hypochondrium exhibits a fullness and swelling not dependent upon the tegumentary tissues and when there is deep seated pain and soreness, which becomes manifest on pressure, we have evidence of inflammation of the spleen; and the pain sometimes extends over the entire abdomen, and has been mistaken for peritoneal inflammation, coughing or sneezing, and a full inspiration is often productive of much suffering; and when accompanying these signs there is considerable constitutional disturbance, a hot skin, a moderately rapid and full pulse, we find indications for prompt therapeutic measures; if we find the arterial excitement very great *Aconitum napellus* may be administered every hour in the 3x dil., ten drops in a glass of water; teaspoonful doses.

TREATMENT.—In *regular practice*, blood letting local or general, revellents and rubefacients, the warm bath, cathartics and a well regulated diet, are recommended; but such treatment is merely palliative; while correctly affiliated Homœopathic remedies will be more likely to affect a radical cure; and among those to be consulted are *Aconite, Bryonia, Arsenicum*, and China; when splenitis accompanies a protracted intermittent, *Arsenicum* and *China* are particularly recommended, 3x dil. as above.

For the hypertrophy of the spleen must be distinguished from engorgement of the blood which disappears with the cause that induced it; while the former is an overgrowth of the viscus which

may remain as a permanent enlargement; vascular engorgement
is quite uniformly present in typhoid and intermittent fevers.

In the opinion of some authors this splenic enlargement during a severe case of intermittent fever affords the strongest evidence that the function of the organ is to assist in the regulation
or proper distribution of the blood; which during the cold stage
of a paroxysm is withdrawn from the surface and circulates more
largely in the internal organs and thus involving the spleen, which
after repeated attacks may become chronically engorged or enlarged.

In highly malarious districts splenic disease of this nature is
very common, and is known to present the following symptoms: a
sallow complexion, and anæmic expression, prone to dropsical
swelling and sometimes to hæmorrhages which are checked with
difficulty, owing to a disturbed circulation partly attributable to
the modified circulation of blood through the spleen.

This is termed the splenic cachexia which accompanies the
engorgement and hypertrophy of the spleen so often witnessed.

Some writers aver that there is a tendency to hæmorrhage
from slight causes as injuries, leech bites; blisters and tissues occasionally ulcerate during a protracted splenic engorgement.

Hypertrophy or Enlargement of the Spleen.

By careful observation, the increase in size is often partial,
involving but a small part of the organ, at other times the entire
organ is involved; the enlargement produces a corresponding fulness in the left hypochondrium, a greater or less degree of hardness,
and dullness on percussion.

We have before remarked that malarious influences are frequently the cause of chronic engorgement; this is so common a
sequence in intermittent fever, that the hardness and swelling has
received the name of *ague cake.*

TREATMENT.—The Allopathic treatment consists of large
doses of Quinine, Sulphate of Quinine from forty to sixty grains
daily for a few days; and an ointment made of Sulphate of Quinine and lard to be rubbed on the groins, and armpits, three times
a day. Mercurial preparations have sometimes been used, but
great caution is required in their use. *Iodide of Mercury* mixed
with bread or a sufficient quantity of white sugar is prescribed in

half grain doses night and morning; this treatment has been far from being satisfactory, in as much as the victims of vascular engorgement of the spleen through this treatment become subject to other difficulties; it is far better to withdraw such subjects from malarious districts and dispense with medication altogether until it is ascertained what a full measure of hygienic influences will accomplish for them.

We have seen anæmic subjects suffering from chronic intermittent fever for two years, complicated with enlargement and induration of the spleen, and after having exhausted the virtues of *Quinia* or Sulphate of Quinine, *Iodine*, and *Mercury*, to recuperate rapidly after these agents have been abandoned, simply by a change of residence from an ague district to one in which no malaria existed.

HOMŒOPATHIC TREATMENT.—The splenic cachexia often manifests itself in persons having a scrofulous diathesis, and may be benefited by *Arsenicum* 3x trit. in three grain doses, to be taken night and morning. *Calcarea* and *Sulphur* may also be consulted in such cases. We have also found the 3x dilution of *China* an excellent remedy for splenitis in persons of an anæmic constitution. China, the 3x dilution, is also indicated where there is pain in the spleen caused by over exercise or running. *Aconite* is indicated for pain in the spleen, when there is considerable arterial excitement and fever.

Bryonia is indicated when every motion aggravates, and also when there are other indications, such as pain, with or without enlargement of the left hypochondrium. *Mercurius iodatus* and *Mercurius biniodatus* 3x trit. in grain doses, may be administered three times a day. The following case may be cited in proof of the therapeutic effect of Sulphur: S.— G.—, aged thirty-six, a resident of Southern Illinois, became the victim of an intermittent fever in the fall of 1878. He was then exceedingly robust and weighed a hundred and ninety-seven pounds. According to the custom in that locality he took a large quantity of Sulphate of Quinine, which broke up the fever for a time; he then experienced another paroxysm which came on in the morning with a severe and protracted chill followed by a violent febrile reaction, and a sweating stage of unusual severity. After being greatly prostrated he took twenty-five grains of the Sulphate of Quinine. The next morning another paroxysm occurred, an hour earlier, attended with much pain and aching, intense thirst, and an exhaustive sweat, after which he was greatly prostrated and resorted again to an increased dose of the Sulphate of Quinine. The third day another paroxysm occurred, very similar to the preceding ones, still farther reducing his system, and for three weeks he suffered from this quotidian, in spite of daily massive doses of Quinine. He then, by the advice of his physician, had recourse to *Arsenic*, one-twentieth of a grain every three hours, for another week, and from the time of the first invasion of the disease until the end of the first month, he had lost thirty-three pounds in weight and began to suffer from a dull, heavy pain and sensation of weight in the region of the spleen, and still the daily paroxysm occurred, sometimes earlier, at other times later in the day.

His complexion became sallow and he suffered exceedingly from gastric derangement and loathing of food. The medication of the *Sulphate* of *Quinine* and *Arsenic* was kept up, until the patient, worn out and feeble, became a walking skeleton. He suffered intensely from engorgement and hypertrophy of the spleen, as was apparent from the external swollen condition of the left hypochondrium.

Under the impression that the patient had taken as much *Quinine* and *Arsenic* as his system would bear, and his bowels being obstinately constipated, he was advised to take a dose of cathartic pills; during the time of their action in moving the bowels he suffered intensely from the pain in the spleen; though very weak and feeble, he still went out a part of each day to attend to business; he continued in this enfeebled condition apparently doomed to chronic suffering. The ague was in his system and from time to time it would crop out in the form of a chill, fever and sweat; he suffered much as the weather grew colder, and there was no let up to the disease even in the return of spring; he had apparently settled down in the habit, created by malarial influence and the excessive dosing with drugs; he seemed neither better or worse, for several months he suffered during the warm weather from the effects of the fever and apparently dragging out a miserable life; in autumn, one year after he was first taken, he grew despondent and came to the conclusion that he would take no more medicine, and on the whole his future prospects seemed dim and his life was a burden, when it was suggested to him to place himself under Homœopathic treatment, and for this purpose he came to Chicago, the December following, and placed himself under our care. He engaged board for a month, in order to try the experiment of a different treatment; when he got settled in his boarding house we made a critical examination of the condition of his health and learned the antecedents of the case; we prescribed *Sulphur* in the 2x dilution, twenty drops in a cup of water, and directed him to take a teaspoonful every two hours; and we put him on a bit of toast, rice, and English breakfast tea at first; we continued this treatment for a week, he then said he felt better than he had at any time during the past year and he felt his appetite returning and he began to crave something more substantial in the way of food; we allowed him beefsteak broiled, with baked potatoes; from this time he had no chills or fever; the ague-cake as he termed it, began to disappear; his hope and expectation revived, and he went on improving from day to day. At the end of the month he was much stronger, the sallow complexion began to disappear, and his appetite for good and wholesome nourishment was normally increased; two weeks after, he had so far recovered that he was intent on returning home; the nutritive function appeared to be restored, and he was rapidly regaining his flesh. A careful examination of the condition of the spleen indicated a decided change for the better, the swelling had nearly disappeared, there was less tenderness on pressure, the induration was scarcely perceptible and he complained of no unpleasantness of weight as he had before experienced in the left hypochondrium. We permitted him to return home after giving him full directions as to diet, and the continuance of his medicine, and a wholesome warning against the use of *Arsenic* and the *Sulphate* of *Quinine* should his ague return. We have in a number of cases found Sulphur a satisfactory remedy to employ against enlargement of the spleen caused by protracted intermittents, and anæmic subjects.

China is a suitable remedy to give after Sulphur. The diet when the splenic cachexia is established may consist of a generous supply of animal food, porter and other stimulants, provided there are no inflammatory or febrile indications.

Atrophy of the Spleen.

This disease is very uncommon, though many cases of its shrinkage have been observed.

Andral describes a case where the spleen was not larger than a billiard ball. In this case it was indurated and all bloodless; and weighed but one ounce; this atrophy is believed to be connected with derangements of the alimentary canal.

TREATMENT.—The treatment in case of atrophy is based upon symptoms indicating that of the primæviæ, or chronic affections of the liver and kidneys, with peritoneal dropsy.

Arsenicum, China, Digitalis, Helleborus niger may be consulted. There are other affections of the spleen, which give rise to no symptoms that would indicate the use of specific remedies.

The Thymus Gland.

Situated at birth in the superior mediastinum; its ordinary weight is said to be about half an ounce, it is an organ more allied to fœtal life and consequently of less interest in its pathological relations. In after years it diminishes and becomes very diminutive in size and ultimately it becomes so small as to be scarcely discoverable. The chief pathological condition of interest is the abnormal size or hypertrophy sometimes met with in this organ. The asthma of children is sometimes referred to this enlargement.

In some instances this gland has been found to weigh from one to two ounces, and so large as to compress the lungs, trachea, and pneumogastric nerve in their downward passage.

Thymic Asthma.

Thymic asthma is sometimes met with in quite young children and requires treatment. In the Allopathic school only a meagre treatment is suggested. The Homœopathic remedies are *Argentum metallicum, Baryta carb.*, Sulphur and their analogues.

Diseases of the Mesenteric Glands.

The mesenteric is a duplicature of the peritoneum which suspends and retains in situ the small intestines; it has many glands subject to serious derangement during the existence of certain diseases described under the head of tabes mesenterica; consists of softening and ulceration of these glands in persons of a scrofulous cachexia; this affection is by no means uncommon; it is allied to tuberculosis, and too frequently joins in breaking down all prospects of relief; remedies are nevertheless called into requisition to afford temporary relief, such as *Arsenicum*, *Calcarea carbonica*, *Baryta carb.*, *Nitric acid* and *Sulphur;* Cod liver oil has been recommended, as long as the patient's appetite will permit; the nutritive system must be supplied by a suitable diet, this may consist of animal broths and if the patient's appetite indicates, a broiled beef or venison steak; warm fomentations such as flannels wrung out of tolerably hot water may be applied over the region of the abdomen when much inflammation is apparent.

CHAPTER XXXII

DISEASE OF THE BILIARY SYSTEM.

Hepatitis or Inflammation of the Liver.

In tropical climates, acute inflammation of the liver is a common affection, it is much less frequent in the temperate zone.

The symptoms which indicate the presence of this disorder are the following: at first rigors and chills usually make their appearance, quickly followed by hot skin, thirst and scanty urine; sometimes nausea, and vomiting, bitter taste, pain and tenderness more or less severe in the right hypochondrium, aggravated on pressure, or by deep breathing, or coughing, pains in the right shoulder, fullness and enlargement of the organ, as may be inferred from the distension of the right hypochondrium; the skin appears sallow; the whites of the eyes have a yellow tinge, the breathing is short and confined to the chest, being performed entirely by the intercostal muscles; there is also a sympathetic cough and vomiting, and the fever sometimes of a typhoid character.

SYMPTOMS.—The symptoms, however, vary in different persons, in accordance with the temperament, age and portion of the gland implicated in the inflammation. A burning, stitching pain in the right side, which extends into the chest under the collar bone, between the shoulder blades, indicates inflammation of the convex side of the liver. When the substance of the gland is affected, the pain is of a dull, tensive character, the urine is of a saffron color, the eyes and skin often have a yellowish hue, the patient complains of thirst and some degree of fever, the bowels are usually constipated. This disease terminates either by resolution or abscess. The former is indicated by diminution of the febrile symptoms, a copious perspiration, etc. When an abscess is indicated, the patient experiences a sensation of throbbing, or pulsating in the part accompanied by, or with the general symptoms of hectic fever. When the abscess discharges, it is sometimes into the stomach, at others, either into the duodenum or colon, or externally through the walls of the abdomen, or by perforation of the chest.

Acute inflammation of the liver is supposed to arise from cold, nervous depression, drunkenness, and even pregnancy, and other causes. In some cases it is seated in the peritoneal covering and resembles pleuritis, and terminates in adhesion to the adjacent parts.

TREATMENT.—The Allopathic consists mainly in the administration of Calomel and saline purgatives. Topical depletion by wet cups over the region of the liver is now generally used.

HOMŒOPATHIC TREATMENT.—*Bryonia* is indicated when there is considerable fever, and the patient is inclined to lie on the affected side, and complains of severe pains when moved. *Mercurius*, after the use of *Bryonia*, is indicated when there is a heavy odor from the breath, and dryness of the mouth and a bitter taste. *Nux vomica* is indicated when there is severe pain in the region of the liver, extending to the back, and when there is sympathetic nausea and vomiting. *Podophyllum* is given when the action of the liver is torpid and secretes less than the normal quantity of bile. *Collinsonia* when there is a jaundiced complexion and yellowness of the inner canthi of both eyes. Pulsatilla, if during pregnancy the liver becomes inflamed. In case of diarrhœa and thirst, *Mercurius* and Arsenicum.

Accessory treatment.—When there is severe pain, the region of the liver may be covered with cloths wrung qut of hot water, with two or three layers or thicknesses of linen. One drachm of the tincture of Aconite may be added to a pint of hot water for the purpose of making a lotion with which to saturate the wet cloths or compresses already applied, and these may be covered with dry flannel.

If the inflammation be of the abscess form, *Hepar sulphur* may be given first, and afterwards *Phosphorus, Conium, Nux vomica,* and Chamomilla.

Enlargement of the Liver.

This disease is occasioned by the distension of the blood vessels and gall-ducts; it is indicated by a fullness on the right side in the region near the false ribs; on assuming an upright posture the patient experiences a sense of weight, and when the part is pressed upon, an uneasy restless feeling besets him; the complexion may be pale, yellow, or sallow, the tongue coated, the bowels constipated, the appetite faulty; and there may be vertigo, vomiting, lassitude, headache and depression of spirits. The pulse is usually irregular, and slow; when the liver is congested, the secretion is for the most part suppressed, the causes that may be enumerated are sudden chills, high-living, and the habitual use of intoxicating liquors; sometimes anger, and other mental influences may so operate upon the biliary system, as well as severe bodily exercise in the heat of the sun. The disease is so common that an indictment is continually found against other tributary agencies.

Hepatitis is an occasional cause of enlargement, persons of a sedentary habit who indulge in excesses at the table are liable to suffer from this disease more than the laboring classes; their feasting on highly seasoned food, in connection with the variety of luxuries prepares the way for the entrance of noxious matters into the portal blood that should never be present in it; the consequence is engorgement of the liver; the laboring classes even may suffer from similar effects from the excessive use of beer and other malt liquors.

Hydatid diseases of the liver are believed to be dependent on the influence of worms or other parasites.

Cirrhosis or hobnailed liver is a chronic inflammation and enlargement of the areolar tissue which covers and pervades the gland, causing induration, and firmness, and ultimately contraction.

This leads to the drawing in of the capsule, which gives to the liver the hobnailed appearance; from the fact of this pathological condition being found in persons who are given to spirit drinking, it has been denominated the *gin-drinker's liver*; the gland is so contracted, that the normal secretion is interrupted and this gives rise to dropsy and a fatal termination.

TREATMENT.—In Allopathy, Mercury is the sheet anchor; saline cathartics are also employed.

HOMŒOPATHIC TREATMENT.—*Phosphorus* may be employed against enlargement of the liver.

Aconite for shooting pains after exposure.

Bryonia for tensive burning, or stinging pains, and in rheumatic persons, *Mercurius, Sabadilla* if the pain be dull.

For biliousness where there is vomiting of bile and mucus, *Nux vomica;* for stimulants and over-feeding, *Nux vomica;* when associated with piles, *Sulphur,* when with constipation, *Mercurius* and *Lycopodium,* particularly if there are white costive stools and depression of spirits; *Iris versicolor* is a valuable remedy for sick headache; and other remedies for biliousness are *Lycopodium, Hepar sulphur, Pulsatilla, Podophyllum, Chelidonium* and *Taraxicum.*

For bilious diarrhœa, when there is a bitter taste and dark stools, *Podophyllum,* when there is vomiting in hot weather give *Iris versicolor.* In simple cases which occur during the summer China; Chamomilla is suitable for children and females when the diarrhœa is caused by teething or passion.

In case of dropsy of the abdomen from cirrhosis, *Arsenicum, Croton tiglium, Nitric acid* and *Nux vomica.* The leading indications for remedies:

For *Aconite* are sudden bilious attacks succeeded by chills and fever, threatening an icturic condition of the whole system. *Arsenicum* on the contrary is indicated in chronic cases with extreme weakness, burning pain, vomiting and exhausting diarrhœa, enlarged spleen and ascites.

Bryonia is indicated for hardness and enlargement of the liver with shooting and stinging pains aggravated by pressure, severe constipation and disinclination for a stool. *Chamomilla* is indicated for bilious attacks in children, brought on by teething, cold or from anger; in females likewise who suffer from bilious attacks in consequence of anger or a cold, this remedy is well suited. *Chelidonium* 3x dil. is indicated for chronic liver disease when there is a thick yellow coating upon the tongue, dull headache, urine thick and of a deep yellow color, and also when there is pain and fullness with constipation. *Mercurius* 3x trit. is indicated for dull pressing pain which prevents the patient from lying any great length of time on the right side. *Mercurius* 3x trit. is also indicated for a bitter taste in the mouth, yellow tinge of the eyes, shivering followed by profuse perspiration, white stools, bowels either constipated or relaxed; in simple cases of jaundice this remedy has a definite action. Nux vomica is the great remedy for inebriates; it may be employed successfully against a torpid liver arising from sedentary habits or nervous exhaustion with constipation, deep red urine, associated with piles.

Nitric acid is suitable for long-continued obstinate cases with jaundice, and especially if organic disease is feared, like abscess or tendency to dropsy. *Pulsatilla* for affection of the liver which becomes palpably manifest during the catamenia. *Macrotin* 3x trit., *Cimicifuga* 3x dil. and *Caulophyllum* 3x dil. are remedies suitable for affections of the liver attendant upon the menopausal period of women.

Accessory treatment.—Rest, with frequent change and absence from the burden of business, domestic cares and broils and the monotonous scenes of household duties, which should be exchanged for hilltop and mountain ramblings. Long hours of mental and physical exhaustion should be abridged by an exchange for dog and gun or the fishing tackle, and tramps through the wildwood in search for game, or for angling in the running streams.

Jaundice.

Icterus or jaundice is a discoloration of the skin, of the conjunctiva and other tissues, dependent on derangement of the biliary secretion. From the different degrees of color this disease has received several terms of distinction, as the black, the green, and the yellow.

Jaundice, in the main, arises from some impediment in the biliary ducts which obstruct the outward flow of bile, the reabsorption of which by the blood in the liver is followed by its diffusion throughout the system by that medium. After jaundice from obstruction has existed some time, suppression supervenes. The function of the liver is to secrete bile from the blood, therefore it may also be occasioned by suppression of the biliary function, and in consequence of which the bile is not eliminated from the blood, but remains with cholestrine in such quantities, as to affect the tissues by reabsorption of the bile which has been properly eliminated, but still retained in the liver and not transmitted to the duodenum. Jaundice may also arise from enervation of the gland, active and passive congestion, disordered hepatic circulation or destruction of the secretive cells of the liver. It occasionally supervenes, and is a symptom both of the acute and chronic inflammation of the liver.

The unmistakable signs of jaundice are yellowness of the skin and of the eyes, whitish fæces, urine having the color of saffron, and communicating a bright yellow tinge to white linen or muslin.

The prognosis of this disease is usually favorable when it is merely a functional affection, but when it depends upon a structural disease of the liver, or comes on suddenly from some mental shock or bodily concussion, it is not so favorable.

In old persons of impaired constitution, even if there is no obvious cause for jaundice, the prognosis is the most unfavorable of all, and particularly when the color of the skin is greenish or approaching the black.

TREATMENT.—In the Allopathic treatment of this disease some cases are believed incurable, while others may recover without any treatment at all.

Mercury in some form is the chief remedy in the treatment of this disease; repeated doses of *Calomel*, the milder cases may require a single dose of five or ten grains, while the chronic cases have required small doses of *Calomel* and *Rhubarb* as each acute manifestation occurs.

HOMŒOPATHIC TREATMENT.—In acute jaundice *Aconite, Mercurius, Nux vomica* and *Chamomilla* 3x. We have found Aconite an effectual remedy for jaundice with symptoms of inflammation, and a distinctly marked pain in the region of the liver; we have derived great satisfaction from the use of Nux vomica when costiveness was a prominent symptom, and when there was considerable tenderness in the region of the liver, from indulgence in stimulants and sedentary habits; *Mercurius* 3x is indicated for that kind of jaundice unattended by pain, but merely from yellowness of the skin and eyes. For the chronic forms of this disease; *Arsenicum, Chelidonium, China, Carbo vegetabilis, Digitalis, Podophyllum,* and some others, each in 3x. The leading indications for *Arsenicum* are great anguish and fear of death; for *Chelidonium,* pain in the region of the liver and right shoulder, deep red, clean tongue, and bitter taste; *China* 3x is indicated when the jaundice is intermittent, or comes on with paroxysms of fever with bilious diarrhœa; when chronic jaundice afflicts those who indulge in the daily use of stimulants, *Nux vomica* 3x is particularly indicated.

Carbo vegetabilis is required when there is coldness of the lower extremities, and the patient complains of not being able to keep warm.

Digitalis is suitable where there is a clean tongue and fre-

31

quent dry retching, soreness and bloatedness of the pit of the stomach.

Podophyllum 2x dil. is particularly indicated when the skin is sallow, and when there is an indication of drowsiness, bitter taste in the mouth, white stools and brown urine; the diet in jaundice must be such as the patient is able to take; from the fact many cases are attended with febrile symptoms, very little food will supply the demand in such cases; the appetite varies in degree, the same as the disease; some will require something substantial, some choose light food, others are allowed to take food under any circumstances; on the whole I think it wise to allow an unmedicinal diet, and as frequently as the patient desires.

Diseases of the Gall Bladder.

Icterus calculosis, is a species of jaundice entirely different from that which we have been describing and requires a totally different treatment; when the gall duct is obstructed mechanically so that the secretion of the liver cannot be secreted, the bile, instead of passing through the ordinary channels to perform its office in the process of digestion, becomes eliminated so as to affect the cutaneous surface; sometimes fever attends the passage of a gall-stone, acute suffering always attends the passage of these concretions which form a mechanical obstruction to the exit of healthy bile when secreted; many old school physicians have resorted to *Opium* in the form of two grain pills to mitigate the suffering of the patient; they have found from experience that *Mercurial* treatment which met their approbation in acute and chronic hepatitis, would aggravate the sufferings rather than afford relief.   In modern times hypodermic injections of *Morphine* have been employed to mitigate the acute pain but neither the *Opium, Calomel,* or hypodermic injection have any tendency to remove the concretion, or cure the patient.   In Homœopathic treatment we have found that a single dose of Arnica 2x dilution would remove the pain after repeated doses of Morphine amounting to several grains had been administered without effect.

In the case of an aged gentleman who had suffered intensely from these mechanical obstructions for six weeks, defying the skill of Allopathic physicians until wearied of their efforts to procure relief; a few doses of the third dilution of *Calomel* in water was followed by complete relief from pain.   Another case of a gentleman suffering from the same difficulty was relieved after four weeks of Allopathic treatment by *China* 1x dilution in water. In our experience with many other cases olive oil in considerable quantities has had a beneficial effect in softening the concretions and favoring their discharge from the duct; we have known from twenty to thirty gall-stones to be excreted in several instances after drinking a cupful of olive oil; we have seen the good effects of *Chamomilla, Colocynth, China, Chelidonium, Pulsatilla*, and *Nux vomica* in the 3x dil. In other cases and nearly in all subjects, when the mechanical obstructions are removed a rapid convalescence follows. The diet when the patient is able to partake of food, should be beef tea and chicken broth; or an emollient farinaceous food.

Diseases of the Pancreas.

It is seldom that this gland becomes involved in disease; we have never been able to diagnose a case of the kind because their existence is not signified by any plain or intelligible signs; carcinomatous deposits, according to some writers, are liable to occur in the pancreas, most always in that extremity which lies next to the bowels; it is alleged that jaundice is sometimes caused by some change in the pancreas obstructing the bile ducts, and sometimes it has produced enormous enlargement of the liver itself and great distension of the stomach, by compressing the duodenum to a degree that has fatally obstructed the passage of aliment through this portion of the intestinal tube.

Pancreatic diseases are believed to be uniformly fatal, and yet when symptoms are such as to lead one to infer the presence of any disease, Homœopathic remedies should be prescribed; when hypertrophy of the liver, in connection with obstruction of the duodenum occurs in connection with enormous distension of the stomach, *Iodine* may exert a specific influence in affording temporary relief. *Arsenicum*, when the patient suffers from extreme debility, sallow complexion, thirst and emaciation, *Arsenicum iodatus* for great prostration and weakness, and finally all the other remedies employed in the treatment of *marasmus*, scrofula, or against a cancerous diathesis.

The accessory treatment and diet are the same as directed in tabes mesenterica and scrofula in general.

CHAPTER XXXIII.

RENAL DISEASES.

The kidneys are subject to functional derangements which result in a variety of changes in the fluid they secrete; before taking cognizance of the organic derangement we will give our experience concerning those of a strictly functional character: first nephralgia; this is generally produced, but not always, by the transit of a urinary calculus from the pelvis of the kidney through the ureters towards the bladder; this is called in common parlance, a fit of gravel.

DIAGNOSIS.—Pain sometimes dull, but more frequently severe, and generally in the loins on one side, descending along the tract of the vessels of the same side, numbness of the corresponding thigh, retraction and some pain of the testicle, a frequent desire to urinate, with more or less gastric disturbance; the urine is usually high colored.

TREATMENT.—The treatment of nephralgia—the application of warm water fomentations to the renal region, and to direct the internal administration of *Arnica, Belladonna, Gelsemium* and *Squillæ.* The leading indications for the use of Arnica are as follows: dull pain in either the right or left kidney, which increases in severity until the patient cries with torture. We have given this remedy in several cases of this kind, under the belief that the suffering was of a traumatic character, as in the passage of biliary calculus after large doses of morphine had been given without effect; this remedy has produced sudden relief and the calculi in a few hours have been found in the urine.

The leading indications for the use of Pulsatilla are a lymphatic temperament, severe colic, attended by sallowness of the skin, an inclination to lie on the face and to draw the knees up so as to press upon the abdomen, the pain is sometimes attended with dry retching, when near the menstrual period. After *Pulsatilla Belladonna* may be given to relieve congestion, which sometimes is a source of nephralgia in females.

Gelsemium is indicated when the pain in the kidney is severe, and extends downward on the side of the affected kidney.

Squillæ is indicated for gravel, when there is pain in the kidney attended with strangury; other therapeutic hints may be had by consulting *Cannabis sativa, Cantharis, Petroleum, Sarsaparilla* and *Sulphur.*

We have found the application of poultices made of equal parts of corn meal and ground flax seed valuable accessory treatment.

Nephritis or Inflammation of the Kidneys,

Which is indicated with severe pressing and pungent pains in the renal region following the course of the ureters to the bladder with dysuria or strangury.

When both kidneys are implicated, which is rarely the case, there is an entire suppression of the urine, or otherwise the urine is hot and high colored. In the male subject the testicle on the affected side is swollen, painful and drawn up and the lower extremity on the same side is often numb, and sometimes spasmodically affected; nausea and vomiting, severe colic and tenesmus usually accompany the disease.

TREATMENT.—Allopathic treatment, venesection and saline purgatives are commonly relied on for giving relief.

HOMŒOPATHIC TREATMENT.—Where there is considerable pyrexia, *Aconite* is indicated, five or ten drops of the third dilution in water, a teaspoonful every hour. *Aconite* may be followed by *Belladonna* 3x, *Cannabis sativa* 3x, *Cantharis* 3x, *Gelsemium*, or *Nux vomica* 3x, in accordance with the symptoms that may indicate their use. In gouty subjects and intemperate persons addicted to the use of alcoholic stimulants, *Colchicum* 3x, *Nux vomica* 3x, *Pusatilla* 3x, and Sarsaparilla 3x, are remedies to be consulted, accessory treatment in this disease may be the same as that recommended in nephralgia.

Albuminuria or Bright's Disease of the Kidneys.

One of the chief indications of the presence of this disease in the kidney is found in the habitual impregnation of the urine with albumen; in healthy urine neither can we recognize its presence in the secretion by mere inspection, it is detected by certain tests, albumen of which we have a familiar example in the white of eggs. It may be solidified by subjecting the urine to a temperature of 160 degrees Farenheit, when much diluted it may require a higher degree of heat to complete the coagulation; we can always discover albumen in the urine by heating it in a small glass tube to the boiling point, if the urine is hazy or cloudy in consequence of the presence of mucus, it will be well to filter the fluid before testing it.   In some cases albuminous urine is turbid from the presence of the lithates, these dissolve as the heat is applied, and the urine first becomes clear, and then as the temperature rises the albuminous opacity becomes apparent. This test, however, is not conclusive, in as much as some conditions or circumstances may prevent the heat from coagulating the albumen, even if it is present, on the other hand it may produce a fallacious appearance of albumen where none exists.   We may avoid this fallacious appearance by testing the suspected urine with Nitric acid, which has the property of precipitating the albumen in the form of a pulp, it will thus detect albumen when the tested urine is alkaline; but *Nitric acid* alone is not an equivocal test of the presence of albumen, for it may occasion a pulpy precipitate of lithic acid when there is no albumen.   There are other tests frequently spoken of and sometimes recommended, but not more certain than that of heat and Nitric acid, which may enable the practitioner to judge with tolerable accuracy of the presence of albumen in the urine recently evacuated from the bladder.   It is quite certain that the presence of albumen in the urine, in many cases indicates a very serious organic disease of the kidneys which has no appropriate name; some call it granular degeneration of the kidney, but the term granular is not always applicable; the disease is familiarly known as that of Bright's disease, named after an eminent physician, who first described its pathology in 1837, under the head of Bright's disease, therefore we must consider this disease of the kidney.

It has been our fortune to treat many cases of this distressing malady. We can better illustrate its nature by a brief allusion to a few unmistakable cases of the disease:

CASE I.   John J.—, Esq., aged 54 years, a man of great activity in political and civil affairs, being one of the county commissioners of Cook county, of the State of Illinois, began to experience severe pain in the cardiac region which interfered with rest and quiet. Sleep departing from his eyes and a derangement of his stomach preventing him from taking food, he called on an eminent physician of the Old School, who made a careful diagnosis and pronounced the gentleman's suffering to be the result of heart disease, and for this trouble this physician treated him for several weeks, and still there was no mitigation of the suffering, no let up, no more inclination to sleep or take food than there had been when he was first called to see the patient. Another physician of the same school was called in counsel, and after the most critical examination of the case, no conclusion was arrived at that implicated the kidneys. There was no pain in the renal region, but an indescribable anguish and pain about the heart, and in the region of the chest. Auscultation and percussion revealed nothing abnormal in the sounds of the heart, and it was exceedingly difficult to account for the great suffering and anguish that the patient had to endure. If there had been any inflammation or other trouble at the seat of the pain, it might have been detected, or had there been serious difficulty in any other locality, a metastasis to the region of the pain might have been inferred, but the physicians utterly failed to make a satisfactory interpretation, so as to determine pathologically the nature of the case. They finally stood aside and requested to be discharged from the case. A third physician was called who recognized in the suffering an insiduous, if not fatal, renal disease. The urine was examined and subjected to several tests. There was nothing that disclosed the nature of the disease from inspection of the urine. It was clear, and apparently free from sediment, some of which was heated in a test tube and found to be full of albumen. A pint of the urine was procured and sent to the laboratory of a chemist who made a specialty of urinary analysis, and, to the astonishment of all, the chemist found albumen in large quantities, as well as evidence of the rapid degeneration of the kidneys. Immediately after this examination it was thought best to give him the tincture of *Senecio aurens* in doses of ten drops every two hours. This remedy did something toward relieving the anguish and want of sleep; after the first twelve hours the patient was able to take a little rest in sleep, and the pain which gave him so much suffering was removed and became apparent in the region of the kidneys. Up to this time there was no sign of dropsy, either local or general, and the only fact we could command to determine the nature of the disease was the albumen in the urine. There now appeared to be an interregnum from suffering, and temporary rest for the patient. In a short time after, the patient's feet began to swell and other signs of dropsy, both general and local, began to be apparent. A steady pain in the renal region, uncontrollable by medicine, was accompanied by hydrocele. So enormous in size was the scrotum when distended, that it interfered with the locomotion of the patient. Another change of physicians ensued and a resort to hydragogue cathartics which were given persistently until the patient was unable to walk, although relief was obtained for the distended scrotum. The case terminated fatally in a few weeks.

The insidious manner in which this disease made its appearance is worthy of note as exhibiting in some degree the difficulty of making a diagnosis from the locality of the suffering without testing a quantity of the urine.

CASE II. Miss Minnie L——, aged 21 years, had an attack of scarlet fever when nine years of age from which she recovered after passing through a painful sequelæ of dropsy. She nevertheless was subject at times to urinary derangements, and the passage of albuminous urine; at the age of fifteen she suffered greatly from this derangement and was apparently cured by the tincture of Terebinthina in drop doses, repeated every two hours for several days. She remained apparently well until she attained the age of twenty years, when she showed signs of the reappearance of the disease. Her parents took her to Europe and employed the best medical skill for the succeeding nine months without any satisfactory result. They returned home with her, and in spite of the most careful medical treatment and good nursing she died in four months after her arrival. A post-mortem examination of the two cases above recited revealed morbid appearances of the substance of the kidney, noting great changes in its structure.

Albuminuria however, does not always indicate organic derangement of the kidney; some cases have been permanently cured by the administration of Homœopathic remedies, *Galium aperine* was given in one case which resulted in a cure, and other cases have yielded to *Senecio aurens, Terebinth, Cannabis, Cantharis* each 3x dil., three times a day, and other remedies, Homœopathic to individual cases.

Diabetes.

Before treating of this dyscrasia of the kidney we will briefly consider that condition which usually precedes it, and is termed ISCHURIA, meaning a complete suppression of the urine as well as those cases in which the urine is secreted, but not discharged from the body; these two conditions are vastly different from each other, the one being dependent upon the inactivity of the kidney in its excretory function, the other simply means a retention of the urine after it is secreted; it will thus be seen that in *suppression* the secretion is suspended, and in retention it may be as active as ever.

Retention of the urine presents itself as a surgical case involving points of great practical interest. But *ischuria* or *suppression* belongs to the physician and is termed *ischuria renalis*, it occurs to persons advanced in life and inclined to corpulency; a celebrated English writer says that the similarity of cases is so marked that one is an exact copy of the other. That we may better understand the nature of the difficulty, we will relate the case of a corpulent, robust farmer, about 60 years of age, who was seized with a chill which somewhat alarmed him because he had not passed water for twenty-four hours; to gratify his desire for an evacuation of the bladder, he prevailed upon his medical attendant, against his convictions, to introduce a catheter, and no urine was found in the bladder, and from the fact that excrementitious matters become eliminated from the blood when suppression does not really exist, it was reasonable to suppose that the impurities generally excreted through the kidneys were suffered to accumulate in the system and to become destructive of its life, and death ensued in this case in about thirty hours.

In cases of temporary suppression of the urine, the first dilution of Terebinthina will quickly afford relief, but in more serious cases should the kidneys remain inactive for twenty-four hours, the patient is in a perilous condition.

In Allopathic practice powerful diuretics and alteratives are relied upon to revive the functions and thus relieve the patient, but this practice more frequently fails than the employment of such Homœopathic remedies as *Terebinth*, *Senecio Apis melliflca*, in the 3x dil. and *Sulphur*, as opposed to this pathological condition.

Diabetes Mellitus.

This is usually a constitutional cachexia, or chronic disease characterized by mal-assimilation of food, and the discharge of enormous quantities of urine, of a pale, sweet and heavy nature, containing something like grape-sugar. The term *diabetes* has been applied to two diseases which resemble each other in the copious secretion of urine, the one is termed *diabetes insipidus*, and the other *diabetes mellitus*, in the former the urine is clear, and contains no abnormal ingredient, its specific gravity is about 1,000 in this disease, the urine is colorless and the patient has much thirst, dry skin, and much physical weakness, but the latter possesses most remarkable pathological features, and in addition to the mal-assimilation of food employed for the nourishment of the body, the carbo-hydrates which enter into the composition of food undergo change and are converted into diabetic sugar, a product incapable of oxydization or of assimilation, and therefore, excreted by the kidneys as useless, and injurious. In the early stage the misappropriation of starchy, and saccharine matter. It is not general, but as the disease increases, it becomes greater; the adipose matter is then perverted and all the carbonaceous elements which should nourish the system, become depraved and useless, and inasmuch as they are not oxydized the temperature falls below the normal standard; then ensues a period of degenerate changes, the albuminous and nitrogenous elements in the food also undergo similar changes, and are unfitted to enter the circulation, so that ultimately very little is left for nourishment, or for the maintenance of the temperature of the body. The sugar is thus increased in quantity. It is maintained that the seat of diabetes is in the *pancreas*, *liver*, and *duodenum*, and that organic disease of the *pancreas* and *liver* causes a disturbance of duodenal digestion.

SYMPTOMS.—Long before the health becomes seriously impaired, the disease makes considerable headway, but when it is fully developed the following train of symptoms becomes apparent, at first in a simple malaise, weakness of the limbs, constant thirst, general debility, frequent micturition, and emaciation; as the disease increases these symptoms become more decided in the lower extremities, and the feet become numb to that degree that the gait is quite unsteady, the tongue is red and fissured, the mouth dry, the appetite voracious, with sinking at the stomach, the bowels are generally constipated, the evacuations are hard, pale and dry, the breath has the odor of apples, seemingly due to a large secretion of glucose, as this increases the odor becomes more observable and less so as the secretion diminishes. The specific gravity of the urine at this stage is 1,050 owing to the fact that all the water drank passes off by the kidneys, the insensible perspiration is diminished, skin becomes dry and harsh, and is frequently the seat of some stubborn cutaneous eruption. Women frequently complain of disagreeable itching of the vulva when suffering from this disease; this symptom is undoubtedly the result of the irritation caused by the saccharine urine. Then follows muscular weakness, diminution of weight and serious atrophy of the muscles and a general sinking of the frame. The gums become soft and spongy, and painful looseness of the front teeth, like unto what is met with in scurvy, pain about the loins, absence of sexual desire and complete loss of sexual power, burning of the hands and feet, accompanying coldness of the extremities; sometimes there is œdema of the limbs, and occasional carbuncles, or boils; from these symptoms the brain may become implicated, manifest in dimness of vision, amaurosis and cataract. The pulse remains normal; as the disease advances it may become complicated with latent pneumonia or phthisis. The temperature is uniformly below the normal standard, ranging from 94 to 97 deg., and very seldom becomes raised. When the disease is complicated by inflammatory difficulties the quantity of urine is increased from the normal standard of two pints in twenty-four hours, to four, six, eight, ten, and even thirty pints, in the same length of time, inducing frequent calls to micturate day and night, producing great soreness or urethritis. As high as four pounds of solid saccharine matter has been discharged in a single day's evacuations of the bladder. From this fact it will be seen that diabetic patients may pass a quantity of sugar in a few months equal to that of their own bodies. The tests applied to ascertain the quality of the urine are, first its specific gravity being increased from 1018 to 1050, and it is passed in large quantities and has a pale straw color and a faint smell like apples, or milk. The test for diabetic urine most readily practiced is to half-fill a test-tube with the urine to be examined, add about two drops of the solution of Sulphate of Copper to make it slightly blue, and then add of liquor Potasse enough to clear it by re-dissolving the precipitate which it at first produces, let it boil up once over a flame, and if it contain sugar there will be a reddish brown precipitate of the sub-oxate of copper, if there is no sugar, the precipitate will be black oxate of copper; several repeated tests of this kind are however required to render the fact apparent that the urine uniformly contains this saccharine matter. One application of this test is not sufficient evidence, because the urine may temporarily contain sugar from some unusual article of diet, neither is excess of urine an infallible sign of diabetes mellitus, because enormous discharges may occur in hysteria, and the insipidous variety of the disease as well as in other disorders.

The most reliable information concerning diabetic urine is obtained by the aid of the Urinometer; when this instrument stands above 1030 we may conclude that sugar is present.

The cause of this disease is supposed to be some dyscrasia of the liver which produces abnormality in the function of digestion, so that the sugar required for the maintenance of the body enters the blood and leaves it again unchanged and is excreted from the kidneys. We refer not merely to the sugar and starch contained in food, the latter of which is converted by the saliva into sugar, but to that always contained in greater or less quantity by the blood, unless the amount is more than one third it is not eliminated.

PROGNOSIS.—The prognosis may be favorable when the patient is corpulent and in easy circumstances and blessed with a healthy residence, and receives early energetic and persevering treatment before the disease matures, but unfavorable when it occurs in infancy, and youth under twenty years of age of a spare habit, careless and neglectful of themselves, and a residence in unhealthy dwellings; when the duration of the disease has been so long that the patient is unable to obtain relief from the constant drain upon the system as to indicate the approach of latent pneumonia or phthisis, or when gangrenous inflammation, or thoracic and intestinal complications set in, the prognosis is very unfavorable. The course of the disease is not characterized by rapid changes, although there are frequent ameliorations and exacerbations, it sometimes lasts for years; in those cases supposed to be cured relapses occur after several months of comparative health and it is not safe to pronounce a case absolutely cured until at least one year has passed since any diabetic symptoms have shown themselves.

TREATMENT.—Blood-letting and opium are among the principal agents employed in Allopathic treatment, together with a diet composed in the main of animal food; all articles of diet containing starch or sugar are carefully excluded.

In Homœopathic practice, the blood-letting and opium, with nearly all the collateral remedies, are believed to be injurious, but experience has confirmed the utility of the diet laid down in allopathic works.

HOMŒOPATHIC TREATMENT.—The Homœopathic medical treatment consists mainly in the employment of *Phosphoric acid* 3x,

Nitrate of Uranium 3x, *Terebinthina* 3x, *Arum triphyllum* 3x, *Helonin* 3x, *Muriate of Quinine* 3x, *Plumbum* 3x, with many other remedies indicated by special symptoms. Phosphoric acid generally relieves and sometimes cures; the symptoms indicating its use are urgent urinating, pain in the loins, emaciation, and great prostration; Nitrate of Uranium has sometimes proved to be efficacious, and some extraordinary cures are reported. In our own experience these two remedies have produced more satisfactory results than any others we have used.

In the case of a young man aged seventeen, troubled with dyspeptic symptoms, and passing a quantity of diabetic urine, equaling in amount to twelve pints every twenty-four hours, after taking Nitrate of Uranium daily for three weeks the digestion improved, the quantity of urine diminished to four pints with the prospect of an ultimate cure. We have also noticed the favorable changes that occur after the administration of Phosphoric acid. Many symptoms indicate the use of Arsenic, as also Muriate of Quinine, and for particular symptoms, Nux vomica, Cantharis, Eupatorium and Purpureum are often required each 3x.

Accessory treatment.—While all articles of diet containing starch or sugar are discarded as injurious, diabetic patients may be allowed fat meat, oysters, fish, eggs, milk, beef soup thickened with wheat bran, and salad with vinegar.

In cases we have treated we have found a drink prepared of gluten, two parts of bran, and a small quantity of butter, made into a soup with skimmed milk, or a bread may be made of the same ingredients minus the milk. We speak from experience in recommending the above diet. Skim-milk alone may be used as a constant drink for diabetic patients. Six pints a day may be allowed with impunity, and in the earlier stage it has had a curative effect. Thus it will be seen that butcher's meat of all kinds (except liver), bacon, ham, dried or cured; poultry, venison, all kinds of shell fish, also all other kinds of fish, either fresh or salted, and broths that are not thickened with flour, bran bread and almost every other kind of aliment free from starch and sugar are allowed in this disease. The ordinary beverages, such as tea, coffee, and cocoa, claret, burgundy, and sauterne, also bitter-ale.

Diabetis Isipidus.

This is simply a chronic diuresis; it is a very rare disorder, but when it does occur it indicates some organic change in the kidneys; large quantities of urine are secreted of a watery appearance which contains no abnormal ingredient; its symptoms are thirst, dry harsh skin and considerable physical weakness.

TREATMENT.—The Allopathic treatment consists of *Opium* or some of its salts.

HOMŒOPATHIC TREATMENT consists of *Aconite* 3x, *Bryonia* 3x, *Pulsatilla* 3x, and *Hyoscyamus* together with *Mercurius solubilis* 3x, *Mercurius vivus* 3x, may be consulted in this affection, and administered in accordance with the symptoms. The diet may be the same as pointed out in the regimen prescribed for diabetis mellitus.

CHAPTER XXXIV.

Cystitis inflammation of the mucous membrane of the bladder, diffuse, serous, adhesive, suppurative or ulcerative, affords the best definition of this disorder.

Acute cystitis is a rare occurrence except that which occurs as a metastasis of gonorrhœa, or from wounds produced by the catheter or instruments in search of calculi, or it may occur occasionally from cold or damp, when exposed to their influence.

SYMPTOMS.—The symptoms of inflammation of the bladder are indicated by pain, sense of weight on pressure, and extreme irritability in the region of the bladder, rigors and often alarming constitutional disturbances; the urine ejected by a sort of spasmodic action as soon as it collects, with straining and generally much suffering, and there may be a discharge of mucus or pus, together with blood.

Chronic Cystitis.

Chronic cystitis is more common than the acute, though sometimes it may be the sequelæ of an acute attack, but more frequently it is the production of calculi, or disease of the prostate gland, or of stricture, etc., but a still more common cause may be the loss of power to evacuate the bladder, or prostatic enlargement. The urine then undergoes such changes that it becomes a source of irritation to the lining membrane of the bladder.

The urea by decomposition is transformed into carbonate of ammonia, and this salt being acid and irritating, so affects the mucous lining of the bladder as to cause a morbid secretion upon its surface. The symptoms of chronic cystitis are a modified form of those pertaining to the acute, and though the pain is less the discharge is generally more profuse. In some cases the discharge is very abundant, and becomes very tough or tenacious on standing, as will appear from the ropy, stringy mucus which follows the urine on emptying the vessel into which it was discharged. The vesical catarrh of the bladder may be distinguished from inflammation of the kidneys by the pain extending upwards toward the loins; while that produced by inflammation of the kidneys extends downwards from the loins to the bladder.

TREATMENT.—It has been the prevailing practice in the old school to resort to general and local depletion, or by exciting diuresis, by the administration of *Nitric ether*, *Spirits of juniper* and other diuretics.

HOMŒOPATHIC TREATMENT, which is varied to accord with the causes and associations. *Aconite* may be prescribed first when the inflammation results from a cold and is attended by febrile symptoms, *Cantharis* 3x, may be administered after Aconite, in case of tenesmus or painful micturition, *Dulcamara* 3x, for those cases which result from exposure to dampness, *Belladonna* 3x, is suitable when there is much nervous irritability. The chronic form of the disease requires *Cantharis* 3x, or *Cannabis sativa* 3x, *Apis mellifica* 3x, in case of habitual tenesmus, *Eupatorium purpureum* 3x, *Kali hydriodicum* 3x, *Pulsatilla* 3x, and *Chimaphila* 3x, are the best remedies for reducing the pain attending profuse discharges of mucus.

Accessory treatment.—Warm fomentations applied to the region of the bladder may relieve the pain in acute cases; when the patients are at rest in the recumbent posture, the warm hip bath, abdominal compresses, and mucilaginous drinks, will frequently favor recovery. The gentle introduction of tepid water into the bladder by the use of an elastic catheter-syringe that will not injure the orifice of the urethra, is sometimes commended.

Urinary Calculi,

Or Gravel, sometimes called stone in the bladder, and less frequently in the kidneys. When the urine deposits a precipitate after it has been voided it is *called* a sediment. When the same is precipitated in the bladder, or kidneys, it is called gravel, and the urine as it passes has a mealy appearance, and when the gravel becomes concrete, and lodges in any of the urinary passages it is called stone, when the urine passed habitually presents any *one* kind of deposit, the patient is said to have a corresponding diathesis, which is characterized by a yellow, red, or pink deposit, or the formation of red gravel. The Phosphatic Diathesis presents the appearance of white sediment or gravel. The concretions differ in character, some being uric, or lithic, some the phospathic and others the oxalic. The lithic deposit is observed in synochal fever, chronic hepatic disease, forming a brick-dust deposit, or coloring matter in the urine. When this exists in large quantities as in more advanced stages, it has received the name of red gravel. We find the lithates more frequently in the urine of robust persons who live high, and suffer from difficult digestion; sometimes they are associated with rheumatism, but more frequently with gout and chronic skin diseases. There sometimes occurs in the same individual the uric acid condition in alternation with gout; where the disease is hereditary and decends from generation to generation, it has been observed that it may assume the form of gout in one generation, and in the next that of gravel, and the next succeeding generation gout again. Thus it really appears that the alternation of the uric acid condition, and gout, is kept up for successive generations. The phosphatic deposit usually depends on a full digestion, and an anæmic or shattered constitution usually manifested in aged persons. The oxalic deposit is found in the urine of those persons possessed of febrile powers of assimilation and subject to nervous prostration, either from excess of work, anxiety, or excessive venery; such persons are usually pale, and victims of hypocondriasis, disturbed sleep, and acidity of the stomach; the particles of oxalate are found formed into crystal, and float in the urine or subside if it be allowed to stand, but only in a moderate quantity.

Renal Calculi.

The most frequent source of stone in the bladder is from calculi found in the kidney, and passed through the water into the bladder, but cannot pass through the urethra with the urine and thus lie in the bladder as foreign bodies, around which the uric acid or urate of Ammonia collects and adheres. These acquire considerable size by constant accretions in the bladder, and form stones which occasion much suffering until an operation for lithotomy reduces them to fine sand which may escape with the urine. These *vesicula calculi* seem to form readily when there

is an excess of insoluble material eliminated in the urine, or
stagnation of urine in the bladder, which sometimes results from
paralysis cystitis, or obstructions in the urethra, and from disease
of the prostate gland.   A stone in the bladder by the mere precipitation and aggregation of ordinary crystaline and amor-
phus deposit except in accordance with a well-known chemical
law which is as follows: Any body, whether introduced from
without or existing within in the form of coagula blood, fibrin,
etc., causes the secretion of an alkaline fluid, decomposition of
the urine, and facilitates the deposit of salts around itself.   This
leads us to inquire into the composition of calculi.   The most
common are formed by the chemical ingredients, uric acid and the
urates with their modifications, the oxalates, uric oxate, while
those which are less common present the varied combinations of
phosphates; other organic matters are sometimes present.   The
phosphoratic calculi are often soft like mortar, the urate hard, the
oxalate harder still.   A stone recently and quickly formed is less
dense than one of long standing or slow in its formation.   The
symptoms of gravel, which are very conclusive, are as follows:
Increased frequency of urinating during the day and less frequent at night, or during rest, pains in the glans-penis during
and immediately after micturition, with a continuous desire to
pass more urine, in consequence of an affection of the neck
of the bladder.   Another symptom is pain low down in the
abdomen, which is due to chronic inflammation of the bladder.
Pus is found in the urine, or, in other words the urine contains
muco-purulent matter; at other times the urine is bloody.   This
usually occurs after much exercise, such as riding on a hard,
springless seat over a rough road, or on horseback.   All attempts
to dissolve stone in the bladder by chemical agents have proved
unavailing and injurious.   The surgical means for removing them,
called lithotomy, has now reached considerable perfection.   For
preventing the formation of stone in the bladder various laxative
waters have been recommended as common diluents with food
taken into the system, and an abstinence from all kinds of food
containing sugar or fatty matters.   Rain-water, carefully filtered,
and made alkaline with a little soda, may be used moderately for
a drink, and a fair amount of exercise in the open air, and judicious bathing is commended.

TREATMENT.—Those who have a predisposition to the formation of stone, and particularly if they have passed calculi with
their urine, require careful treatment with remedies, as well as
careful regimen, to correct the tendency. It is regarded as useless
to remove a stone if remedies aid in the expulsion of sand or
gravel, and also correct the tendency to such formations. Under
medical treatment many patients have recovered who formerly
passed small calculi, and have entirely ceased to do so. To begin a
correct treatment all avoidable causes must be removed, generous
living, indulgence in stimulants and insufficient exercise on the one
hand, and excessive work, and over indulgence of all kinds on the
other; a moderate amount of abstinence from animal food is advantageous, fruits and vegetables of a succulent character are
commendable, frequent draughts of pure cold water, and a milk
diet are also recommended: if dyspeptic symptoms are present they
must be met by such remedial measures as are called into requisition in the treatment of dyspepsia, a residence in a locality
where pure soft water *cannot* be produced favors the production
of calculi.

With medicines Allopathically, consists of warm enemas,
purgatives, of an anti-saline character, and in addition venesection and the application of wet cups near the region of the pain.

HOMŒOPATHIC TREATMENT.—For renal calculi, LYCOPODIUM,
3x, CANTHARIS, 3x, PODOPHYLLUM, 3x, CANNABIS, 3x, and PUL-
SATILLA, 3x, if there are spasms attending the passage of renal
calculi, *Aconite* 3x, *Chamomilla* 3x, *Gelsemium* 3x, and *Nux
vomica* 3x, very warm hip baths or fomentations for the early
symptoms of stone in the bladder, *Cannabis* 3x, *Mercurius* 6x,
Cantharis 3x, *Macrotin* 6x, *Eucalyptus* 3x, and other preparations such as *Citrate of Lithia*, have been employed to
advantage, *Senecio aurens* 3x, is supposed to increase the secretion
of the kidneys and facilitate the passage of the red sand in the
urine through the ureters; the pain attending stone in the
bladder, and also the micturition may be greatly alleviated by
Phosphoric acid 3x, *Nux vomica* 3x, and *Belladonna* 3x. The
hæmorrhage may be arrested by *Eucalyptus* 3x, *Arnica* 3x, or
Hamamelis 3x. It is impossible, however, to gain any relief except that which is temporary, without a resort to a surgical operation. When there is a large stone which has been increasing in
size for years, the most favorable use of mucilaginous drinks and

medicines cannot give the relief which will be afforded by the
skillful hand of the surgeon.

Hæmaturia.

Hæmaturia signifies bleeding from the urinary organs. The
urine is altered in color when there is bleeding consecutively with
its passage; sometimes it has a bright red tinge, at other times
it assumes a dark hue, brown like coffee, sometimes its color
approaches to blackness. When we find the urine to have either
of these characteristics we at once come to the conclusion that it
derives its peculiar tint from the blood that is mingled with it.
But the color is not a test of the presence of blood, certain
articles of diet will impart a red color to the urine, as for instance
the *prickly-pear* or *indian-fig*, *beet-root*, *logwood* will also produce
the same effect; *rhubarb* and *senna* give to the urine in case it is
alkaline, a blood-red color. The natural color of the urine inclines toward redness independently of any mixture of blood.
When blood mixed with urine causes it to assume a black appearance it is partially owing to the action of some acid acting
chemically upon it. *Black urine*, though very rarely, according
to some writers, may be caused by the presence of a peculiar
principle called Melanic acid; with this exception almost all the
urine of a very dark or black color is owing to the presence of
blood acted upon by various causes. When blood is present in a
considerable quantity it sinks to the bottom of the vessel and
may be readily recognized. A very small quantity of blood is
observed to alter the transparency of the urine causing it to
assume the appearance of a dark brown or cherry-color. A pinkish color of the urine may subside under the action of heat, but
if blood be present the heat will not cause it to disappear from
observation. Another test for a mixture of blood and urine, is
that it reddens a piece of white linen that is dipped into it.
Another that the precipitation of a brownish sediment by raising
the suspected urine to a boiling temperature which leaves the
urine transparent; but the best test of all is by the use of the
microscope, which will enable one to discover the blood corpuscles turgid or collapsed, when diffused through the
urine, or collected at the bottom of the vessel, but these tests
merely enable us to ascertain the presence of blood in the urine
without settling the question concerning the disease which has

given rise to the hæmaturia. The blood emerges from the urethra but it may be poured out at any point of a long and somewhat complex tract of mucous membrane. It may have proceeded from one or both of the kidneys, from each or either ureter; from the bladder, prostate gland, or the urethra.

Hæmaturia, is rarely if ever idiopathic, it is therefore incumbent on us to inquire what local affection of the urinary organs may give rise to hæmorrhage, and how to interpret the symptoms, whether it is owing to the presence of urinary calculi in the ureters or by the accumulation of the calcareous deposits in the kidneys which by change of position may lacerate or lay open by ulceration some of the smaller vessels in contact therewith, and when a calculus descends into the bladder it may give rise to hæmorrhage first from the kidneys, then from the ureters, and lastly from the bladder which it enters and wounds or irritates, and from the urethra in the last stage of its progress from the body; if the concretion is formed in the bladder and does not descend from the kidneys, there is some liability to hæmaturia which in many cases gives rise to a suspicion of stone in the bladder.

A distinguished writer observes that urine of a deep coffee color manifestly mixed with blood is rarely passed unless it is the effect of a stone in the urinary passages; should there be a fungus growth either in the kidney, or bladder, blood may proceed from either, especially if these growths are malignant, in which case the prognosis will be unfavorable.

Hæmorrhage may take place from the surface of the bladder from chronic disease, when not cancerous it may be distinguished from that which comes from the kidneys by its coming in clots, and not diffused through the whole urine; there is another phenomenon which indicates hæmorrhage from the kidneys, which is the discharge of shreds or fibres with the urine that contains the blood, these are the chief diagnostic signs of hæmaturia.

When there are no symptoms referable to the kidney, and pure blood is discharged from the urethra, either in drops or in a stream and mixed with urine, it is viewed as a local hæmorrhage from the urethra. It is presumed that hæmorrhage comes from the kidneys or from the upper portion of the urethra when it is preceded, by or at the same time is accompanied by, a sensation of heat, or weight, or some degree of pain in the region of the kidneys, but more particularly if these feelings are confined to one side of the body.

TREATMENT.—The Allopathic treatment for hæmaturia is not so specifically directed against this symptom as against the general disease of the body of which this may be a prominent symptom.

Sometimes, however, the bleeding is so profuse or so long continued as to require some measures of restraint, when the bladder is filled with blood a large eyed catheter may be employed, with an exhausting syringe and by the aid of tepid water the bladder may be evacuated, when it has been thoroughly washed out, a solution of alum may be injected to exert styptic influence against further hæmorrhage, a mild solution of *Acetate of lead* is administered by the mouth, with a view of guarding against farther bleeding, having a styptic influence. *Gallic acid*, has also been recommended for the same purpose, these drugs imbibed into the circulation are supposed to act favorably in closing the open vessels from whence the hæmaturia proceeds.

HOMŒOPATHIC TREATMENT.—The Homœopathic remedies employed are *Aconite* 3x, *Belladonna* 3x, *Cantharis* 3x, *Senecin* 3x, *Hamamelis* 3x, *Mezereum* 3x, *Eucalyptus* 3x, etc.

Aconite 3x, is indicated when there is considerable fever, full and bounding pulse, and more or less pain attending the hæmaturia.

Belladonna 3x, is indicated when the signs of active congestion are present.

Cantharis 3x, when the hæmaturia is accompanied by tenesmus of the bladder.

Senecio aureus 3x, when the hæmaturia proceeds from the kidneys, and the blood discharged is of a dark color resembling the dregs of wine. In a case of hæmaturia where pure blood was discharged from the urethra, *Galium aparinum* 3x, gave prompt relief to the patient which seemed to be lasting. Eucalyptus 3x, gave prompt and permanent relief in a case of hæmaturia of long standing; aside from these remedies are Chimaphila 3x, Erigeron 3x, Trillium 3x, and Coccus cacti 3x, which may be consulted in special cases for this symptom.

CHAPTER XXXV.

ACUTE OR INFLAMMATORY RHEUMATISM.

Acute rheumatism is a very common, painful, and sometimes a very perilous disease, and in some respects the chronic form of the disease is equally severe. The two species apparently merge insensibly into each other, the chronic form being a sequelæ of the acute, in many instances, though not always, for it sometimes occurs in persons who have had no preceding attack of the acute form.

Rheumatism appears to be an inflammation of the fibrous tissue, and may manifest itself in any part of the body where this tissue exists. Other tissues at times are evidently indicated. The synovial membranes sometimes become implicated from an inflamed fibrous tissue about the joint, and in many cases the serous surface of the pericardium, and the endo-cardial membrane are liable to be affected with inflammation in the acute form of rheumatism, but in all cases it is probable that the fibrous texture is primarily affected, the pericardium being a fibro-serous membrane and fibrous tissue being interposed between the folds of the serous membrane in the cardiac valves, invites the rheumatic inflammation in this direction. It is, therefore, evident that rheumatism is essentially an inflammation of the fibrous tissue which commonly seizes the fibrous parts around the larger points of which the ligaments and tendons are made up. The same is true in reference to the parts connected with the motion of the heart. This inflammation, when confined to the fibrous tissue, is not regarded in the light of common inflammation, because it does not eventuate in the effusion of plastic lymph, or suppuration, or gangrene. When suppuration in very rare cases occurs, it is because the rheumatic inflammation extends to contiguous textures and must then and there run through the ordinary course of common inflammation.

The areolar tissue around the joint may thus inflame and suppurate. In some cases the inflammation of the synovial membranes may be so intense as to cause the formation of pus, but

when the inflammation extends to the serous tissues in and around
the heart, the product is the same as that of the textures elsewhere in the body.

Acute rheumatism then consists in the heat, redness, pain and
swelling of the tissues entering into the structure of one or more
of the larger joints, and frequently of several at the same time,
or in rapid succession, with an inclination to shift from one joint
to another, or to certain internal organs, and especially to the
membrane of the heart, and generally with acceleration of the
pulse, and fever. This tendency to change its location is usually
termed metastasis and is an interesting feature of the disease.
The inflammation and heat will appear in one joint suddenly and
quickly disappear from another previously affected. At other
times it will extend its march, invading fresh joints without leaving or diminishing the suffering in those first affected. In this
way all of the body may become affected, involving even the
smaller joints of the wrist and fingers, ankles and toes.

In truth, acute rheumatism is a blood disease. Some *toxical*
agent in the blood is carried by the circulation from the center to
the periphery of the body, and by some kind of elective affinity
this poisonous material falls upon the fibrous tissues, visiting,
and quitting them in a capricious manner apparently without any
uniform law.

The migratory character of the inflammation, shifting from
one texture to another, and from one of the larger joints to another, commences with a high fever of an inflammatory character,
full bounding pulse, flushed cheeks, headache, profuse acid perspirations which distress and weaken the patient, these perspirations bring no relief from suffering. The tongue is coated with
a dirty white fur, its tip and margin are red, a brick dust sediment is deposited in the urine, which is saturated with acid.

Rheumatic fever differs from the inflammatory in not being
liable to run into the typhoid form, the mind is for the most part
clear unless the heart becomes affected, which lateral condition is
sometimes attended with violent delirium; this latter symptom
often misleads the practitioner by directing his attention to the
head when the dangerous force of the disease is being expended
in the chest. This delirium may be caused, not by inflammation but
by a simple disturbance through sympathy with the cardiac disorder; the *toxical* materials in the circulation vary in kind and

quality, as well as in their effects upon the animal economy; the joints are exquisitely tender and painful; the fibrous tissues around the joints become acutely painful when inflamed, and pressure increases the pain and the inability to move his joints renders him perfectly helpless, or in other words creates in his mind a fear of moving, or being moved; the loss of power is not a palsy, but a loss of will and the fear of exertion. In this condition the touch of the doctor, the heavy tread of the nurse, the approach of a friend, and the playful antics of the cat, or dog, are dreaded to a degree that apparently places the patient in a perpetual fear of being hurt. There are several varieties of rheumatism spoken of as the synovial, diffuse or fibrous, occasionally there is œdema of the lower extremites, when the disease commences in or near the knee joints involving the fibrous tissues about them, but if the inflammation is confined to the synovial membrane, the knee joint may swell by reason of the distension of the membrane without it becoming œdematous, the local differences, therefore, between the two forms of the disease, consist in swelling without fluctuation and, with this phenomenon, when the rheumatism is strictly fibrous or diffuse in the fibrous variety of rheumatism, the fear runs high, the suffering is great, and the perspiration profuse. In the synovial rheumatism the fever is less intense, and after the swelling takes place there is comparatively little pain.

What is the cause of acute rheumatism? It is believed to be in the main exposure to cold combined with moisture, the perspiration becomes checked by this agent which probably exercises its injurious influences in preventing the elimination through the skin and other emunctories of the poisonous material as it forms, thus leaving it to accumulate in the blood. The predisposition consists of this poison in the blood, without which it would never occur; no exciting cause can produce the rheumatism unless the predisposing influence of poisonous material in the blood were present.

Acute rheumatism is principally a disease of youth, and seldom occurs later in life than forty years of age; we have repeatedly seen it in children three or four years of age; and the complication of heart disease is more liable to occur at this tender period; after the age of puberty the danger of cardiac complication is not so great.

TREATMENT.—In the treatment of this painful disorder, bleeding has been regarded one of the chief measures for affording relief from suffering. For internal administration in the old school practice, the use of saline purgatives, *lime juice*, and the *acid* of *lemons*, are among the chief resorts, and in case of heart complications *Digitalis*, is freely given.

HOMŒOPATHIC TREATMENT.—*Aconite* 3x, may be given at once after the invasion of the disease, or as soon as the rheumatic fever becomes manifest, *Bryonia* 3x, when the pains are lancinating, or sticking, and become worse on the least movement or relieved by rest. *Belladonna* 3x, is chiefly indicated when the patient is sleepless at night. *Guiacum* 3x, may be employed when there is little or no perspiration upon the surface and when the patient requires to be moved every few minutes, *Cactus* 3x, when the disease is principally confined to the heart, *Caulophyllum* 3x, when the disease is most apparent in the wrists and fingers, with much swelling, and when the disease shifts from the back to the nape of the neck with rigidity of the muscles, *Cimicifuga* 3x, for articular rheumatism of the lower extremities, with much swelling, *Colocynth* 3x, when the pain is mostly confined to the hip joint, *Colchicum* 3x, is indicated for moderate swelling, with a pale redness of the affected part, burning, tearing or jerking pains, unsteady and shifting, with intermingling chilliness, and flushes of heat when sitting near a hot stove, Metastasis with stitches and tearing in the chest and region of the heart, during respiration, strong and fluttering beating of the heart, profuse and sour smelling sweats, especially indicated for this remedy. *Nux vomica* 3x, for pain in the back and loins in connection with other indications of a rheumatic suffering. *Pulsatilla* 3x, for rheumatism in lymphatic patients with but *little* swelling or redness of the affected parts, *Rhus toxicodendron* 3x, has swelling and redness of the affected parts, pains, drawing and tearing, a feeling of lameness which motion relieves, and also by warm applications. *Sulphur* 3x, in chronic rheumatism, or for the secondary effect of acute rheumatism, constant on the top of the head, frequently followed by weakness and faintness. *Veratrum album* 3x, when the rheumatic resembles those from a blow or bruise, and the warmth of the bed aggravates, feels better from getting up and walking about. *Veratrum viride* 3x, when the pains are most prominent in the left side, left shoulder, head and knee, and for cardiac symptoms.

The accessory treatment for inflammatory rheumatism consists measureably in the necessary ablutions to promote cleanliness. Lukewarm or tepid water applied with a sponge to the entire surface of the body, especially after the profuse, characteristic perspirations attendant upon the disease. Affected joints may be wrapped in cotton-batting. The clothing may be changed frequently and especially as it becomes saturated with the acid exudations from the skin. To quench the thirst, *lime juice* or *quince jelly* in water, and in some cases where other beverages than water or black tea are desired, raspberry vinegar and lemonade may be useful.

Gout.

Gout is a disease which closely resembles rheumatism and yet it is distinct from it. From its liability to attack the joints, it has been termed arthritis, but not being confined uniformly to the joints, but occasionally attacks both feet and hence it has received the name of podagra.

SYMPTOMS.—The attack begins most commonly after midnight. The patient after retiring at a seasonable hour falls asleep in usual health without suspecting what is to be his fortune before morning, is awakened by a sudden pain in the first joint, or ball of the great toe, or perhaps in other parts of the foot, of the heel, instep or ankle. As an attendant with the approach of pain there is a general chilliness or cold shivering which gradually disappears as the pain gets worse, and is succeeded by heat. The pain increases in violence, and becomes intolerable, and is spoken of by the victim as the height of human suffering, amounting to a torture. It is a grinding, crushing, wrenching pain, or a burning sensation, as if a hot iron was applied to the joint. In short, the suffering attendant on gout is superlative in a degree, and in comparison with which scarcely any other grade of human torture can equal. The pain is always attended with extreme restlessness, and the affected joints are exceedingly tender. In the extreme cases the patient cannot bear the weight of the bed-clothes upon the affected limb. The patient is so sensitive that he can bear nothing like a footstep or a jar in the room. He is so restless, and so bent upon securing relief, that he changes from side to side, hoping that he may obtain it. After a while, during, or about the middle of the night, the pain remits, sometimes gradually, and sometimes so suddenly that he thinks he has been relieved by the change of position. He falls asleep in a gentle perspiration. The next morning when he awakes, he finds the part which has been so painful, red, swollen, tense and shining, surrounded by some degree of swelling and by turgid veins. The same series of symptoms recur in a less severe form for several days, and the swelling subsides, the redness ·fades, and the cuticle of the part that had been affected peels off.

Such is the picture which reveals to us an attack of *gout* in an adult with nearly all its forms.   It is said that *rheumatism* is blood disease, and that the poison eliminated from the system is charged with acetic acid, and that which is eliminated from poisoning by *gout* is or partakes of the nature of lithic acid.

It is undoubtedly hereditary in a majority of cases, but it may be acquired. Very many can trace the disease in themselves to hereditary taint. The victims are robust men who live luxuriously and indulge freely in the use of wine and malt liquors. Animal food taken in excess of what is required by persons of sedentary habits, are liable to contract the disease even if it is not hereditary, for the excess is readily converted into uric acid, or lithic acid, which combines with morbific matter and finds its way to the feet. The free use of wine, such as port, sherry, or Teneriffe is thought to favor the production of *gout* more than alcoholic stimulants or malt liquors. Gout differs from the rheumatism in several particulars; in *gout* the blood is impregnated with uric acid, in rheumatism with lactic, or acetic acid. In an attack of the former the smaller joints of the fingers are first implicated, while in the latter the larger joints are for the most part affected.

TREATMENT.—Diet forms an important feature in the common treatment of gout, by some the employment of garlic and alterative doses of the tincture of *colchicum.*

HOMŒOPATHIC TREATMENT in a febrile attack of *gout* is best met with *Aconite* 3x and afterwards when the fever is subsided, *Colchicum* 3x, is the Homœopathic remedy.

If the disease is confined to the foot, covering the part with cotton batting beneath a bandage of oil silk, to protect the joint is valuable as a local application. *Bryonia* 3x, is called into requisition when the slightest motion is attended with pain; when the pain is steady, sharp and shooting *Belladonna* 3x;

Colchicum 3x is indicated when the kidneys are evidently implicated and when palpable quantities of urea and uric acid are found in the urine; it is also a polychrest in its range of action and a source of great relief from gouty pains, manifest in several localities at the same time. This remedy as used in Allopathy practice is an irritant, cathartic, emetic, and diuretic, and when we find in connection with *gout* that the bowels are lax, the stomach irritable and the flow of urine copious, *Colchicum* must be regarded as a valuable Homœopathic remedy for *gout* or *rheumatism*.

J. H. P—, aged 34 years, was seized in the month of April with severe vomiting, urgent diarrhœa, dryness and burning of the throat, excessive heat in the abdomen, and colic, great depression of the circulation, and suppression of the urine. All of these symptoms are characteristic of toxical doses of *Colchicum* 3x. This attack was one of a series which he had experienced for many years, and each had been succeeded by some form of *gout*. *Colchicum* in the third decimal dilution gave prompt relief to his last attack, which, with the exception of local applications, was treated exclusively with this remedy. His recovery was satisfactory, and for quite a number of years he has not suffered from the malady. *Rhus tox.* 3x, *Pulsatilla* 3x, *Actea racemosa* 3x, *Ledum* 3x, and *Senecio* 3x are remedies that may be required in the treatment of acute arthritis; for the chronic form of the disease, *Aurum muriaticum* 3x, *Calcarea carbonica* 3x, *Hepar sulphur* 3x, *Phosphorus* 3x, *Phosphoric acid* 3x, and *Sulphur* 3x, may be consulted. The diet in all cases should be confined to amylaceous or starchy food.

CHAPTER XXXVI.

THE SKIN AND ITS DISEASES.

A healthy skin imparts to the touch the sensation of an agreeable temperature, moist and emollient; it is remarkable for its elasticity and smoothness, and any departure from this standard is indicative of disease. A harsh, dry, burning heat of the skin either indicates fever or the presence of inflammatory stages of internal disease. A bluish tint of the skin indicates heart disease. A yellowish tint biliary derangement. An irritable condition of the nervous system is often the source of a circumscribed blush of the cheeks while excessive moisture or sweating upon the surface may indicate the presence of organic lesions or violent functional derangements. The skin is liable to many diseases.

Erysipelas.

It is scarcely possible to give an accurate description of all the phases which this disease assumes. It has been common to include under this term every kind of inflammation of the skin characterized by shining redness upon the surface, but in our consideration of the subject a distinction is proper to be made between erysipelatous inflammation and the actual characteristics of the disease. Acute erysipelas for the most part is preceded by severe pain in the head, chills, and a decided febrile reaction tending to the tegumentary tissues of the face and the head, which become inflamed, red, and swollen, by reason of subcutaneous inflammation and infiltration into the cellular tissue; sometimes the swelling increases to an extent that implicates the entire face, attended with much tumefaction of the features. In some cases the swelling is so great as to close the eyes, while the nose and the lips become so swollen and sore as to conceal the natural expression of the face; every natural feature for a time becomes obliterated and the swollen lips, nose, cheeks, and head temporarily assume a monstrous appearance.

A milder form of erysipelas is often preceded by a general

lassitude and depression of spirits and protracted rigors, followed by an accelerated pulse, thirst, headache, wandering pains in the back and limbs, and general restlessness, or it may make its appearance without any promonitory symptoms except fever, or after wounds and injuries, or it may occur after an acute attack of pneumonia; when the eruption makes its appearance it is in blotches which are characterized by burning or a pungent sensation.

The most malignant form of erysipelas is that which evinces from the start a strong disposition to terminate in a gangrenous form; the inflammation is confined mostly to the subcutaneous cellular tissue, the swelling is indurated, and the skin is of a reddish or a purple color; large vesicles filled with an acrid pus form on the surface, presenting a sluggish tendency and gangrenous.

The accompanying fever, in this form of erysipelas, is of a typhoid character. The muscular and nervous tissue are below the normal standard; delirium and coma are generally present, suppuration and gangrene generally result.

Erysipelas neonatorium is confined mostly to infants; and the upper part of the body, although the lower part of the body in the first instance; the character of the attack depends much upon the constitution and predisposition of the patient, although commonly the inflammation is of a high grade, the swollen part is very painful and tender, disposed to suppurate and slough; the duration of the attack varies from two to four weeks.

Erysipelas sometimes prevails as an epidemic, and whole neighborhoods become affected by it. The exciting causes of erysipelas are exposure to extremes of temperature, and want of proper kinds of food, nearly all cases are attended with biliousness, and gastric derangement, with constipation.

In many cases the disease is complicated with other disorders; it varies in intensity; the sufferer may lie quietly in bed, apparently conscious and rational until the swelling diminishes and the ability to open the eyes returns, frequently delirium, and when followed by coma, the patient is in a dangerous condition, which sometimes proves fatal. When death takes place, it has been found that serous fluid exists in the arachnoid cavity, or in the cerebral ventricles; when erysipelas recedes from the surface, inflammation of some internal part, or of the brain is liable to follow; cases of this kind are rare, but the extension of the disease the supervention of delirium and coma, while the inflammation continues, is a common occurrence, and in this way there may be a fatal termination by effusion within the head, and coma.

It is said that erysipelas sometimes affects the throat and suddenly proves fatal, and this is accounted for by reason of the submucous tissue of the glottis and epiglottis being filled with serum or pus which closes the chink of the larynx, the swelling being analogous to what takes place externally when the enormous swelling of the eyelids, lips, and face is owing to the infiltrations of serous fluid into the subcutaneous areolar tissue, or membrane.

The disease may prove fatal also by gradual loss of strength and exhaustion, without any stupor, or severe suffering, or delirium, or any fatal signs except feebleness of the pulse which becomes weaker and weaker, the surface becomes cold and ultimately the heart ceases its action. It is believed by many that erysipelas is contagious and may spread from person to person, especially in certain places when there are predisposing causes to the disease.

TREATMENT.—In Allopathic practice *Bark*, and *Wine*, are used to keep up the strength of the patient in many instances, while in others depletion, and especially when surgically treated.

HOMŒOPATHIC TREATMENT.—*Aconite* 3x, is recognized in the febrile stage when the patient complains of much heat upon the surface with a full and bounding pulse; *Bryonia* 3x, is indicated when there is nausea and apparent struggling to eliminate the disease; *Belladonna* 3x, when there is severe pain in the head, and a tendency to the eyes, and face, and also when there is neuralgic pains shooting from one locality to another. *Calcarea carbonica* 3x, in persons of a scrofulous diathesis, *Cantharis* 3x, when there is an erysipelatous eruption which consists of blebs or blisters upon the cutaneous surface; *Carbo animalis* 3x, when the tumefaction seems to be indurated, *Hepar sulphur* 3x, when there is a determination of the inflammation to particular localities, with throbbing as if suppuration were taking place. Other remedies as *Rhus tox.* 3x, *Rhus venenata* 3x, *Veratrum viride* 3x, etc.

For gangrenous erysipelas *Arsenicum* 3x, *Hyoscyamus* 3x, *Lachesis* 6x, *Sepia* 6x, *Carbolic acid* 3x, *Sulphuric* 3x, etc.

For chronic erysipelas *Nitric acid* 3x, *Graphites* 6x, *Calcarea carbonica* 6x, *Sulphur* 6x, *Arctium lappa* 3x, and others.

The accessory treatment consists of covering the surface with rye flour to protect the surface from irritation.

Impetigo.

This is a common disease of infants; it is often severe and contagious; it has been described as an inflammatory pustular eczema. The characteristic symptoms are an eruption of small semicircular flattened pustules which appear in clusters, the pustules running together and forming a thick and moist incrustation. It usually attacks the ear, the nose, scalp, and face; the eruption with its yellow, tenacious secretion sometimes covers the face as with a mask and extends to the scalp, discharging a tenacious matter, matting the hair so that it forms a sour smelling mass; beneath this incrustation the surface is red, and tender. This form of the disease has been termed porrigo or milk crust.

TREATMENT.—It is believed that this disease is dependent upon a poor diet. Scrofulous diathesis and infectious irritations of the skin, various external applications such as cleansing and healing washes, have been recommended by Allopathic practitioners; the objection to this treatment is its tendency to cause a retrocession of the eruption and thus pave the way for some internal disturbance of the brain.

HOMŒOPATHIC TREATMENT is preferable and attended with less danger. *Viola tricolor* 3x, may be successfully employed in the treatment of this disease, and likewise *Arsenicum* 3x, *Tartar emetic* 3x, *Antimonium crudum* 3x, and *Kali bichromicum* 3x. When the scabs get thick and hard they should be moistened by a little fresh butter, or other oily substance and then they should be removed by emulcient poultices made of bran or linseed-meal. Carbolated vaseline may be lightly applied.

Acne.

This is a chronic inflammation of the sebaceous glands and hair follicles caused by a retention of sebaceous matter, which becomes manifest in the form of an eruption of hard nodules and

33

pustules of various degrees of redness; it usually occurs at the age of puberty and frequently is a source of annoyance for one or two years.

The acne punctata is simply a pointed eruption containing sebaceous matter which may be squeezed out in a cylindrical form, resembling a small maggot.

The remedies in general for this eruption are Arsenicum 3x, Causticum 3x, Natrum muriaticum 3x, Nitric acid 3x, Sepia 3x, Sulphur 3x, etc. For the acne rosacea, which occurs in older persons, especially in women in whom the catamenial function is imperfect, exhibits a bright redness, and disfiguration of the face, which may be much aggravated by improper food and stimulants.

TREATMENT.—This form of the disease disfigures the countenances of both men and women, and is what is termed rosy-drop, or grog-blossom. Various resorts have been tolerated, such as alkaline, and mercurial solutions have been recommended for bathing the affected part, but this practice is now generally discarded, while depurating measures, and an unstimulating diet, together with total abstinence from alcoholic stimulants, is enjoined.

HOMŒOPATHIC TREATMENT.—The Homœopathic remedies for internal administration are Carbo animalis 3x, Kreosotum 3x, Veratrum album 3x, Rhus tox. 3x, etc.

The acne rosacea sometimes results from interrupted circulation and congestion not necessarily connected with alcoholic stimulants, the cause of the whole difficulty being congestion of the sebaceous follicles resulting from various internal and external agencies.·

Erythema.

By the term erythema is understood inflammatory redness of the skin which manifests itself in the form of a blush without swelling or abrasions of the surface. There are several varieties of this affection, named according to their characteristics. When there is a blush on the surface of an œdematous swelling it is called erythema læve. A fleeting, patchy redness is called erythema fugax. A redness with a well-defined circumference is designated erythema marginatum. When it consists of small red spots varying in size from a pin's point or head, it is termed

erythema papulatum. This particular form of the difficulty
becomes pale from pressure and usually passes away in a few
days with a slight desquamation. It is sometimes associated with
the rheumatic diathesis and usually occurs in young persons.
There is erythema tuberculatum and erythema nodosum, which
are varieties of the same disease. The former are more aggravated forms than that which precedes, and the latter a still
greater augmentation of similar symptoms. Chronic erythema
is sometimes an accompaniment of some inveterate form of dyspepsia or gastric derangement and frequently is a source of much
discomfort. There is seldom any burning, or itching, or heat, as
in erysipelas, for which it is sometimes mistaken.

TREATMENT.—The Allopathic treatment is usually restricted
to saline cathartics and in the more aggravated form to blood-
letting.

HOMŒPATHIC TREATMENT requires Belladonna 3x for the
simple redness, and the e. papulatum when attended with fever,
and the flushing of the face from excitement, Aconite 3x. For
the other forms consult Apis melif. 3x, Rhus tox. 3x, Kali bich.
3x, Nux vomica 3x, Bryonia 3x, Arsenicum 3x, Ranunculus bul.
3x. It is recommended that the patient exercise in the open air
after and between meals, and that excitement or over-exertion
should be avoided. The free use of cold water internally, and
externally for ablutions, internally for a diluent for the simplest
kind of food.

Urticaria or Nettle Rash.

This annoying disease has sometimes been classed among the
exanthemata, but not being contagious, and liable to frequent
repetition in the same person, there seems to be nothing justifi-
able in classing it among the exanthemata. In general the
eruption consists of what from analogy are called wheals, that is,
of little solid eminences of irregular outline, generally rounded
or oblong, and either white, or red, or both red and white. The
eruption is usually attended with some heat, and very little pain.
There is an indescribable itching and stinging, with tingling in
the affected parts, and great irritation. In fact, the appearance
of the skin, and the effect upon the surface, is almost the same
as that produced by nettles rubbed upon the skin. On this ac-

count it has been termed nettle rash, or urticaria, which is a significant term relating to the effect of nettles.

TREATMENT.—It has been regarded a trivial disease, but one of great annoyance, and in Allopathic practice efforts have been made to expel the poison from the system by emetics and cathartics.

HOMŒOPATHIC TREATMENT has usually acted promptly in relieving the patient from the itching, stinging, and burning that constitute the main features of the disease. These remedies are Apis mellifica 3x, Arsenicum 3x, Sulphur 3x, Urtica urens 3x, and other remedies prescribed in accordance with the symptoms. Accessory measures, such as warm baths, softened with a little bicarbonate of soda, are particularly recommended.

Prurigo,

Is a cutaneous affection having some analogy to urticaria in the sensations accompanying it, and it often proves to be a terrible melancholy affection. There is little or no change in the appearance of the skin when in health, and yet the critical inspection will detect a papular eruption of the same color as the skin itself. The itching is greatly aggravated by heat and exposure to the air, and consequently is very distressing when the patient is undressed for retirement at night. The perpetual inclination to scratch, if indulged in, tears away the summits of the papulæ, permitting the exit of a watery fluid mixed with blood, and this concretes into small black scabs or scales. This kind of prurigo is quite uniform in its effects upon different persons.

In that form of the disease termed prurigo farmicans the itching is combined with other painful sensations which are described differently by different subjects. The feeling is like the creeping of ants or the stinging of insects, or as if hot needles were thrust into the skin. The prurigo senilis occurs in old persons and is a very persistent annoyance to them, as it sometimes effectually destroys all comfort during the remainder of life.

TREATMENT.—In the first place great care should be taken to thoroughly cleanse the surface of the body, the diet and regimen should be rigidly plain, no rich sauces, gravies, hot condiments,

pickles, radishes, horse radish or any other acrid or medicinal
condiments should be allowed.

There are but few local applications that have ever been
known to produce any beneficial effect in this disease. It has
been the custom to besmear the body with various kinds of ointments and lotions, carbolated and non-carbolated, metallic and
vegetable, savory and unsavory, but no form of skillful application of these agents have been of service, yet due credit may be
given to a distinguished professor and author of therapeutics, in
London, England, for having discovered the therapeutic action of
Aconitum napellus when used as a lotion, or when used in the
form of the officinal Aconitine ointment, which he found to his
great satisfaction, capable of producing speedy and perfect relief.
Another gentleman has discovered that a weak solution of the
Chloride of Soda has been of service. The internal remedies are
Arsenicum 3x, Hepar sulphur 3x, Dulcamara 3x, Mercurius 3x,
Nitric acid 3x, Opium 3x, Pulsatilla 3x, Petroleum 3x, Sulphur
3x, and other remedies may be studied with reference to the cure
of this formidable disease.

Scabies.

Scabies or the itch. Like prurigo this disease is often worri-
some to the patient in consequence of perpetual itching. It is an
eruptive difficulty and believed to be contagious, or more properly speaking infectious. It is not producible from the exhalations from the body, or susceptible of being conveyed by the atmosphere. It can only be propagated to such persons as touch
the diseased patient, or some substance which has been in contact
with his diseased skin. Certain parts of the skin are more liable to
the disease than others, it is most frequently manifested about the
wrist, between the toes, and the flexion of the joints, or it may
spread all over the body, involving every part of the trunk and
extremities, but is seldom if ever seen upon the face. The eruption
is at first papular, but soon takes the vesicular form, presenting a
number of pointed watery heads. When the inflammation is
aggravated by filthy and intemperate habits, or by scratching, the
vesicles are liable to become pustules, and this has been the reason why some authors have been pleased to term scabies puru-
lenta or pocky-itch.

In this stage large pustules may be seen filled with yellow viscid matter standing on an inflamed base. Unless acquainted with these variations or changes there is a liability to mistake the diagnosis; other pustular diseases may assimulate this form of scabies to which the offensive name of itch may be given unjustly. The disease proper is usually considered, though not in all cases justly so, a disgrace to those who have it, for it is well known that the disease is fostered and propagated in the most disgraceful places, where poverty, vulgarity, and filth predominate, nevertheless the most delicate and cleanly may contract the disease by innocent contact with some article of clothing which has been infected, and it may go on indefinitely through life unless proper curative means are employed. It never gets well of itself.

The most singular fact in relation to this disease, is its connection with a peculiar insect, denominated the *acaris-scabia*. The existence of this insect has been subjected to frequent affirmations and denials, but the vexed question has been scientifically settled by unmistakable demonstration of the presence of the e living itch-insects, not having been found, however, in every vesicle. Some have searched in vain for the acaris, because they have not known exactly where to look for it, and because the insect is so small it may have escaped detection. It is scarcely visible to the naked eye, but under a microscope it has seemed to be a most formidable monster having six or eight legs. It is believed that this insect is the veritable cause of scabies.

It is maintained that the vesicular fluid alone, if inoculated, will produce disease, whereas the transportation of the acaris has always excited the eruption. This would indicate that the disease is only curable by such means as will cut off and destroy the generation of these itch mites.

Remedial measures which will change the condition of the nutritive system, and thus prevent the unhealthy process which develops the acaris, must be essential to this disorder.

TREATMENT.—From time immemorial Sulphur has been regarded as a specific for the itch, and the presumption has been that it kills the acaris. It has been applied externally in the form of an ointment composed of Sulphur and lard, by no means agreeable in smell and cleanliness. The objection to the profuse application externally of the Sulphur ointment, is its liability to cause a retrocession of the eruption, to the detriment of the constitutional health, and thus furnishing the foundation for various forms of chronic diseases.

HOMŒOPATHIC TREATMENT for scabies consists, first, in ablutions for the promotion of cleanliness, daily washing with warm water and castile soap, and the daily internal administration of anti-psoric remedies. Sulphur 3x, Hepar sulphur 3x, Calcarea carbonica 3x, Lycopodium 3x, Mercurius solubilis 3x, Rumex crispus 3x, and other anti-psoric remedies furnish a group from which to select the curative agent for the various forms of the disease. The rightly selected remedy, administered at proper intervals is likely to so change the condition of the system, and establish a healthy recuperative action which will cut off the sources of the eruption, and the effect seen upon the surface must therefore cease.

Eczema, or Herpes.

Herpes are the various forms of tetter. It is an eruptive disease, characterized by burning and smarting, and sometimes corroding on the surface. It is sometimes dry, and at others humid, and then again the eruption is furfuraceous, or bran-like in appearance. Itching is a characteristic sensation, sometimes a prickling, and the eruption is red, at other times nearly white.

TREATMENT.—The prevailing treatment for herpes has been external applications, an ointment being used composed of the red oxide of Mercury and lard. Some danger, however, attends the free use of this ointment.

HOMŒOPATHIC TREATMENT is preferable in all cases. When the eruption is attended by burning and itching, Arsenicum 3x trituration may be given twice a day and also when the eruption is dry, Calcarea carbonica 3x, Rhus tox. 3x, Sepia 3x. Where eruption is humid, Graphites 6x, Hepar sulphur 3x, and Lycopodium 3x. When the chief symptom is itching, Agaricus 3x, Alumina 3x, Bovista 3x, Clematis 3x, Graphites 6x, Mercurius 3x, and Petroleum 3x. For furfuraceous tetter, Calcarea carb. 6x, Sepia 6x, and Sulphur 3x. When the tetter exhibits a red appearance, Clematis 3x. When the eruption is scabby, Dulcamara 3x, Graphites 6x, and Hepar sulphur 6x. When scaly or squamous, give Phosphorus 3x. When the eruption presents the appearance of scurvy, it indicates the use of Alumina 3x, Calcarea carb. 3x, Dulcamara 3x, and Rhus tox. 3x. Cleanliness and frequent ablutions of warm water avail but little in the worst forms of this disease. Eczema differs in appearance from herpes by being painful and uniformly humid. The remedies for internal administration are Arum triphyllum 3x, Arsenicum 3x, Aurum muriaticum 3x, Dulcamara 3x, and Natrum muriaticum 3x. The application of fine wheat flour is frequently a source of relief to the patient.

Pemphigus.

This is a vesicular eruption, with or without fever. It consists of vesicles varying in size from a split pea to a chestnut.

These blebs are filled with serous fluid resembling in some degree that of a fly-blister or a scald.

The disease exists in both the chronic and acute form. Acute pemphigus is attended with fever and requires Belladonna 3x, Cantharis 3x, Dulcamara 3x or Lachesis 6x, Rhus tox. 3x, and Sulphur 3x; a selection made from this group in accordance with the symptoms will affect a speedy cure.

The chronic form of pemphigus may continue for months and even years one set of vesicles while another is leaving continously. The remedies found to be the most useful are Arsenicum Graphites 3x, Hepar sulphur 3x, Staphisagria 3x, and Sulphur 3x. It is always preferable for the patient to subsist on a generous but non-medicinal diet.

Lepra.

Leprosy; in this disease there is a thick, rough, swollen, disorganized skin with rose colored tuberosities or white spots with scaling of the epidermis.

The skin is covered with crusts or scabs discharging from intermediate places a fetid or corrosive ichor, this is called the Lepra Orientalis.

The whole surface of the body is covered with crusts or scabs, and corrosive ulcers, excessively painful and destructive to the entire cutaneous surface.

TREATMENT.—This disease is treated by Allopaths with different unguents externally applied, such as Sulphur ointment and those made with the red oxide of Mercury and Unguentum.

HOMŒOPATHIC TREATMENT.—Ablutions of warm water softened with bicarbonate of soda for the purpose of cleansing the surface; remedies internally administered are Alumina 3x, Arsenicum 3x, Carbo animalis 3x, Carbo vegetabilis 3x, Causticum 3x, Graphites 3x, Petroleum 3x, Sulphur 3x, and other dermic remedies.

Impetigo.

Impetigo is a pustular eruption which manifests itself in clusters, and as they ripen coalesce, dry up and form crusts; there are various forms of impetigo which come under the same general description and are subject to the same general treatment.

TREATMENT.—For therapeutic hints, Arsenicum 3x, Belladonna 3x, Causticum 3x, China 3x, Dulcamara 3x, Graphites 6x, Hepar sul. 3x, Lachesis 6x, Rhus tox. 3x, and Tartar emetic 3x, may be consulted.

Psoriasis.

Psoriasis is like a dry scald, or scaly tetter, characterized by a rough, scaly condition of the epidermis, which is usually cracked, and of a reddish color.

TREATMENT.—The remedies to be consulted are Arsenicum 3x, Calcarea 3x, Clematis 3x, Graphites 6x, Lycopodium, 30x, Mercurius 3x. We have found that infantile psoriasis can be cured in most cases with Calcarea 3x, Mercurius 3x, and psoriasis labialis with Calcarea 3x, Mercurius, 3x, Natrum muriaticum 3x, and Silicea 6x.

Psoriasis Palmaris.

This disease will generally yield to Graphites 6x, Petroleum 3x, Sepia 3x and Sulphur 3x.

Psoriasis Scrotalis.

This disease will generally yield to Causticum 3x, Petroleum 3x, and Rhus tox. 3x.

In all diseases involving the dermic tissue, all oily substances such as butter, gravies, etc., should be carefully excluded from the diet.

Furunculi, or Boils.

It is a very common, as well as a very teasing pustular disease of the skin. At first there is a slight degree and extent of hardness to be felt, a tender spot just beneath the surface, which soon begins to look red, and a small swelling arises, which gradually increases in size from that of a pea to a walnut.

It ripens by a slow process of suppuration, and assumes a conical shape, white or yellow at the tip just before the cuticle gives way, after which the pain subsides and the trouble is soon over. The only sequelæ which remains is a visible mass of dead areolar tissue, which is usually called the core. This has to be expelled, after which the cap-like cavity soon fills up, and the trouble is really over. These little tumors frequent the buttocks, armpits, the thighs and the nape of the neck. They may occur anywhere when there is a constitutional tendency. They may come in crops or series from any kind of irritation; sometimes a piece of soap plaster applied to the skin is followed by a persistent series of boils.

TREATMENT.—Poultices of flax-seed, slippery-elm, brewer's yeast, and many other emollient substances are applied externally while daily doses of Citrate of Magnesia are taken internally.

This treatment is now superceded by the internal administration of Aconite 3x, Arnica 3x, Belladonna 3x, in the first stage; and by Hepar 3x, and Nitric acid 3x, in the suppurative stage; and Lycopodium 6x, Phosphorus 3x, and Sulphur 3x, to hasten the cure and prevent their return.

Anthrax or Carbuncle.

This is a malignant boil which presents a livid, or blackish, deep-seated and painful spot or tumor, differing from a common boil in its not having any central core, and from its tendency to terminate in gangrene instead of suppuration.

TREATMENT.—The internal remedies to be resorted to immediately are Arsenicum 3x, Muriatic acid 3x, Secale 3x, Kreosote 3x, and Carbolic acid 3x. For infectious carbuncle, China 3x. For phthiriasis, Arsenicum 3x, China 3x, and Staphisagria 3x.

Purpura Hæmorrhagica.

The symptoms are dark blue or purple spots in the skin of various sizes, resembling petechia, accompanied with frequently returning hæmorrhages from the nose, gums, palate, and other organs of the body; the disease is attended with great prostration but no fever. The spots which appear through the transparency of the skin, are the oozing of blood from some of the small subcutaneous vessels which are being diffused and give the appearance of purple spots on the skin.

TREATMENT.—Against this pathological condition Arsenicum 3x, China 3x, Sulphuric acid 3x, Kresote 3x, and Rhus tox. 3x, may be consulted.

Scorbutus, Scurvy.

The symptoms of this disease are spongy, swollen, itching, and bleeding gums, with putrid breath, looseness of the teeth, pale, bloated countenance, livid spots on the skin, swelling of the extremities, weak respiration, and great debility. In the course of the disease there are frequent hæmorrhages from the nose and mouth, the gums, and other organs, with increasing debility, fainting fits, ulcers on the feet, and lower extremities, which sometimes become gangrenous.

TREATMENT.—We have found Carbo vegetabilis 3x, Mercurius 3x, Muriatic acid 3x and Staphisagria 3x, the most efficient remedies in the treatment of this disease.

The diet must be of an anti-scorbutic tendency. Raw potatoes have long been regarded as a good preventive of scurvy, as well as a good therapeutic agent. It is truly said that this esculent freely used on shipboard will invariably protect the crew against this disorder. Other succulent vegetables and fruits are also held in high regard by those who have given special attention to the subject. It has been observed that the most common occurrence of scurvy is in the camp, or prison, or on board of ships where the diet has been such as to exclude the various esculents, and especially potatoes.

CHAPTER XXXVII.

EXANTHEMATOUS DISEASES.

This class of fevers are usually contagious and sometimes epidemic. They are attended by an eruption, and are therefore called eruptive fevers. They begin with the usual febrile symptoms, and at a definite period an inflammatory eruption begins to make its appearance, sometimes covering the entire surface of the body. This applies with more or less exactness to the several species of the eruptive fevers, to which your attention is now called. We will begin with scarlatina.

DIAGNOSIS.—The diagnosis of this disease is as follows: Fever, with greatly accelerated pulse, attended with soreness of the throat, and painful deglutition, scarlet redness of the skin, particularly in large, smooth, and glassy spots, or a miliary eruption in scarlet patches of an indefinite size.

The eruption generally appears from three to four days after the fever commences, and usually continues four, five, or six days, when it disappears with desquamation of the epidermis. Such are the usual pathognomonic symptoms, yet the disease has many anomalies, and is the most deceitful of all the eruptive diseases. It is believed to be of an erysipelatous character, and sometimes very malignant. It is subject to metastases to the brain, ears, eyes, etc., and is liable to be followed by dropsical effusion.

Three varieties of this disease are generally recognized, viz.: Scarlatina simplex, scarlatina anginosa, and scarlatina maligna.

Scarlatina Simplex.

The scarlatina simplex, or simple scarlatina, is the mildest form of the disease, and may run its course in seven or eight days and terminate in health. It usually commences with a chill, nausea, and vomiting, which is followed by a febrile reaction, accelerated pulse, sore throat, and bright scarlet eruption.

The fever in this variety is simply inflammatory, attended with considerable vascular excitement.

Scarlatina Anginosa.

This disease begins also with a chill, retching, and nausea, which is followed by a febrile reaction having a typhoid tendency. The eruption is more tardy in making its appearance, and is of a paler hue. The parotid and sublingual glands become inflamed and swollen. The tonsils and vellum-palati become intensely inflamed, and suppurate, and a fetid odor exhales from the mouth; at the same time there may be a sanious discharge from the nose, of an acrid character. The patient most frequently lies in a stupor, or in a comatose sleep.

Scarlatina Maligna.

Scarlatina maligna comes on with chilliness, violent vomiting, great prostration, sunken countenance, which appears pinched and death-like; the eruption upon the surface is seen in patches, very dark in color, and an offensive odor exhales from the mouth and nose; the fever in this variety is distinctly typhus and the prognosis is always unfavorable.

TREATMENT.—The treatment of scarlatina simplex. Is mainly with Aconite 3x, Belladonna 3x, and Pulsatilla 3x.

Aconite 3x, during the stage of invasion, followed by Belladonna 3x, to relieve the sore throat and headache, and Bryonia 3x, to eliminate the eruption, and Pulsatilla 3x to promote the healthy desquamation.

Treatment for scarlatina anginosa must be in accordance with the symptoms. Aconite, when there is great arterial excitement with full and quick pulse. Belladonna 3x, after Aconite when the throat is inflamed and there is severe pain in the head and nausea. Mercurius 3x, after Belladonna 3x, when the parotid gland is swollen and there is a fetid odor from the mouth. Arsenicum 3x, when there is great prostration, thirst and inclination to vomit. Hepar sulphur 3x, when the parotid and sublingual glands are much swollen, throbbing and painful, as if suppuration was about taking place. Baryta carb., when the tonsils are badly swollen. If malignant, give Arsenicum 3x, or perhaps Kreasote 3x, or Lachesis 6x; if the patient is comatose give Opium 3x, and Phosphorus 3x, or perhaps Belladonna 3x, and Lachesis 6x. If the eyes seem red and inflamed and the face flushed, give Belladonna 3x. The patient should be kept in a well ventilated room, somewhat darkened and of a temperature about seventy degrees.

Scarlatina maligna is the most aggravated form of this disease and will require Ammonium carb. 3x, Arsenicum 3x, Hyoscyamus 3x, and Lachesis 6x. When there is great prostration and low, muttering delirium, Arsenicum 3x, Belladonna 3x, and Phosphorus 3x; a pinched expression of the countenance, Muriatic acid 3x. When there is coma and pulmonary spasms, Belladonna 3x, Ipecac 3x, Opium 3x; for sanious or acrid discharge from the nose, producing excoriation at the base of the nose and the corners of the mouth, Arum triphyllum 3x.

If when the eruption is coming to the surface there should be a retrocession, Bryonia 3x and Sulphur 3x. For sleeplessness, Aconite 3x, Coffea 3x and Phosphorus 3x. For difficulty in passing urine or strangury, Cantharis 3x, Conium 3x, Nux vomica 3x and Rhus tox. 3x. When the symptom of vomiting is prominent and persistent with great thirst, Nux vomica 3x and Veratrum alb. 3x. Scarlatina is reckoned among the many blood diseases and the symptoms are indicative of the struggle which nature is making to rid the system of the materes morbi which characterize zymotic diseases.

The prognosis is usually favorable in the simple variety, which rarely proves fatal. In the anginose form, which is believed to result from some hereditary taint if under a vigorous anti-psoric treatment, a favorable prognosis may be made in the majority of the cases, while some suffering from a malignant sequel may terminate fatally.

Scarlatina maligna strikes a prostrating blow at all the vital forces and the patient sinks under the influence of a low typhus which forbodes the greatest danger and renders recovery doubtful. Accessory measures in the treatment of all forms of the disease consist in the most careful nursing and ventilation, cleanliness and washing of the mouth and throat, and the preservation of the proper temperature for the patient; the utility of the clinical thermometer in testing the status of the animal heat is of the greatest importance.

Morbilli. Rubeola. Measles.

The first invasion of this disease is in the form of severe catarrh and more or less inclination to cough, considerable fever which is believed to be infectious; after a while a crimson rash makes its appearance on the surface and during its elimination there is usually an inflammation of the mucous membrane of the organs of respiration.

In times past the disease was confounded with scarlatina, but there is a well marked difference which we shall eventually show. When the measles receive proper treatment, the disease is unattended with danger, but with improper treatment many cases prove fatal.

Children are usually the subjects of its attack, but it frequently occurs in adults with greater severity. It is a contagious disease and often prevails epidemically. As a rule persons once attacked with the measles are not liable to a second attack. The disease is so highly contagious that no susceptible person in the same room or same house with an infected person is likely to escape taking the disease. In large establishments or schools when a case of the kind occurs it is difficult to effect an isolation that will prevent the spread of the infection in such places. In families who have never had the disease, when one becomes affected the whole household incurs the risk of taking the infection.

It is believed that the germs of the disease can be carried in the clothing, packed in boxes, or from the bed clothing used with persons suffering with the disease.

The duration of the disease is divided into stages. The period of incubation is from ten to fourteen days. The precursory fever may last a longer, or a shorter period. The eruptive stage lasts about three days, and then follows the period of desquamation, or decline of the disease. The early stage of the disease is indicated by symptoms not much different from those of a common cold, such as sneezing, red, swollen and watery eyes, discharge from the nose, a hoarse, harsh cough, languor, fever, and sometimes vomiting and diarrhœa.

SYMPTOMS.—The symptoms usually increase in severity, until the fourth day of the eruption, which first appears on the face, and then on the neck and breast, and soon after on the whole body. The eruption consists of slightly raised red spots, which multiply and coalesce into blotches, varying in form, particularly on the face, which often appears to be considerably swollen. It is always favorable when the eruption is abundant, and less so, when the eruption is scanty, and more difficult of elimination. The eruption is generally two or three days coming out, and remains out two or three days, and then fades gradually away, sometimes attended with diarrhœa, which should not be interfered with as it usually proves beneficial.

Through improper treatment in the early stages of the disease, catarrhal inflammation of a serious character, may be entailed affecting the bronchial tubes, and sometimes the substance of the lungs, even after the period of desquamation. The cough attendant upon bronchial irritation, remains as an unpleasant sequel. Sometimes pneumonia, bronchitis and laryngeal inflammation of a dangerous character occur as a sequel of a certain variety of measles, characterized by the eruption being of a dark purple color.

The chief difference between measles and scarlet fever, consists in the presence of prominent catarrhal symptoms, and of a watery discharge from the eyes and nose in the former, and in the absence of these symptoms in the early stage of the latter. The eruption of measles is of a pinkish red color, while that of scarlatina is of a light scarlet color.

In measles the eruption is rough to the sense of touch, while in scarlet fever the eruption presents no inequalities, and is so minute as to impart a uniform red color to the skin. There is also a perceptible difference in the appearance of the eye, which in measles is usually watery, while in scarlet fever the eye has a peculiar brilliant stare, and appears to glisten with a peculiar lustre.

The desquamation of measles consists in the throwing off of a fine bran like substance, while that of scarlet fever is thrown off in large patches, especially from the hands and feet.

The sequelæ of measles are diseases of the lungs, eyes, and skin; while dropsy and glandular swellings are the most frequent sequel of scarlet fever.

TREATMENT.—The common practice in measles has been a resort to stimulating hot drinks to eliminate the eruption; while cooling drinks have been given to allay the febrile symptoms.

We have found by experience that this practice is objectionable, because of the susceptibility of the patient to the slightest variation of temperature and cold, which enhances the catarrhal symptoms and renders them more formidable.

HOMŒOPATHIC TREATMENT of the primary fever requires *Aconite* 3x in connection with a warm sponge bath carefully administered. In all cases of well marked febrile symptoms at the outset, *Aconite* 3x is necessary to control inflammatory action during the progress of the disease, a dose every two or three hours. This remedy has proved so valuable that some practitioners regard it essential as a curative agent in all the stages and even the sequelæ of the disease.

Bryonia 3x may follow Aconite 3x in a febrile stage, to counteract imperfect elimination of the eruption in case of suppression, or retrocession of the same. Belladonna 3x is indicated for sore throat and difficult deglutition, dry spasmodic cough, headache, inflammation of the eyes, drowsiness, inquietude and tendency to delirium.

Veratrum viride 3x is indicated in the febrile stage, when engorgement of the lungs or convulsions are feared.

Pulsatilla 3x is indicated when the cough is more towards evening or during the night, with rattling of the mucus in the air passage and expectoration of a yellowish or whitish color, and a similar discharge from the nose.

This remedy is also indicated for nose bleed, catarrhal derangement of the stomach and diarrhœa, and in case of suppressed eruption followed by troublesome sequelæ of various kinds of a persistent character.

Pulsatilla 3x has been given with extraordinary and beneficial results in obviating the secondary disorders.

Ipecacuanha 3x and *Tartar emetic* 3x are indicated when there is much retching and vomiting and cough, when the eruption is *pale, imperfect* or irregular, attended by a dry, hollow cough, pain in the chest with nervous or typhoid symptoms.

Phosphorus 3x, is indicated especially, when the sequel manifests a pneumonia, during the decline of the disease; *Sulphur* 3x, may be given as a preventive of secondary symptoms. The treatment of the sequelæ must be in accordance with the symptoms. For the dry, hollow and spasmodic cough that is frequently entailed after an attack of measles, we have found Drosera 3x, an invaluable remedy; for gastric derangement, and particularly that of the digestive function, Pulsatilla 3x, is indicated.

Macrotin 3x, is also a suitable remedy for feeble digestion, and also for diarrhœa.   For inflammation of the eyelids after an attack of measles, and for redness from congestion of the small vessels of the sclerotic coat, *Sulphur* 3x, may be given first and afterward *Belladonna* 3x. For deafness during the catarrhal stage Aconite 3x, may be given first, afterwards Dulcamara 3x, or Gelsemium 3x.   `

If the deafness becomes chronic, Calcarea carbonica 3x, and Baryta carb. 3x, especially, if there is enlargement of the tonsils, accessory measures in the form of water bathing, and the introduction of a small quantity of Glycerine into the ear.

Sulphur 3x, Belladonna 3x, Mercurius 3x, and Chelidonium 3x, may also be called into requisition.   To quench the thirst in all stages of the disease, including the sequelæ, moderately cold water is the most suitable beverage; the diet must be regulated according to the indication of the appetite.

Varicella or Chicken Pox.

During infancy and childhood a trifling, infectious fever, with vesicular eruption, frequently occurs. It sometimes, though rarely, affects those of advanced age. It is similar in appearance to small pox, for which at first it may be mistaken, but it differs from this disease in the fever which attends it being later, and in the vesicles being pointed in the centre, and becoming filled with a watery fluid, about the second or third day. This fluid is never converted into yellow matter, as in small pox. The disease also differs in the rapidity of its course, as it may pass through all its phases in five or six days. The vesicles dry up, forming crusts, from the third or fourth day, and pass of without any permanent cicatrices or scars. The characteristic odor of small pox is never present. In addition to the term chicken pox, it has been termed swine pox and water pox.   •

TREATMENT.—If there are no complications the disease is self-limited. Aconite 3x, is useful in the febrile stage, after which Rhus tox. 3x, will hasten a cure. If headache acompanies the disease, with flushed face, and sore throat, Belladonna 3x. In case of intense itching, Apis mellifica 3x. The patient should be kept warm if the disease occurs during cold weather. A milk diet, or perhaps a little milk toast is the best. Owing to the mild character of the disease there is seldom ever any entailment of other disturbances.

Variola, or Small Pox.

The most formidable of all the exanthemata, is small pox. It presents such disgusting features, as well as frequently fatal results, it has been dreaded by all classes of society. Some even have regarded it the most filthy and offensive of all the eruptive diseases. The symptoms of the various stages are first, malaise, a sense of weariness, and soreness, severe pain in the head, as if it would fly to pieces, an indescribable pain in the back, and not unfrequently there is a ptyalism, and an offensive odor from the mouth.

Small pox is an infectious disease, and the time from the exposure to the appearance of the eruption may be from nine to twelve days; in some cases the period of incubation is not so long. In connection with the headache and pain in the back there is usually soreness in the throat, and more or less gastric disturbance; just before there is any sign of the eruption the fever is intense, the arterial excitement is very great, and the temperature is from 102° to 103°. The febrile odor is very marked, and sometimes the patient is delirious.

The eruption is first seen upon the face and exposed parts of the body; its appearance first is in the form of small red points, and has been mistaken both for scarlet fever and measles.

During the eruptive fever the little points first seen enlarge greatly and assume the pustular form and are filled with pus.

The eruptive stage generally continues three or four days. When the eruption is fully developed the pustules begin to wither and dry up, forming incrustations or scabs; there are three forms in which the eruption makes its appearance, one of which is termed discreet, because the eruption becomes manifest in pustules each of which is distinct without coalescing together. Another variety is termed the confluent because the pustules coalesce and run together; and still another is termed coherent, where the pustules are numerous and enlarge their margins so as to cohere with each other. The discreet form of the disease is considered less dangerous and the severity of the symptoms is not so great. The confluent form is more severe and dangerous, because the attack upon the vital condition of the system is attended with great prostration.

The coherent form is more severe than the discreet, but runs its course in about the same length of time. The premonitory symptoms of each variety differ but little except in severity. The eruption is of a different character from the vesicular eruption of varicella, in as much as its action upon the skin is more serious, and the inflammatory process extends deeper and is liable to disorganize to a certain extent. The varicutis to a degree is disorganized, and is left in a pitted condition after desquamation has taken place.

TREATMENT.—The treatment which is required in the early stage of the disease is such as required in other febrile difficulties. For the headache, pain in the back, and fever, *Aconite* 3x may be given first and this remedy may be followed with *Nux vomica* 3x, when it becomes manifest that the fever is of an eruptive character. Bryonia 3x, may be given to hasten the elimination of the eruption. Tartar emetic 3x, may be given after Bryonia 3x, to aid in completing the eruptive process. When the eruption is fully upon the surface, measures should be taken to prevent pitting.

We have found that a resort to Glycerine with which to cover the entire eruptive surface, and persistently used until desquamation begins, has proved to be salutary; a mixture of charcoal and lard has been successfully employed in the same way in confluent cases threatening pitting; great benefit has been derived in puncturing the pustules in their ripe stage with the point of a lancet and then making an application with a camel hair brush of the styptic colloid. The employment of *Tartar emetic* 3x, for internal administration, until desquamation begins, is generally followed by rapid convalescence, and a very trifling amount of pitting supervenes.

Pulsatilla 3x, to aid a healthy desquamation is generally approved. When the patient appears to suffer from extreme prostration we have given *China* 3x, with good effect.

In adults when recuperation appears to be retarded by reason of low fever, Brandy may be given in teaspoonful doses in water for a time, and then Rhus tox. 3x may be given to allay this variola fever.

The patient should be supplied with a light nutritious diet as soon as his appetite returns and he expresses a desire for food.

There is still another variety of variola which is characterized by hæmorrhagic diathesis. The symptoms in the main are similar to those we have detailed, and in addition there is violent nosebleed and hæmorrhagic rash.

This variety is more persistent; the vomiting and nosebleed are its marked features until the eruption is perfectly eliminated.

In Jousset's Clinical Medicine a remarkable case of this variety is reported.

The eruption first made its appearance upon the upper and anterior part of the thorax and was decidedly hæmorrhagic, characterized by many little spots of echymosis.

This eruption runs into larger patches, some of which are red, others black with intermediate tints.   In a fully developed case of this kind the prognosis is unfavorable.

Jousset gave *Phosphorus* in the sixth dilution, which arrested the nosebleed when the temperature in the evening was 104°; he continued the Phosphorus with good results until the ninth day, when the patient was evidently convalescent; and according to the experience of Prof. Ludlum, Phosphours 3x is a reliable remedy for the treatment of variola in subjects who have suffered from purpura and evidently of a hæmorrhagic diathesis.

Varioloid or Modified Small Pox.

In persons that have been vaccinated successfully it is supposed that true variola becomes greatly modified and is of a milder and more discreet form; nevertheless the victims of varioloid suffer from similar aches, and pains and fever, but of less severity. The eruption is of a discreet variety; and frequently but few pustules comparatively are observed upon the face, neck, and chest; the general impression prevails that varioloid is simply a modified form of variola, originating from the same infection, modified by the prophylactic power of vaccination; it is not usually dangerous, as it seldom proves fatal.

TREATMENT.—The treatment employed in the various stages does not differ essentially from that of the genuine small pox.

CHAPTER XXXVIII.

Continued Fever.

Febrile diseases, are by many, believed to be contagious, and to a certain extent they are so when produced by an animal poison.

There are many poisons which are not communicable from person to person, and yet they cause diseases, sometimes of a deadly character.

A vitiated atmosphere is unquestionably the source of much febrile disorder. Malaria, or bad air when inhaled, permeates through the body, and exerts its influence upon the solids and fluids of the various tissues. A sense of weariness, indifference, and inclination to keep quiet, are often the primary indications of malarial influence. Supervening upon these, a frontal headache, somewhat severe and stupefying, is often observed.

The tongue exhibits a dirty or brownish coating, with great derangement of the sense of taste, and general antipathy to food. The pulse becomes full and somewhat accelerated, and the temperature of the body slightly increased. These symptoms are more or less persistent, and gradually increase in severity. The skin becomes hot, the breath is heavy and feverish, and the secretion of the kidneys usually highly colored, and in a majority of instances these symptoms continue from day to day, with little change except in severity, until a crisis occurs, which may be in seven, nine, eleven, thirteen or fifteen days, and then a copious perspiration follows, the violence of the headache ceases, and the force and frequency of the pulse abates. A new train of symptoms now becomes apparent; a diarrhœa frequently sets in, there is coolness of the surface, stupor comes over the patient, who is prone to lie in a comatose state, and apparently free from acute suffering.

These symptoms continue until another crisis occurs; which either causes the patient to sink lower or ends in a general break

up of the disease. When the diarrhœa continues and finally runs
into a bloody flux the prostration is so great as to render the prognosis unfavorable, but when the diarrhœa gradually diminishes
and warmth is restored to the surface, and the stupor and comatose symptoms disappear and the coating of the tongue clears off,
and the patient's inappetency in a measure subsides, and a moderate amount of food can be taken with impunity, the prospect
of the patient's recovery is greatly brightened; when the portal
system becomes greatly congested, and is suddenly relieved by
copious discharges of blood, the strength of the patient declines
rapidly and if the hæmorrhage is not speedily arrested the countenance becomes pinched and sunken, and the prospect of reaction from this condition is by no means promising. It will
be seen that in the first stage of the disease, the fever is inflammatory and continued until the first crisis occurs; the
second stage which ensues is decidedly of a nervous character,
and may indicate serious internal derangement and ulceration of
the mucous coat of the intestines. It is then termed congestive
and requires a difference of treatment from that of the first stage.
When a disease assumes the most malignant form it becomes putrid, and exhalation from the patient's body becomes correspondingly offensive.

TREATMENT.—The treatment of this form of continued fever
must be in accordance with the symptoms. In the first stage
when the pulse is full and bounding and the headache is very severe, the bowels constipated; In Allopathic practice, depleting
measures are resorted to, with mild or saline purgatives.

HOMŒOPATHIC TREATMENT.—But in Homœopathic practice, the
condition of the patient is taken into consideration, and remedies
are affiliated in accordance with the symptoms.

Aconite 3x, when the skin is hot and the pulse full and bounding, and there is considerable heat in the head, thirst and a feverish breath.

Belladonna 3x dil. follow *Aconite* 3x, when there is intense pain
in the front of the head affecting the eyes, and when the patient
is unable to bear the light. If there is a heavy sickening odor
from the breath, Baptisia 3x, may follow Belladonna 3x. These
remedies have sometimes aborted the disease, and their use has
been followed by a breaking up of the symptoms, by warm perspiration and a rapid convalescence. In case of failure and a ner-

vous prostration ensues, Bryonia 3x, is called into requisition. In case of stupor or coma, and other manifestations of nervous symptoms *Rhus tox.* 3x, may follow Bryonia 3x.

In case diarrhœa sets in, *Mercurius sol.* is suitable to follow Rhus tox. 3x. If this should mitigate the diarrhœa and restore warmth to the surface, the indications are favorable; but if the diarrhœa should persist and the discharges from the bowels be offensive and the patient be greatly prostrated, *Arsenicum* 3x, may follow Mercurius 3x. In case the abdomen is distended and tympanitic, *Carbo vegetabilis* 3x, may follow the Arsenicum 3x. Any attenuation of these remedies above the third decimal may be employed when indicated; much depends upon the accuracy of the affiliation.

Nitric acid 3x, is one of the best remedies against hæmorrhage from the bowels; it may be administered in the third aquatic dilution, and the doses may be repeated every one or two hours.

Accessory means.—Well ventilated apartments and critical attention to cleanliness, the patient should be supplied with a moderate amount of food, according to the indications afforded by the appetite; it is not well to compel the patient to partake of food, when the appetite is entirely suspended, which is usually the case in the earlier stages of the disease. Ablutions of warm water softened with a little bi-carbonate of soda are for the most part beneficial; frequent use of the tooth brush and tepid water with which to wash the mouth is useful in preventing the collection of sordes upon the teeth.

Intermittent Fever.

By the term intermittent is understood a fever which occurs in paroxysms either daily or on alternate days; with a complete intermission or freedom from febrile symptoms, from the termination of one paroxysm to the beginning of another.

There are usually three stages in each paroxysm, the cold or chilly stage followed by the hot stage, and terminating in the sweating stage.

Previous to the commencement of the paroxysm the victim labors under a degree of depression; feels languid, and is disposed to yawn frequently, at length a chilliness comes over him which is characterized by coldness of the extremities and general chilliness and shuddering, sometimes the shivering is so great as to cause the whole body to shake with the cold; as a rule there is intense thirst during the chill, which lasts a longer or shorter period. This stage is attended with depression of the pulse and a bluish appearance around the tips of the fingers, while at the same time there is a pinched expression of the countenance, and the patient complains of severe pain in the back and loins, and sometimes, of general restlessness and aching of the whole system.

After a time there is a reaction from this cold and depressed condition which is first indicated by a cessation of the shivering and a manifest rising of the pulse and warmth upon the surface.

This stage augments in violence until the entire surface of the body comes under the influence of a feverish heat, the pulse then becomes full and rapid, the thirst more intensified, with severe pain in the head, frequently attended with gastric derangement.

This is termed in common parlance the hot stage, inasmuch as the whole system, including the head, trunk and extremities are under the influence of an extreme feverish heat; this stage is generally.followed by copious sweating of a colliquative character, and so abundant as to cover the body with a dripping perspiration, and so extreme as to render the clothing about the patient wet with the exhalation, after which the sweating gradually subsides until the paroxysm is over.

The patient then is found to be free from fever, the pulse becomes apparently normal, without thirst and without other abnormal symptoms except the deterioration of strength and languidness from having passed through such a purgatory.

A quotidian intermittent is indicated when these paroxysms occur every twenty-four hours with an entire intermission of fever during the interim between them and occurs most commonly in the spring. The tertian intermittent has a paroxysm every forty-eight hours and occurs generally in the spring or autumn. The quartan intermittent has a paroxysm at an interval of every seventy-two hours and commonly occurs in the autumn.

The paroxysms often occur at the same hour of the day, but this is by no means a uniform rule.

When they occur at an earlier hour than is expected it evinces a more stubborn resistence to the effect of remedies. When they occur later each day, it evinces the gradual improve-

ment of the patient. It has been observed that the paroxysms are
shorter when the cold stage is the most persistent and protracted.
It has also been observed that the shorter the interval the longer
the paroxysm.

The quotidian generally has the shortest cold stage, and the
paroxysm is correspondingly protracted. As there is a longer interval between the paroxysms in the tertian form, the cold stage
is longer and the paroxysms when they occur are somewhat
abridged in duration, the interval between being seventy-two
hours; being longer is indicative of greater severity and length
of the paroxysm when it occurs. There are other forms of intermittent fever which occur about every five or eight days; these
different forms of intermittent fever exhibit in some degree a
regularity in the occurrence of the paroxysms, but there are cases
of two paroxysms, one in the morning and the other in the
evening and are termed double quotidian. The double tertian
has a paroxysm every other day in the morning, and on alternate
days a lighter paroxysm occurs in the evening. It is observed
also that paroxysms occur without regard to regularity when the
patients are surrounded by certain influences, such as dampness
and cold winds and the depressing effects of the sun's rays in midsummer.

All forms of intermittent fever, it is believed, result from
malaria. In all localities of marshy or undrained alluvial soil,
there is evidently a condition of the atmosphere which favors
the generation of intemittent fevers. For many centuries
we have had examples of the deadly influence of malaria in
such districts, and in proportion to the extent of these marshy
or undrained districts, is the severity of the disease. In the
northern part of the temperate zone, where valleys and lowlands
are not so profusely watered, malarial influences are not so depressing to the vital forces. In the valleys of the Cumberland,
Susquehanna and Schuylkill, in Pennsylvania, an annual return
of intermittents is expected. The same is true of the northern
part of the State of Indiana and many localities in the valley of
the Mississippi.

The slightest modification of the atmosphere by lithial influences, wafted upon the wings of the wind, is liable to result in
some form of ague.

TREATMENT.—In all localities where intermittents prevail,

massive doses of Peruvian bark or its alkaloids, have been relied on to excite a tonic condition of sufficient force to resist the effects of malaria, and to act as a febrifuge when the fever occurs. The massive doses which have been administered, have in some instances, resulted disastrously. The indiscriminate and excessive use of this drug, are in some cases disastrous and therefore objectionable.

It must be conceded nevertheless, that in many marshy districts the employment of Acetate and Sulphate of China 3x is indispensable.

In recent cases when the symptoms are well defined and take place in their regular order; and the paroxysms terminate in comparative health, Chin. sulph. 3x.

China 3x is indicated when the following symptoms are present: drowsiness after a meal, sinking, empty sensation with little appetite or desire for food; soreness or swelling of the liver or spleen, watery, slimy or bilious diarrhœa; extreme sensibility to currents of air, irritable disposition and depression of spirits. The Sulphate of China may be used instead of the *China* for similar symptoms, but not in massive doses. The first, second or third decimal trituration may be used in grain doses and repeated every three hours during the apyrexia and if there should be a recurrence of the paroxysm, the same may be repeated after each succeeding paroxysm in the same manner until there is a breaking up of the disease, or in case of no satisfactory change, four grains may be dissolved in four ounces of water acidulated with one drop of Sulphuric acid, a dessert spoonful of the mixture to be given every four hours as before.

Arsenicum album in the third trituration may follow in grain doses every three or four hours if necessary, when the paroxysm is attended with severe pain in the head, and rigors, a few doses of *Belladonna* 3x may be given at intervals of one hour until the headache ceases.

Our experience in the treatment of ague of the quotidian type with these remedies has been exceedingly satisfactory, and we have found no excuse for employing a more concentrated form of the remedies. *Carbo vegetabilis* 3x is indicated when the cold has greatly predominated, we have seen its decided action in preventing a recurrence of the disease; we have seen its curative

action in protracted cases after much quinine has been administered to the patient, we have also found *Cedron* 3x a valuable
anti-periodic in uncomplicated intermittents, when the paroxysms have regularly appeared at the same hour of the day; and
especially when the paroxysms are attended with neuralgic
suffering.

For chronic intermittents with vomiting before and during
the chill, great thirst and sores about the mouth, we have frequently seen the salutary effects of *Natrum muriaticum* 3x.

In those cases where there is nausea and vomiting without
thirst, with a thick coating upon the tongue and a yellowish color,
we have seen the beneficial effects of *Ipecacuanha* 3x; there are
many other remedies that may be called into requisition in the
treatment of the various forms of intermittents; but the manifest
symptoms must guide in their selection, and in all cases the critical observance of the symptoms during the progress of the disease, must suggest the remedies to be employed.

Dumb Ague.

We have had considerable said about a dumb ague or marked
intermittent, but in truth it is more of a medicinal or drug disease or sequel of mismanaged intermittent; in some localities
endemic intermittents have been treated to excess with *Quinine*
and *Arsenic* and pronounced cured, when in fact the observable
shivering chill is merely smothered by these drugs and the patient
suffers from cold extremities, occasional headaches and fevers,
which are evidently the typical effects of the drugs.

This has frequently been termed *dumb ague* or marked intermittent.

TREATMENT.—To treat the disease in this form successfully,
requires *Sulphur* 3x, *Natrum muriaticum* 3x, and *Mercurius* 3x;
the latter remedy is especially indicated in hepatic derangement,
sallow complexion, loss of appetite, yellowish coating upon the
tongue, bitter taste in the mouth.

Sulphur 3x, is indicated for dryness of the skin, inclination
to coldness of feet and persistency of coldness upon the surface.

Nitric acid, 3x when there is a sensation of fullness in the
right hypochondrium and discharges of bloody matter from the
bowels and in all cases where there is evidence to justify the con-

clusion that the patient is suffering from the protracted use of Quinine or Arsenic; Sulphur, Potassium and Mercurius vivus of the third decimal trituration, administered three or four times a day, will prove sufficient to antidote the mischief.

We once had a patient from southern Illinois, who had suffered for two years or more with a tertian ague, and who, from an apparently robust, plethoric and vigorous constitution, had become emaciated, sallow and uncomfortable, from indurations of the spleen and liver, together with an interrupted nutrition. When he came under our care, we recognized in his case the effect of perpetual drugging with Quinine. He had been taught that it was impossible for him to subsist without daily doses of from twenty to twenty-five grains, every day. We ordered the discontinuance of this practice, and substituted the third decimal dilution of Sulphur, to be taken twice a day, and directed the patient to secure well-ventilated apartments, and to resort to a sponge bath of warm water, saturated with common salt. In less than a week he began to improve rapidly, and in three weeks an entire change came over his system. He suffered from no more chills, he regained his appetite, and was apparently free from suffering. He improved from day to day, and at the termination of the sixth week, we discharged him cured, and he returned to the scene of his labors, where he fully recuperated, and has remained in perfect health ever since.

Irregular Ague.

In some constitutions there is a proclivity to irregular paroxysms of ague, because the predisposition is so strong that the most trivial exciting cause may provoke chilliness, and a febrile reaction will immediately follow. We have seen many persons who suffered from this constitutional peculiarity, but it is extremely variable in regard to symptoms, and the degree of severity. It is impossible, therefore, to point out a uniform treatment with remedies, inasmuch as the symptoms may differ greatly in each individual case, and remedies must be affiliated accordingly.

TREATMENT.—The accessory or dietetic treatment, however, is much the same. Such patients should be subject to an unmedicinal diet, as generous as the appetite may indicate. They should be supplied with fresh air, warm clothing, and freedom from extremes of temperature, and dampness, as much as possible.

A gentleman aged sixty, of nervous temperament, could never sit by a window even in the warmest weather without contracting this peculiar suffering. He would first begin to sneeze and then to yawn and stretch his limbs, and then he would experience in rapid succession chilliness and heat; for several hours he also suffered from thirst, more or less nausea, and burning at the pit of the stomach.

Arsenicum album in the sixth trituration wrought a change in his constitution and rendered him less amenable to these trifling exposures, nevertheless he remained extremely impressible to draughts of cold air. We gave him Baryta carb., the sixth decimal trituration three or four times a day, and under the influence of this remedy, this impressibility passed away and afterwards he happily experienced complete relief from this proclivity.

In other cases we found Phosphorus 3x, an admirable remedy to cou teract this impressibility.

Carbo vegetabilis and *Carbo animalis* in the thirtieth dilution exerted a curative influence, when night sweats were of common occurrence, and especially where dull aching pains, and general restlessness contributed to the discomfort of the patient.

Hectic Intermittent.

In some persons of feeble constitutions, subject to cough and other pulmonary diseases and particularly when attended by an irritable pulse, we have noted the daily occurrence of chill and fever. The former would consist of rigors, coursing down the back, followed by a febrile reaction which became manifest by a flushed face, circumscribed redness of one or both cheeks, acceleration of the pulse, labored respiration, heat in the palms of the hands and burning sensation of the feet; these symptoms with others less prominent, would indicate a hectic dependent upon some local dyscrasia, either in the lungs, liver or some other internal organ.

It is usually dependent upon tuberculosis and is characteristic of tubercular consumption; emaciation in consequence of a feeble nutrition is usually apparent. After the paroxysm passes off a clammy perspiration usually follows and lasts the entire night.

TREATMENT.—The remedies employed most successfully in the

treatment of hectic fever are Arsenicum 3x; when there is great prostration, thirst and watery papescent stools, when the cough is persistent, and the expectoration muco-purulent, Stannum 3x, is a remedy that will prove to be beneficial. Calcarea carbonica in the thirtieth dilution we have seen act beneficially.

Lycopodium, thirtieth dilution, entirely obviated the fever and acted favorably, in the diminution of the bronchial purulent expectoration.

The accessory treatment for hectic fever is mainly dietetic, in connection with a residence in the most favorable climate.

That of Colorado is regarded the most favorable for patients subject to hectic fever. In some cases when emaciation has taken place, and the fever has become manifest, a residence in Minnesota, near the head waters of the Mississippi, has wrought a favorable change; the fever has subsided, and the regaining of flesh has been apparent.

When dependent upon tubercular disease the fever may subside in a dry atmosphere much more apparently than in a humid one. A dense atmosphere is regarded more favorable for promoting strength and invigorating nutrition than a rare or sultry one.

Remittent Fever.

In certain localities where dampness and decaying vegetation produce malaria, there is reason to believe that this operates disastrously in the production of febrile diseases.

We have already treated briefly of intermittents originating from this cause; the only difference between intermittent and remittent fevers is the entire intermission of febrile symptoms between the paroxysms of the former and the mere remission of the febrile symptoms without an intermission in the latter.

The symptoms of remittent fever are for the most part biliary derangement, pain in the head; with continuous febrile symptoms characterized by morning or evening exacerbations, nausea, and sometimes vomiting of biliary matter.

At first the patient feels weary and is inclined to inertia, he loses his appetite, complains of a bitter taste in his mouth, his tongue is furred, the sclerotic coat of the eye is tinged with yellow, the face exhibits a sallow appearance, and the patient complains of chilly sensations; immediately after the skin be-

comes hot, the pulse accelerated, and there is a gradual increase
of fever until it reaches the climax of the paroxysm, and then the
fever gradually subsides, with a gradual diminution of the force
and frequency of the pulse, and a mitigation of temperature of
the skin, and yet there is no entire cessation of the fever until it
begins again to increase and approach another climax to undergo
a similar diminution as in the preceding paroxysm; these alternate elevations and depressions in remittent fever may continue
from seven to fourteen days before a complete intermission between the paroxyms occur. And then the disease becomes intermittent, with daily or tertiary paroxyms, according to its peculiar
type.

TREATMENT.—When the gastric symptoms prevail in intermittent fever, and there is much vomiting of matters from the
stomach; if there is considerable excitement, and a full bounding
pulse, with constipation of the bowels, the prevailing practice has
been to give the patient an emetic and follow it with a dose of
Calomel and *Rhubarb;* but this practice has been of late very
greatly modified.

HOMŒOPATHIC TREATMENT.—The Homœopathic treatment of
the disease we have found to be more effectual.

Aconite 3x, may first be given when the fever is high, and
the pulse full and frequent. The remedy will sometimes allay the
vomiting, and relieve the fever and reduce the force and frequency
of the pulse; but should the vomiting continue and be attended
with considerable retching, *Ipecacuanha* 3x may be given to allay
the irritability of the stomach; *Nux vomica* 3x may follow, when
the bowels are constipated and there is simultaneous pain in the
head and back.

In lymphatic temperaments and especially in females, we have
found *Pulsatilla* 3x more effective in relieving these symptoms.

Belladonna 3x, when there is severe pain in the head affecting the eyes, and when there is occasional sensations of chilliness.

Bryonia 3x, when there are glairy vomitings, and when the
patient is disposed to remain quiet, finding that moving about
aggravates the gastric irritability, and also when there is a sensation of heat in the stomach.

We have found these remedies for the most part sufficient to
correct the derangement observed in gastric remittents when the

secretion of bile is abundant and there is continuous vomiting of biliary matters, with more or less pain in the right side.

Mercurius 3x, after Aconite may be given and repeated frequently until there is a decided change.

Podophyllum 3x, after Mercurius, acts beneficially in such cases.

When there are no complications in bilious and gastric remittents, the remedies named will in most cases be sufficient; when they run into the intermittent form, the remedies employed in their treatment are *Arsenicum* 3x, when there is great thirst during the paroxysm and when there is simultaneous shivering and heat.

China 3x, may be administered in the interim between the paroxysms, and remedies during the succeeding paroxysms must be selected in accordance with the symptoms, in order to bring the disease to successful termination.

Natrum muriaticum 3x, Nux vomica 3x, Mercurius sol. 3x, Macrotin 3x, Podophyllum 3x, Pulsatilla 3x, Rhus tox. 3x, and Sulphur 3x, may be consulted.   In all cases the symptoms must be the guide in the selection of remedies; and this remark holds good in case of complications, such as colic, diarrhœa, and other derangements which may occur in the course of the disease; when there has been a hard chill in the morning, with great thirst, through all stages of the fevers. Vomiting frequently precedes the chill and the fever simply remits and the patient has cold hands and feet, stupefaction and heat, obscuration of sight and fainting, fever blisters on the lips, loss of appetite.

Muriatic acid, 3x, may be given in water, ten drops in a glass, a dessert spoonful every hour when the paroxysm has mitigated. Nux vomica 3x, trit. may be given in two grain powders when the chilliness is irregular, with aching in the limbs, yawning, thirst and protracted febrile reaction, every two hours. When remittents are attended with great drowsiness and diarrhœa, anxiety, heat of the face, *Pulsatilla* 3x dil. may be prepared and administered as above.

Rhus tox. 3x, is valuable in remittent fevers, when before the attack there is burning in the eyes, increase of mucus in the mouth, a dry, annoying cough, during the cold or chilly stage, and when the febrile reaction brings out the nettle rash, etc. Rhus tox. 6x dil., ten drops in a tumbler of water, and a spoonful every two hours.   As soon as the paroxysms have a visible intermission, a few doses of China 3x, may be given to mitigate or ward off succeeding paroxysms.

From the fact of remittent fevers being generally associated with biliary derangements, they are usually considered under the head of " bilious remittent," and in addition to chills and reactive fevers, which gradually decline almost to an intermission, and then return again into the various stages of remittent paroxysms,   there are bilious vomitings, sallow countenance, bitter taste in the mouth, and a thick bilious coating on the tongue. These symptoms indicate the use of Mercurius vivus 3x trit., two grain powders, repeated every third hour, or, perhaps, Nux vom. 3x trit., given every afternoon in the same manner.

When the gastric symptoms predominate, Ipecac, Nux vom., Puls., Bry., Cham., Eupatorium, Lobelia and Tartar emetic; either when indicated may be administered ever third hour, in the 3x dilution, or fifteen drops in a tumbler of water, a spoonful at a time.

When the bilious symptoms predominate, Acon., Bry., Arsenicum, Cham. and Sulphur, each in the 3x dilution.

When there is evident irritation of the mucous membrane of the stomach and bowels, Bell.,China, Mercurius, 3x trit.,Rhus tox., and for any signs of invermination or worms, Cina., Cinnabar, Spigelia, Terebinth and Sulphur.   Each remedy when selected according to the symptoms, may be administered, ten or fifteen drops of the 3x dil., in a gill of water, in dessert spoonful doses, every two hours.

Non-Malarious Congestive Fevers.

The precursory stage of congestive fever is characterized by irritability, restlessness, and aversion to mental and bodily exertion, and also vertigo, giddiness and apprehension from the slightest exercise.   The pulse is often below the natural standard.   Now the symptoms will be modified according to the part of the body or organ, which sustains the violence of the attack.   If this be the brain, the patient will complain of headache, oppression or tightness in the head, with contracted or dilated pupils, confusion of ideas, slow pulse, coma, paresis, and convulsions.   When the attack is upon the bowels, there is usually an anxious, or distressed expression of countenance, eyes sunken and glazed, more or less nausea and vomiting, bowels tender on pressure, and burning hot. The extremities are cold, tongue thinly coated with a whitish or reddish fur, a constant desire on the part of the patient to be moving about, restless and uneasy, alternations of diarrhœa and constipation, and finally, stupor, spasms, and stertorous breathing. If the congestion occurs in the lungs, there will be rapid and obstructed breathing, intermittent and iregular pulse, cough, face and skin purple from imperfect decarbonization of the blood, pains in the chest and surface cold. In all these congestions, the mental energies of the system sink below the normal standard. The pulse is slow and feeble, and the function of the lungs imperfectly executed.

CAUSES.—Excessive cold, and sudden changes of temperature, drinking copiously of cold or iced water when the body is in a heated condition, and also, from low living, insufficient clothing, overexertion of body and mind, sudden news, disappointment, fear, mortification, and depression of spirits.

TREATMENT.—For febrile congestion of the brain, Belladonna, Acon., Opium, Hyos., Cuprum, 6x, Conium, Lac., each in 3x dil., ten drops dissolved in a gill of water, a teaspoonful every hour. For congestive fever of the bowels, Ipec. 3x, Ver., Nux vom., Bry., Arsen. For congestive fever of the lungs, Bry., Acon., Phos., each 3x dil., Lach. 6x, Stibium 3x, Rhus tox., prepared and administered as above. Congestive fevers often attack the system suddenly and with great violence, and if not soon arrested run on to a fatal termination. As soon therefore as the right Homœopathic remedy is selected for the treatment of severe cases, it should be repeated frequently, until a decided impression is made upon the symptoms. If there is a failure for a time, increase the strength of the remedies.

Irritative Fevers.

This variety of fevers, is believed to be idiopathic, and arises from causes of irritation that have nothing specific or peculiar in their mode of action. The most trifling cause may induce over excitement in one or more of the functions. The nervous communication to different parts of the system, may throw all the functions into a state of derangement which will be capable of sustaining itself for some time after the direct cause of excitement is gone. This fever does not depend on the continuance of any local disease, but having originated from a cause ever so trifling it goes on by independent action to its natural termination. This termination may be in an hour or two, or several days, but when it runs on for five or six days, it is probable there is some local inflammation existing in the stomach or intestines. This fever attends dentition of children, and is excited by this process.

TREATMENT.—When dentition is the cause of irritative fever Cham. 3x, in saturated globules may be administered, three or four at a dose, and repeated every two hours. When this fever produces profuse ptyalism or drewling Merc. 6x, dil. in globules may be given as above, when there is nausea and vomiting and even diarrhœa. When the irritative fever is characterized by restlessness, Acon. 6x, dil., ten drops in a glass of water, dessert spoonful doses every third hour until relieved. When the head and hands are hot and face flushed, change to Bell. 6x, prepared and given in same manner.

Infantile Remittent Fever.

This is a disease peculiar to childhood and originates from unhealthy and indigestible food in addition to the irritation of teething, invermination, repelled eruptions, and the too rapid drying up of old sores, and discharges of any kind. This disorder affects the stomach and intestines most generally, and in some instances the brain and lungs seem to participate in the disorder, and in whatever locality the disease spends its force, there are usually remissions and exacerbations. The disease makes its appearance with symptoms like those of an ordinary fever. Slight chills, thirst, and wandering pains in the back, bowels and limbs, together with great restlessness. In the febrile reaction, the child appears to suffer in the stomach and intestines, which are painful, tender on pressure, while there is either constipation or diarrhœa. The stools are usually dark and offensive, as in case of deficiency of bile. There is a burning thirst with vomiting of liquids when swallowed. A whitish fur covers the tongue which is red at the edges. When this inflammation is permitted to progress, without appropriate remedies, ulceration, and other lesions may occur in the digestive tube, which are likely to lay the foundation for disorder of the brain and lungs. The causes of this derangement are exposure to extremes of temperature, improper food, worms, suppression of eruptions and accustomed evacuations, and the injurious effect of drastic medicine on the bowels.

TREATMENT.—The Allopathic treatment for this disorder is the employment of calomel, and quinine, followed by purgatives.

HOMŒOPATHIC TREATMENT consists in the judicious affiliation of remedies indicated by the symptoms. Ipec. 3x, Merc. 3x, Puls. 3x, Nux v. 3x, Calc. 6x, and in case the brain becomes affected Bell. 3x, Bry. 3x, Nux v. 3x, and Opium 3x, each in dil., 15 drops in half a goblet of water, dessert spoonful doses every third hour; if the selection from this group of remedies proves insufficient, a change to Sulphur 3x, trit., Calc. 3x, trit., Ars. 3x, trit. and Silicea 30x, trit., may prove more effectual. If worms be the cause of the difficulty, Cina. 3x, dil., Spigelia 3x, dil. may be called into requisition.

Inflammatory Continued Fever.

Continued fevers may arise from functional derangement or inflammation. Those that arise from functional derangement are less dangerous, being caused by overloading the stomach with crude indigestible food, irregular habits, insufficient clothing and habitual intemperance in the use of tea, coffee and tobacco.

TREATMENT.—In Allopathic practice, mild doses of Calomel and Rhubarb are the main resort.

HOMŒOPATHIC TREATMENT, which is altogether preferable, is Aconite and Nux vom. in the sixth attenuation, will speedily bring about a cure.

If the functional form is neglected, inflammation or congestion may follow as a sequel, but the inflammatory continued fever, which we are now considering, is a more dangerous, and deeper seated affection.

The general symptoms are hot, dry skin, rapid and full pulse, dyspnœa, thirst, nausea, depression at the pit of the stomach, restlessness, a coated and dry tongue, but the symptoms connected with the organ are those which are characteristic of the disease. If the inflammation implicates the membranes of the brain, the face becomes flushed, and the eyes exhibit a fiery red appearance, sparkling and protruding, staring and distorted, the pupils contracted or dilated. There is, at this stage, an unnatural expression, and furious delirium, and there is at the same time, a full, bounding pulse, greatly accelerated, and, as the disorder progresses, a sopor, and muttering delirium, and sometimes twitchings and convulsions supervene. When the lungs are attacked, there is anxious and oppressed respiration, somewhat rapid, with shooting pains in the thorax, a troublesome cough, and difficult expectoration, pain and soreness becomes apparent at every inspiration. There may be other symptoms that are characteristic of pulmonic inflammation. If the inflammation attacks the membrane which covers the stomach and intestines, we have the signs which would indicate the presence of this affection, such as nausea, vomiting, pains in the bowels, augmented by pressure, red tongue, and an anxious countenance, bowels hot and swollen.

The causes of synochal fever are extremes of temperature, overexertion, and errors of diet. These fevers often succeed neglected, or badly-managed fevers, from functional derangement, especially in cases where some organ has before been debilitated, and in this manner become predisposed to inflammatory action.

It is generally conceded that inflammation seldom occurs in perfectly healthy parts. When exciting causes co-operate with predisposing conditions, they give rise to functional derangements which are easily remedied. When any structure or organ is suffering from preternatural irritation, a powerful predisponent, which invites an attack of inflammatory fever, is present, which requires but a few additional morbific influences to induce its full development.

TREATMENT.—The Allopathic treatment is anti-phlogistic, consisting of depletion and saline purgatives.

HOMŒOPATHIC TREATMENT is preferable as being applicable to each organ of attack.

Cerebral inflammatory fever requires Bell. 3x, dil., Opium 3x, dil.; Stramonium 3x dil. in alternation with Aconite 3x, may be found essential. When the pulmonary tissues are inflamed frequent doses of the third dilution of Bryonia, Tartar emetic 3x, Ipecac 3x, and Phos. 3x. When the stomach and intestines are the seat of the difficulty one or more of the following medicines may be employed in the third or sixth decimal attenuation, and given in drop doses in water, repeated every hour, two hours or three hours according to the severity of the case.

When the fever results from atmospheric changes, or follows a sudden check of perspiration, Gelsemium in the 3x dil., drop doses, repeated every hour, will relieve the patient and cure the general irritability, confusion of the head, flying pains, and soreness of the throat. The usual irritation of the nasal cavities, heat of the face, suffused eyes, frontal headache, pain in the back and limbs, soreness of the muscles, chills rendered worse by motion, the skin feels hot and dry; all indicate the use of Gelsemium. As also do the following symptoms: restlessness, quick pulse, full and tense, with thirst and sleeplessness. A few doses of the 12x will often produce a drenching perspiration, and a long continued sleep; and when the patient arouses he finds himself relieved of all suffering except prostration.

The Homœopathic preparation of *Mercurius vivus*, is a most successful remedy in synochal or inflammatory fever, when given in the 6x, trit., about a two grain powder repeated every two hours.

Nearly every case of typhoid or even typhus fever commences like inflammatory continued fevers, but terminates after a week or ten days, in a copious perspiration and discharges from the bowels, followed by great nervous prostration. Aconite in the first stage, when the pulse is full and bounding; and indeed a selection of remedies with great care and affiliation, according to symptoms, in the first or inflammatory stage, might obviate the severity of the future course of the disease.

DIET.—It is believed by many that fevers of every variety are but normal struggles to throw off offensive matter from the vital domain and to better effect this end the appetite generally is greatly diminished, or lost, to denote that nutrition is partially if not entirely lost; or in other words, the organic functions are in some degree suspended in order for reparation to take place. Great concern is usually manifested by friends when the patient cannot eat liberally of good food. But to thrust food upon fever patients when their appetite refuses it, is liable to add to the burthen already existing, therefore the diet should be exceedingly light, and supplied in no greater quantities than is demanded by the capacity of the system to dispose of it.

Typhus Fever.

In modern times the word *typhus* signifies a low nervous fever. The word itself is employed to denote general stupor or a disease that burns with a concealed and smothered flame.

The symptoms that denote the commencement of the disease are lassitude, debility, sense of fatigue, a beclouded memory, slight chills, alternating with flushes of heat, dull, stupefying pain in the head and back and limbs, loss of appetite, depression of the spirits. These symptoms continue for a longer or a shorter period, the patient not feeling sick enough to take to his bed, or well enough to attend to ordinary business affairs; restlessness soon ensues, especially at night, delirium soon sets in which obliges him to keep his bed from debility. His tongue, which at first is coated with a thin white coating, becomes dry, dark through the center, and cracked as the disease advances; the old fur passes off leaving a glazed appearance on the surface of the tongue which is unusually red. The eyes become suffused as the disease progresses, and the countenance loses its natural expression. The muscles are weak and tremulous, a viscid saliva collects and dries upon the lips and teeth. The surface acquires a dingy color, defective vision, subsultus tendinum, partial loss of hearing, involuntary discharges from the bowels and bladder and inclination to slide down to the foot of the bed, a constant picking of the bed clothes, low muttering delirium, and finally coma and convulsions. There will be some modification of the symptoms in the course of the disease in accordance with the severity of the attack, and the part most seriously implicated, together with the plan of treatment pursued.

TREATMENT.—Judging from the opinions expressed by the most experienced practitioners of the old school, the usual course of treatment has not only been unsuccessful, but partially injurious. This has been so palpably manifest to the best Allopathic physicians that they reached the ultimate conclusion that all cases of typhus would fare better if left to cure themselves.

Others of modern acquirement maintain an idea of the necessity of moderate stimulation from the commencement of the disease. By others again, this practice is repudiated.

HOMŒOPATHIC TREATMENT.—The Homœopathic remedies employed are Bry. 3x dil., ten drops in a half tumbler of water, tablespoonful doses every two hours. The indications for the use of this remedy are difficult respiration, dry mouth and tongue, pulse variable, and extreme debility, drowsiness during the day, and flightiness at night. If there are any indications of a sub-synochal character, Bell. 3x dil., may be prepared and administered the same as directed for Bry.

Opium 3x trit. may be given in two grain doses repeated every two hours, when the face is dark red or brownish, hot and bloated. When the pupils are dilated and immovable, the lower jaw relaxed and hanging, lethargic sleep and much snoring, mouth and eyes open.

Rhus tox., when there are petechial spots, blue circles round the eyes, pointed nose, vitiated secretions in the angles of the mouth, in the 3x dil. may be administered the same as directed for Bry. This remedy alone is not a specific for typhus fever, but is Homœopathic in its application to many symptoms.

Merc. viv. when there is great weakness and rapid declining of strength, profuse perspiration, fainting fits, numbness of the limbs, cramps and convulsive movements with great trembling, agitation and uneasiness of body and mind, this remedy has been successfully employed. Camphor in drop doses of the tincture has been successfully employed in the treatment of low nervous fever, when the temperature of the body is lowered, the sensibility depressed, and the vital powers greatly diminished. In case of apathy or general stupor, dry and cracked tongue, with the teeth covered with black sordes, frequent and dry cough, persistent delirium or dull mutterings, twitchings of tendons, glassy eyes, great hesitancy in replying to questions, involuntary aqueous stools, cold perspiration on the face and hands and pit of stomach, feeble, frequent and intermittent pulse, Phos. acid 6x dil. in drop doses has proved eminently successful. For like feebleness attended with hæmorrhage from the bowels, Nitric acid greatly attenuated is an effectual remedy; four drops of the chemically pure, in a gill of water, may be administered in dessert spoonful doses every hour.

Typhus Abdominalis.

This form of typhus particularly affects the abdominal viscera and has many symptoms in common with those which are manifest when other localities are affected. As for instance, there is fullness and pain in the head, vertigo and dizziness. At times the countenance appears flushed and bloated, throbbing in the temporal arteries, and visible pulsation of the carotids, palpitation of the heart, dryness of the mouth, mental apathy, constipation or diarrhœa, with tenesmus, persistent moaning, illusory visions or gloomy forebodings.

TREATMENT.—For most of these symptoms Bell. 3x dil., ten drops in a gill or water, may be administered in spoonful doses every two hours until there is a change in the symptoms. For fullness and pressure in the head from within outwards, aggravated by motion, buzzing in the ears, hardness or acuteness of hearing, rheumatic pains in the back and loins, worse on movement, drowsiness by day, delirium by night, Bry. 3x dil. may be prepared and administered the same as Bell. The abdominal typhus is an exceedingly dangerous disease, and liable in the last stages to assume a putrid character, Arsen. and Carb. veg. may be given in alternation in many instances. This practice has wrought a favorable change. In case of a sickening odor from the breath, Baptisia tinct. 3x dil., drop doses in water, has produced a desirable change in the condition of the patient. There are various forms of typhus fever that have been considered with reference to distinguishing marks, as putrid typhus, contagious typhus, or petechial typhus, but it is seldom that any one of these forms is found to be distinct or unmixed, because the brain, nervous system, lungs and abdominal viscera partake to a greater or less extent of the general disturbance, resulting of course in a great diversity of symptoms which must be the guide in the employment of remedial agents.

Typhoid Fever.

The general symptoms of enteric fevers are as follows: severe pain in the forehead and occiput, of a throbbing or shooting character, vertigo, dry cough, increasing in severity, and augmenting the headache. The patient suffers from prostration and fatigue; these symptoms are generally followed by alternations of rigors and febrile heat which finally ends in a continuous dry burning heat, and hot skin, the pulse from the commencement is accelerated, full but not tense, usually from a hundred to a hundred and twenty per minute. In a majority of cases there is a rush of blood to the head, redness of the face, noises in the ears, tongue either clean or coated with white fur which subsequently assumes a dryness, with impaired taste. There is frequently great pressure in the region of the heart or in that of the spleen.

The patient has no appetite. The bowels are either constipated or loose, the evacuations are fluid and of a yellowish or greenish appearance. In a later stage these evacuations are mixed with flakes or with blood, griping pain in the bowels, and often with burning pain in the anus. In a more advanced stage there is pressure in the abdomen with rumbling in the region of the large intestine. The urine is scanty, and after standing a short time deposits a copious sediment of a dark muddy appearance, gradually diminishing in quantity. Later in the disease the lips, teeth and tongue are covered with a very dry brown sordes, and the patient longs for water and suffers from loss of flesh and strength.

As the disease advances nervous symptoms become more prominent, and the patient becomes delirious and inclined frequently to get out of bed.

From the commencement of the disease the nights are very restless, even when the patient lies in somewhat of a stupor. This uneasiness is apt to increase with the delirium until a sopor ensues which generally terminates in absolute unconsciousness. The tongue is then very dry, the pulse becomes weaker and greatly accelerated; the breathing becomes labored and hurried. A characteristic of this condition is a kind of purpura on the skin. Small red spots appear on the surface, some of which are tumefied. They sometimes come out on the abdomen, and extend over the limbs, varying in color from a pink to a bluish red. The symptoms change in the latter stage; the skin becomes cooler, expectoration becomes difficult, and what is thrown off is mixed with streaks of blood.

CAUSES.—The causes of this fever may be found among the various determining influences which leave their impression on the nervous system, such as malaria, insufficient food and clothing, which are the precursors of intestinal degeneracy, which results in septic and contagious poisons, defective sewerage, badly ventilated closets, and general want of ablutions. A sponge bath of tepid water, saturated with a little bisulphate of soda, is a commendable accessory treatment, as well as a valuable prophylactic measure for the benefit of those in the room who are obliged to be about the patient.

The term typhoid applied to this fever, signifies a disease like typhus, and although there are many symptoms in the one disease that resemble those of the other, yet the *typhoid*, or more properly the enteric, is an essentially different disease. The causes of these fevers are different, and suggest a difference in the regulations of the sanitary measures.

The enteric or typhoid fever is slightly contagious in comparison to that of the typhus. The tendency to a fatal termination is not so marked in the average cases of typhoid, as in the great majority of the *typhus* cases. The treatment of these two palpably distinct diseases must be regulated accordingly.

The stage of invasion differs materially, and it is in this that practitioners should accurately note the discriminating points. In typhoid or enteric fever, a shorter period of malaria precedes a heavy, dull, but severe pain in the head. In the typhus there is a keen sense of weakness with but little pain, and the victims often persist in attending to the business of their occupations much too long for their good. Rest is essential; rest in bed may have a conservative effect in keeping up the strength, and in moderating the progress of the disease.

Children rarely suffer from enteric fever, especially before they merge from the period of infancy, and in persons advanced beyond the age of forty-five or fifty years. Nearly fifty per cent. of the cases occur between the ages of fifteen and twenty-five. Persons over thirty, are less liable to take the disease than when younger, and still more seldom do persons, from forty-five to fifty. The brain is chiefly affected in typhus. But in the enteric the bowels are chiefly affected. The evacuations are watery and colored, the mucus membrane of intestinal canal, often becomes congested, and sometimes there is hæmorrhage, ulceration and tumefaction of the abdomen.

The causes of typhoid or enteric fever are bad drainage or vitiated drinking water, as from a drain leading into a well; decomposing animal matter, etc.

The true typhus arises from destitution, overcrowding, with defective ventilation as in that form termed *ship fever*. This disease is contagious and spreads by reason of this fact. While relapses are rare in this disease after convalescence they frequently occur in the enteric fever especially when it becomes epidemic.

TREATMENT.—We attended briefly to the treatment without an attempt to systematise in a preceding portion of this article; we will now give what is a reasonable epitome of Homœopathic treatment. For febrile symptoms Acon., 3x, dil., Bryonia 3x, dil., Gels., 3x, dil., 10 drops of either in a gill of water. For the cerebral symptoms, Hyos., 3x, dil., Bell., 3x, dil., Veratrum vir., 3x, dil. For uremic symptoms, Terebinth 3x, dil., either in drop doses repeated hourly. For sleeplessness, Coffee 3x, dil., Bell., 3x, dil., Gels., 3x, dil., for stupor, Opium 3x, dil., Rhus tox, 3x, dil. For symptoms implicating the lungs, Phos., 6x, dil., Bry., 3x, dil. For extreme prostration, Ars., 6x, dil., Phos., 6x, dil. For paræsis, Nux vom., 3x, dil., Rhus tox., 3x, dil. For putrid symptom, Bapt., 3x, Carbo veg., 3x, trit.

Aconite 3x, dil., is specially indicated for thickly furred tongue, foul taste, thirst, dull pain in the head, sense of weight and soreness in the bowels, dark and foul urine, restlessness and depression of spirits. This remedy should be given early in the disease before the brain is seriously involved, and when the fever is at the highest pitch.

Baptisia 3x, dil., should be given in drop doses, when there is a putrescent odor from the mouth and a thick, dirty coating on the tongue.

Gelsemium is indicated for strange sensations in the head, neuralgic pains, and the twitching of certain muscles.

Hyoscyamus, Bell., and Stramonium for severe pains in the head, distressed expression of the face, brown tongue, noises in the ears, deafness, derangement of sight, delirium and a desire to escape or hide from some imaginary evil. *Hyoscyamus* 3x, dil., drop doses repeated hourly, is an excellent remedy in this disease; *Bell.*, 3x, dil., drop doses every hour against congestion, picking the bed clothes; Opium 3x, dil., for stertorous breathing, low muttering delirium or stupor.

Arsenicum 3x trit., for sunken countenance and eyes; dry and cracked tongue, burning thirst and involuntary diarrhœa.

Rhus tox. 3x dil., for nosebleed, discharge of fetid urine, involuntary bad smelling evacuation from the bowels.

Acid muriatic 6x dil., in drop doses, repeated every hour, is capable of effecting a beneficial influence in an advanced stage of the disease when there is extreme dryness and parched appearance of the skin and a complete loss of muscular power.

Nitric ac. chemically pure, four drops in a full tumbler of water will be found exceedingly salutary against hæmorrhages from the bowels, and may be given in spoonful doses occasionally throughout the disease.

We have treated many cases of enteric or typhoid fever, and have always affiliated our remedies to meet the symptoms from day to day. We have also when practicable, enjoined on the friends the placing of the patient in a large, well-ventilated room that will admit a plentiful supply of fresh air, cool but not cold. When cases occur in close and crowded rooms, we stipulate, as a condition of vital importance, that all such patients should be removed to suitable places for the enjoyment of hygienic influences, and in addition we have directed frequent changes of personal and bed linen, and change of posture to avoid congestions and bed sores, and the giving of food in small quantities at regular and frequent intervals.

We have also recommended disenfectants and cleanliness as of paramount importance. It would be advisable to give the patient a sponge bath, with water impregnated with phenic acid, at least once a day. Five drops of pure Carbolic acid in a quart of water makes a disinfectant solution for sponging the patient. But without fresh air we have found chloride of lime, chloride of soda and all the vaunted antiseptics of little use in the sick room. Hyoscyamus and Baptisia are believed to be good prophylactics for those in attendance either upon patients suffering from some form of the *enteric* or typhus. They should avoid the breath exhaled from the diseased subject. Nurses should not be over-worked or wholly deprived of rest in bed or of frequent walks in the open air. The diet should be generous, as a wholesome preventive in connection with fresh, invigorating air.

Relapsing Fever.

This is a form of continued fever, sudden in its invasion, taking about a week and terminating abruptly in excessive perspiration. The victims are generally in the lowest ranks of life, ill-fed, in filthy over-crowded rooms or houses.

TREATMENT.—The symptoms are quite as severe as those of a sudden invasion of typhus, and to guard against relapses the Hypo-sulphite of Soda has been employed successfully in three grain doses. In other respects the disease must be treated in accordance with the symptoms. China 3x dil., Podophyllum 3x, as well as Ars. ?x dil., may be consulted. Camphor and Nux vom. are believed to be good prophylactics.

Careful nursing is required, light nutritious food should be liberally supplied, with all the hygienic supplies mentioned for the treatment of enteric fever.

Yellow Fever.

This fever for short has been styled the Black vomit. It is a specific acute, continuous fever accompanied with jaundice, internal hæmorrhages, black vomit and black stools, pain about the epigastrium, severe headache and delirium. It is a tropical fever and must not be confounded with fevers of a malarial type. It is a specific disease and described as a pestilential infection and malignant scourge. The late Dr. Hering maintained that Carbo veg. was a specific and should be administered in the crudest form capable of being imbibed into the system.

It has prevailed in the Southern States and West Indies, and the mortality has been frightful. Its origin is supposed to be from the rapid decomposition of vegetable matter in the tropics and its duration is brief and its most fatal period is from the fourth to the sixth day. It comes on with a violent chill and follows rapidly with intense fever, burning, dry, hot skin, excruciating backache. and pain in the head and limbs.

TREATMENT.—In Allopathic practice massive doses of Calomel and Quinine have been relied on, but the success of this treatment has been unsatisfactory.

HOMŒOPATHIC TREATMENT in skillful hands has greatly reduced the mortality. Camphor tinct., drop doses every half hour in the first stage, followed by Bell. 3x dil., in the second stage, Ars. and Crotalus in the third stage.

Dr. Taft, who several years ago resided in New Orleans, was very successful in the treatment of this disease. In the cold stage he gave Camphor in drop doses every ten minutes.

It was our fortune to have several severe cases in Philadelphia at the time the epidemic was raging so fatally in Norfolk, Va., and we found Camphor indispensable in the first stage, when the patient was suffering from one of those terribly painful aching chills that sometimes would come on in the night without warning. Its primary effect is to reduce the animal temperature, and this is but temporary and therefore a frequent repetition becomes necessiry, after employing the Camphor in the first stage. Acon. 3x dil., in drop doses during the hot burning febrile reaction. Ipecac for the vomiting, in drop doses, of the 3d dil. immediately after each spell; and to meet the congestive tendencies, give Bell. 3x dil., in drop doses hourly. This treatment can be extended to the second and third stage. In addition to the above, consult the following remedies in the 3x dil. and select according to the symptoms. Drs. Holcomb and Davis, who had charge of the Mississippi State Hospital at Natches, relied on making a selection from Ars., Lach., Crotalus, Mercurius, Colocynth and Veratrum in the lowest attenuation. Their success eclipses that of the most skillful physicians of the old school. Dr. Taft in New Orleans was so successful in the treatment of yellow fever that the old thorough treatment was cast into the shade. China, Rhus tox. and Carbo veg. also enter largely into his treatment, 1st, 2d and 3d attenuations.

DIET.—Arrow root, in water, black tea with a little sugar and cream in it, in the first stages. Small bits of ice may be taken into the mouth to relieve the thirst.

The Plague.

Some pathologists have classed this disease with malignant typhus, which in many respects it resembles, the only phenomens which distinguishes it being the different buboes and carbuncles which manifest themselves on the surface of the body, and yet by many it is regarded nothing more than a genuine typhus fever, rendered peculiarly severe, putrid and malignant by the atmosphere, and other influences in those regions where it has prevailed.

As in the most formidable cases of typhus, maculæ, petechiæ, diarrhœa, hæmorrhage from the bowels, etc., generally supervene in the last stage, in addition to the buboes and carbuncles. The conclusion is inevitable that the plague and these cases in the light of pathological science are identical.

But in this country, so far from the localities where this disease has prevailed, our knowledge is so limited, being simply derived from imperfect descriptions, that it would be useless for us to attempt to detail the symptoms.

TREATMENT.—But if from the information we have gathered, we may be allowed to judge of its nature, we should unhesitatingly recommend a treatment similar to what has been found useful in typhus, Ars., Mur. acid, Nit. acid, Baptisia, Mercurius, Hep. sulph. and Sulphur.

Dengue Fever.

This is known as an ephemeral continued fever, an epidemic and perhaps infectious fever, having an eruption like measles, cerebral headache, and severe rheumatic or neuralgic pains in the back and limbs, joints and trunk, which give to patients a stiff and awkward gait; on this account it is also called dandy fever.

This fever is seldom fatal; it lasts eight or ten days, or longer. Patients suffering from this fever are liable during convalescence to suffer from relapses. But one attack of the disease is said to leave no predisponent behind, and consequently the patient is exempt from future attacks.

This disease has prevailed in the Southern States and West Indies. It has been styled the break bone fever in Philadelphia and Virginia, and an eruptive rheumatic fever elsewhere. It is known as the dandy fever in the West Indies and Louisiana.

DIAGNOSIS.—The attack comes suddenly, commencing with vomiting, headache, pains in the back, limbs and joints, but no rigors or chills. The joints become swollen and painful; the lymphatic glands of the neck, axilla, groins, and testes, pain in the eyeballs. The skin soon becomes hot and dry, the pulse varies from rapidity to infrequency, small and feeble, the face is flushed, the appetite is lost, while there is great thirst; the eyes are red and watery, the tongue is red and clean; the bowels are torpid, violent cramps in different parts of the body sometimes occur. The fever remits about the third day, and then returns with pain in the back and limbs, accompanied by an eruption; this appears in the form of a scarlet efflorescence, first on the palms, then on the whole body, affording some relief from the fever. There is no uniformity in the eruption; sometimes it simulates measles, scarlet fever, chicken pox or herpes, often with an apparent mixture of the whole. If there are no complications the complaint gradually subsides in a week or ten days. There is however an unpleasant sequel, the patient suffers from neuralgia and rheumatic pains and is physically and mentally depressed.

TREATMENT.—The Allopathic treatment consists of Calomel and Rhubarb, with palpable doses of Sulp. Quinine.

HOMŒOPATHIC TREATMENT consists in the employment of Aconite 3x, dil., drop doses every two hours, for the inflammatory symptoms; for rheumatic swelling of the joints with tenderness and pain, Bry.; Rhus., prepared and given as directed for the acute; *Clematis* for pains, and swelling of the testes; Gel., for developing the eruption; Veratrum album, for cramps; Phyts., Ars., Sulph., are good remedies during convalescence, each in the 3x, dil. Eupatorium, 1x, dil., for the breakbone symptoms.

CHAPTER XXXIX.

THE NERVOUS SYSTEM.

It must be conceded that a very great proportion of the diseases incident to mankind, have their seat in the nervous system; —it is therefore requisite that the general nature of the functions of the nervous system should be well understood, in order to be able to learn accurately the nature of the interruptions to which they are subject from disease.

The mind evidently is connected with the nervous system on the one hand, while the contractile and sensitive parts are connected with it on the other. It may fairly be presumed then, that the inmost powers of the physical system are to be sought for in the nervous centers, and the nerves proceeding from them. It is therefore thought advisable to present a concise view of the anatomy and physiology of the nervous system, as an introduction to a consideration of the diseases incident to it.

The nervous system is divided into two parts; one portion is denominated the *cerebro-spinal system*, and the other is termed the ganglionic system; and though each possesses many properties common to both, yet each has a distinct office to perform in the animal economy, and to promote this end each has a certain peculiarity of structure, and mode of action corresponding to its range of influence.

Bichat denominated the cerebro-spinal system, " *the nervous system of animal life*," because it includes all the nervous organs through which sensation, volition and mental manifestation, the peculiar characteristics of animals, become apparent. This system includes the brain and spinal cord, and all the nerves proceeding from them, together with the several ganglia seated upon these nerves or that form a part of the substance of the brain.

The same author denominated the ganglionic system, the *nervous system of organic life*, because it performs a mediatorial office between the animal and organic functions. This system extends from the cranium to the pelvis, along each side of the vertebral column; it consists of a double chain of ganglia con-

nected by nervous cords, from which nerves with ganglia proceed
to the viscera of the thorax, abdomen and pelvis. From the nature of its distribution it will be observed that it has less immediate connection with the mind, either as communicating sensations, or receiving the impulses of the will; and by its peculiar
mode of action it will be seen that it has a closer connection with
the processes of the organic functions than the cerebro-spinal system, and moreover by its peculiar attachments and relations to
this system, it would seem to be the channel through which all
that is really peculiar to animal life may exert a controlling influence over the processes of organic life, to render them subservient
to the animal kingdom.

It is only in the higher orders of animals and in man, that
these two systems seem to be so distinct, and yet so harmonious
in their separate modes of action. The differences between them
are not so very essential, since their composition may be said to
be the same. Their actions differ in degree, and for different objects,—yet the kind of action as well as their modes of action are
essentially the same.

In the lower animals all the nervous functions are performed
through a single system, corresponding with the cerebro-spinal
system of the vertebrate animals; and even among this class
many of the functions which are controlled in the warm-blooded
by the ganglionic nerves, are controlled in the cold-blooded by
the pneumogastric cerebral nerves.

In noting the peculiarities of the inorganic and the organic
world the fact becomes apparent that the powers and processes that
control in the inferior orders of nature become subservient to
processes of a higher grade in the higher orders; for example, the
physical forces of the mineral kingdom, that under all circumstances
and conditions control the inorganic elements, are no less the property of the vegetable kingdom, but here they become subject to the
processes of organic life, which usurp complete control in the
vegetable kingdom; and further, the processes of organic life that
control in the vegetable kingdom are assumed and controlled by
those which are still higher in the animal kingdom; for as every
thing in the mineral kingdom becomes fashioned into the image
and likeness of the vegetable, so every thing in the vegetable becomes fashioned into the image and likeness of the animal. It is
by the superinduction of the nervous system in animals and in

man that all the processes carried on in the inferior kingdoms of nature become subservient to the controlling influences of animal life. A system therefore so important, and one that particularly characterizes the elevated position of man in the order of creation, demands the most careful consideration, and the following order may be observed in the investigation of the structure and function of the nervous system.

1st. *Elementary structure of the nervous system.* The two nervous systems are made up of *nervous centres* and *nerves.* There are two kinds of structure entering into their composition, *vesicular* and *fibrous;* both of these structures are regarded absolutely essential in the formation of the simplest nervous system.

In the nervous centers the vesicular and nervous matter are mingled together in masses, and wherever these two kinds of matters are found, and the vesicular matter is mingled with the fibrous, it may be inferred that the generation of nervous force takes place and it must be regarded a nervous centre. The mingling of the vesicular matter with the fibrous in masses is found in the brain, spinal cord, and the several ganglia; these therefore are the nervous centres of the nervous system. Nervous force being generated in the nervous centres, requires as a matter of course, appropriate channels to convey it to the periphery of the animal body, and these channels are the *nerves,* which are constructed entirely of the fibrous nervous matter, and distributed in the several parts of the body, for the purpose of conveying nervous force to them, or of transmitting to the nervous centres the impressions made by stimuli. Impressions or conditions are simply conducted along the nerve fibres; they may be made to deviate from a direct course in the nervous centres, and be reflected, diffused or otherwise disposed of. The particular structure of nerves is of minute fibres or tubuli filled with nervous matter arranged in bundles of parallel or interlacing fibres; and these bundles are connected by intervening fibro cellular tissue in which the blood-vessels of the nerves ramify; a layer of the same tissue also surrounds the whole nerve, and constitutes its *neurolemma* or sheath.

There are two kinds of nerve fibres observed mingling in most nerves throughout the body. One kind is the most numerous in the nerves of the cerebo-spinal system, and the other the most numerous in the sympathetic system.

The fibres of the nerves of the cerebo-spinal system consist of tubules of simple membrane, remarkably pellucid, within which is contained the proper nerve substance, a transparent oil-like material, which gives to each fibre somewhat the appearance of a perfectly transparent glass tube filled with a fluid of a corresponding character. This is the appearance of the recently fresh fibres, but after a little time elapses after death, these same fibres change their appearance so as to render it quite evident that their contents are composed of two different materials, the internal or central part occupying what is termed the axis of the tubes, becomes grayish, while the outer or cortical portion becomes opaque and grumous, as if from a kind of coagulation; at the same time the transparent cylindrical tube is exchanged for an opaque double contour, the outer of which being formed by the sheath of the fibre and the inner by the margin of curdled medullary substance. Little masses of granular material soon begin to collect, which distend some portions of the tube, and cause others to collapse, so as to impart a bended appearance to the structure instead of their former cylindrical form.

By reason of the marked difference produced upon the contents of the nerve fibre when exposed to the same conditions, the opinion has been entertained, that the central and circumferential portions of each nerve fibre differ in their essential characteristics. The central portion has on this account been named by some the *axis cylinder*, and by others the *primitive band*. The outer portion is usually described under the name of the *white substance* of Schwann, which gives to the cerebro-spinal nerves their peculiar white aspect. When the nerve tubules are pressed, their contents readily pass from one portion of the tubular sheath to another, being extremely soft. The size of nerve fibres varies from $\frac{1}{14000}$ to $\frac{1}{2000}$ of an inch in diameter, the smallest being found in the fibrous matter of the brain and spinal cord.

The *fibres of the second* kind, are found abundantly in the trunks and branches of the ganglionic nerves, and they mingle somewhat with other fibres in the cerebro-spinal nerves. They differ from the fibres of the first kind: 1st, in being only about one-half to one-third the size. 2d. They have not the double contour, as have the first and fourth, their contents are apparently uniform. 3d. They wear a yellowish-gray aspect, instead of the peculiar white aspect of the cerebro-spinal nerves. These characteristics render it probable that they differ from the other nerve fibres in not having the outer layer of white or medullary nerve substance; their contents are seemingly composed throughout of the substance corresponding with the axis-cylinder, or primitive band of the larger fibres.

There appears to be a third kind of fibre intermediate between the two above described, having somewhat the peculiarities of both—which perhaps may be sufficiently indicative that the two kinds of nervous fibre may not be so essentially different as to ·lead to the supposition that a material difference, either in their office or mode of action, must inevitably be maintained.

Every nerve fibre proceeds uninteruptedly from its center or origin, to its destination, without branching, anastomosing or forming any direct union whatever with the substance of any other fibres, and it matters not whether its destination be at the periphery of the body, another nervous centre, or the same centre of its origin.

Bundles of fibres may lie in apposition with each other and run together in the nerves, but they never unite; where the bundles appear to anastomose there is no union of the fibres, but only an interchange of fibres between the fascicula or bundles. It will therefore appear that the central extremity of each fibre is connected with the peripheral extremity of a single nervous fibre only, and this extremity is in direct relation to only one point in its nervous centre, whether this point be in the brain, spinal cord, or other nervous centre. It is therefore plain, that all the nerves distributed to the periphery of the body, are represented by corresponding parts of the large nervous centre; that each nerve is represented by its corresponding centre, and that each of the millions of primitive fibres which are distributed to the peripheral points of the body, is represented by a corresponding point in either the one or the other of the nervous centres; each nerve may proceed from its ganglion and each fibre from its vesicle—thus presenting the sublime view of a centre within a centre, corresponding, 1st, to all the nerves, and 2d, to each separate nerve, and 3d, to each separate fibre of which the nerves are composed.

The nerves at certain parts of their course, form what is termed *plexuses*, in which they anastomose with each other and exchange fasciculi ; the object of such interchange of fibres is apparently to give to each nerve passing off from the plexus, a more extensive connection with the spinal cord, as this would evidently be the case, by communicating with other nerves. The most familiar examples of the communication of nerves in forming of plexuses, are found in the brachial and lumbar plexuses. The brachial is formed by the intermingling of fasciculi from the last four of the cervical nerves, and the first dorsal. It will be perceived from this intermingling, that the parts supplied with the brachial plexus become more extensively related to the nervous centres and more extensive sympathies.

The nerve fibres have a *central termination* in the nervous centres, and a *peripheral termination* in the parts which they supply.

The nerve fibres are said to form a delicate *terminal plexus* as they approach their final and minutest distribution in the several tissues, in small nerves or bundles, which divide, break up, and give off the primitive fibres to be disposed of in various ways, in different tissues. It is difficult to describe the manner in which they terminate, several different modes have been noted, as follows :

1. They terminate in *loops*, each fibre after issuing from a branch in a terminal plexus, runs over the elementary structures of the containing tissue, then turns back and joins the same or a neighbouring branch in which it proceeds back again to the nervous centre; examples of this arrangement are found in the internal ear, papillæ of the tongue, papillæ of the skin, and some other tissues.

2. They terminate in *plexuses* in certain serous membranes, as in the arachnoid of the brain and spinal cord, and other serous membranes.

3. They terminate by *free ends*, as in the *retina* and in the pacchionian corpuscles of the skin.

4. They terminate according to Wagner, by the large nerve fibres suddenly breaking up into numerous branches, anastomosing and forming a net-work, giving off branches which seem to become lost in the substance of the tissue in which they are distributed.

The above constitute the chief modes of the peripheral termination of the nerve fibres; but their *central termination* is in vesicles in the nervous centres, as before stated. These vesicles or *nerve* corpuscles have a variety of shapes, and are described as the *simple stellate* or *caudate*, etc. *The function of the nerve fibres* is simply to convey or conduct nervous impressions, and this is of a two-fold character. First, any impression made upon their peripheral extremities, or any part of their course, they convey to the nervous centres; and it is for this reason, that the mind through the brain is able to take cognizance of external objects. Second, they serve to convey impressions from the brain and other nervous centres to the parts where the nerves are distributed.

These impressions appear to be of at least two kinds; such as excite muscular contractions, and such as influence the organic functions, secretion, nutrition, etc.

To fulfill the two-fold office of nerve fibres, two distinct sets of them are provided in both the cerebro-spinal and ganglionic systems; and in general terms they are called *afferent* and *efferent*.

The *afferent* are those which conduct impressions from the periphery to the centre. In the cerebro-spinal system, they are termed *sensitive*. The *efferent* are employed to transmit central impulses to the muscles, and are termed *motor*, as belonging to the *nerves of motion;* both of these offices of the nerve fibres, appear to exercise influence in functions of secretion and nutrition.

Nerve fibres appear to possess no power of originating impulses to action, or of generating nervous force; they require to be stimulated in order to enable them to manifest their peculiar endowments. The property which the fibres actually possess is that of conducting impressions; this property has been named *excitability*, but it always requires the application of some stimulus to produce this property. Those nerves which convey sensations to the brain, are stimulated by external objects acting on their extremities; and those connected with locomotion or motion, are acted upon by the will, or by some force generated in the nervous centers. Almost everything that interrupts the pressiveness of the nerves, may in some sense be regarded a stimulus. But it is to be observed that a stimulus applied to the motor fibres will produce motion, but if the same stimulus be applied to the nerves of sensation, or rather to the fibres of the sensitive nerves, sensation will be produced. It is not necessary to enumerate the various stimuli that will give rise to excitability; in general terms it may be said to be mechanical irritation, chemical stimuli, electricity, magnetism, etc.

Nerve force moves with inconceivable velocity along the nerve fibre; in a moment, in the twinkling of an eye, a single mandate of the will controls all the motive fibres of the body and any impression from any source whatever made upon the peripheral extremities of the nerves of sensation, is as rapidly conveyed to the nervous centres.

Mechanical irritation so violent as to injure the texture of nerve fibres may prove an obstruction to nerve force, so that a stimulus applied to the nerve more distant from the nervous center than the injured spot, will fail of producing sensation; and any injury done to the fibres of the motor nerves operates as an obstruction to the mandates of the will, in producing muscular contraction, more distant from the nervous centre than the point of injury.

It must be observed also, that no nerve fibre can convey more than one kind of impression; a motor fibre can only convey motor impulses, or such as contribute to motion in contractile parts, and a sensitive fibre can only convey such an impression as may produce sensation if propagated to the brain. The fibres of the nerves of the special senses can only convey their peculiar sensations; as, the optic that of light, and the auditory that of sound. Neither the rays of the former, nor the sonorous vibrations of the latter, can influence the nerves of common sensation, but other stimuli which may be productive of pain when applied to the nerves of special sense, may produce morbid sensations of light, or sound, or taste, according to the nerve on which the impression is made. This fact is important in a pathological point of view, as a correct interpretation thereof may often aid in forming a more accurate idea of diseased action.

Impressions conveying sensations may be made upon any point of a nerve; thus when parts are deprived of sensibility by compression or division of the nerve supplying them, irritation of the portion connected with the brain still excites sensation as sensibly as if connected with the peripheral portion. This accounts for the violent pain sometimes experienced from a paralyzed limb, when the limb itself is totally insensible of any impression; the sound part of the trunk of the nerve in connection with the brain being irritated, while that portion distributed to the limb is void of any sense or feeling. When a nerve is divided, there is no possibility of any impression made upon its cutaneous extremity being conveyed to the brain, but the same sensations which were before produced by external impressions may result from internal causes. This accounts for the fact that when a part of the limb is amputated, the remaining part of the nerves which were distributed to it, gives rise to sensations, which the mind refers to the lost portion; as for instance, when the stump and divided nerves become inflamed, the patient complains of pain as if felt in the part removed. When the stump is healed, after a hand or foot has been amputated, the sensations commonly felt when these limbs are sound, even to the extremities of the fingers and toes, are still felt.

There are many interesting facts illustrative of the peculiar characteristics of the nerves which might be cited in addition to the above, but our object being to consider the general physiology of the nervous system with reference to diseases incident to the same, we will pass to a consideration of the *function of the nervous centres*.

As before remarked, every nerve and every fibre terminates in a centre. All parts of the nervous system which contain ganglion corpuscles, or vesicular nerve substance—the brain, spinal cord, and the several ganglia which belong to the cerebro-spinal and ganglionic systems, the term *nervous centre* is applied.

Each of the nervous centres has a distinct function to perform in the body that bears a direct proportion to the number of nerve fibres that connect it with the various organs, and with the other nervous centres; but there are general properties common to all nervous centres.

All nervous power or force is believed to be generated in the nervous centres, whether it be the impulse by which the muscles are excited to action, or the force that maintains and controls the organic functions; but this is only true in a dependent or qualified sense, for the brain does not issue any impulse only when it is impressed by the will or stimulated by impressions from without. Neither do the other nervous centres impart any power only as it is called out by previous impressions. For example: the ganglia connected with the organic functions do not give out the nervous force necessary to the contractions of the intestines, only as stimulated by substances already in the intestinal canal.

It is the specific office of the nervous centres throughout the body, unquestionably, to variously dispose of or to transfer the impressions that reach them through their many centripetal nerve fibres. All impressions are conveyed to the centres along the simple course of the fibre and communicated, but they are *perceived* only in the brain.

To illustrate more fully what is understood by *conduction in or through nervous centres*, the following example may be cited: food taken into the stomach acts as a stimulant, producing a certain impression on the nerves in the mucous membrane of the organ; this impression is conveyed through them to the adjacent ganglia of the sympathetic system; ordinarily, this would call forth a force from the ganglia that would result in a movement of the muscular coat of the stomach and the adjacent parts; but if the food should contain any thing detrimental to the interests of the economy, a sharper irritation than the food is capable of imparting may be conducted through the nearest ganglia to others more remote and more distant, causing an influence to be sent back upon the organic functions that either paralyzes their efforts or enhances their activity to a degree that draws forcibly upon the vitality of the system. Irritation may be conducted through all the sympathetic ganglia, and farther to the ganglia of the spinal nerves, and through them to the spinal cord, whence may react that kind of motor impulses sometimes witnessed in the abdominal and other muscles, producing cramp. From the spinal cord, the same impression may be sent to the brain, and to the mind itself in a reverse direction. The mind may act on the brain, and send its influence from them to the cord, the ganglia of the spinal nerves, sympathetic ganglia, and back so far as to exert its influence upon the stomach and neighboring parts.

The nervous system in man, composed as it is of nervous centres and nerves, is so connected in all its parts as to produce the most intimate relation between the motive and sensitive fibres. The sympathetic system when in health may receive normal impressions without a palpable conveyance of them to the sensorium, as may the normal operations of the sensorium take place without producing any perceptible modification of the organic functions; but any unnatural impression made upon either may sensibly affect the other.

Impressions may be *transferred, diffused or reflected;* as for instance, an *impression* made upon the nerves of the hip-joint, may be conveyed to the spinal cord, and from thence to the central ends of the nerve fibres of the knee-joint, and through these the transferred impression is conducted to the brain. This accounts for the mind taking cognizance of the disease as existing in the knee instead of the hip. Sometimes, however, the primary impression is conveyed from the hip, and then the pain is felt in both the hip and the knee. An impression is said to be *diffused,* when it is received at a nervous centre, and diffused to other fibes in the same centre, produces sensations over an indefinite area; hence result various kinds of impressions, denominated *sympathetic.* Sometimes such sensations are referred to every part of the body. *Reflected impressions* are such as are communicated from sensitive to motor fibres; as for instance, light falling upon the retina contracts the iris; and more extensively, when an irritation in the larynx conveyed to the sensorium brings all the muscles engaged in expiration into coincident action.

In order to apprehend more conclusively the nature of diseases pertaining to the nervous system, a more thorough acquaintance with the nature of these various kinds of impressing is requisite, and the reader is recommended to works on the nervous system, that he may become as familiar as possible with its physiology; our space will only permit an outline view.

The specific functions of various portions of the nervous system commend themselves for careful consideration.

The cerebro-spinal nervous system includes the brain, medulla oblongata, the spinal cord, the nerves going from them; and the functions in general of these several portions must be well understood in order to note with any degree of accuracy an interruption of them. From what has been stated, it will be perceived that the nervous system is not only the essential instrument of vital association but of vital endowment, and therefore present in every part of the body. The nerves may be divided into three classes, as follows:

First.—The cerebral, or the sentient and voluntary.

Secondly.—The true spinal, or excito-motory.

Thirdly.—The ganglionic, or the nutrient and secretory.

Without pursuing the physiology of the nervous system farther, as preliminary to the consideration of the diseases incident to it, we will remark, that it will be necessary to have frequent reference to the physiology of the parts where the disease is manifest. We will first consider the characteristics of the various diseases incident to the nervous centres.

CHAPTER XI.

The nervous centres of the cerebro-spinal system are each protected with coverings or meninges, which often become the seat of disease; these will be duly considered in the following pages. The nervous centres often become the seat of congestion, which may be considered in the following order: 1st, of congestion, or hyperæmia of the cerebrum; 2d, of the cerebellum; and 3d, of the medulla spinalis.

Congestion, or Hyperæmia of the Cerebrum.

By congestion is understood an accumulation of blood in the vessels of some portion of the centre, and when it occurs in the cerebrum the following symptoms are apparent: when slight, there is merely pain in the head, vertigo, confusion and disposition to sleep; the intellectual faculties may not be disturbed, sensibility and the power of motion may remain unimpaired; at other times, there may be retarded movements, or the reverse, an incessant desire to be moving, and sometimes, though seldom, accelerated movement, may result. Formication is sometimes felt on one or both sides of the face, and in the limbs.

The *pulse* is full and strong, very tense and vibratory; the temporal and carotid arteries beat violently, although the pulsations of the heart may betray nothing abnormal.

The *face* generally becomes red; the *eyes* injected; and sometimes *epistaxis* succeeds these indications.

Sometimes fever attends these symptoms, and at other times they are unattended by any febrile excitement.

The hyperæmia may continue for a short or longer period, recurring frequently, and sometimes at regular seasons, as for example, every evening; or at more distant intervals, as spring and autumn. When it is extensive, the patient sustains a sudden loss of consciousness, and falls down as if deprived of life. He may remain in this condition for a length of time, deprived in a great measure of sensation, volition and mental manifestation. Death may take place in a very short time, or restoration may speedily ensue; some slight impairment of the intellect may be apparent for a short time, the speech may be somewhat affected, and not unfrequently the sight or hearing becomes temporarily impaired. This disease having been described frequently as *a form of apoplexy, determination of the blood to the head*, etc., may be distinguished from that which is termed hemiplegia, on the account of there being only an ephemeral debility, either general or partial, and not permanent paralysis, as is the case when there is an arterial, cerebral hæmorrhage. Paralysis of the entire side of the body may take place from hyperæmia of the cerebrum, but it differs from that which takes place from hæmorrhage in the cerebrum in being of short duration only. There are, however, some exceptions to this rule, as cases of permanent paralysis have occurred from a mere congestion of the blood vessels of the cerebrum, without the slightest traces of there being any evidence of hæmorrhage. This form is generally attended with convulsions and ephemeral paralysis of important organs, as the tongue.

Sometimes persons are attacked several times a day with *rush of blood to the head*, impairing for a short period the functions of sensibility and locomotion, and sometimes the difficulty may be indicated only by intellectual disturbance, with scarcely any impairment of sensibility or mobility. In this case the delirium is intense, and the patient may exhibit immense muscular power. Death, for the want of nervous supply to the respiratory apparatus, sometimes takes place suddenly, when this symptom supervenes, the face appearing florid and swollen, and at times livid and black.

CAUSES.—The causes of hyperæmia or cerebral congestion are various; sudden changes from the extremes of temperature, or exposure to a very cold atmosphere, may be recorded among the prominent causes; anything that produces irregularity of action of the blood vessels of the brain, may produce hyperæmia in that viscus, and anything that interrupts the general circulation may also occasion the difficulty. Copious blood-letting, and other debilitating losses such as are brought about through hæmorrhages, may also be recorded among the causes that impede the circulation, and result in cerebral congestion. Over doses of Opium, Alcohol, Belladonna, and other narcotics, may also be recorded among the causes.

TREATMENT.—The remedies the most suitable for cerebral congestion are, Aconite, Arnica, Belladonna, Bryonia, Chamomilla, China, Ferrum, Graphites, Ipecac., Mercurius, Nux vom., Opium, Pulsatilla, Sepia, Sulphur, Veratrum, and Zincum.

When the determination of blood to the head is accompanied by a full bounding pulse, flushed face, or the patient complains of fulness and oppressive weight in the forehead, with sensation as though all the contents of the skull would gush through the forehead, or when there is heat in the forehead and redness of the face, *Aconite* 12x dilution, a drop every hour until relieved.

When there is rush of blood to the head, with burning heat in the head, the body being cool or not usually warm, *Arnica* 6x dil., drop doses.

When there is cerebral congestion, with internal and external heat of the head, with distension and throbbing of the cerebral arteries, attended with loss of consciousness, *Belladonna* 6x dil., drop doses.

When in bilious temperaments there is great fulness of the head, with pressure in the direction of the forehead, or pressure from within outwards or the reverse, attended with drowsiness in the day time and slight wandering, and when the symptoms attending the hyperæmia become aggravated by motion, *Bryonia* 6x dil., drop doses.

When there is rush of blood to the head, with beating in the brain, attended with inquietude, moaning and tossing, and particularly when the patient has complained previously of semilateral drawing and tearing in the head, *Chamomilla* 6x dil., drop doses.

Rush of blood to the head, with heat and fulness in the head, in exhausted persons, or in those who have sustained severe losses, *China* 6x dil., drop doses every hour in water.

In persons of feeble constitution, who are subject to alternate constipation and diarrhœa, with headache and painful pressure when in the open air, periodical throbbing headache when attacked with hyperæmia of the cerebrum, *Ferrum* 3x trit., two grains every hour.

When there is mere headache, vertigo, confusion, and a tendency to sleep, without loss of sensibility and the power of motion, and also a humming in the ears and perspiration about the head, *Graphites* 6x.

In cases where the hyperæmia is succeeded by vomiting and aversion to every kind of food, bitter taste in the mouth, pressure in the head, or headache of the most violent character, and vomiting at the same time, with violent distress in the stomach, *Ipecacuanha*.

In bilious temperaments somewhat subject to arthritis or gout, where the subject is prone to nocturnal fevers or disposition to perspire, vertigo in the evening, and headache as if it would fly to pieces, with fulness or hyperæmia of the cerebrum, *Mercurius*.

When there is an increased desire to be moving about, and formication on one or both sides of the limbs and face, irascible and irritable, or very drowsy, severe headache after eating, and rush of blood to the head, with humming in the ears, *Nux vomica*.

When there is felt a heaviness of the head, and stupefaction or headache, aggravated by moving the eyes, or congestion of blood to the head, attended with drowsiness and violent throbbing, *Opium*.

In females subject to painful menstruation and frequent attacks of hyperæmia, *Pulsatilla, Sepia*. These remedies are also well suited to alleviate rush of blood to the head in feeble constitutions and mild dispositions of either sex. When the subjects are of a psoric habit, or possess any hereditary taint, *Sulphur* may precede the use of either.

Bubbling or throbbing headache, caused by rush of blood to the head, especially in the morning, *Sulphur*.

When the rush of blood to the head has been caused by fright, and the head feels as though it would burst, *Veratrum*, and also *Aconite* and *Chamomilla*.

Hyperæmia in scarlatina, *Zincum*.

Aside from the remedies named above, the following may be considered:

When there is headache when sitting, as if there is fulness of the blood-vessels and throbbing in the vertex, and twitching on the forehead and temples, itching in the eyes or vertigo as from intoxication, *Agaricus muscarius*.

For headache in the forehead from staying in a close room, with feeling of weight when turning the eyes, *Agnus castus*.

. Rush of blood to the head, affecting the eyes and nose, and headache as if the hairs were pulled out, pressure in the forehead and bleeding at the nose, augmented during a walk in the open air, *Alumina;* also when the rush of blood is preceded or followed by weak memory and inability to think, *Alumina;* attended with nausea, drowsiness in the day time, vertigo ..nd painful pressure and humming, as if the contents of the skull would issue through the forehead, or as if the head would split, burning in the eyes, *Ammonium c.*

When the rush of blood occasions headache deep in the brain, with sensation as if the head were larger, *Bovista.*

Congestion of the blood to the head, attended with icy coldness in and about the head, tendency to start, obstinate, despairing mood, chilly internally, *Calcarea carb.*

Rush of blood to the head with throbbing in the head, red and hot cheeks, and headache as if a stone were lying on the head, *Cannabis.*

Rush of blood to the head with humming in the ears, and hard of hearing, the occiput feels enlarged, *Dulcamara.*

Painful rush of blood to the head when first commencing to move, *Fluoric acid;* when brought on by mental emotion, *Ignatia;* when brought on by stooping, *Lachesis;* with intense heat in the head, *Nitric acid;* when attended with shocks in the head, *Spigelia;* when there is stupefying pressure of the whole brain, *Ruta graveolens.*

The general function of the cerebral hemispheres being intimately related to the mind, one of the main evidences of their being implicated is the greater or less impairment of the mental manifestation, such as dullness, stupor, loss of mind and memory, delirium, etc. Nearly all cases of hyperæmia, will be indicated to a greater or less degree by some of these phenomena. It is well known that any severe injury to the cerebrum, or sudden pressure by severe rush of blood to the head, may instantly deprive a man of all power of mental manifestation, and that congenital deficiency of the cerebral hemispheres is attended with corresponding feebleness of the intellectual powers.

GENERAL TREATMENT.—During an attack of hyperæmia of the cerebrum, whether the patient is severely afflicted or not, it is better for him to lie with his head low, and if subject to frequent attacks to subsist upon a moderate diet easy of digestion.

The author from many years' experience commends the

higher dilutions and triturations. Hence the 12x to 30x, drop doses every two hours, or two grains of the trituration every three hours until a change.

CHAPTER XLI.

CONGESTION, OR HYPERÆMIA OF THE CEREBELLUM.

The cerebellum is a segment of the encephalon, about which there has been entertained different views. In the opinion of the phrenolgist, it is the seat of sexual love, and were this the exclusive function of the organ it would be easy to detect any local difficulty appertaining thereto. But other physiologists from a variety of experiments, have come to adverse conclusions.

Flourens, experimented in such a way, as to lead him to regard the function of the cerebellum to be the co-ordinator of muscular movements; in removing the cerebellum of birds by successive layers, he found on removing the most superficial, that feebleness and want of harmony of the movements were the consequence. When he reached the middle layers the animals became restless without being convulsed, their movements were violent and irregular, but their sight and hearing were perfect. By the time the last portions of the organ were removed, the animals had entirely lost their power of springing, flying, walking, standing and preserving their equilibrium. When an animal in this state was laid upon its back, it could not recover its former posture, but it fluttered its wings and did not lie in a state of stupor; it saw the blow which threatened it and endeavored to avoid it; volition, sensation, and memory, therefore were not lost, but merely the faculty of combining the actions of the muscles, and the endeavors of the animal to maintain its balance were like those of a drunken man. Similar results were obtained by a repetition of the experiment on different classes of animals, from which *Flourens* inferred that the cerebellum belongs neither to the sensitive nor to the intellectual apparatus, and that it is not the source of voluntary movements, although it belongs to the motor apparatus; but it is the organ for the co-ordination of the voluntary movements, or for the excitement of the combined action of the muscles; comparative anatomy confirms this view, inasmuch as in each of the four classes of vertebrata, the

581

species where natural movements require most frequent and exact combinations of muscular actions are those whose cerebella are most developed in proportion to the spinal cord. On the account of the strength of the evidences, the view of *Flourens* has been generally adopted. But another hypothesis is started by *Foville* that the cerebellum was the seat of the muscular sense, that is, of the sensation derived from muscles, through which the mind acquires that knowledge of their actual state and position which is essential to the exercise of the will upon them. This hypothesis will explain the facts elicited by *Flourens*, perhaps, quite as well as his own inference. But in the absence of perfect physiological knowledge we deem it proper to make use of uncontroverted facts, as far as developed. From the foregoing it might be supposed that complete *congestion* or *hyperæmia* of the blood vessels of the cerebellum would destroy the combination of muscular movements, not destroying the power of the muscles, but occasioning the loss of the power of the will in properly adjusting and controlling them. As the development of the cerebellum is evidently associated with the strength of the muscular system or rather the combined action of the muscles, a partial congestion might be attended with a want of harmonious movement, which difficulty would be increased, as the congestion became more general. We have met with the following cases, which perhaps may serve as a partial delineation of the symptoms that might arise from congestion of the blood-vessels of the cerebellum.

CASE I. A female of bilious temperament, in full possession of consciousness, complained of a sensible fulness at the base of the brain without any definable pain; when she attempted to move her head, she would complain of its going in a direction which she did not contemplate; she manifested a disposition to put forward her chin and throw her head back involuntarily; when she attempted to walk she could exercise the muscles of the lower extremities without being able to control their direction. In attempting to put her hand to the head, she would move it without control in various ways; in short she appeared to know what movements she desired. but could not co-ordinate her muscular movements, so as to effect what she desired. There was also a convulsive twitching of the chin towards the left shoulder. It may be remarked that this lady had previously suffered from attacks of rush of blood to the head, causing her at times, to remain insensible for hours. She had been subject to severe mental disturbance, her pulse was full but not tense, her digestion appeared to be undisturbed, and the usual secretions appeared to be normal. She had been in this condition for some weeks previous to the time I saw her, and at times I learned her respiration had been labored and difficult. Although the symptoms were the only guide for the treatment, I could not avoid the inference that there was hyperæmia of the blood vessels of the cerebellum, which perhaps affected sympathetically the contiguous portions of the base of the brain. She had been subject to Allopathic treatment on former occasions, and her system had evidently been mercurialize l, her *pulse* was somewhat accelerated and evinced a general irritability of the system.

TREATMENT.—The first remedy employed in this case was *Sulphur* 18th, repeated every twenty-four hours for a week; little or no change was produced during the time. *Nux vomica* 6th was then administered for several days with little marked effect, except that she appeared to shudder as from cold. *Conium* 6th was next employed, and after two days the patient could articulate more distinctly, but in other respects, there was scarcely any improvement. *Pulsatilla, Sepia, Belladonna and Aconite*, were severally employed with but little effect. The patient appeared to emaciate, and slight febrile symptoms, and night sweats set in. *Graphites* 30th, was employed for four or five days, three globules daily without effect, after which, *Stannum* 30th was given, which seemed to produce a marked change in the condition of the patient. The twitching of the chin towards the left shoulder ceased, the night sweats passed away with the fever, the sensation of fulness from beneath the occipital suture also became relieved, and from this time the patient gradually recovered.

CASE II. A gentleman about thirty-five years of age, an attorney at law, of sanguineo-bilious temperament, complained at first of severe pressure and pain, at the base of the back part of the head, which was followed by complete loss of power in controlling the movements of the body. When he attempted to walk, his movements would be various, evincing a complete absence of all power to combine the muscular movements necessary in walking. The mental faculties of this gentleman remained unimpaired, there was no perceptible tenderness of the spine, his speech remained perfect, but whether from habit or the effect of the disease, there was a constant inclination to draw up the shoulders, with the head thrown backwards. This man was under the treatment of several of the most eminent Allopathic physicians, for several years. He was treated with moxas, setons, and other topical measures, with no effect whatever. His brother being an eminent Allopathic physician, was his chief medical adviser, and of course debarred him from a trial of Homœopathic treatment. This patient became the father of children during his affliction, but he never recovered. This case is cited because it came under the observation of the writer when a student, and also because there are symptoms, which if properly interpreted might indicate a chronic hyperæmia of the cerebellum.

CASE III. A gentleman of bilious temperament, aged thirty, a merchant by profession, became afflicted with a severe pain in the occiput, which afterwards ceased, leaving a sensation of weight and fulness in the back part of the head near the neck, and a partial derangement of muscular action in walking, which rendered it necessary for him to have the support of another when he ventured the experiment. When the writer first took charge of this case, he found the patient in full possession of his intellectual faculties, with a good appetite, and normal condition of the digestive organs, and regular daily evacuations, and this had been the case, from the best information that could be obtained, from the commencement of his sufferings, a period of thirteen months. He was at first under Allopathic treatment, under which he had to endure a resort to severe topical measures.

TREATMENT.—Sulphur was the first Homœopathic remedy given in this case, followed by *Phosphorus*, each in the sixth dilution; under this treatment, he appeared to rally for awhile, and there seemed to be some promise of complete recovery, but after awhile he relapsed into his former state. *Graphites* 3d, was given without effect. *Conium* 6th appeared to be of service for a while, as also did Belladonna and Bryonia, but soon after an apparent improvement from the use of any remedy he would soon relapse. His friends perceiving that no permanent good resulted from Homœopathic treatment after three months, placed him at a *water cure* establishment, where he was faithfully attended to for four months, during which time he lost about forty pounds in weight, with no improvement of his general health, after which he gradually sank away and died. During his whole illness, his sexual instincts remained without being impaired, and his wife bore him a son one year after he was taken sick. There was no post mortem examination of this case, which is much to be regretted.

CASE IV. A man who died about forty; the following facts were elicited from a post mortem examination: complete congestion of the blood-vessels of the cerebellum, partial congestion of the blood-vessels of the cerebrum. For some weeks previous to death, the patient was averse to exercise, reeled and tottered when he attempted to walk, his bowels were so completely torpid that he had no natural evacuations.

The above cases are sighted, merely for consideration, because they appear to be illustrative of the effects of hyperæmia of the blood-vessels of the cerebellum; but it is by no means certain that this important segment of the encephalon, was the source of all the phenomena detailed. When its physiology is better understood, it is not at all unlikely that we shall be able to detect with greater accuracy, its implication by disease from the manifest symptoms.

The only indications for treatment of diseases implicating the nervous system, are the symptoms; and it strikes us, that as rush of blood to the cerebrum, if not sufficiently severe to interrupt sensation, is accompanied by severe pain and fulness in the sinciput, so a similar hyperæmia of the cerebellum, may give rise to pain, etc., in the occiput, and in the absence of anything more definite, the following indications for the use of remedies when there is pain in the occiput, may be of service:

When there is dull pain in the occiput, accompanied by general febrile symptoms, full bounding pulse, vertigo when rising from a recumbent posture, with reeling, as if intoxicated, *Aconite.*

If the pain is felt in the occiput from concussion, which is sometimes produced by jumping upon the heels when the lower extremities are stiffened from muscular exertion, and not duly flexed, *Arnica.*

In cases where there is aching in the back part of the head, extending to the forehead, with dread of becoming delirious, tearing pains behind the ears, with heat in the head, and tearing, crampy pains, and twitchings and spasms in the muscles, *Ambra grisea.*

Headache in the occiput when making a wrong step, or from a loud noise, accompanied with rigidity in the joints, as if the tendons were too short, or when there is paralytic weakness and languor, *Ammonium muriaticum.*

When there is oppressive pain in the occiput, towards the nape of the neck, and a disposition to feel chilly, and nocturnal twitchings of the muscles all over the body, heaviness in the whole body, emaciation, especially in scrofulous persons, *Baryta carb.*

In cases where there is rush of blood to the head, especially in the occiput, with beating in the brain, and worse in bad weather, accompanied with weakness of the joints and coldness, generally in the afternoon, *Borax.* If also accompanied by sensation as if the head were larger, *Bovista.*

Pain in the occiput, extending to the right side of the head, with eructations and inclination to vomit, congestion of blood to the occiput, and heat in the back part of the head, numbness of single parts, and especially in psoric constitutions, *Calc. carb.*

When the head inclines backwards from a crampy pressure in the occiput, and especially if in sensitive persons, the victims of silent grief, and inclined to weep, *Ignatia.*

Aching in the occiput, especially when walking, in a vexed mood, accompanied by stitches in the ears, and humming as if from rushes of blood, *Kali carb.*

Rush of blood to the occiput, with sensation as if the head had grown larger, and heaviness of the head, pain worse in the open air, *Manganum.* Sensation of pressure in the occiput, *Magnesia muriatica.*

Rush of blood to the head, tensive, spasmodic drawing in the head, especially the occiput and nape of the neck, and especially when attended with hypochondriac and hysteric anxiety, with palpitation of the heart, *Moschus.* Heaviness of the head, especially in the occiput, and particularly if the symptoms occur during a paroxysm of intermittent fever, *Natrum muriaticum.*

For fulness of the head, especially in the occiput, with stitches all through the head, or rush of blood to the head, with heat in the back part of the head, *Nitric acid.* This remedy is best suited to syphilitic subjects, when there is a tendency to caries of the bones or rickets.

Rush of blood to the head, with humming in the ears, and heat and pain in the occiput, arising from a sudden cold, *Nux vomica.* Throbbing headache in the occiput, and sensation as if everything in the head were alive, *Petroleum. Sepia* is especially suitable for females, when suffering from rush of blood to the head, and beating headache, especially in the occiput, heat in the head, and particularly when stooping. *Spigelia,* is suitable for painfulness of the occiput, with sensations of stiffness as if gone to sleep in the nape of the neck, and when the pressure in the head is worse when stooping, or when there are shocks in the head when walking in the open air. When the head is drawn backwards with convulsive motions, *Stramonium. Sulphur* is especially indicated, when there is a rush of blood to the head early in the morning, with a feeling of fulness in the head, especially in the occiput. It is particularly indicated, when there is heat in the back part of the head, and drawing and tearing through the head, with a bubbling or throbbing headache, or tingling, roaring and humming in the head, and heat caused by the rush of blood. There are other remedies that act directly upon the occipital region, well calculated to relieve anything like congestion of the cerebellum, which is probably attended in its incipient stage with more or less pain in the occiput.

DIET.—During treatment, should be light but nutritious.

Congestion or Hyperæmia of the Spinal Cord.

It is by no means probable, that congestion of the blood-vessels of the spinal cord, ever becomes general, although certain portions may become implicated, and under such circumstances, the organs to which the nerves proceeding from these portions are distributed, become to a greater or less extent implicated.

If congestion occurs in the superior or thoracic portion of the cord, the superior portion of the trunk is affected; but if the same occurs in the region of the sacrum or lumbar vertebræ, the abdominal portion of the trunk becomes affected.

SYMPTOMS.—Congestion of the blood-vessels of the spinal marrow, if located in the dorsal portion, may give rise to oppressed respiration, dyspnœa, sometimes cough, increased sensibilities of the tissues of the lungs, and increased or diminished sensibility of different parts of the frame; increased or diminished mobility of the upper extremities, and paralysis. If the congestion occurs in the lumbar region, various phenomena occur, with reference to the abdominal organs. There may be paralysis of the bladder, and other organs, constipation as well as pain, in the region affected. The difficulty may terminate spontaneously, after a short or longer duration, or it may become chronic, or end in death.

CAUSES.—Supposed to be the same as affect the organism in producing other congestions.

TREATMENT.—The treatment of hyperæmia of the spinal marrow, is nearly the same as that for other local congestion.

When there is an indication of congestion in the dorsal region, affecting the function of the lungs, and the muscles of the upper extremities, with sensation of heat over the region of the dorsal vertebræ, *Aconite* may be given and repeated several times, and afterwards *Belladonna*, if the Aconite fails of affording complete relief.

When there is pain and heat in the back or spine, that has been occasioned by contusion or mechanical injury, affecting the organs of respiration, as above, and there is a full pulse, and the patient complains of feeling sore in the affected region, and particularly if there is anything like paralytic weakness in the thoracic extremity, *Arnica* and *Hypericum* may afford relief.

If the difficulty occurs in females of lymphatic temperament, of mild or sensitive disposition, or if attended with anything like derangement of the menstrual function, *Pulsatilla* has been known to afford relief.

Note.—All the remedies named in the treatment of the diseases of the nervous centres should be given in the 6x or 10x dil., except otherwise expressed.

In a case of apparent congestion of the blood-vessels of the lumbar portion of the medulla, which was characterized by pain and heat in the lumbar region, obliging the patient to lie on the back for the sake of ease, and also affecting the abdominal muscles with a paralytic weakness that interrupted all efforts for the evacuation of the bowels or bladder, *Belladonna* afforded relief, and *Nux vomica* completed the cure. The patient was of sanguine temperament, aged about twenty-five years.

In the case of a male, aged forty-two years, of leuco-phlegmatic temperament, where there was pain and heat extending from the sacrum to the inferior dorsal vertebræ, attended with loss of power in the lower extremities and the muscles of the abdomen, *Nux vomica* afforded partial relief, and *Conium* completed the cure.

Attending congestions of different portions of the medulla spinalis, which in most cases, will be denoted by heat and pain in the region, different groups of symptoms may arise, which will require corresponding Homœopathic remedies. *Aconite, Belladonna, Nux vomica, Rhus tox., Bryonia, Sulphur, Calcarea,* and many other remedies will be found serviceable, if otherwise indicated.

When individuals are subject to attacks of hyperæmia of the nervous centres, too much care cannot be exercised to avoid all excitement, and total abstinence from all intoxicating drinks cannot be too strongly recommended. Regular exercise is recommended, and even enjoined, and, also a moderate diet, with only a small portion of fluid, in order to avoid repletion of the vessels.

To facilitate the return of blood to the extremities, patients should not be suffered to remain too long in a horizontal position, and during attacks of hyperæmia of the encephalon, it would be as well for the head to be slightly elevated. The extremes of heat and cold should be avoided as much as possible, and too much sleep is to be avoided, as having a pernicious tendency.

As in the employment of remedies, symptoms must be the guide, and as every remedy in all probability, acts directly upon some specific locality, there cannot be too much care exercised, in the study and right interpretation of the symptoms, and the proper affiliation of the remedies.

CHAPTER XLII.

INFLAMMATION OF THE NERVOUS CENTRES.

Although the nervous centres have numerous anatomical divisions, and each performing specific functions, yet the researches of physiologists have not been sufficiently extensive to enable us from symptoms to locate the precise seat of inflammations, as they take place. In general, we can distinguish inflammation of the encephalon, from that of the medulla spinalis; but it is not always easy to determine between that of the cerebrum, cerebellum, and medulla oblongata, and when we have decided in general terms, that the inflammation is encephalitis or myelitis, there is no means of being positive whether it affects the medullary substance, or the membranes that invest it. In the treatment, therefore, of inflammations of the nervous centres, the symptoms must be the guide.

As the intellectual faculties are supposed to be seated at the periphery of the brain, it has been supposed, that much delirium accompanying other signs of inflammation, indicates that the seat of the inflammation is in the meninges or peripheral portion of the brain.

On the other hand, somnolency, convulsions, and want of power over the apparatus of voluntary motion, have been regarded as indications of deeper seated inflammation; we will therefore proceed to describe the symptoms of

Encephalitis.

SYMPTOMS.—The encephalon being the seat of sensation, volition, and mental manifestation, an attack of inflammation will modify these faculties to a greater or less degree, according to severity and extent, as well as in accordance with the seat and character of the inflammation;—hence, some cases will be characterized by violent delirium, augmented by every impression made upon the sensorium; the slightest noise may bring on a paroxysm. This, at times, continues throughout the whole duration of the disease, but when it is about terminating fatally,

590

coma takes its place. There is usually sleeplessness and great restlessness. In other cases, patients appear morose, and unwilling to be disturbed. In some cases the intellect remains unaffected. The earliest symptoms, are violent excruciating pain in the head, increased by light or noise, at times the skin is unusually sensitive,—the sight and hearing depraved; flashes of light, detonations and singular noises are heard. At a later period, the senses become less acute. Vomiting may mark the onset of the disease; sometimes the bowels may be deranged; at other times, the concentration of the forces to the encephalon are so great that complete constipation is the result.

The presence of encephalitis may also be indicated by disordered motion, and much agitation, tremors, convulsions, and paralysis; sometimes, these symptoms may be general,—at other times, only partial, implicating certain muscles.

Respiration is more or less affected; sometimes labored, hurried, and not unfrequently stertorous, when the inflammation is severe.

Encephalitis in children, may often come on insidiously; the child may be dull and restless, the pupils may be contracted, and there may be sensibility to light and sound, and more or less headache. These symptoms should always enlist the attention of the physician, or before he is aware, convulsions, or some other positive signs of encephalitis may occur. Sometimes, inflammatory fever and congestion precede encephalitis, or violent delirium may be the only indication of its presence. But this symptom may exist when there is merely fever without the actual existence of encephalitis; disordered bowels in children during febrile affections, are often attended with slight delirium, which is sympathetic, rather than actual inflammation of the encephalon.

As a general rule encephalitis in the first stage is indicated by exaltation of the functions of sensibility and in the second and final stage the patient sinks into insensibility, coma or paralysis, with dilated pupils that do not contract on the approach of light.

Sometimes the disease destroys in a day, at others it is protracted and passes through several stages and ends in restoration to health or gradual sinking away. Often in cases of recovery, some of the functions are liable to remain permanently impaired;

strabismus, deafness, and dementia, have been the most commonly observed.

CAUSES.—There are numerus causes that may bring on encephalitis; external violence, falls producing concussion of the brain, a fall of considerable force upon the breech or feet, may induce it, though it may be weeks before the inflammation supervenes, exposure to the hot sun, too free an indulgence in the use of stimulants, as wine or alcoholic drinks, excessive mental exertion, teething in children, and febrile diseases generally, may determine themselves to the head and produce encephalitis.

TREATMENT.—The remedies employed in the treatment of this disease, are for the most part, Aconite, Arnica, Arsenicum, Belladonna, Bryonia, Chamomilla, Cuprum metallicum, Hyoscyamus, Ignatia, Ipecacuanha, Mercurius, Nux vom., Opium, Pulsatilla, Phosphorus, Petroleum, Rhus tox., Sulphur, Sepia, Stramonium, Spigelia, Tart. emetic and Veratrum.

When there is an exaltation of the senses, and a dread of light and noise, and considerable headache, which appears to be increasing in severity, and there is any disturbance of the nutritive functions, heat in the head, full, quick pulse, and general febrile condition of the system, *Aconite* should be administered at short intervals until relief or change.

Where the symptoms of encephalitis supervene upon a fall or blow, producing symptoms of the brain, and particularly when there is a pressing headache in the forehead with heat in the head; the body being cool or naturally warm, jerking, tearing or stitches in the head, tingling around the eyes, empty eructations and inclination to vomit, *Arnica* may be administered and repeated at intervals of one or two hours until amelioration or change.

If there is a beating pain in the forehead, excessive anxiety and chilliness, or general coldness, followed by fever and vomiting, or with indistinct chilliness and heat, with humming in the ears, burning in the hypogastrium, and great thirst accompanying the usual symptoms of encephalitis, great prostration or sudden and excessive debility, and especially if the pain in the head is ameliorated by cold applications, *Arsenicum* may be used with advantage.

In the commencement of an attack when there is severe, excruciating pain in the forehead and vertex, attended with vomiting and burning thirst, pains in the orbits, and violent aching through the eyes, ringing and roaring in the ears, feeling of distension and throbbing in the head, delirium, somewhat violent, coming on from the excitement of noise or light, and e pecially if these symptoms occur from a sudden cold, attended with redness of the skin, bloated face, *Belladonna* may be used in alternation with *Aconite*. And also if the delirium and wakefulness is followed by *coma*, *Belladonna* may still prove of service repeated at intervals of two or three hours.

In cases where there is severe gastric derangement at the commencement, and burning in the stomach during motion, and great fullness of the head, and excruciating pain, pressing in the brain, either from within or outwards, or the reverse, aggravated by the slightest motion, or when the encephalitis is of a typhoid character, *Bryonia* may be given at intervals of one or two hours until the bilious vomitings cease, or there is occasion for change of remedy, and also when the pain in the head is confined to one side, attended with vomiting, and followed by delirium, and when. there is a short or hurried respiration and delirious talk about business at night, and heat in the head and face, and fever of a typhoid character, *Bryonia* in alternation with *Aconite* may be administered at intervals of two hours.

Encephalitis supervening upon the teething of children, attended with an irritable and sensitive condition of the nervous system, vomiting of greenish matter from the stomach with tendency to topor, or half-sleep or sleeplessness, screaming, starting and tossing, or moaning when asleep, and heat in head, redness of the conjunctiva, and spasmodic closing of the eyes, or distention of the eyes, *Chamomilla* may be given at short intervals, or when vomiting of greenish matter from the stomach precedes convulsions, and when the convulsions are succeeded by *coma*, *Cuprum metallicum* may be given at intervals of four or six hours until amelioration or change; and, also, when the child exhibits a pale complexion, spasmodic distortions of the face, blue lips, and unsteady motion of the eyeballs, *Cuprum* will be found of great service.

Cuprum is also of great service in inflammation of the brain of adults when the cerebrum is chiefly affected, when there is severe vomiting attending the delirium, and especially when the

patient in the commencement of the attack complains of bruised
sensation in the head.

When there is drowsiness and loss of consciousness with delirium about one's affairs, or when there is singing, murmurs and
laughter, picking the bed clothes, starts and screams, *Hyoscyamus.*

If the patient is disposed to weep, with frequent paroxysms
of crying and sobbing as if the heart would break, *Ignatia,* and
also in the commencement of an attack when the patient complains of headache, as if from a nail in the brain, and when the
head inclines backwards with convulsive movement of the eyes
and lids.

If the attack comes on with coldness of the hands and feet
with intense excruciating pain in the forehead, and nausea and
vomiting, pale face, convulsive twitching of the facial muscles of
the lips, and aversion to every kind of food, constant gagging,
sobbing breathing, and where there is a peevish, fretful delirium,
and also where there is looseness of the bowels with dysenteric
stools, and frequent paroxysms of pain in the bowels, *Ipecac* may
be given with some hope of affording relief, and also in the commencement of an attack, when there is a violent distress in the
stomach and pit of the stomach.

When encephalitis supervenes upon gastric and bilious difficulties from the abuse of Cinchona or Quinine, and particularly
when in the commencement of the attack there is a violent pain
in the head as if it would fly to pieces, or tearing, burning, headache followed by delirum and intolerance of light, profuse lachrymation, stitches in the ears, burning and smarting of the eyes,
pale complexion, inflammatory fever and disposition to perspire,
Mercurius may be given every three hours until a change in the
symptoms.

In cases occurring in sanguine and choleric temperaments
subject to hæmorrhoids, when the pain in the head comes on from
cold, or intense mental application, or from the use of wine and
other intoxicating drinks, *Nux vomica* and *Arsenicum* may be
used with advantage.

In deep-seated inflammation, characterized by coma or low
muttering delirium and convulsions, general torpor of the nerves,
sleep with half consciousness, coldness of the skin, or, at
times, burning heat of the body with redness of the face, pulse

full and slow, *Opium* may be given and repeated at intervals of four hours.

Cerebral inflammation in young girls near the age of puberty that appears to result from the struggle of passing into the menstrual period, may be controlled by the use of *Aconite* and *Pulsatilla*, and especially if there is a tendency to convulsions and frequent attacks of epistaxis. If signs of hyperæmia precede the encephalitis, *Belladonna* may be administered, to be followed with *Pulsatilla*, and especially if the attack is preceded by jerking and tearing and drawing in the muscles, or if it occur from suppression of menses, or after frequent attacks of rush of blood to the head.

Encephalitis attending acute diseases, such as scarlatina or small pox, attended with redness of the eyes, face pale and sunken, bloated face, with constant gagging, and disposition to vomit, dryness of the throat, disposition to coma, *Phosphorus*, repeated at intervals of an hour may be employed with advantage.

Petroleum may be used when there is a severe throbbing pain in the occiput with excessive languor, loss of memory, and coldness of the hands and face.

In cases of typhoid fever where there is great prostration and cerebral inflammation, indicated by coma and delirium, inflammation of the eyes, and derangement of the kidneys, *Rhus tox.*, and particularly when there is any erysipelatous tendency, this remedy has been found of great service.

In psoric constitutions where inflammation of the brain has been brought on by suppressed eruptions, *Sulphur* may be repeated every twenty-four hours until a change.

Encephalitis characterized by sleep that is almost natural, but with jerking of the limbs, moans, tossing and mental absence after walking, or when there is a fixed look and desire to withdraw in a slow and timid manner, or to run away with cries and fear, violent feverish heat, redness of the face, and moisture on the skin, *Stramonium*.

Spigelia and *Cina* have both been found useful where there is vomiting with clear tongue; these remedies are particularly useful for children subject to worms, and also when the disease is superinduced upon invermination. In the commencement when there is severe pain in the head from the least exercise, aggravated by noise and shocks in the occiput.

Tart. emetic is indicated when the attack comes on with violent straining, retching and vomiting of acrid and acid matters or mucous from the stomach, and when this is followed by painful pressure in the eyes, oppressive constrictive headache, as if the brain were agglomerated into a ball, and followed by delirium or stupor as if the inflammation were deep seated.

Veratrum, Viola odorata, and Viola tricolor are severally remedies that may be consulted for cases of inflammation *of the encephalon.* The remedies best suited to deep seated inflammation, where the intellect remains entire or only slightly impaired are, *Sepia, Spigelia, Sulphur* and sometimes *Arnica, Phosphorus and Arsenicum.*

Hygienic Treatment.—Patients suffering from encephalitis, should, if possible, be placed in a well-ventilated apartment, where the air can circulate freely through the room, and the room should be in a perfectly quiet place, so as to shut out the noise from the streets and from other sources; the windows should be darkened so as to exclude the light, in a great measure, although it would be well, during the day, to admit a moderate degree without subjecting the patient to the action of a glare of light at any time.

All perfumery, of every description, should be kept out of the room—no cologne, whisky or alcohol, in any form should be allowed about the patient, and flowers or green plants should be entirely excluded from the room.

It has been recommended to put ice to the head of encephalitic patients, without exercising any discrimination, but this practice has a pernicious tendency, and without doubt, the chances for a cure are more frequently diminished than augmented by the practice; and this would seem reasonable from the fact that cold applications not only abstract the heat, but effectually close the pores, so as to interrupt the necessary exhalations from the surface. Experience assures us that cold applications to the head when perspiring, throws the fluids escaping from the external surface back upon the mucous and serous surfaces, producing severe nasal catarrh, and hastening the formation of water in the sub arachnoid cavity, or causing the inflammation to merge into hydrocephalus more rapidly than it otherwise would. In deep-

seated inflammation the practice is entirely to be discarded, but
when the disease is mainly confined to the membranes, it may
prove of service. The use of warm water, applied by saturating
cloths, has been found by those who have tried the experiment,
much more serviceable. We have witnessed a number of cases
where the application of warm fomentations afforded speedy
relief after the use of remedies and cold applications had failed of
producing any perceptible good results. We have recently seen
a cure of coma of several days standing, speedily effected by the
application of warm fomentations to the head.

A child of Mr. A., aged three years, had been ill ten days
with cerebral inflammation, which was characterized by furious
delirium, at first, and afterwards by deep coma and speechless-
ness. Up to the time when we first saw the little sufferer, cold
applications had been made to the head by his Allopathic attendant. We prescribed *Belladonna* and the use of cloths saturated
with warm water, upon the head, and the little patient in twelve
hours became aroused from the *coma*, and soon manifested signs
of recovery.

In case the bowels are constipated in encephalitis, so that no
natural evacuation takes place, an *enema* of moderately cold water
may be employed, and especially if there appears to be any fulness
or hardness or distension of the bowels. But cathartics should
never be used, because the irritation they occasion is likely to
cause a sympathetic action of the brain, tending to aggravate
rather than diminish the existing difficulty.

DIET.—Nothing but thin gruel should be allowed during an
attack of inflammation of the brain, and this should be given a
spoonful at a time and frequently; very weak chicken-soup may
sometimes be substituted for the gruel, and in case the patient
manifests unmistakable signs of convalescence, it is better to still
continue a very light diet for some time, gradually increasing from
gruel to something more substantial.

Inflammation of the Spinal Cord.—Myelitis.

The spinal cord appears to be a continuation of the brain
down the spinal column, and like the brain itself, is subject both
to acute and chronic inflammations. These two forms, however,
do not differ materially from each other in their characteristic
symptoms, therefore the disease may be described as follows:

SYMPTOMS.—Disorder in the movements, pain in the region of the spine wherever the inflammation occurs, various effects produced upon the muscles, sometimes sprains, permanent contractions, involving either one or several of the muscles; sometimes with paralysis and sometimes without, in the parts which receive their nerves from the affected portion of the cord. When the meninges are only implicated, it is believed that nothing more serious occurs than a spasm; but when the cord of the medulla is the seat of inflammation, paralysis will generally attend the difficulty. The pain felt in some portions of the spinal column, is generally augmented, when the patient moves or bends the spine. It may also be augmented by percussion—a jar may also be sensibly felt. But pressure upon the vertebræ or spinous processe can afford but little aid in detecting the inflammation.

Sometimes the pain extends down the back and extremities, in the course of the great nervous trunks, and either is intermittent, or continuous; not unfrequently the pains appear like rheumatism or neuralgia, and on this account, these affections have been erroneously mistaken for spinal inflammation.

Sensation is sometimes destroyed in the parts that receive the nerves from the inflamed portion of the cord; or if not wholly destroyed, it seems very much impaired, as indicated by numbness or formication in the fingers and other portions of the extremities, and these symptoms may appear more and more distinct, until total insensibility results.

The digestive system may be more or less impaired; at times there is difficulty in swallowing. The reflex nerves coming from the inflamed medulla, thus affect deglutition, and may be regarded as one of the early indications of myelitis. The function of digestion is more or less retarded, and as a consequence, usually accompanies the difficulty.

The circulation is greatly affected, when the disease is active; but myelitis may exist in a considerable degree, without causing any very striking departure from the normal condition of the pulse.

When the upper portion of the cord is involved in the difficulty, the function of respiration is more or less disordered. Inspiration becomes difficult, or almost impracticable. The diaphragm becomes the subject of irregular spasmodic contraction, occasioning constant hiccough, gradually tending to asphyxia.

When a lower portion of the cord is affected, the urinary and genital organs lose their power, so that retention of urine and impotence result. Or in some instances the reverse may take place; the genital organs may be greatly excited, and the ability to retain the urine may be lost.

In pregnant females, the power of contraction in the uterus is sometimes lost, while at other times its contraction is stimulated, and the delivery is easily effected.

Inflammation of the spinal cord and its membranes, presents many symptoms in common with neuralgia, hysteria, and the various phenomena that writers have classed under the head of spinal irritation.

Sometimes inflammation of the spine may continue only a few days, at other times it becomes chronic, and impairs the nutrition of the whole system. In most acute attacks, there is reason to hope for a favorable termination, although in some severe case, the inflammation may extend to the brain and destroy the patient.

CAUSES.—The causes of myelitis are related to those of encephalitis; blows, falls, or mechanical injuries of any kind, may occasion it. It may arise from cold, or any influence that deranges the capillary action.

Those cases that have terminated fatally, present the following post mortem appearance: injection of the vessels, tumefaction, suppuration and induration; and sometimes the continuity of the cord had been destroyed by the softening and breaking down which the disease had occasioned; previous to the fatal termination, those parts supplied with nerves from the diseased portion of the cord, were completely paralyzed.

TREATMENT.—The remedies employed in the Homœopathic treatment of this difficulty, are Aconite, Arsenicum, Belladonna, Bryonia, Causticum, Cocculus, Digitalis, Dulcamara, Ignatia, Lachesis, Nux vomica, Pulsatilla, Rhus tox. and Veratrum.

Arsenicum, when there is a violent burning pain in the back, aggravated by contact. Tearing or drawing pain in the back, between the scapulæ, and great prostration and difficult inspiration. When there are general febrile symptoms accompanying the pain in the back, and other symptoms, such as paralysis or numbness of the extremities, *Aconite* may be called into requisition.

When there is stiffness of the nape of the neck, paralysis, and stiffness of the arms, heaviness and lameness of the lower extremities, short, hurried respiration, danger of suffocation when swallowing, and pressure at the chest, retention of urine, or involuntary emission of the urine, spasms or convulsions in plethoric subjects, and severe pain in the dorsal region of the spine, *Belladonna.*

When there is pain in the small of the back, and painful stiffness, not allowing one to stand erect, or pain in the small of the back as if bruised, when at rest, crampy, contractive pain over the whole back, gastric difficulties and constipation, involuntary urination, fatigued sensation in the lower extremities, and pain in the back from the slightest motion, *Bryonia.*

If there is paralysis, chorea, and contraction of the tendons of certain muscles, and painful stiffness of the back, dull, drawing and tearing pains in the arms and hands, contraction of the fingers, rigid feeling in the joints of the legs and feet, palpitation of the heart, *Causticum.*

For lancing, drawing or tearing by turns, and continuing in the extremities, as if in the bones, sensation of constriction of the internal organs, pains which appear on one side only, spasms and convulsions of the extremities and whole body, paralysis, especially hemiplegia; weak, exhausted trembling, want of animal spirits, and other derangements, attendant upon inflammation of the spinal cord, *Cocculus.*

When the patient is subject to gastric affections, cold hands and feet, and great nervous debility, pale face, and drawing pain in the small of the back, after a cold; also when there is increased action of the heart, tension and stiffness of the cervical muscles, *Digitalis.*

When inflammation of the spinal cord proceeds from a cold, attended with drowsiness in the day time, internal uneasiness, difficulty of speech, and paralysis of the tongue; or when attended with diarrhœa, violent pains in the loins, lameness of the arms, etc., *Dulcamara.*

When there is evident inflammation of the cord, attended with vertigo, deep sleep, spasmodic yawning, opisthotonos, convulsive twitchings of the arms, and convulsive jactitation of the lower limbs, *Ignatia*.

If there is weakness and inability to support the back, with weakness of the knees, and sense of suffocation, by reason of difficult inspiration, *Lachesis*.

In plethoric persons, when there is inflammation of the cord, and pain in the back and small of the back, as if bruised; oppression of the chest, as if from a load, and sometimes a forcible, racking cough, *Nux vomica*.

When there are present the general symptoms of inflammation of the cord, attended with itching of the spine, feverish sopor, hypochondria, ill humor, especially in damp, foggy weather, palpitation of the heart, semilateral headache, abdominal spasms, retention of the urine, constipation, flatulent colic, tenesmus of the bladder, pain in the small of the back and back, curvature of the spine, tension and drawing in the lower extremities, *Pulsatilla*.

If there are unmistakable indications of spinal irritation, with rheumatic and arthritic tensions, drawing and tearing in the limbs, erysipelas, spasmodic yawning, oppressive fulness of the head, drowsy after eating, anxious oppression of the chest at night, tremulous feeling about the heart, bruised feeling and pain in the small of the back, opisthotonos, rheumatic stiffness of the nape of the neck, curvature of the spine, *Rhus tox*.

When there is general weakness of the body, in connection with spinal irritation, and rheumatic tearing pains in the limbs, abdominal spasms, oppressed respiration, severe pain in the back and particularly in the small of the back, alternate constipation, and prostrating diarrhœa, and sometimes paralysis of the lower extremities, *Veratrum*.

It is an excellent remedy after Nux vom.

There are many other remedies that may be consulted, in the treatment of this disease. The habit of resorting to blisters or moxas, should be discarded.

DIET.—The digestive organs should not be severely taxed during treatment for spinal irritation, or inflammation of the spinal cord. The digestible meats in moderation, may be used during the treatment for the chronic variety of the disease, in other respects, a simple farinaceous diet is sufficient.

Cerebro-Spinal Meningitis, Spotted Fever.

This disease has prevailed epidemically in several localities in the United States. When it appeared many years ago, it was regarded as a malignant form of typhoid congestive fever and was treated with stimulants.

SYMPTOMS.—A severe chill, not anticipated by any previous indications, occurs in the commencement of the attack, much like that of an ague. The cold stage is not succeeded by the usual febrile reaction, but on the contrary the cold stage gradually continues for a long time, and the patient sinks into a stupor from which he seldom recovers. In a brief period after, the muscles are observed to be rigid, the pupils of the eyes become insensible to light, or touch. The surface of the body is exceedingly sensitive to the touch, the head is drawn back, the teeth set, inspiration is forcible, producing a hissing sound, as if by great effort through the closed teeth, the patient is blind and deaf, children are liable to merge from the stupor into convulsions. The stupor increases with the augmentation of the disease; large spots rise on the skin apparently forming black blisters. The patient frequently lingers for some days, stricken with paræsis of the lower extremities, blindness and deafness. In some cases the patient revives a little and exhibits signs of convalescence which soon pass off and he sinks more profoundly into the stupor and death soon occurs. In a few cases a protracted typhoid fever may set in, and the patient after a faithful course of Homœopathic treatment recover.

CASE. A son of Mr. K. aged fifteen years, attacked suddenly with a chill, followed by a stupor and convulsions from which he emerged deaf, blind and speechless and the case was regarded in all its features hopeless. Stimulants were used freely, and Belladonna 6x dilution in water, a teaspoonful every half hour. This prescription was made by the writer who was called to counsel in the case at a distance of sixty miles. The boy was critically cared for by a competent nurse. After returning from the visit, the first news anticipated was that death had ended the same. Four months after, the father with this son, to my surprise, came into my office. It appears from the time the Belladonna was prescribed, convalescence continued.

From the fact that purple spots appear on the skin after a case has terminated fatally, it formerly took the name of spotted fever and its prevalence in any locality was regarded an alarming scourge. It is evidently a congestive disease, non-contagious, but in those localities where autumnal intermittents have prevailed, it yields to epidemic influences. Stimulants must be used freely in the treatment, Aconite 6x dil., every half hour, Belladonna 6x dil. should follow Acon.; Arsenicum 6x dil., Bryonia 6x dil., Nux vom. 6x, China, each in the 6x dil., ten drops in a glass of water, may be given in teaspoonful doses every thirty minutes when indicated.

CHAPTER XLIII.

ANÆMIA OF THE NERVOUS CENTRES.

By the term anæmia, is understood a paucity of blood in any part, and when applied to the nervous centres, means a paucity of blood in those regions. It has been remarked by some writers, that either a superabundance or paucity of blood in the vessels of the nervous centres, will give rise to nearly the same phenomena. For instance, at one time, coma and convulsions evidence a congested state of the encephalic vessels; at another time, this may supervene upon excessive losses, when it must appear palpably manifest that these vessels have been partially emptied of their contents. From this fact, it may be inferred that anæmia of the nervous centres may result from general paucity of the blood, which of course may be occasioned by diarrhœa, or long protracted disease of any kind, or severe vital prostration. We may suppose such a condition of the nervous centres to occur in acute fevers, such as scarlatina, or severe inflammatory fevers of any kind, that are characterized by hyperæmia in some of the visceral organs, and consequent deficiency in the vessels of the brain.

SYMPTOMS.—Such as characterize extreme loss of blood, tottering, unable to stand, tremors, convulsions similar to epilepsy, may severally indicate anæmia of the nervous centres, provided they occur in females recently delivered, or who have sustained an immoderate uterine hæmorrhage; or in males who have sustained great losses either in consequence of local hæmorrhages or severe diarrhœa. This latter disturbance often empties the blood vessels of the greater proportion of fluid which they contain, and of course detracts from the sustenance they afford to the nervous centres, and induces that peculiar condition which we term anæmia; central apoplexy has resulted from severe losses of blood.

There are other symptoms that excessive loss of blood may produce, by causing anæmia of the nervous centres, which are to be viewed as the more remote effects of the difficulty, or rather the reaction, which may supervene in a few hours: as for instance, a female that has been almost drained of blood by flooding, in a short time afterwards, may experience headache, flushed face, beating of the temporal arteries, which cannot be allayed by depletion. Not unfrequently after such losses severe headache is met with, or severe oppression in some part of the head, with intolerance of light and sound, sleeplessness, slight delirium, with or without palpitations—all of which may be ascribed to anæmia of the nervous centres.

In persons who have died of convulsions, after having sustained severe losses of blood, the post-mortem appearances accord with the condition of the system. The encephalon is found to be pale, the vessels containing only a small portion of blood, and it is affirmed that the vesicular matter partakes more of this character than the fibrous.

TREATMENT.—The medicines that have the most decisive tendency to relieve the effects of anæmia of the nervous centres, are Carbo veg., China, Ferrum, Hepar, Ipecac, Kali carb., Natrum mur., Nux vomica, Phos. acid., Sulphur, Veratrum.

Carbo veg.—After severe diarrhœa, when there is weakness of memory, slow ideas, oppressive headache, and general weakness, coldness and chilliness and restlessness, pains and heaviness of the limbs, etc.

After severe losses of blood, when there is headache, loss of memory or weakness of the memory, and loss of strength, dullness of the head, vertigo, *China.*

If after a severe fever, or other acute suffering, in which the circulatory system has sustained considerable loss, there is debility, weakness of the memory, headache and heaviness of the limbs, and with all a paleness of the complexion, and general languor, Ferrum and China may both be employed.

If the body has been drained of the animal fluids by purgatives, and especially mercurials, so as to produce anæmia of the nervous centres, which is denoted by weakness of the memory, lightness of the head, vertigo, and noises in the head, *Hepar* may be found useful.

If, after severe losses, as in case of parturition, there is headache, and nausea and sickness at the stomach, *Ipecac,* or if in case of hysteria or hysteric headache, *Kali carb.,* especially if there is vertigo with nausea.

In case physical and mental prostration and emaciation, produced by losses from onanism or over sexual indulgence, especially when there is anything like paralysis or hysterical affections, or epileptic convulsions, weak memory, unable to meditate, vertigo, with jerks in the head, and inability to collect one's senses, *Natrum mur.*

In sanguine and choleric temperaments, that have sustained severe losses from hæmorrhoidal affections, followed by indications of anæmia in the nervous centres, such as headache, weak memory, hysteric affections, great prostration, almost amounting to paralysis, dread of motion, emaciation, and congestion of some of the internal organs, *Nux vomica.* China may also be employed in cases of this kind, and also Sulphur, should Nux vomica fail of procuring decided relief.

In case of frequent debilitating emissions, being the cause of anæmia of the nervous centres, *Phos. acid* may be employed with advantage; and also this remedy may be employed when the same results from diabetes or prostrating diarrhœa, and discharges of grey stools, or involuntary and undigested.

Sulphur may be employed with advantage, when there is evident anæmia resulting from scarlatina.

Diet and Regimen.—In all cases where there is anæmia of the nervous centres, the recuperation of the system is the grand end in view, and to effect this, great caution must be exercised to supply the system with the kind of nourishment it requires, and such as it is capable of receiving. Immediately after the system has sustained losses, the diet should be nutritious, but composed of gruels and soups, such as will not be much of a tax upon the digestive organs. The diet may gradually be increased in strength until that which is decidedly substantial may take the place of that which is less so. All condiments, except salt, should be entirely prohibited.

Apoplexy—Hæmorrhage in the Nervous Centres.

When a determination of blood to the nervous centres causes a rupture of some of the vessels, there is hæmorrhage in them, that gives rise to what is termed apoplexy. This term, however, has been applied to congestions, where no hæmorrhage takes place. Hæmorrhages may take place in different parts of the nervous centres, giving rise to various phenomena. 1st. They

may take place at the external surface. 2d. They may take place
in the cavities. 3d. They may take place in the nervous matter.

1. When it occurs in the external surface from the meninges,
it may be seated between the dura mater and the skull, or between
the dura mater and arachnoid. The symptoms in such cases may
be those of compression, such as sudden loss of sensation, volition,
and mental and moral manifestation. Some writers have termed
this meningeal apoplexy, but these cases are believed to be of rare
occurrence.

2. When hæmorrhage takes place in the cavities there are
also such symptoms as would denote compression, sudden loss of
consciousness, volition and sensation, and not unfrequently
paralysis.

3. But in the greater number of cases hæmorrhage takes
place in the very substance of the brain, either in the cerebral
hemispheres or in those of the cerebellum, although seldom in the
latter.

SYMPTOMS.—Many of these are premonitory, indicating
merely hyperæmia before described, sometimes, however, these
premonitory symptoms are entirely wanting; where the hæmorrhage has actually taken place, it commonly induces symptoms
not easily mistaken; there is complete loss of sensation, motion
and mental and moral manifestation, prior to the hæmorrhage
there may be headache, vertigo and confusion, with numbness or
sense of creeping in some parts of the surface, especially in those
of the fingers and toes; the vision may be depraved, spots or
sparks may appear before the eyes, and also appearance of cobwebs or flashes of light; sometimes the hearing is impaired, inton-
ations or singular sounds, tinnitus aurium or susurrus, and the
sense of taste and smell may also be impaired, but the two last
senses rarely afford any symptoms that can guide us. These
symptoms exist also in congestion, and may continue for days and
even weeks and then pass away, but when they occur from actual
hæmorrhage they rarely disappear, and the impairment of the
senses permanently remains. When the attack has been sudden,
all attempts to arouse the patient to sensation will prove insufficient, and when the immediate apoplectic effects disappear, the
sensibility of the part affected with loss of motion does not return. Sensation may sometimes be restored, but motion not till
after the elapse of a long time, if ever.

In severe cases, not only the encephalic, but the spinal nerves lose their impressibility, so that the contact of any body with the lining membrane of the mouth, or of the œsophagus induces no muscular contraction. The sphincters, too, which belong to the true spinal system in their real relation, suffer a loss of power so that the several reservoirs discharge their contents involuntarily, also the conjunctiva which receives the fifth pair of nerves, which convey both sensation and motion to the part, becomes impaired so that contact with the finger will produce no irritation.

The sight at first may be entirely destroyed, and remain so until sensation returns, and then perhaps it may be restored to one eye, while in the other it remains lost. This will in nearly all cases be the eye upon the paralyzed side.

Loss of motion or paralysis is the almost universal effect of hæmorrhage in the nervous centres. It was shown under the head of hyperæmia that general paralysis may result from mere congestion of the nervous centres, which passes off as the congestion is removed. The paralysis, however, that follows hæmorrhage generally comes on suddenly, concerns only one-half of the body, and remains more or less for the rest of the patient's life.

Andral mentions some rare cases of cerebral hæmorrhage where there was no paralysis, that proved fatal however, mobility remaining to the last. A post-mortem examination disclosed large clots at the posterior portion of the right cerebral hemisphere; other authors have cited similar cases.

The degree in which paralysis is manifest varies, sometimes it is complete from the first; at others, the first indication may be a mere heaviness of the limb, or inability to grasp objects, but generally these symptoms go on augmenting, until complete hemiplegia is the result. These symptoms may be looked upon as being the forerunner of hæmorrhage, which an early precaution may sometimes avert.

It seldom happens that all the limbs become paralyzed from hæmorrhage, though we may infer that such would be the result if it takes place in both cerebral hemispheres, or if that of one side is such as to compress the other. In this latter instance if the patient survives, the clot may be diminished by absorption so that the compression may be removed, and mobility may be restored to one side.

It has usually been observed that hæmorrhage in either hemisphere will produce paralysis of the opposite side, generally of both the upper and lower extremities, though sometimes of but one only. The face, too, becomes implicated, and the muscles are paralyzed, the angle of the mouth is drawn upwards by the sound muscles of the opposite side.

Anatomists have anxiously sought for an exposition of this general law of decussation, and it is generally admitted that at the portion of the spinal cord at which the medulla oblongata unites, there is a crossing of the fibres of the anterior pyramids, or of those conected with motion, by which the fact, it is believed may be explained. This will undoubtedly explain the general features of the phenomena. But this will not account for the face of the affected side being paralyzed on that side, but this may be explained from the fact, that the nerves supplying the face are derived from a portion above that point where the decussation takes place.

Hæmorrhage into the cerebellum produces symptoms not unlike those resulting from the same in the cerebral hemispheres, and this fact has given rise to the interesting questions in physiology concerning the decussation of fibers of the corpora restiformia.

Hæmorrhage into the spinal cord may also produce paralysis of both upper and lower extremities, according to the seat of the effusion; where hæmorrhage has occurred in one of the anterior cords hemiplegia has resulted on the same side of the lesion. The symptoms of spinal apoplexy are however observed.

When a hæmorrhage in the encephalon occurs, other voluntary muscles besides those of the limbs are affected with paralysis, as those of the eyelids, the tongue, the movements of which become so lost as to impair the power of speech.

Many attempts have been made to make the paralyzed portion the index of pointing out the precise seat of the hæmorrhage, but although the researches have been arduous, there has yet been véry little of a satisfactory character elicited.

When paralysis has once occurred, especially in the extremities, it may gradually improve and yet never disappear, though in many instances it remains stationary. The nutrition of the limb is always more or less impaired, when the paralysis entirely disappears; it is probably owing to the entire absorption of the clot that has produced it, in which event the continuity of the nervous matter is restored so that the nervous action can be propagated through it.

In most all cases an attack of hæmorrhage is preceded by some sign of intellectual disturbance, the mental acts are sluggishly executed, the patient is drowsy, scarcely able to keep awake, or otherwise there is great restlessness and unusual mental excitement; the former symptoms however, are the most frequently noticed. Not unfreqently varied hallucinations occur, which however may be indicative of other lesions. Some object may impress the sense of sight which the patient cannot rid himself of for months; this however occurs not so much as a precursor as that of an effect of previous cerebral disturbance; similar hallucinations occur in the other senses. Sounds are often heard as of voices calling to the individual, which have no existence only in his imagination. After these hallucinations occur and have existed for some time, unless the individual takes timely warning and uses every precaution, he is attacked with all the symptoms of encephalic hæmorrhage.

In some unusual cases the mental faculties are not much impaired, though generally the reverse is the case. When the effusion takes place in the cerebral convolutions, the mental faculties are so much impaired as to produce imbecility, and when other portions of the encephalon are the seat, compression alone may impair the mental powers to a greater or less extent.

It has been observed that hæmorrhage even in the spinal marrow has so reacted upon the encephalon as to impair the mental manifestation in a considerable degree.

If due credit is accorded to some singular facts which are found detailed by eminent authors, large portions of the cerebral hemispheres have been lost or injured without the mental manifestation being destroyed. This would seem to indicate that the seat of the mental endowment was nearer the base of the brain than has been generally imagined.

In some cases only the memory seems to be impaired, and no cognizance whatever of recent events is taken; only one event sometimes will be retained in the memory. All the phenomena that occur as the result of hæmorrhage in the nervous centres can-

not be referred to, although such must afford an interesting subject for research.   The nervous centres being the primary seat of
vital endowment in the body, cannot receive too much attention,
as something new and interesting is continually being developed,
that requires constant attention.

The final result of cerebral hæmorrhage is generally fatal;
after the first attack the individual is liable to the second, which
almost always occurs sooner or later, and so on the third, and it
is only in some rare cases that recovery takes place so completely
that the patient dies of some other disease.

CAUSES.—Those detailed as producing hyperæmia or congestion of the encephalon, may operate to produce hæmorrhage,
therefore, they need not be repeated.   It may be remarked, however, that the difficulty occurs frequently in the torrid zone,
where the subjects are exposed to the intense heat of the climate.

The aged are more predisposed to the difficulty than the young.
It is much more common after forty years of age than before,
males are more predisposed than females.   There is reason to believe also that a particular conformation derived hereditarily may
have some influence as a predisposing cause.   Several instances
are recorded, strongly tending to prove that it has occurred as a
family disease.   There are numerous cases that might be cited, to
prove that there is a predisposition sometimes impressed on the
organism, which may be developed by some slight exciting cause.

TREATMENT.—It is believed that the treatment of this formidable disease, with Homœopathic remedies, will prove successful
in many cases where the ordinary Allopathic treatment would
prove useless, if not injurious.   It must be by noting accurately
the premonitory indications, that timely treatment will prove
availing in averting an attack.   Therefore it is proper to make a
division of the treatment.   1st.   The treatment which is required
during the first premonitions; and 2d. That which is required
when the hæmorrhage has actually taken place.   The former has
been sufficiently detailed, under the head of hyperæmia of the
nervous centres, and need not be again repeated.   The latter
requires, for the most part, *Aconite, Arnica, Belladonna, Nux
vomica, Pulsatilla and Sulphur.*

Aconite is the first remedy to be employed in sudden and
violent attacks, when there is full bounding pulse, or general
arterial excitement, loss of consciousness, and complete prostra-

tion, with flushed or swollen face. *Arnica*, when there is general paralysis, following a severe blow upon the head, indicating a hæmorrhage in the nervous centres. *Belladonna*, when there is violent beating of the temporal arteries, followed by paralysis, or attended with paralysis of the face and limbs. *Nux vomica* is well suited to bilious, sanguine, or nervous temperaments and is indicated when the patient vomits, and has no power of motion. *Pulsatilla* may also be called into requisition in complete apoplexy, when it occurs in persons of mild disposition, with entire loss of consciousness and speech, bluish red hue of the face, when there is violent palpitation of the heart, suppressed pulse. This remedy is better suited to the lymphatic temperament.

When the first symptoms have passed away, leaving partial paralysis, or paralysis of certain parts, Nux vomica, if there is paralysis of the left side. If only paralysis of the face, tongue and the muscles employed in deglutition, Belladonna, and afterwards, in psoric constitutions, Sulphur may be employed advantageously. When there are signs of recuperation, or disappearance of the symptoms that usually attend hæmorrhage in the nervous centres, the administration of remedies should be discontinued, so long as the patient appears to recover.

DIET.—The diet should be very simple, and free from any thing that would seem to indicate a tax upon the digestive function. Rice or other kinds of farinaceous gruel, would be indicated at first, before any mitigation of symptoms takes place. Afterwards, as soon as the patient can take it, meat soup may be allowed; and if the system sufficiently recuperates to bear it, something more substantial may be permitted. In the treatment of this affection, it is customary to resort to violent friction upon the paralyzed members; but this is seldom attended with benefit. It may, however, be of some use to resort to dry rubbing with the hand, for the purpose of keeping up a vigorous circulation in the extremities. Pouring cold water upon the head, is another measure often resorted to, and may be attended with some benefit, especially if actual hæmorrhage has not taken place.

Softening of the Nervous Centres.

SYMPTOMS.—The principal symptoms that indicate softening of the nervous centres, is pain, fixed to some locality, that appears to be of an unyielding character. It is not an unusual occurrence for the pain to be unaccompanied by any acceleration of the pulse. When the softening occurs in the cerebral hemispheres, the intellect becomes more or less impaired, and sensation and motion are not so well accomplished as in health. Sometimes both are deranged or obscured, although sensation at times may be augmented, while motion on the opposite side to the hemisphere affected is impossible. A common attendant on softening of some portions of the brain, is paralysis. Sometimes, however, instead of the limbs being affected with paralysis, they are more or less contracted and rigid.

It is, however, impossible to say that the symptoms detailed above are invariably an indication of softening, as they in general may attend other diseased conditions; and not much can be said about treatment, with reference to the pathological condition, as the symptoms must be the guide.

CAUSE.—Softening may arise from inflammation, or it may arise from failure of the circulation from arterial disease.

TREATMENT.—The remedies employed in accordance with symptoms that may give rise to fears of softening, are Belladonna, Nux vomica, Sepia, and Sulphur.

When there is severe pain in either cerebral hemisphere, that seems to be fixed and continuous, impairing the mind, and causing rigidity of the muscles of the extremities, *Belladonna* may be used daily for a week. If there is no mitigation of the pain, or relief of the other symptoms, and especially if there is any indication of paralysis, *Nux vomica* may be used daily for a week, provided there is no mitigation of the symptoms before the week passes away—in which event, it is better to discontinue the remedy. When there is pain fixed to a single spot, impairing motion, so that the patient cannot move about, Sulphur may be given and repeated every forty-eight hours. *Calcarea* may also be employed for other indications. (*See Hyperæmia of the cerebrum, cerebellum, and spinal cord.*)

Induration of the Nervous Centres.

This affection may exist in connection with hyperæmia, as the consequence of inflammation; but as there are no symptoms by which we can accurately determine this condition, aside from other difficulties that may be associated with it, the treatment must be according to symptoms, which may or may not be the consequence of such a lesion.

Accumulation of Serous Fluid in the Nervous Centres.

As the nervous centres are enveloped by a serous membrane, which passes into the cavities, which like other serous membranes may be the seat of watery secretion, œdema or dropsy may result from the accumulation of such secretion.

Effusion is regarded as the result of inflammation, or rather as one of its terminations. Encephalitis has been regarded the source of hydrocephalus, or dropsy of the brain. It may also result from hyperæmia, no matter how produced, by transudation occurring through the coats of the over-distended vessels. This is probably the way in which *serous apoplexy* occurs, and the same symptoms may be present, as are seen in connection with hæmorrhage in the nervous centres; so that it is difficult to distinguish between the two. Either may exist alone, or both may exist at the same time. When this serous accumulation supervenes upon acute inflammation, it is the *hydrocephalus acutus* of writers; but sometimes the chronic stage is met with, especially in persons of more advanced age, in whom sensation, motion and intelligence have severally become impaired. The stupidity of the insane has sometimes resulted from chronic œdema of the brain. Whenever a serous effusion takes place in the brain, it produces compression, and manifests nearly the same symptoms as are found in connection with hyperæmia, or *hydrocephalus acutus*.

When the fluid accumulates in the spinal sheath, as is sometimes the case in infants, the spinous processes are cleft, or there is what is termed *spina bifida*, so that the membranes protrude, and the compression is diminished.

It has been remarked, that acute hypercrinia of the encephalon is often the consequence of inflammation, or of hyperæmia. The symptoms are often so obscure, that we cannot determine precisely the cause of the compression; but the accumulations of fluid which occur in a more chronic form, generally exhibit their existence by unequivocal symptoms in the bony coverings. The serous fluid, if contained within the cranium, distends the parieties of the cranium, causing the head at times to acquire an enor-

mously large size, constituting the chronic hydrocephalus, or
dropsy of the head.

TREATMENT.—As the accumulation of serous fluid in the nervous centres may present a varied phase, as well as many degrees
of severity, many remedies may be called into requisition. The
remedies for the most part employed are Aconite, Arnica, Arsenicum, Belladonna, Digitalis, *Helleborus niger*, Hyoscyamus, Mercurius, Nux vomica, Pulsatilla, Rhus tox. and Sulphur.

When there is acute pain in the head, and vomiting, with
acute febrile symptoms, Aconite may be administered every three
hours. When the pain and inflammation has been produced by
concussion, giving rise to symptoms that indicate compression
from serous effusion, *Arnica* may be substituted for *Aconite*, and
repeated every three hours, until some mitigation of the symptoms is witnessed.

When there is a small quick pulse, and frequent disposition
to vomit, dry, white tongue, heat in the head, stupor and great
prostration, *Arsenicum*.

When there are the following indications of serous effusion,
viz., great heat in the head, bloated and red face, strong pulsation
of the arteries of the neck, severe pain in the head, and inclination to bury it in the pillow, or moving the head from side to
side, frequent flushes of heat, eyes sparkling, and protruding with
wild expression, contraction or dilatation of the pupils, drowsiness, etc., *Belladonna*. When there is intense action of the heart
and arteries, attending the usual symptoms, Digitalis. When
there are convulsions, loss of consciousness, or inarticulate speech,
redness of the face, fixed look, white coating upon the tongue,
dry and parched skin, thirst, and picking at the bed clothes,
Hyoscyamus. Mercurius is suitable to employ, after *Belladonna*.
Pulsatilla in females, when there has been an interruption of the
menses. *Rhus tox.* may be administered, when the signs of effusion become manifest, during an attack of erysipelas. Sulphur
may very generally be employed in chronic effusion of serum into
the nervous centres, especially with Belladonna and Mercurius.

The calling of the attention merely to serous effusions in the
nervous centres, producing hydrocephalus, serous apoplexy, etc.,
is by no means for the purpose of inducing the habit of treating
the disease from the name, but to point out a pathological condi-

tion that may exist, in connection with certain symptoms, which of course must be the guide in treatment.

DIET, when under treatment, must be exceedingly simple, farinaceous gruels for the acute form, and also light and nutritious food for the chronic.

Morbid Formations in the Nervous Centres.

Although morbid formations may and do take place in the nervous centers, we have no symptoms demonstrative of their presence, except such as may denote other diseased conditions. It is, nevertheless, a fact that *adipous, fibrous,* and osseous formations do occur in the nervous centres.

Tubercular, scirrhous, and encephaloid transformations, have been known to exist, but the symptoms produced by them, are at best equivocal, and can afford no certain indication to distinguish them from other chronic lesions of the nervous centres. Paralysis, convulsions, or meningeal inflammation may result from some of these transformations, and the same may arise from other causes, and as the treatment in both cases would be in accordance with symptoms, but little practical importance is attached to a mere pathological view of the matter.

TUBERCLES may be indicated by impairment of sensation and motion, but as this may arise from other causes, it cannot be regarded as pathognomonic.

Scirrhous and encephaloid productions, less common than tubercles, can only be suspected as to their existence during life, although their size may vary somewhat, as well as the position they may occupy in the nervous centres.

Calculi, or calculous secretions have been found in the nervous centres, the greater proportion in the cerebral hemispheres, and yet no symptoms have been manifest during life that could determine their existence. Therefore, in the treatment of unknown difficulties, the symptoms alone must be the guide. When certain symptoms indicate unerringly certain lesions, both the lesions and the symptoms connected with them may be taken into account in the treatment; but when the symptoms simply indicate a difficulty in determinate, they may as accurately point out the true remedial agents to be employed, as if the nature of the precise formations corresponding with the symptoms were known. Other formations than those that we have named, have been found on dissection, in the nervous centres; facts elicited from post-mortem examinations, seldom afford any other satisfaction than a knowledge of what has been in connection with the symptoms previous to death. When we note a symptom weunavoidably connect it with a cause, and although post-mortem appearance may not be so available in a practical point of view as ante-mortem appearance or symptoms, yet there often results a satisfactory solution of fatal difficulties, by a resort to autopsy, that would otherwise inflict upon the mind wearisome states of suspense, as well as fruitless conjecture.

CHAPTER XLIV.

We have been considering diseases of the nervous system
thus far, of an organic character, which generally produce lesions
discoverable on dissection; and we have yet to consider many important affections, which unquestionably are the result of an irritation of the nervous centres, although no lesions are found to
confirm the fact. These affections are manifest in disordered sensation, volition and mental manifestation. The term *neuroses* has
generally been applied to denote affections of this character.

Augmentation of Sensibility.

It sometimes happens that one or more of the special senses
becomes so quickened as to take cognizance of impressions that
would otherwise be unobserved. All the senses are subject to this
kind of exaltation. As for instance, in the example of the sense of
sight, the patient may be unable to discern objects distinctly in the
light of day, but as twilight and even the darkness of the evening approaches, objects can be readily discerned. This difficulty
may be caused by remaining a long time in a dark place, as in
mines. The sense of hearing may be so much exalted as to render the patient unable to bear the least noise. Both exaltation
of the sight and hearing generally accompanies encephalitis and
various cerebral diseases.

The sense of smell, from some morbid action, may become
exalted in the most remarkable manner. The degree of exaltation has been such as to enable the subject in some cases, to
readily distinguish persons in the dark. *Cloquet* relates a
remarkable exaltation of this sense in one suffering from fever,
who was unable to tolerate the disagreeable and overwhelming
odour of copper, which was found to have been exhaled from a
pin which had accidentally dropped in his bed. In cases of decided
and strange antipathies to certain animals, the sense of smell has

been so augmented, as to detect their presence when unobserved by others.

The sense of taste also, by certain kinds of diseased action, becomes immeasurably exalted, though seldom in comparison with the other senses.

The sense of touch also becomes very much exalted, sometimes, however, confined to a single part, at others, it extends entirely over the cutaneous surface (*hyperaphia*), and is so excessive, that the individual is unable to bear the slightest pressure. This diseased condition is frequently met with in persons suffering from neuralgia, and frequently it may be regarded one of the most prominent symptoms of that affection.

Supersensitiveness of touch may in some instances be regarded as a premonitory indication of encephalic disturbance, more frequently manifest in persons of extreme impressibility.

Instances are sometimes met with, where individuals are so highly impressible, as to be disturbed by the slightest impression made upon any of the senses. Such persons are usually termed "nervous," and are found among the subjects of the mesmerist.

That there are various degrees of impressibleness is evident from the fact that some persons are more sensitive than others. Some will faint when any unusual impression is made upon the senses, others will perceive on the account of an exaltation of common sensibility, the minutest changes in the atmosphere, so as to be disagreeably affected. Some persons suffer almost intolerably from slight ailments, that would hardly be noticed by others.

CAUSES.—Excessive impressibility of the nervous system may result from various causes. Long continued mental exertions may give rise to it, or any other circumstance calculated to exhaust the nervous system, such as want of sleep, great fatigue, or excessive evacuations of any kind, and abstinence from excitants and stimulants to which the system has been habituated.

TREATMENT.—Where extreme irritability or impressibility appears to be connected with an apparent cause, this, of course, will have to be removed, in order to ensure a cessation of the effect. The hygienic treatment to be observed, when the patient's strength will admit of it, is exercise and traveling in the open air,—and also by moral discipline of the mind,—a wholesome nutritious diet, and frequent change of scene.

The remedies employed in the Homœopathic treatment, are Aconite, Belladonna, Bryonia, Calc., Conium, Hepar sulph., Drosera, Hyoscyamus, Lycopodium, Nux v., Opium, Pulsatilla, Sepia, Sulphur.

In *nyctalopia*, where the patient is unable to see by day, but readily distinguishes objects by night, *Aconite, Belladonna,* Conium and Hyoscyamus are remedies that may be consulted.

In *hyperacusis*, or morbid exaltation of the sense of hearing, so that slight noises become almost unbearable, *Aconite, Belladonna, Cham., Coffea, Lycopodium,* and *Nux vom.,* may be consulted.

In *hyperosmia*, or morbid augmentation of the sense of smell, Barytes carb., Belladonna, Hepar sulph., Lycopodium and Sulphur may be found useful in removing the difficulty.

In *hypergeusia,* or morbid sensibility of the organ of taste, *Calcarea, Lachesis, Carbo veg.*

In *hyperaphia,* or excessive acuteness of the touch in general, or in other words, extreme impressibility, Nux vom., Opium, Pulsatilla, Sepia and Sulphur.

In persons of lymphatic temperaments, highly susceptible to cold or depression of spirits in cloudy or damp weather, *Pulsatilla.* Great sensitiveness to pain may be overcome by *Mercurius.* Or if mercurial drugs have been the cause, Sulphur and Hepar sulphur may be employed. The solution of the remedy will in most cases depend upon the general condition of the system, and the nature of the disturbance that has given rise to the difficulty.

Diminution, or Deprivation of Sensibility.

Anæsthesia, or loss of general sensibility, is a condition of the system that may be induced by some morbid condition of the nervous centres; sometimes it is only partial, at others it is complete. At times only one side is affected in this way, while the other appears to be in a state of hyperæsthesia. When there is complete loss of sensibility, the contact of boiling water or hot sealing wax will produce no pain.

CAUSES.—Tumors pressing upon the nerves; interfering with their continuity; poison of lead, and other obscure causes may give rise to the lesion.

TREATMENT.—The principal remedies employed in the treatment of this difficulty, are *Acon.*, *Arnica*, *Nux vom.*, *Pulsatilla*, *Calcarea* and *Sulphur*.

When there is acceleration of the circulation; febrile heat; dry tongue and thirst attending the diminution or loss of sensibility in a part, *Aconite* may prove effectual in removing the difficulty.

When sensation of a part has been impaired by a blow or concussion or some mechanical injury, *Arnica* may be employed.

When loss of sensibility supervenes upon rush of blood to the head in plethoric persons, Aconite. If in females, it occurs at or near the menstrual period, *Pulsatilla*. If the loss of sensibility be recognized in one arm, while at the same time there is an augmentation of sensibility in the other, *Aconite* and *Nux vomica*, or perhaps *Calcarea* and *Nux vom.* may be employed in alternation at intervals of six or twelve hours.

When there is a total loss of sensibility in the lower extremities, *Sulphur* and perhaps *Conium*.

In case of the difficulty being produced by the poison of lead, *Sulphur*, *Hepar sulp.*, *Nux vom.*, and other remedies may be employed, while at the same time, the patient should quit his occupation in lead and allow sufficient time for his system to recover from its effects.

In nearly all cases of loss of sensibility, whether confined to a part or the whole surface, external friction may be demanded, douches of warm or tepid water, and sometimes of cold water, and also electricity may be successfully employed in cases of the kind.

Perverted Sensibility.

All the senses are subject to varied disturbances that arise from obscure causes. Only one of the special senses may be involved at a time, and this to a degree that amounts to an entire perversion of its normal use.

Paraphia, or perversion of the sense of touch, may be so manifest as to convey constantly, erroneous impressions in regard to shape, size, consistence, weight and temperature of bodies.

Purageusia, or perversion of the sense of taste, may be so apparent as to allow of the most disgusting objects to be taken as food with the highest relish. This condition is sometimes at-

tendant on pregnancy, and also in chlorotic patients, who sometimes fancy slate pencils, charcoal, pipe clay, ashes, etc., in preference to articles that are eatable and relished in health. To
change this condition, Antimonium crud., Bryonia, Cocculus,
Ipecac, Nux vom., Oleander, Petroleum and Pulsatilla may be
consulted.

Parosmia, or perversion of the sense of smell, may be such
as to render what is disagreeable in health, perfectly agreeable;
sometimes the olfactory nerve is so affected as to produce illusory
smell, that may be obviated by appropriate remedies: as for
instance, when there is illusory smell of brandy, Aurum is the
remedy. When as of something burnt, Anacardium, Aurum,
Graphites, Nux vom. When produced by catarrh, Pulsatilla,
Sulphur. When of cheese, Nux vom. Of coffee, Pulsatilla. Of
lime or chalk, Calcarea, Magnesia carb. When disgusting, Cantharides. As of spoiled eggs, Calcarea, Magnetus Polus Anticus.
When depraved, so as to render assafœtida agreeable, Aurum,
Bell., Phos. When illusory of gunpowder, Calc. Of herring,
Agnus castus, Bell. Of burnt horn, Pulsatilla. Of manure, An-
acardium, Calcarea, Veratrum. Of musk, Agnus castus. Of
pitch, Arsenicum, Conium. Of pus, Senega. When putrid,
Arum, Bell. Of smoke, Sulphur, etc.

Paracusis, or perversion of the sense of hearing, presents
itself in various forms, but mainly connected with diseased conditions. When there is a sensation of hissing, Graphites, Kreosotum. Of humming, Ammonium carb., Belladonna. Of reports, Graphites, Kali carb., Staphysagria. Of ringing, Ambr.,
Calc., Con. Of roaring, Aconite, Aurum, Barytas, Belladonna,
China, Crocus. Of thundering, Graphites, Platina. When any
of these symptoms are prominently attendant upon diseased conditions of the system, they may be taken into account in directing the remedy to be employed.

Paropsis, or perverted vision, may be so marked as to produce many strange anomalies, as *diplopia*, or double vision;
Hemiopia, or seeing one-half of objects; and *pseudoblepsia*, or
seeing objects that have no existence. Many of these are symptomatic of various diseases of the nervous system, and may be
made to disappear by the treatment of these diseases, in accordance with the totality of the symptoms. For double sightedness,

Bell. and Cicuta. For hemeralopia, Bell., Hyoscyamus, Mercurius, Stramonium and Veratrum. For pseudoblepsia, Calc., Drosera, Ignatia, Mercurius, Natrum mur., Lycop. For feeble sight, Anacardium, China, Cin. For short sightedness, Conium, Lycopodium, Nitric acid. Far sightedness, Con., Hyoscyamus. For other particulars different remedies are applicable.

CHAPTER XLV.

CEPHALALGIA, HEADACHE.

Headache may be general or confined to a single part of the head, and not unfrequently arises from varied disordered conditions. There are indeed so many varieties of the disorder arising from such a multiplicity of causes, and symptomatic of many different morbid conditions, that a perfect knowledge of the pathological condition of the system attending it, is impossible; and therefore the only guide in treatment must be the symptoms. We may, however, derive much aid in the treatment, when either the remote or proximate cause is apparent.

CAUSES.—As before remarked, the causes are various. Headache may be attendant on febrile diseases; it may result from debauch, fatigue, nervous excitability, constitutional infirmity, indigestion, improper or unsuitable articles of diet and almost any other disturbing agency.

TREATMENT.—The principal remedies employed in the treatment of the different varieties of the disorder are Aconite, Arnica, Arsenicum, Belladonna, Bryonia, Chamomilla, China, Coffea, Digitalis, Dulcamara, Ferrum, Graphites, Hyoscyamus, Kreosotum, Lachesis, Mercurius, Nux vom., Natrum mur., Opium, Pulsatilla, Rhus tox., Sepia, Sulphur, Veratrum, Zincum, etc., etc. An analysis of the remedies to meet the various symptoms and conditions, requires minute observation. From the 12x to the 30x should be employed.

When headache arises from taking cold, Aconite, Bell., Nux vomica, especially if there is fever, pain in the back and limbs.

Headache in the afternoon, Bell., Lycopodium.

Headache in the cold air, Coffea, Ferrum; in the open air, Calc., Caus., Chin.; in warm air, Iodium.

When there is a sensation as if the head would split, Aconite; when arising from a fit of anger, Nux vom., or with getting angry, Dulcamara; when attended with apprehension, Fluoric acid.

Headache arising from disorder of the bowels, Graphites. Plumbum.
Headache ascending from the nape of the neck, Sanguinaria.
Headache relieved by falling asleep, Anacardium.
Headache extending down the back, Natrum mur., Phos., Puls.
Headache with backache, Sabina, Veratrum.
Headache as if the brain were pressed together, Arnica.
Headache as from a band around the head, Merc., Stann.
Headache in arthritic persons, Bell., Colocynth, Nux vom.
Headache from bending forward, Spigelia, Staphysagria.
Headache with bloated feeling, Bell.
Headache arising from loss of blood, Chin., Cocculus.
Headache in the bones of the head, Aurum, Mercurius, Sulphur.
Headache with desire to bury the head in the pillow, Bell., Hyos.
Headache arising from debauch, China, Nux vom., Lachesis.
Headache caused by chagrin, Bryon., Cham., Ignatia.
Headache with sensation of burning, Mercurius.
Headache with chilliness, Lachesis, Nitric acid.
Headache during paroxysms of coughing, Nux vom.
Headache continuing day and night, Rhus tox.
Headache from drinking coffee, Cham., Ignat., Nux vom.
Headache as if it would fly to pieces, Bell., Bry., Merc., Sil., Sulp.
Headache from mental exertion, Aurum, Calc., China, Nux vom.
Headache abating in the evening, Natrum mur.
Headache with sensation of hammering, Ferrum.
Headache caused by grief or fright, Ignatia, Phos. ac., Opium.

When headache is attended with fever, and in the forehead with heat in the head and heaviness, Aconite.

If produced from fatigue, brought on from over-exertion, Arnica. If produced by alcoholic drinks, attended with derangement and burning in the epigastrium, Arsenicum.

If confined to the forehead, as if there is hyperæmia, and pain as if the head would split or fly to pieces, pain in the orbits, with closing of the eyes, *Belladonna;* and also where there is hemicrania, *Belladonna.* If attendant on severe gastric derangement in rheumatic patients, great fulness and heaviness of the head, with digging pressure in the direction of the forehead and when the headache is worse when moving about, *Bryonia.*

When there is headache during sleep, or early in the morning on waking, as if the head would fly to pieces, or rush of blood to the head with beating in the brain, *Cham.*

When there is headache from suppressed catarrh, or bruised sensation of the brain, with sleeplessness—headache as though the head would fly to pieces, with heat and fulness of the head, at night, or worse in the open air, or aggravated by contact, and especially if the headache supervenes upon the loss of blood or diarrhœa, *China*, and also if the roots of the hair are sensitive to contact and a general soreness of the integuments of the head, *China.*

For headache, attended with excessive painfulness and irritability of the body and mind, aversion to the open air, or arising from intoxication on wine, or from excessive emotions, or supervening upon an attack of measles, or for hemicrania as from a nail in the parietal bone, *Coffea.*

For attacks of pressure in the forepart of the head during mental exertion, stitches in the temples and forehead externally, vertigo, with trembling, *Digitalis.*

When there is internal uneasiness, dry heat and burning in the skin, or fever after a cold, attended with stupefying headache, confined only to some spots, the occiput feels enlarged, or when attended with rush of blood to the head with humming in the ears and hard of hearing, the headache aggravated by motion and talking, *Dulcamara.*

For headache on the vertex with a painful pressure when in the cool, open air, and the eyes red with burning and the scalp is painful, *Ferrum.*

For headache confined to the occiput, chronic dryness of the skin, pressure in the eyes, oppressive constriction and tension in the occiput, *Graphites.*

In headache, as if from concussion of the brain, stupefying, attended with spasmodic closing of the lids, or double vision, or headache arising from inflammation of the meninges, hydrocephalus, and a shaking of the head to and fro, *Hyoscyamus.*

For headache in rheumatic or scrofulous patients, attended with weak memory, tearing day and night with flushed heat in the face, sleeplessness and throbbing in the forehead, *Kreosotum.*

When the headache arises from exposure to the sun, or abuse of mercury, or from intoxication, attended with nausea, or when coupled with nausea, *Lachesis.*

For tearing, burning headache, burning and smarting of te eyes, *Mercurius.*

If the head becomes painful early in the morning or after eating, increased by motion or bending forwards, attended with nausea, and especially in drunkards, *Nux vom.*

For headache and weak memory, attended with heaviness of the head, and painful, as if it would fly to pieces, or as if compressed, especially during mental exertion, *Natrum mur.*

Headache produced by congestion of blood to the head with violent throbbing in the same, or headache aggravated by moving the eyes, or like oppressive tightness of the whole head, *Opium.*

Headache caused by the abuse of mercury, a cold, or by derangement of the stomach in consequence of eating fat, or pain upon one side of the head with nausea and vomiting, and pain as if the brain would be torn, or from rush of blood to the head, with stinging beating in the brain, when stooping or studying, and headache after lying down in the evening or early in the morning, *Pulsatilla.*

Headache immediately after eating or after drinking beer, or when moving the arms, throbbing in the occiput, painful tingling in the head, or oppressive fulness and heaviness, as if the brain would issue through the forehead on stooping, *Rhus tox.*

For morning headache, weak memory, dulness of the head and hemicrania with nausea, and vomiting; semilateral headache, after lying down preceded by weight in the head; beating headache, especially in the occiput, or when occasioned by rush of blood to the head, with heat in the head when stooping, pressure in the eyeballs and especially if attended with depression of spirits or sadness and even anxiety, *Sepia.*

Headache nightly, with feeling of fulness and weight in the head, especially in the occiput, and also if attended with weak memory or melancholy, or vertigo when sitting, or early in the morning, or coldness of the outer head or irritable drowsiness in the after part of the day and a good deal of chilliness at night, *Sulphur.*

For hemicrania with nausea and vomiting, or with painful stiffness in the nape of the neck, or with eneuresis or oppressive headache with pain in the stomach, considerable tendency of blood to the head, cold sweat upon the forehead, *Veratrum.*

Headache attended with drawing in the occiput, vertigo and inclination to fall to the left side, pain in the forehead, temples and occiput, worse after dinner; oppressive headache early in the morning in the forehead with dullness in the temples and occiput, and sometimes attended with pressure in the eyes, *Zincum*.

Headache being produced by so many disturbing agencies and being connected with so great a variety of conditions that a great variety of remedies will be required, and in all cases a careful adaptation of the remedy according to the group of attendant symptoms, will be necessary.

DIET AND REGIMEN—When suffering from headache arising from any cause whatever, it is necessary to guard and protect the function of digestion by adhering strictly to a plain but nutritious diet, and moreover unless the disorder is attendant upon such conditions of the system as forbid it, the patient should frequently be supplied with a fresh, invigorating atmosphere and should be restricted to regular habits, in eating, drinking, sleeping, etc.

Sick Headache.

Ordinary sick headache is characterized by rending pain at the top of the head, with violent retching and vomiting. It appears to be essentially nervous, inasmuch as the circulation does not appear to be affected.

CAUSES.—Sick headache appears to be a constitutional infirmity with many, and comes on at irregular periods from trivial exciting causes; sometimes an attack is brought on by looking at any dazzling object, by too tight ligatures about the head, or by a comb pressing powerfully upon it. Hemicrania, which is one of the forms of sick headache, is not unfrequently attended with hysteria and is peculiar to hysterical individuals, and on this account is sometimes termed *hysteric* or *hysteric nail*, from the sensation having been compared to that of a nail driven into the scalp.

Hemicrania in many cases returns periodically, like the paroxysms of an intermittent fever; by some it is regarded a form of neuralgia. *Piorry* regards it neuralgia of the iris, because fatigue of the eye brings on the difficulty, and operations upon the eye will produce vomiting, the same as in hemicrania; as the difficulty is common to all ages, it is believed to be hereditary, or that a decided predisposition may be laid in the organization.

At times an attack of hemicrania is preceded by deprivations of vision and audition and the stomach exhibits signs of derangement by the presence of nausea and vomiting of an acid matter. At other times the attack comes on without any preceding premonotions, and is excessively severe, being confined to one side of the head, affecting more especially the forehead and the temples. Although during an attack there is no encephalitis, the encephalon, nevertheless, is quite sensitive to light and sound and even the skin of the parts affected is unable to bear the slightest touch. The intellect is rarely disturbed, though strange perversions of senses are occasionally witnessed. In most cases the stomach is disordered, but the circulation remains in a normal condition.

During a severe attack there is profuse lachrymation upon the side affected, and sometimes the secretory organs are so much deranged by the attack as to occasion jaundice. The duration of the paroxysms vary from two to four or six hours. The periods of their occurence are very irregular, sometimes only once a year, at other times every week or two weeks.

TREATMENT.—The remedies for the most part employed in the treatment of sick headache, are Bell., Bry., Cham., Calc., Ignatia, Nux vom., Pulsatilla, Iris versicolor, Sepia, Sulphur. Those which are the most applicable in hemicrania, are Bryonia, Calcarea, Graphites, Mercurius, Spigelia, etc., 12x attenuation.

Belladonna will be applicable to those cases that are marked by severe rending pain in the vertex and forehead, attended with severe vomiting, and also in hemicrania where the pain is confined to a single spot, and affecting the eye, and attended with nausea and vomiting.

Bryonia is suited to those paroxsms where there is vomiting of bilious matters, aggravated by motion, and also into hysteric headache or hemicrania, attended with vomiting and lying down.

Chamomilla, when there is hemicrania in children, attended with vomiting of greenish bile, and general restlessness of the whole system.

Calcarea carb., when the hemicrania is simply attended with eructations and inclination to vomit, icy coldness about the head, especially on the right side.

Ignatia, when there is headache as from a nail driven into the brain, with inclination to vomit, lessened by bending the head forwards, and when there is hemicrania, aggravated by stooping, coffee, noise and odors.

Nux vomica is suitable when there is pain and fulness of the head, and nausea in the after part of the day, and also in hemicrania, with nausea and sour vomiting, and when worse in stormy weather.

Graphites, when there is hemicrania, with nausea and sour vomiting, worse when moving the head, as when riding in a carriage.

Cocculus, when there is inclination to vomit, and bruised feeling in the bowels, and convulsive trembling of the head, pressure and bruised pain in the eyes, headache and vomiting resembling seasickness.

M-rcurius viv., when there is violent, rending headache, as if the head would fly to pieces, and bitter vomiting, resulting in jaundice, and when the pain is aggravated by warmth in the bed, tearing headache on one side, and also tearing, burning headache, and bitter vomiting, especially when the pain is confined to the temples, very suitable for persons of pale complexion, jaundiced hue of the skin, with dim, dark-looking eyes.

Pulsatilla, when there is sick headache in persons of mild disposition and lymphatic temperament, hemicrania with nausea and vomiting, semilateral headache and nausea, at or near the menstrual period, aggravated by lying down, or when the headache has been caused by the abuse of mercury, or previous derangement of the stomach, and when it is especially worse in the evening, and when there is sweat on the hairy scalp and in the face.

Iris vers., when there is semilateral headache, and severe beating in the head and an irritable condition of the stomach and bowels; frequent nausea, retching and vomiting.

Spigelia.—Headache and vomiting, aggravated by the least exercise; boring and digging, tearing headache during motion; shocks in the head and bilious vomiting, or nausea and retching; burning pain at the forehead and temples, as far as the eyes; pain in the orbits; pressure on the eyeballs, especially when turning the eyes, and when there is vertigo and nausea.

Sepia is one of the best remedies for sick headache in the morning, or semilateral headache in the evening; dullness of the head; hemicrania, with nausea and vomiting, and stinging and boring pains; beating headache, with nausea and eructations; headache, with deathly sickness, and pressure upon the top of the head; pressure in the eyeballs. This remedy is especially suited to those of pale face, with blue margins around the eyes, or yellow or sallow complexion, having the appearance of jaundice, and especially when headache is attended with eructations, mostly sour, or bitter, or foul, or tasting of the ingesta after breakfast. It is suitable for hysterical females suffering from uterine weakness, and prone to paroxysms of sick headache.

Sulphur is one of the most efficient remedies in sick headache, when there is a feeling of fulness and weight in the head, or when the pains are so violent as to cause fainting fits or hysteric spasms, and especially when the pain is most felt when the body is at rest; and also when there is chronic headache, and occasional nausea, and a throbbing headache, mostly with heat in the head; or stitching headache, especially in the forehead; and also when the paroxysm is succeeded by yellowness of the skin and schlerotica; and when the headache is worse in the open air; and finally, when the paroxysms are characterized by coldness of the forehead and the scalp.

When sick headache frequently affects those who are suffering from prolapsus uteri, Sulphur may be employed first, and followed by Sepia, if in feeble constitutions; or it may be followed by Belladonna in robust or plethoric females.

Platina will be found a successful remedy when the headache comes on, gradually increasing and then decreasing, with a numb feeling in the head, and on the vertex; and when there are pains in the sides of the head, as from a plug; or when there is compressive pain in the forehead and temples, roaring in the head; and when there is a cold feeling in the eyes, objects seem smaller than they are; and also when there is burning and redness of the face, burnt feeling on the tongue; and especially when the headache supervenes upon protracted menstruation; or when there is debility of the menses, attended with short breath, constrictive oppression of the chest and palpitation of the heart; and when, during the headache, there is constrictive pain in the pit of the stomach.

Aurum is also a remedy especially suited to females when there is burning in the forehead; cold feeling on the top of the head, and beating in the left side of the forehead, and when there is sadness and weeping, and inclination to suicide; or when the sick headache attends a prostrating leucorrhœa, and is preceded by palpitation, pulling and cutting pain in the region of the heart, and when there is burning and stinging in the palmar and plantar surfaces.

Arsenicum will be found a useful remedy, when there is beating pain in the forehead, with inclination to vomit, and in hemicrania, when there is burning, tearing pains in one side of the head, and acrid vomiting and intense thirst.

Many other remedies may be consulted with reference to the cure of this inveterate lesion.

Sometimes cold applications to the head during a severe attack may be permitted, such as cloths, dipped in cold water, and perhaps too, when there is any indication of hyperæmia, tepid water, or that which is quite warm may be applied in the same way.

The *diet* and *regimen* for persons addicted to sick headache, should be restricted; they should refrain from the use of stimulants entirely, such as coffee, green tea, wine, ale, or alcoholic drinks, and from all fat or greasy food. Plain toast and black tea, bran bread, mutton and beef, with a sparse quantity of the vegetable aliments, should chiefly constitute the diet, and when practicable, exercise in the open air is commended.

To relieve suffering is the aim and design of the physician, and no common ailment, whether of body or mind, can fail of requiring his strictest attention, and in the treatment of a malady so commonly prevalent as *headache*, but little advantage will be realized from the treatment unless certain rules and regulations are strictly adhered to. It is for the medical practitioner to point out these rules and require strict attention to them. In order that a clear idea may be had of what is meant by strict attention to certain rules, the following may be specified:

1. If headache seems to be dependent upon difficult digestion, the greatest regularity should be observed in relation to the meals. The most nutritious and digestible aliments should be used, and great care should be exercised to masticate every particle before taken into the stomach.

2. The quantity of food should be restricted to what the

digestive organs can take care of, without being burthened, and none but light food should be taken to retire to rest upon.

3. If any of the allowed aliments are ascertained to be the cause of bringing on a paroxysm, or of producing any aggravations, such articles should be prohibited.

4. If any known practice appears to produce headache, let it be discontinued, if possible. Sometimes a person's labor or employment may disagree with his health, as indicated by continual headache when in the discharge of his duties; of course, a change of employment is recommended when it is practicable.

5. If headache arises from drinking wine, ale, beer or any other stimulating beverage, abstinence from the use of these articles should be an imperative rule.

6. Should headache succeed the too free use of tobacco or coffee, tea, or any other stimulant, abstinence from their use until the health becomes established, should be regarded an imperative rule.

7. When persons appear to suffer from constitutional sick headache, it is the duty of the practitioner to seek out the most favorable measures for affecting a change in the system, that it may obviate the suffering—as for instance; all irregularities should be guarded against, such as in eating, drinking, exposure, sleeping, etc.

8. In prescribing remedies, the practitioner should first study his case well and be critical in the selection of his remedy, and then he should persevere in the treatment, allowing of no derelictions on the part of the patient, until the effect has been satisfactory, and in this way a change may be effected in the system, and the headache may be effectually cured, and on the contrary, any relaxation on the part of the patient will only retard the efforts of his physician, for no constitutional changes can be effected without a persistent change of regimen.

Headaches of a mild character, and when the subjects are able to keep about, may often be mitigated by gentle exercise in the open air, and particularly if they are purely nervous in their character, and not dependent upon febrile difficulties; but the exercise should be regular and not violent, for in feeble constitutions nothing is better calculated to produce headache than a degree of exertion beyond the patient's power of endurance. Many females when they go into the streets to walk, are led by a fondness of novelty and change to prolong their exercise to a degree that defeats the legitimate object for which it is intended. In all such cases the practitioner should be critical in prescribing proper restrictions, and particularly when headache is dependent on other chronic lesions, easily aggravated by over-exertion. Headaches attended with fever require rest in healthy departments, free from an adulterated atmosphere, or sickening odors of any kind.

CHAPTER XLVI.

ECLAMSIA—EPILEPTIC SPASMS.

UNDER this head is included the epileptiform convulsions of children which occur during dentition: 2d, Those that occur during gestation, or during parturition:

1. Convulsions of Children.

Prior to two years of age, it is quite common for children to be affected with this difficulty—for the infantile frame, during this period, is extremely impressible, and any exciting cause, such as the irritation arising from dentition, may readily occasion convulsions.

SYMPTOMS.—Sometimes without any apparent dullness or any previous indication, these convulsions may take place; but more commonly, the child will show signs of indisposition for a longer or shorter period previous, and then the child falls suddenly down in a state of insensibility, agitated with convulsions, twitchings of the muscles of the face, and those of the upper and lower extremities; the eyes are turned up, the face becomes livid, and there is at times, slight foaming at the mouth, though seldom.

The unconscious state varies in its duration; when the paroxysm is slight, it may continue but a few minutes, but generally the duration is longer, and the child gradually recovers its consciousness, though sometimes it remains dull and lethargic for hours. The first paroxysms rarely terminate fatally, but the pathological condition of the system may be such that fit will follow fit until death relieves the little sufferer. Our bills of mortality show, that a large portion of infants fall victims to this difficulty.

CAUSES.—There exists, undoubtedly, in some children, a peculiarity of constitution that predisposes them to the disease. This peculiarity may be hereditary, or, it may arise from some congenital debility. *Andral* mentions an instance of a family of five children, all dying with convulsions, where the antecedents

of the family had never known anything of the difficulty. But as
the nervous system is unusually impressible, under the age of two
years, it is not difficult to trace the disease to some irritation,
either intestinal or from dentition, that may in most cases be the
cause of the difficulty. It has been observed, that children having
a prominently developed cerebrum, are more subject to convulsions than others; and this is probably the case; for this development would seem to indicate a fully developed nervous system,
and, of course, more susceptible to impressions or shocks from
irritation, than those less developed. When very young children
are observed to be unusually precocious, with tendency to blush
or turn pale suddenly, and under the influence of the most
trifling causes, there is reason for exercising due care with
them, for such may be regarded exceedingly liable to convulsions.

Dentition is the most frequent cause of convulsions in children—the irritation produced in the nerves distributed to the
gums, being propagated to the nervous centres, and reflected to
the muscles, which are thrown into convulsions. Indigestible
food in the stomach of a child, may also prove an exciting cause
of this difficulty, and even food perfectly digestible, in too large
quantities, may have a similar effect, particularly where there is
a predisposition to the disease.

Intense mental emotion, such as fright or great terror and
severe bodily pain may likewise be reckoned among the exciting
causes. Fever will always affect some children in this way, probably on account of the hurried circulation which it occasions. A
constitutional tendency to hyperæmia on the part of some children,
occurring at certain seasons, during the first four or five years of
life, proves the source of convulsions, which often excite the
apprehension of parents as to the final result; but as the frame
has acquired more vigor—becomes more developed, the difficulty
as well as the tendency has disappeared.

Most children that die of convulsions, afford no evidence
from autopsy of disorganization of the brain, at least so far as
examination has been made.

TREATMENT.—A disease exhibiting so much of an alarming
character, requires decisive and very prudent treatment. If there
is just grounds for suspecting the cause, the treatment, of course,
will be with reference thereto. The resort to the warm bath at
first when the convulsion has made its appearance, may in a

majority of cases be commended; but its effects are only palliative and should be followed up by the administration of well chosen remedial agents.

The remedies that have proved the most effectual in the treatment of convulsions in children are Belladonna, Cantharis, Causticum, Chamomilla, Cina, Ignatia, Nux moschata, Nux vomica, Phosphorus, Platina, Stramonium, Sulphur, etc.

In children of obstinate disposition, given to crying and howling as from rage, who manifest anguish and restlessness before the spasm, and who have convulsive motions and spasms of single limbs, and of the whole body, and who appear to have considerable heat in the head, flushed face, wild and wandering looks, or half-open, protruding, or staring eyes, *Belladonna*.

In some cases, where children from the irritation of teething, become troubled with urinary difficulties, especially such as are of yellow complexion, or pale face, with tendency to erysipelatous eruptions upon the cheeks, and when the body appears to be exceedingly sensitive all over and when the spasm appears to come on from strangury, *Cantharis*.

For children of unsteady gait, and constantly liable to fall down, who are full of fear at night, and liable to spasms from irritation of the stomach, either from over-eating or from indigestible food, and in children of large abdomen and habitual or chronic constipation, involuntary emission of urine, with numbness of single parts, contraction of single limbs, convulsive motions and twitchings, *Causticum*.

For the most part, when spasms in children arise from the irritation of teething, affecting both the internal and external organs—especially when the child lies insensible changing its color frequently, with cough, rattling, yawning and stretching; or, when the spasm seems to come on violently in children, or new born infants, and especially when there has preceded the spasm a feverish condition of the system—very restless—moaning and tossing about; and also, if in new born infants the spasm has been preceded by violent crying, or if after, they lie in sopor, or half-sleep, *Chamomilla*. Another indication for the use of Chamomilla is screaming, starting and tossing about during sleep. This remedy seems to be particularly adapted to children, when the whole nervous system is very irritable and sensitive, predisposing them to spasms or convulsions. Frequent fevers and bowel complaints often deteriorate the feeble frame of infants during dentition, so as to bring about an excessive nervous irri_ tability, Chamomilla has been found one of the most useful nd effective remedies to meet these conditions.

When the spasm appears to be general, twisting the head and trunk in every direction, with striking about of the limbs— occasional violent jerks through the whole body, more particularly perceived in the hand and epigastric region, with stamping of the feet, jerking of the head upwards and backwards, and particularly if the child has manifested any symptoms of a vermicular affection, *Cina*.

Ignatia may be employed to cure children of eclamsia, when the spasms come on from teething, fright, or mortification.

Nux moschata is a valuable remedy for eclamsia in children —better suited to those of feeble constitution and scrofulous diathesis, frequently troubled with diarrhœa from debility, and violent palpitation of the heart.

Nux vomica seems best suited when the eclamsia has been brought on by cold or indigestion. When eclamsia appears to set in when the weather changes, in children afflicted with great nervous debility and contraction of single limbs, and especially when there is a tendency to rush of blood to the head, or the patient is suffering from some gastric complaints, *Phosphorus* may prove an efficient remedy.

Platina will be found a valuable remedy in cases of extreme debility, where the eclamsia does not appear to result from any local irritation, but from general debility and prostration of the nervous system.

Stramonium has been administered with great apparent benefit, in eclamsia, especially if there has been any suppression of cutaneous eruption, or when the spasm has been brought on by fright.

Sulphur is a remedy often called into requisition for children of strongly marked psoric constitutions, and in many attacks of eclamsia, where other remedies appear to be indicated. a single dose of Sulphur may prove of service.

There are other remedies, such as Aconite, Arnica, Mercurius, Pulsatilla, Veratrum, etc., that may be consulted in the treatment of eclamsia in children.

DIET.—It is requisite that the digestive crgans should be

guarded with great care; and when parents are aware that their children are predisposed, or are habitually inclined to eclamsia, the physician should enjoin upon them the duty of withholding all sweet meats—such as preserves, candies, etc. etc., and all substances of difficult digestion. The food should be of a pultaceous character—such as will sufficiently nourish the child without being a severe tax upon the digestive organs.

2. Eclamsia in Pregnant and Parturient Females.—Clonic Spasms.

Females either in the pregnant or parturient state may be attacked with convulsions decidedly of a hysterical character, but those most frequently met with in these conditions are epileptiform. The average number of females thus affected is not great; according to Churchill and others, not more than one in six hundred.

SYMPTOMS.—The symptoms that usually characterize convulsions at the latter period of utero-gestation, and during parturition are, with the exception of the *aura epileptica*, essentially those of epilepsy. It is also observed that similar premonitory symptoms in other respects are witnessed. In the convulsions, however, that occur during the latter period of gestation and during parturition, there is evidence of a greater vascular hyperæmia, as indicated by the tumefaction of the face and the injection of the blood-vessels of the tunica conjunctiva. Sometimes an intense pain in the forehead has been described as an important premonitory symptom, and also a severe pain in the stomach. The difficulty, however, sometimes comes on without warning; the pupils become dilated, the face tumid, the conjunctiva injective, and the patient temporarily convulsed; the respiration at first is irregular, the teeth being closed, the respiration forming the frothy secretion is at first hissing, but afterwards almost suspended. The paroxysms are usually short, lasting only a few minutes, the convulsions exhibiting less and less violence, gradually subside, and at variable periods after, the disordered movements cease, and the patient becomes quiet; but usually with a pulse much accelerated. Frequently consciousness is entirely restored, leaving the patient with headache and great debility. But in more unfavorable cases the consciousness is not restored, and the confused condition of the intellect remains apparent. In other cases there is total insensibility, with stertorous respiration.

It has been observed that there is usually a return of the convulsions after an uncertain interval, and then will succeed another interval. This alternation may take place several times in the course of twenty-four hours.

When convalescence is the result, recovery may take place very gradually; the patient remaining in a state of coma for some time, and when there has been considerable modification of the functions of the encephalon, the patient may continue deaf or blind, and even motionless and speechless.

In some cases of a fatal termination, the patient may lie in a comatose state for some time, and ultimately sink away and die, with an exhibition of symptoms greatly resembling those of apoplexy.

In some cases the disease manifests a fatal character from the very onset, and the patients never speak or show the most obscure indications of reason or sensation. They apparently sink at once into an apoplectic sleep and die.

Those cases of convulsion occurring during labor, are apt to engender abdominal inflammation, if not carefully guarded against by the practitioner.

Puerperal convulsions are always regarded of an exceedingly dangerous character. Dr. Churchill collected statistics that would go to prove that about one in every four cases proves fatal; and even when the patient recovers, there is no assurance seemingly, that she will not be more liable to similar attacks in her after pregnancies.

CAUSES.—It would seem from facts elicited by observation, that the causes are not always apparent. The seat of the irritation may be in the uterus, stomach or bowels, from whence it acts upon the great nervous centres, producing the convulsions. It has been ascribed to mental emotions, rush of blood to the encephalon during uterine contractions, to the use of stimulants during pregnancy, and at the time of parturition, and by some the cause is assigned to atmospheric influence, but in a majority of cases the causes are obscure. Post mortem appearances of the encephalon seldom disclose anything to rely upon as the cause, though in some instances the vessels have been turgid with blood, and in others serum has been found effused in the ventricles, or in the cavity of the arachnoid.

TREATMENT.—For Homœopathic treatment of eclamsia in pregnant and parturient females, the following group of remedies may be consulted: Argentum, Belladonna, Cantharides, Causticum, Chamomilla, Cicuta, Helleborus niger, Ignatia, Nux moschata, Nux vomica, Phosphorus, Platina, Stramonium and Sulphur.

In epileptiform attacks, during pregnancy, when the patient ʾ has complained of pains as if bruised, especially in the small of the back and the joints of the lower extremities, raw and sore pains of the internal organs; and when the patient is subject to anxiety and lowness of spirits, vertigo, with obscuration of sight, pain in the occiput, stupefying pressure in the fore part of the head, paroxysms of compression in the brain with inclination to vomit, and burning in the pit of the stomach when standing, bleeding of the nose, heartburn, etc., *Argentum.*

When the spasmodic attacks are attended with stiffness of the whole body in highly excitable temperaments, and particularly if the spasms occur during parturition, and the patient has clenched hands, or, when the attack appears to rise from rush of blood to the head, *Belladonna.*

When the patient is faint, weak, and excessively sensitive all over, with trembling desire to lie down, and is threatened with convulsions, or even if convulsions do occur during pregnancy, and especially if there is retention of urine, or spasmodic pains in the bladder before the attack, and there has been a complete loss of appetite and aversion to food, and burning eructations, increased by drinking, or when there has been any inflammation of the kidneys, *Cantharides* may be consulted.

Causticum may be employed with advantage when there is convulsive motions and twitchings, and spasm—and when coffee appears to aggravate the sufferings, and when there is an intolerable restlessness of the whole body; and when the patient is melancholy and disposed to weep, full of fear at night, and complains of stitching pain in the temples, pressure in the eyes, roaring or buzzing reports in the head, and particularly in the ears.

Chamomilla is one of the best remedies that can be called into requisition, for spasms in pregnant or lying in females, subject to debility and nervous restlessness; it will be found unusually applicable to the various ailments of females, during the delicate period of gestation, and also during parturition.

Cicuta has been regarded a useful remedy for spasmodic pain of various kinds during pregnancy and parturition. It has been successfully employed when the patient has been attacked with general convulsions, and also, when the patient has complained of jerks through the head, arms and lower limbs, resembling electric shocks.

Helleborus niger may be consulted when the patient manifests an œdematous condition of the lower extremities, and great debility and convulsions supervene, and a convulsive movement of the muscles; and also when the patient manifests a silent melancholy, or excessive anguish as if she would die.

Ignatia for confused feeling in the head with sensation of suffocation, convulsions, spasmodic and compressive pains.

Nux moschata, when the patient is subject to fainting fits, hysteric paroxysms and convulsions, either during pregnancy or parturition—and particularly if she manifests excessive languor, either in the knees or small of the back, and drowsiness before or after the spasms.

Nux vomica, when there is a gastric and bilious derangement and congestions, and tendency to convulsions; convulsions or spasms followed by paralytic weakness. This remedy is the most suitable for females of sanguine or choleric temperaments, subject to much nervous irritability, and rushes of blood to the head.

Phosphorus may be found useful, when there is a complication of chest affections, and a tendency to catarrhal fevers and lung complaint. This remedy is for the most part to be consulted as an adjunct to those well suited to spasmodic difficulties, when the symptoms that indicate its use are present.

Platina is especially suitable for females, subject to frequent trembling and palpitation of the heart, excessive debility and uterine weakness, attended with spasms without loss of consciousness, and also, when there is mental derangement after a convulsion, and when there is involuntary weeping and extreme anguish about the heart, with fear of approaching death, or general lowness of spirits.

Stramonium, when there is trembling of the limbs during labor, and convulsions with loss of consciousness.

Sulphur, when there is some impairment of the senses, such as deafness, loss of sight; and also, when the memory is impaired, after the patient has suffered from convulsions.

It has been suggested that females, suffering from eclampsia during pregnancy, should be as exempt from irritations of every kind as possible, and in a darkened room away from the noise; and that they should not be allowed the free use of watery drinks, and but little food of any kind.

Epilepsy.

This disease has a striking resemblance to eclampsia; it manifests itself in paroxysms, sometimes periodically, but generally at irregular periods.

SYMPTOMS.—The premonitory symptoms are usually such as foretell nervous affections in general. One or more of the senses may be depraved; flashes of light or dark spots before the eyes, tinnitus aurium, vertigo, confusion, or slight mental aberration, headache, numbness of some part of the body, as a finger or toe; a disagreeable itching or formication; palpitation, or irregularity in the action of the heart, with violent pains in the chest; vomiting occasionally. Most writers have described a peculiar sensation, denominated the aura-epileptica, as a premonitory symptom. It is said to be a sensation originating in the extremities, as if the air were passing upwards to the heart or brain, and when it reaches either of these centres of vital action, the patient immediately falls deprived of consciousness and the paroxysm commences.

' But whether there has been any procursory symptoms or not, the epileptic falls suddenly, sometimes uttering a distressing cry, deprived of all sensation, volition, or mental manifestation of any kind. Sometimes the patient will moan when the attack comes on; at other times he will run or jump, and move about rapidly before he falls.

French writers distinguish this disease into three varieties.

1st, *Grand mal*, when the patient falls in perfect epilepsy.

2d, *Petit mal*, when there is vertigo, confusion and partial convulsions.

3d, *Absence*, when there is no convulsion, but simply loss of sensation and intelligence.

It would seem, however, that this distinction depends entirely upon the severity of the symptoms.

When the symptoms are severe, the face appears tumefied and livid, the eyes turned up and fixed, the pupils dilated or contracted, and immovable; the jaws are so firmly brought together as sometimes to injure the tongue. The convulsions are for the most part general, affecting all the voluntary muscles, though sometimes those of one side are more affected than those of the other. The inspiratory muscles likewise participate in the convulsions; the respiration becomes hurried and laborious; short inspirations, frequent and loud. Sometimes the circulation does not appear to be affected, though generally it is much disturbed; at times the respiration seems temporarily arrested. The violence of the distortions does not usually last many minutes, before it begins to diminish. The redness of the face disappears, and the face becomes pale; perspiration begins to appear upon the surface, and the patient manifests great prostration and is generally devoid of consciousness, completely comatose, with loud respiration.

After an indefinite length of time, the patient begins to recover, still complaining of a confusion, lassitude, pains in the head and limbs, and ignorant of what has occurred except from the injuries he may have received during the paroxysm.

Sometimes a furious mania succeeds, which may last for several days. This has been termed mania epileptica, or epileptic delirium.

The paroxysms of epilepsy may sometimes occur only once in a year, but more frequently they occur as often as once a month, and sometimes every week; and, occasionally every day and even at shorter intervals. The more frequently they occur the less violent may be the symptoms; the paroxysms not being fully formed. Sometimes there is merely a loss of consciousness, or a slight exhibition of convulsions in the muscles of the face.

When the disease is confirmed, the attacks commonly come on during the night, shortly after the patient has gone to sleep; and he awakes in the morning with no knowledge of his having had an attack, except from the feelings of languor and lassitude with which he finds himself afflicted.

The horizontal position assumed on going to sleep, is supposed to facilitate the flow of blood to the head by the arteries, and thereby occasion the difficulty; but it seems quite as reasonable to suppose, that some modification of the nervous centres themselves during sleep, may favor the epileptic condition.

PROGNOSIS.—In a majority of instances, epileptics have ultimately fallen into idiocy, but when the difficulty occurs prior to the age of puberty, it may terminate in health. The evolution that takes place at this period in the system may change the morbid condition, and the disease may disappear under Homœopathic treatment. Cures have been wrought at other and more advanced periods of life, but in many cases after a duration of years, other maladies supervene, under which the patient sinks. Death seldom occurs during a paroxysm, unless it results from congestion of the brain, or from the severe depression which the violence of the disease has produced upon the system, rendering it totally unable to rally.

CAUSES.—Young persons are more subject to epilepsy than adults, and females more than males, from which it might seem that feebleness or delicacy of the constitution may render the system more liable to the disease. It is maintained by some that epilepsy is a hereditary disease, but there are doubts of this being true; although in some instances, perhaps, the disease may be hereditarily transmitted.

When there is great mobility and irritability of the nervous system, atmospheric heat may develop the disease.

Among the exciting causes may be reckoned, mental application and emotion, frights; tickling the soles of the feet or sides of children has been known to bring on the disease; overpowering odors, venereal excesses, great fatigue, vermicular affections, and repercussed eruptions, are also classed among the exciting causes.

Meyer supposes that epilepsy may be epidemic in schools of young misses, who have not attained the age of puberty. One being attacked, he asserts, was followed by the same difficulty in others, who were of highly excitable temperaments. Some have supposed that the condition of the moon may exert some influence of the kind, but this superstitious notion is entirely wanting in confirmation.

Disorders of the intestina. cand. are common exciting causes; paroxysms frequently occur after aliment of an improper character has been taken into the stomach.

Marshall Hall supposed all convulsive diseases to be affections of the true *medulla spinalis*, and he ranks epilepsy among the centric convulsions, which may be induced by any disease within the spine.

Post mortem researches have disclosed no anatomical characteristics peculiar to epilepsy, although the inference is, that some inappreciable modification of the nervous centres may occasion the disease.

TREATMENT.—During the paroxysm much cannot be done, it must have its course; but when there are premonitory symptoms, well chosen remedies may ward off, or materially lighten the attack. The disease is by no means to be regarded as incurable when it occurs previous to the age of puberty, nor yet when it arises as a sympathetic affection.

Its occurrence after the age of puberty, as a constitutional or hereditary infirmity, forbids the hope of a speedy cure. It having been of long duration, would argue that it is difficult to bring about a cure. Treatment, however, under the most discouraging circumstances, may prove useful in lengthening the intervals between the attacks, and also in mitigating the violence of the attacks when they occur.

The remedies generally found most useful in the treatment of this malady are Aconite, Arnica, Argentum nitricum, Belladonna, Calcarea, Causticum, Cicuta, Cuprum, Hyoscyamus, Ignatia, Nux vomica, Opium, Silicea, Stramonium and Sulphur.

Aconite, when there is a full bounding pulse, in the commencement of an attack, and also, when the subject is of a plethoric habit, and of sanguine temperament, and particularly if there is feverish heat about the head, and vertigo.

Arnica, when before the attack there is a disposition to yawn, and the patient seems wearied and fatigued; and also, when the attack has been excited by a blow or fall. This remedy is also useful after the convulsion has passed off, when the patient feels sore and fatigued, with a sensation in the extremities, as if bruised..

Argentum nitricum.—This remedy has been used between the attacks, when the epilepsy has been complete; when there is a sensation as if the limbs would go to sleep, and when very weak and weary as if worn out and exhausted. It also may be administered during an epileptic attack when the convulsion is violent, producing a paralysis of the extremities; and when there is much tenacious mucus in the mouth, or else when there is a dry tongue; and particularly when the face exhibits a sunken, pale or bluish appearance, and the patient looks sick and exhausted.

Belladonna, at the commencement of an attack, when there is a crawling and torpor in the upper extremities, jerking of the limbs, especially of the arms; convulsive movements of the face, eyes and mouth, rush of blood to the head with vertigo; bloatedness or redness of the face, or, on the other hand, paleness and coldness of the face, with shivering and dread of light, with fixed look of the eyes, dilated or contracted pupils; or when the eyes are convulsed, obstruction of the throat, rendering the patient unable to swallow; foaming at the mouth, involuntary discharges from the bowels and of urine, oppression of the chest, and anxious respiration; great tendency to a recurrence of the fits from the most trivial excitement or contradiction, loss of consciousness, sleeplessness after the fit, great restlessness and tossing about, or lethargic sleep with grimaces and smiles, and waking with starts and cries.

Calcarea, when the fits occur in children of a scrofulous diathesis, or from suppressed eruptions, and the attack commences with severe headache, confined mostly to one side of the head or the occiput. This remedy may also be employed in the treatment of females subject to attacks of sick headache, ending in epileptiform convulsions. It may be followed with *Pulsatilla* or *Belladonna*.

Causticum, when there are convulsive motions and twitchings, contractive or burning cardialgia, and epileptic spasms; and particularly when there is preceding the attack a violent headache from getting heated; spasmodic tension of the brain, and oppressive headache and twitching of the upper lip, pressure and burning in the eyes, distension of the abdomen, and involuntary emission of urine, and constip tion of the bowels.

Cicuta, when there is vertigo, as if the patient would fall, spasmodic affections of various kinds, general convulsions and epilepsy in parturient or pregnant females. It is suited to females of pale faces, with cold extremities, subject to scurvy, suppurating eruptions upon the skin or hairy scalp, and in front or behind the ears, violent thirst, burning pressure at the stomach and anxiety at the pit of the stomach, frequent thin stool, and frequent urging to urinate, jerking and twitching of the arms and fingers.

Cuprum, when the commencement of the fit is in the fingers and toes, or in the arms, or retraction of the thumbs; and when there is loss of conciousness and speech, salivation, sometimes of a frothy character, eyes and face red, when the fits occur at the menstrual period.

Hyoscyamus, when the face is bloated, and when there is a bluish color of the lips, foam at the mouth, prominent eyes, convulsive movement of certain limbs, or of the whole body, violent tossing about, retraction of the limbs, renewal of the fits in attempting to swallow the least portion of liquid, cries, *grinding* of the teeth, loss of consciousness, involuntary and unnoticed emission of the urine, cerebral congestion, deep and lethargic sleep, with stertorous breathing.

Ignatia, when the attack is brought on by grief; convulsive movements of the limbs, eyes, muscles of the face and lips, throwing of the head; retraction of the thumbs, bluish or red face, or red on one cheek and paleness on the other, or redness and paleness alternately, frothing at the mouth, spasms in the throat and larynx, with threatening of suffocation, difficult deglutition, loss of consciousness; frequent yawning or drowsy sleep, great anxiety, and deep sighs between or before the attacks, daily paroxysms.

Nux vomica, when there are shrieks, throwing back of the head, trembling or convulsive jerks of the limbs or muscles; re newal of the paroxysms after contradictions and disappointments, or from anger; unnoticed emission of urine and passing of fæces, sensation of numbness of the limbs, vomiting, profuse perspiration, costiveness, ill humor during the intervals between the paroxysms.

Opium, when the fit occurs at night, or in the evening, throwing back the head, or violent movement of the limbs, particularly the arms; loss of consciousness, clasped hands, and deep somnolency after the paroxysm or fit.

Silicea, in chronic epilepsy, may be useful after *Calcarea*, when the fit occurs at night.

Stramonium, when there is throwing back of the head or convulsive motion of the limbs, and especially the upper portion of the body and the abdomen; haggard and pale face, stupid ex-

pression, bloated appearance of the countenance, red face, unconscious, insensible, and sometimes cries and screams, etc., etc., when
the sight of brilliant objects, or contact brings on the fits. This
remedy may be used after Aconite or Belladonna, or in alternation,
with Calcarea or Sulphur.

Sulphur, when the aura epileptica is manifest, which is
denoted by sensation, as if a mouse were crawling over the muscles.

When the patient is attacked, he should be placed in a horizontal position, and such precaution should be taken as will obviate any injury that may result from the violence of the convulsive movements. It is always commendable to insert something
between the jaws, to prevent the tongue from being bitten. If
in males, the cravat should be loosened or removed, and the clothes
also should be made loose about the chest. If in females, the
lacings of stays and corsets should be removed; cold water may
be sprinkled over the face, especially when the breathing is much
affected by a spasm of the muscles concerned in respiration.

DIET AND REGIMEN.—There are few things more pernicious
than a resort to stimulants for persons subject to epilepsy; for it
is seldom that more can be effected by their use than a mere temporary relief, while a positive injury is inflicted upon the depressed nerves, and an obstacle is thrown in the way of recuperation. The patient should be restricted to a plain diet, easy of
digestion; food should be taken only in moderate quantities. A
generous diet may be allowed to persons whose digestion is good
and whose systems are weak and exhausted and require substantial nourishment; great care, however, should be exercised not
to overload the stomach, and between the paroxysms excesses of
every kind should be avoided, and above all, excessive exertion
that is likely to weary the whole system and predispose it for an
attack.

CHAPTER XLVII.

CHOREA, ST. VITUS' DANCE.

This distressing disease, usually denominated *St. Vitus' Dance*, is unquestionably peculiar to the nervous system.

SYMPTOMS.—Irregular and uncontrollable movements of different muscles or portions of the body, and sometimes, though rarely, the whole of the body may be implicated. It has been noticed that the left half of the body is affected more frequently than the right, from which it would be inferred that the right hemisphere of the brain is implicated. The affection is not always so extensive; sometimes the muscular motions are limited to a certain part, as to the face, one arm, or to a single muscle. The motions are both strange and fantastical, as for instance, the most singular grimaces and contortions are witnessed, when limited to the face; stammering is also the result when the muscles concerned in articulation are affected. Sometimes the respiratory muscles and those of deglutition are involved in the difficulty, and it has been affirmed even, that the muscles of the alimentary canal and the bladder may be so implicated as to cause an involuntary discharge of fæces and urine.

It is not usual for the mental faculties to be much impaired unless the disease persists for a long time; under such circumstances the individual may become fretful and capricious, and sometimes, though rarely, there may be some indications of idiocy.

Andral maintains that the nutritive functions are not impaired, but others have observed an unusual torpor of the digestive organs.

During sleep the symptoms are less marked, and sometimes they appear to be entirely suspended. It has also been remarked that a fit of passion will frequently suspend the symptoms.

The disease seldom comes on without some precursory sign, although in some instances it comes on suddenly. The patient often etrays great irritability of temper, disordered digestion, palpitation of the heart and other nervous indications, as well as twitching of the muscles of the face, extremities, etc.

The duration of the affection is uncertain, sometimes it may last for a few days only, at other times it may continue for months, and even years, even to the end of life, unless some great revolution takes place in the system, as at the age of puberty under such circumstances the disease may eventuate in health; though frequently it takes another form, such as epilepsy, etc. It is believed from observation, that Homœopathic remedies may often exert a salutary influence in controlling the disease.

CAUSES.—The disease is common to childhood, and for this reason it may be regarded as one of the predisposing causes. It has been observed in the *Hospital des Enfans* of Paris, that during a period of ten years one in two hundred of the children admitted become affected with *chorea*, from which it may be inferred that the disease is not very common. Professor Reese, of New York, is of the opinion that the disease in this country, from some cause, is more frequent than formerly. It prevails the most between the ages of six and fourteen.

Some writers have reckoned among the exciting causes that of masturbation; but as the disease usually occurs previous to the age of puberty, this idea appears to be erroneous. A greater number of females seem to be affected with the disease than males. According to the observation of *Rufz* in the hospital before alluded to, there were three females to one male; similar observations have been made by other pathologists.

Some pathologists maintain, that a scrofulous diathesis is favorable for the development of the disease, and that it occurs more frequently in rickety children than others; but other authorities maintain that there is no perceptible difference in the constitutions of those affected and those not affected.

It has not been satisfactorily determined by observation whether the constitution, temperament or complexion exert any influence whatever, either as a predisposing cause, or a protection against the disease.

The disease may be transmitted from the parent to the child.

Among the *exciting causes* we may enumerate powerful mental emotions, as fright, or rage, gastric difficulties, and intestinal disease.

As the disease rarely proves fatal, it is difficult to point out the specific pathological changes that may result from it, or that may occasion the peculiar symptoms; consequently it is impossible to locate the seat of the disease or the nature of the affection; different writers have variously located the difficulty in some portions of the nervous centres; some maintain that both the brain and spinal marrow are implicated; others that the disease arises from a morbid condition of the base of the brain, and yet others that it arises from the medulla oblongata; but the majority of observers are not satisfied of there being any morbid appearances in any of the nervous centres, calculated to throw much light upon the pathology of the disease.

A general derangement of the functions of the nervous system is about all that any pathologist has been able to discern.

TREATMENT.—It is evident from the foregoing description of the disease, that nothing is presented as a guide for treatment but the symptoms. It is to these, then, as in all other cases, that the attention must be directed, in determining upon the remedies to be employed.

The remedies usually employed in the treatment of chorea, are: Arsenicum, Belladonna, Causticum, China, Cicuta, Cocculus, Coffea, Crocus, Cuprum, Dulcamara, Hyoscyamus, Ignatia, Iodium, Nux vomica, Pulsatilla, Rhus, Sepia, Stramonium, Sulphur, Zincum.

Arsenicum may prove useful when the disease afflicts persons of extreme debility that are subject to coldness and disposition to lie down, starting of single parts when falling to sleep, and when the patient is very much emaciated, and has uncontrollable twitching of certain muscles, and excessive prostration.

Belladonna.—Suited to plethoric subjects, addicted to pain in the head, or rushes of blood to the head; when there is convulsive motion or twitching of the limbs, or muscles of the face; or when the patient is subject to stammering; and when any of the limbs or muscles are subject to uncontrollable movements. *Belladonna* cured chorea of a year's standing in a girl twelve years of age, of plethoric habit, and sanguine temperament, who had no control over the movements of her arms and lower extremities, and who had previously been subject to severe pain in the head, and occasional twitchings of the muscles of the face. The same remedy has also been found useful when the disease has been brought on by fright or terror.

Causticum.—In subjects very much emaciated, this remedy has been found serviceable in the cure of *stammering*. *China*, in feeble constitutions. *Cicuta*, *Cocculus*, *Coffea* and *Crocus* are remedies that may be employed in highly excitable temperaments, and *Cuprum* is well suited to the condition of the organism that favors chorea, in nearly all cases. A gentleman of extensive experience remarked to the writer, that he had met with several cases of the disease that *Cuprum* appeared to cure, after other remedies had failed. Indeed, he remarked that he had found *Cuprum* 30th so effectual, that he had been nearly convinced that it was the specific remedy for the disease in all cases.

Dulcamara.—In cases brought on by a cold, and also in cases that appear to have resulted from suppressed eruptions.

Hyoscyamus.—When there is great contortions of the face, eyes and limbs, head thrown back, or drawn to the left side, oppressed respiration, wild and staring expression, convulsive laughter, of weeping, and twitchings of the muscles, delirium, small pulse and sunken features.

Ignatia.—When the subject is sensitive and prone to weep. *Iodium*, in persons of a scrofulous diathesis, affected with chorea.

Nux vomica and *Pulsatilla* may be employed, if symptoms of chorea have arisen from constipation, or accumulations of fæcal matter in the intestines, most suitable for sanguine and lymphatic temperaments. *Rhus*, if the symptoms set in after erysipelas, when the patient is yet weak and feeble. *Sepia*, in hysterical subjects; *Silicea* and *Sulphur*, as well as *Lycopodium* and *Calcarea carb.*, when the symptoms have followed the drying up of cutaneous eruptions. *Stramonium*, when the features are sunken, and the patient has small, quick pulse, and is subject to anxiety and delirium. *Zincum*, when there is painful soreness of the muscles, and visible twitching of the muscular fibres, worse towards evening.

DIET AND REGIMEN—The fresh air of the country is always to be commended to patients suffering from chorea. The diet should be simple and nutritious, free from irritating condiments. All stimulating drinks should be forbidden, and the patient should be as far removed as possible from exciting scenes, and children especially should be surrounded by such a combination of circumstances as will both amuse them and promote their enjoyment in a quiet manner.

Nervous Apoplexy.

This form of apoplexy, ranged under the neuroses, presents but little difference in the symptoms from those of serous apoplexy. It is generally preceded by nervous symptoms, tremors, convulsive movements, depraved condition of the senses of sight and hearing, more or less confusion, stupor, vertigo or delirium. The attack usually comes on suddenly after some powerful mental emotion.

The *symptoms* are ordinarily such as attend hæmorrhage into the encephalon; total or partial loss of sensibility and motion, with stertorous breathing, slight convulsive movements and general paralysis. The paralysis that takes place from hæmorrhage in the nervous centres, it will be remembered, is mostly confined to one side; but in nervous apoplexy both sides are affected alike, or nearly so. If it should appear on one side in a greater degree for a time, it may increase alternately to the same or a greater degree on the other; and at the same time the symptoms would be more numerous than usually attend cerebral hæmorrhage.

When symptoms of apoplexy have occurred several times, and have been of short duration, and have passed away without leaving behind them any evidence of compression, it may be inferred that the difficulty is nervous apoplexy.

The duration of the disease is generally short. It frequently appears and disappears in nearly the same moment. The disease usually terminates suddenly, being accompanied in some cases by copious discharge of watery urine, belching of wind, and also discharge of flatus from the abdomen, through the rectum.

Some cases of recovery after a season of complete paralysis have been recorded.

CAUSES.—The causes of nervous apoplexy are believed to be sudden and powerful mental emotions; and the disease usually occurs in hysterical and hypochondriacal persons. It is said to be more frequent in adult males than females, and also in those excluded from the open air, as being more impressible subjects.

TREATMENT.—Since it is apparent that powerful mental emotions are sufficient to produce the disease, it is manifestly requisite, when it does occur, to adopt every reasonable measure for removing the cause. If any subject has been known to irritate and perplex the mind, that has worn upon the system, depressed the powers of the encephalon, it is quite evident that the powers of the heart and blood-vessels may be impaired at the same time. A condition favoring the occurrence of the disease may also result from the use of tobacco, or other pernicious habits; it is requisite that these should be overcome or suspended, if possible, because it would hardly seem probable that a tendency to a disease of the kind could be overcome, so long as these very exciting causes remain.

The Homœopathic treatment of nervous apoplexy will require nearly the same group of remedies as other forms of the disease. If produced by protracted grief, *Ignatia* may have a good effect; *Belladonna*, if in sanguine temperaments, subject to headache; *Nux vomica* is also a remedy that may prove particularly serviceable when over exertion of the mind has been the exciting cause, and particularly if there is general paralysis without any apparent convulsive movements. *Sulphur* may also be consulted when the function of the brain has become so impaired as to produce derangement of the action of the heart and arteries. *Pulsatilla*, *Sepia*, *Zincum*, *Platina* and *Calcarea* are also remedies that may be consulted in the treatment of this disease.

DIET AND REGIMEN.—It seems very reasonable to suppose that persons subject to anything like nervous apoplexy, should be restricted to the simplest kind of diet, that is, such as will tax the digestive organs but little. Fresh air is also commendable, and also the enlisting of the attention by the introduction of pleasant subjects for conversation, and in short a resort to any judicious measures for diverting the mind from any subject that apparently impairs the function of the brain.

Catalepsy.

This disease of the nervous system, classed among the neuroses, consists of such a condition of the nervous centres as results in a tonic contraction of some of the muscles, so that the limbs retain the position they had prior to the attack, or in which they may have been placed during the attack.

Along with the attack, the mind and all the senses are for the time completely dormant.

SYMPTOMS.—There is considerable complication of the symptoms of catalepsy. Sometimes there are prodromic indications of an approaching attack, such as palpitation of the heart, yawning and stretching, cramps and cephalalgia, but, at other times, the patient is suddenly attacked with general or partial rigidity of the muscles, and a total loss of consciousness. The limbs are not thrown about as in ordinary convulsions, but they usually remain as placed before the attack comes on, the eyes are fixed, and usually directed upwards and forwards. The respiration may remain free, unless the disease attacks the muscle concerned in respiration, then this function may be so interfered with as to render it almost imperceptible. The same may be remarked of circulation. The pulse may continue of nearly the normal character, or it may become so feeble as to be difficult of detection. The limbs for the most part continue flexible, but stiff when an attempt is made to move them. This is not always the case, for in rare cases they become perfectly rigid, and will retain any position in which they may be placed.

The face is somewhat flushed, and the skin usually warm. In very rare cases, the mind remains unimpaired, but in the greater proportion of cases the paroxysm causes an entire suspension of the sensation and intellectual action, so that nothing whatever that occurred during the paroxysm is recollected. Neither has the skin any sensibility; it may be pinched or pricked without the patient experiencing any pain; light will not contract the pupil of the eye, and the hearing is entirely suspended.

The attacks vary in duration; sometimes they are transient, and pass off very soon; at other times they continue for hours, and even days, presenting one of the forms of *trance*, it is supposed, which has been described by authors.

CAUSES.—It has been observed that persons subject to catalepsy, possess a highly impressible nervous system, and on this account the affection has been the most frequently noticed in hysterical subjects, and most authors regard this affection only as a variety of hysteria. This being the case, we must look to mental agency as constituting the most apparent exciting cause of the difficulty.

TREATMENT.—This disease being so nearly allied to other neuroses, and especially to hysteria, of which this is regarded as a variety, that we may defer the consideration of the specific treatment till we have considered this disease.

Hysteria.

This description of neuroses is so named from its supposèd origin, in connection with the uterus. But this idea is not generally received at the present day, although it is probable that some morbid condition of this organ may often prove an exciting cause. Many cases occur in males, as well as females, and this circumstance alone would negative the idea of there being necessarily any such connection.

SYMPTOMS.—These are so various that it would be utterly impossible to enumerate them, or even describe them even in a general way. There is scarcely any disease which hysteria cannot simulate, and yet there are symptoms that may be regarded peculiar to the affection. As in other neuroses we may expect to find hysterical subjects highly endowed with nervous symptoms, unusually impressible, easily excited to laughter and crying in alternation, without any assignable cause, and to great variations, as to their spirits, sometimes severely depressed, and at other times unusually elevated, accompanied by a greater or less degree of hypochondria. These symptoms, with the sensation of a ball ascending in the throat, inducing a feeling of suffocation, sometimes fill the patient with fearful forebodings. This sensation of the ball is what is termed the *globus hystericus*. Attending this difficulty is also severe palpitation and occasional dyspnœa, headache, constipation, and a copious secretion of limpid urine. These may be regarded as symptoms that characterize hysteria in a mild form, and when they occur suddenly but little doubt is left of the attack being that of hysteria.

In other cases these symptoms may precede spasms, which are of an exceedingly violent character. Ladies attacked with this form of the disease, even of feeble frame and delicate muscles, will sometimes be so severely affected as to require the exercise of great strength to keep them in bed, the trunk of the body being twisted in all directions, the limbs being moved so forcibly as to defy all efforts to control them; the hands become so forcibly clenched as to resist all attempts to straighten the fingers. It will be seen that this form of the disease differs in nothing from what we described under the head of catalepsy, which we stated was but a variety of this affection.

As patients recover from the severe forms of hysteria, the fits

42

of laughing and crying often recur with distressing hiccough. The intelligence often remains undisturbed, and this shows the wide distinction between hysteria and epilepsy, but when the disease takes the form of catalepsy, both the intellectual and moral faculties are grossly perverted at times, so that obscene manœuvres are often persisted in by the patient, utterly at variance with the usual character and habits.

The severe form of the disease may continue for a longer or shorter period; recovery usually takes place in a few hours, and the patient is restored to her former condition, feeling fatigued on account of the extra exertion to which she has been subjected, and perhaps some degree of lethargy, which gradually disappears. *Dr. Samuel George Morton*, who bestowed considerable attention to this disease, described as a particular diagnostic sign of hysteria, a peculiar gnawing pain situated immediately below the left breast, in a hollow formed between the cartilages of the fifth, sixth, and seventh ribs, and generally so circumscribed that it may be covered by a penny; the seat of pain is believed to be in the intercostal nerve.

To a young practitioner an attack of this disease, if severe, appears most formidable, yet the prognosis is always favorable. An uncomplicated case of hysteria seldom if ever proves fatal. When such is the case, the disease has evidently been the exciting cause of some other mischief implicating some of the vital organs. This undoubtedly has been the case in some instances. The writer once had under his charge an irritable and troublesome patient accustomed to forebode evil about almost all the affairs of life, who was subject to attacks of hysteria every little while, of the most formidable character; after many severe attacks her frame began to sink, and she finally appeared to sink away and die from a worn-out and exhausted condition of the nervous system. Hysteria may merge into epilepsy; under such circumstances the knowledge of the former hysterical condition may render this latter difficulty somewhat obscure, and not easy to diagnosticate.

The occurrence of the paroxysms of hysteria are somewhat irregular, as they may be developed at any time when an exciting cause is present.

The tendency to the disease may disappear under the changes that take place in the system during the progress of life. The disease usually occurs previous to the middle age, and it has been observed that persons rarely suffer from it after thirty or forty years of age. When protracted, the system may become so impressible as to allow the slightest circumstances to develop a paroxysm, or induce a fainting fit, or severe palpitation of the heart.

CAUSES.—The description which we have already given of this malady would argue that it is an unusual impressibility of the nervous system which constitutes a predisposition to it. Sometimes this predisposition is congenital and natural, at other times it is acquired. It may exist in both sexes, but for obvious reasons it is more frequently met with in females. Any morbid condition of any of the organs that will superinduce this impressibility, may be reckoned among the exciting causes. At the commencement of menstruation, as well as at the regular periods after, the nervous system of the female may become very impressible. At such times a more trivial exciting cause may give rise to hysteria than at other times when the system is stronger and less impressible. Sudden and powerful mental emotions are the most common exciting causes, when these occur at periods when the whole system is rendered highly impressible from the causes above named.

Hysteria being properly a disease of the nervous system that presents peculiar phenomena without betraying any organic derangement or lesions, of course leaves us without a knowledge of the precise pathological condition of the nervous centres. Nothing has been elicited from autopsy to throw any further light upon the nature of the disease than can be inferred from the symptoms. It has been inferred, however, by prominent writers upon the subject, that many of the protean forms of hysteria are referable to irritation of the *medulla spinalis*, especially its dorsal portion.

TREATMENT.—The treatment of hysteria may be divided into that which should be called into requistion during a paroxysm, and that which is requisite during the intervals, for the purpose of obviating the predisposition to them.

The remedies that may be employed are Agnus castus, Asarum Europæum, Aurum, Belladonna, Bryonia, Calcarea, Causticum, Cicuta, Cocculus, Conium, Ignatia, Lachesis, Moschus, Nux moschata, Nux vomica, Platina, Pulsatilla, Sepia, Stramonium, Sulphur, and some other

Agnus castus and *Asarum Europæum* are remedies that in some cases may prove very useful. When there is excessive sensitiveness and sadness, with apprehension of impending death, *Agnus castus* would seem to be indicated; and in persons of nervous excitement and mirthfulness, subject to stupefying drawing or pressure in the head, mostly in the temples, *Asarum* is preferable.

Aurum is well suited to females sensitive to pain and given to melancholy and desire for death, and when the paroxysms are preceded by anguish and inclination to suicide, and also when the patient is prone to despair or is quarrelsome, and complains of headache, as if bruised by blows, when exciting the mind until it becomes confused.

Belladonna is suitable when the paroxysm is preceded by severe pain in the head, as if there is hyperæmia of the bloodvessels of the cerebrum, and when the face appears flushed, the eyes red and swollen, and when the senses are unusually excitable, and when there is sadness and hypochondriac lowness of spirits, anguish, restlessness, or raging mania. This remedy is well suited to cases of catalepsy, in persons of sanguine temperament. *Bryonia*, in those of a bilious temperament, afflicted with hysteric spasms, given to crying, fulness and heaviness of the head, with digging pressure in the direction of the forehead.

Calcarea, when there is dizziness or dullness of the head, vertigo and headache, or hemicrania, with eructation and inclination to vomit, constriction of the throat, sensation of swelling at the pit of the stomach. *Causticum*, when the paroxysm is preceded by melancholy and weeping, with apprehension, anxiety, vertigo, oppressive headache, stitching pains in the temples, jerks and shocks in the head, good deal of mucus in the mouth. These two remedies are suitable for persons of a scrofulous diathesis, or subject to eruptions.

Cicuta, when there is trembling of the limbs, and general convulsions, or catelepsy, and spasmodic pains of various kinds, and mania, laughing, and foolish gesticulations, staring of the eyes, pale face, and froth at the mouth, jerking and twitching of the upper and lower extremities.

Cocculus, when the attack is preceded by vertigo, as if intoxicated, and the patient is given to sadness. *Conium* is useful in hysterical complaints, especially in unmarried persons subject to faiuting fits, or irritation of the spinal marrow, and particularly when there is general languor, with desire to laugh, out of spirits, indifferent, lazy and irritable. This remedy is also suitable when the hysteria seems to be connected with derangement of the uterine functions and constipation of the bowels.

Ignatia, for females of extreme sensitiveness, and disposed to weep; paroxysms come on with irresistible inclination to weep and go off with sobbing, and when the hysteric spasm comes on after eating, with hiccough, and when there is empty and weak feeling at the pit of the stomach, abdominal spasms, sensation of a ball in the throat, alternately with a sad and weeping mood, headache, with inclination to vomit, or as if a nail were driven into the brain; spasms after fright and mortification, and for general hysteric debility and fainting fits.

Lachesis, when the attacks come on with shrieks, and are preceded by a strange feeling in the throat, deep-seated headache, with nausea, fearful foreboding, fear of death, excessive moaning, mental alienation after chagrin, vertigo, with headache, especially before the menses, shortness of breath, gnawing hunger, sensation of suffocation in the wind-pipe, icy cold feet and hands.

Moschus, when there is fainting and debility, especially at night, and particularly in hysteric females at the menstrual period, and when the menses appear too early and too profuse, and also when there is constriction in the wind-pipe, suffocating, spasmodic constriction of the chest, burning in the hands, and uneasiness in the lower extremities.

Nux moschata, when there is a disposition to laugh at every thing, headache above the eyes, worse during motion; difficult menstruation, oppression of the chest, fainting fits and hysteric spasms, with excessive languor, especially in the knees and small of the back, with drowsiness, mania or headache, with sense of looseness of the brain when shaking the head; pains in the back and small of the back, as if bruised and lamed by blows.

· *Nux vomica*, when the hysteria appears to be connected with disordered digestion, fainting turns after dinner, paralytic weakness of the limbs; it is suitable for sanguine and choleric temperaments, subject to gastric derangements and bilious complaints, excessively sensitive to external impressions, irascible and irritable.

Platina, when the paroxysms of hysteria are unattended with loss of consciousness, excessive debility, spasmodic yawning, headache gradually increasing and decreasing, numb feeling in the head, burnt feeling of the tongue, constrictive feeling of the chest, and when the hysteria seems connected with uterine derangement.

Pulsatilla is evidently one of the best remedies that can be resorted to in hysteria in young females at the age of puberty, when it may result from the exceedingly impressible condition of the system, which this critical age is apt to engender. *Sepia* is a remedy that is equally useful for the complaint in females subject to paroxysms of sick headache, afflicted with prolapsus uteri, and prostrating leucorrhœa.

Stramonium, for cataleptic stiffness of the whole body and other kinds of spasms, attendant upon suppressed eruptions or secretions, and when there is coldness of the whole body, and when the spasms are not attended with loss of consciousness. *Sulphur* may be called into requisition in psoric constitutions, in changing the condition of the system that favors the development of the disease.

As remarked in the description of the disease, hysteria may present so great a variety of symptoms as well as resemblances to other affections, that it is difficult to point out a treatment that will answer the demands of the system under all circumstances. During a severe attack of hysteria, the remedies selected may be administered frequently; during the interval between the attacks remedies must be selected to meet the condition of the system, so as to overcome the predisposition and obviate, if possible, the recurrence of the attack, or to materially lighten them, should they recur, and it should be an invariable rule to remove all exciting causes as much as possible. Nothing is more to be commended, when practicable, than walking or riding in the open air, for this course will tend to strengthen the nervous system and fortify the patient against the disease.

DIET.—The diet should be plain but nutritious, free from stimulants, such as coffee, wine, strong tea and malt liquors; bathing is also to be commended as a necessary means of refreshing and invigorating the system.

NOTE.—Where signs of plethora exist during an hysterical fit, *Aconite* may be administered every thirty minutes till the

patient is relieved, and during the interval, if the pulse is full and
bounding, a dose of this remedy may be taken every day.   If the
bowels are constipated, *Nux vomica* or *Lycopodium* may be substituted for the *Aconite*, until this difficulty is relieved, and particularly if there is torpor of the intestines, and during this time
the patient should subsist upon a low diet and persist in regular
exercise.

On the other hand, when the habit is languid, *Ferrum* may
be administered during the attacks, and in the interval this remedy or *Stramonium* may be given in daily doses in connection
with a more generous diet, provided the digestive function is not
materially impaired.

Sulphur in the evening, and *China* in the morning, will
prove useful in feeble and psoric constitutions in fortifying the
system against the recurrence of the disease.

Tetanus and Trismus, Opisthotonos, Emprosthotonos.

This formidable malady, when general, consists in a permanent contraction of all the muscles, without alternations of relaxation; when partial, only some of the muscles are implicated.

This disease is termed trismus, or lock-jaw, when the lavator
muscles of the lower jaw are the seat of contraction.

It is termed opisthotonos, if seated in the extensors of the
body, so that the body is bent backwards.

If the body is thrown forward it is termed emprosthotonos,
and pleurosthotonos or lateralis if the body is bent to one side.

SYMPTOMS.—If the disease arises from a wound, the patient
usually manifests great impressibility of the nervous system, with
convulsive condition of the muscles of the neck and jaws.

In most cases the disease commences with permanent contraction of the masseter and temporal muscles, so that it is impossible to exert sufficient force to depress the lower jaw.   At
times the difficulty extends no further for several days; then the
muscles of the neck may become implicated, and finally those of
the trunk and limbs.   Opisthotonos is the most common form of
the disease, but it may assume any of the other forms.

The body, during the violence of the disease, resists every
attempt to move it; the muscles are hard and drawn into knots,
after awhile there is some diminution of the spasm, and the mus-

cles may become partially relaxed and admit of some motion, and even allow a temporary use of the muscles of deglutition in the prehension of liquids; but a remission of this kind is very generally followed by a more severe spasm.

Death is a common result of this disease, and it appears to be induced by asphyxia, the mechanical operation of respiration being interrupted. The mind sometimes remains unimpaired, and the senses may remain almost to the last moment. The circulation generally becomes accelerated.

The most fortunate cases are those of trismus, or lock-jaw. Those less so, present the form denominated opisthotonos, and these are sometimes so severe that the sufferer can only rest on his heels and occiput. Not unfrequently the muscles of the abdomen and the diaphragm are affected with irregular spasms, occasioning severe suffering.

It has been regarded a favorable indication if the pulse does not exceed 110 per minute on the fourth or fifth day of the disease, but this appears to afford a slight foundation for favorable prognosis. Sometimes the skin feels hot, and presents a temperature far above the ordinary elevation.

The disease sometimes terminates in a few hours, but at other times it may last several days, weeks or months. *Andral* states the average duration to be four or five days.

The *prognosis* of the traumatic form is usually unfavorable, though under Homœopathic treatment it is probable that many cases may be cured.

CAUSES.—A predisposition in the nervous system, which, when met by a sufficiently exciting cause, brings on the disease. The disease being more common in warm climates, leads to the inference that an elevated temperature of the atmosphere may be classed among the exciting causes. Bathing in cold water, when the body is warm with perspiration may also bring on the disease.

The pathological condition of various organs, such as inflammation of the intestines, or any irritation in the alimentary canal, as well as intense mental emotion, may give rise to it. Certain drugs also are known to produce tetanic convulsions, when administered to persons in health; *Nux vomica*, *Strychnine*, and *Brucine*, are of this class. But in many instances the disease may occur without any assignable cause.

The precise change in the organism, or the organic cause or condition in the nervous system that favors the occurrence of tetanus, is not known, as no post mortem facts have been elicited that will warrant any conclusion as to what lesions, if any, may have existed, calculated to develop the disease. *Eccentrically*, it has been demonstrated that tetanus can be developed from injuries or irritations, at a distance from the medulla spinalis, but not, however, without some kind of morbid change being produced in this centre, or otherwise tetanus would not result.

It is by no means probable but that tetanus may be developed *centrically*, that is, from some morbid change in the spinal marrow not all dependent upon an irritation in some remote part of the system.

That which is developed *eccentrically*, and called the traumatic tetanus, is by far the most common; the irritation is first induced in the terminal extremities of the nerves—it is thence extended to the medulla spinalis, and whether this condition of the medulla be one of irritation or inflammation, has been a question not yet settled. In a large number of observed cases, there has been considerable engorgement of the blood-vessels of the meninges or of the medulla itself, disclosed on dissection, but this appearance may be accidental and disconnected from the disease. Since, therefore, the intricate nature of tetanus is unknown to us, we must be governed by the symptoms in the treatment of the disease.

TREATMENT.—The treatment of tetanus Homœopathically, may prove successful in some instances; under Allopathic treatment but little success attends the efforts of the practitioner. In the multitude of experiments that have been made by drugs upon systems suffering from this disease, it might seem reasonable to suppose that some have been hit upon having a Homœopathic action. Such undoubtedly is the case with regard to *Strychnine, Hydrocyanic acid, Canabis indica*, etc.

Arnica, Belladonna, Cannabis indica, Hyoscyamus, Lachesis, Nux vomica, and Pulsatilla, are among the Homœopathic remedies employed in the treatment of the disease.

Arnica has been particularly indicated when the disease has been produced from irritation arising from local injury, which is by far the most dangerous form of the disease. It may be used both internally and externally. This form of the disease, termed traumatic tetanus, may be arrested by treating external irritations, by applying the tincture of *Hypericum*. The same remedy taken internally may have a good effect.

Belladonna in sanguine temperaments, is one of the most useful remedies for that form of tetanus brought on by a cold, or the lockjaw. It is also useful after *Arnica* in traumatic tetanus. The indicating symptoms are sensation of constriction in the throat, with tightness in the chest, grinding of the teeth, spasmodic clinching of the jaws, distortion of the mouth, foaming, interrupted deglutition, and removal or aggravation of the paroxysms on attempting to drink.

Cannabis indica is known to produce symptoms resembling *tetanus*, when taken in large doses by persons in health, and for this reason it may prove valuable as a remedy in the treatment of the disease. Hyoscyamus may be used in connection with *Belladonna*, particularly in trismus. Lachesis in *opisthotonos*, and also *Stramonium*, *Opium* and *Rhus tox*. From the fact that Nux vomica acts upon the medulla spinalis, this remedy may be usefully employed in the treatment of this disease in *sanguine* and *bilious temperaments*. Pulsatilla may be employed in persons of a mild disposition and lymphatic temperaments.

Mercurius viv. in trismus of an inflammatory character, with swelling of the angle of the lower jaw, and tension of the muscles of the throat and neck from cold.

Sometimes it will be difficult to administer remedies, in consequence of the jaws being so tightly clenched, except by olfaction, or simply bathing the lips with the medicine in solution, or perhaps in the form of an *enema*.

DIET.—The diet will of course be necessarily simple, as it will be difficult for the patient to take much except in the form of a liquid. Powerful stimulants have been called into requisition as palliatives, such as laudanum, black drop and brandy, but under Homœopathic treatment these should be discarded as obstacles in the way of a cure. The use of a flesh brush upon the surface of the skin may prove useful, but the application externally of revellants of any kind, whether in the form of sinapisms or ammoniated lotions, are believed to be pernicious. The use of cold, or even tepid baths is not clearly seen, and therefore they should be employed with great caution.

CHAPTER XLVIII.

RABIES, HYDROPHOBIA.

The term "hydrophobia" literally signifies a dread of water, which is recognized as the chief characteristic of the disease produced by the bite of a rabid animal. Water, however, is not the only thing the sight of which throws the patient into convulsions, for it has been observed that mirrors or polished bodies may have the same effect. *Andral* maintains that something closely resembling the disease may be occasionally met with in hysteria, and in some febrile affections accompanied with excessive nervous impressibility. The disease bears a close resemblance to tetanus.

SYMPTOMS.—First, those which occur before convulsions take place as follows: After an indefinite interval has elapsed from the time of the infliction of the bite, uneasiness is felt in the wound, which occasionally is re-opened, though under some circumstances no local inconvenience is felt at all. At the same time the patient complains of dullness and sense of heaviness in the head, is low spirited, and restless at night, often disturbed by terrific dreams, the appetite fails, and there is an indescribable dread in the countenance. These symptoms may occur from mere dread, without the positive existence of hydrophobia.

In the second stage the symptoms are by no means equivocal; this is termed the characteristic stage, the invasion of which is denoted by the patient being attacked with a kind of convulsive shuddering, and very soon after with real convulsions of the muscles of respiration and deglutition. *The pneumogastric nerve* in the larynx, as well as a portion of the fifth nerve in the face or fauces, appear to be subject to great impressibility, which is reflected upon the muscles of the pharynx and larynx, and the most distressing dysphagia or dyspnœa results. The convulsions come on in paroxysms, more and more frequent, and constantly increasing in intensity until death ensues.

Hydrophobia.

The sight of water, flashes of light, or polished surfaces, and sometimes the least noise, will bring on an attack of the most horrible spasm of the muscles of the pharynx and larynx. Any attempt on the part of the patient to overcome this dread of water is attended with unutterable anguish and the most distressing corporeal effort. The muscles of the face are thrown into violent agitation, and those of the throat and trunk contract so forcibly, as to threaten suffocation. These attacks at first, last but for a short time; but subsequently they occur with violence, and somewhat prolonged; the intervals between the paroxysms become shorter and more disturbed. The intellect, in a majority of instances, remains sound, and frequently the patient will utter warnings to those around him to keep out of his way lest he may bite them, or otherwise do them an injury. Ultimately, the whole system becomes agitated, the face red, the eyes sparkling, the pulse small and contracted, and the convulsions which occur at this stage are of the most inveterate character. Agony and terror seem to be depicted upon the countenance; a frothy saliva flows from the mouth. The muscles of the stomach and intestinal canal participate in the difficulty, and there is constant vomiting, with hiccough, and a cold, clammy sweat breaks out from every part of the cutaneous surface; the vital powers diminish, the pulse is scarcely perceptible and intermittent; the respiration becomes difficult, and the patient, amidst unutterable sufferings, sinks and dies.

The duration of the disease is not always the same. Sometimes it proves fatal in twenty-four hours, and at other times it may continue for three or four days, or a week; but the average duration of the disease before the patient sinks, is from fifty to sixty hours.

CAUSES.—The original cause of the disease in animals is not known; it is believed to be spontaneous, but when one becomes affected by it, others may become the victims, by having the virus communicated by its bite. It is not known that the disease ever arises spontaneously in human beings, or even in animals, except those of the canine race.

Some authors have maintained that genuine hydrophobia may be induced by powerful impressions, made upon the nervous sys-

tem; and it is probable that many of the symptoms of rabies may
be present in some cases of hysteria and monomania; as for instance, in these diseases, the nerves of deglutition and respiration
may be excessively impressible at the sight of liquids or mirrors,
but the strong resemblance of these symptoms to hydrophobia
does not argue their identity. They differ from them as not being
dependent upon any lesion of the nervous centres that may not
end in a restoration of health: whereas, the symptoms induced
by the bite of a rabid animal are in most cases fatal.

Other authors have maintained that the symptoms following
the bite of a rabid animal, and already described as characterizing
hydrophobia, are essentially those of hysteria, and altogether
dependent upon the imagination; but this view of the case is nega-
tived by the fact, that children so young as not to be suspected of
being under the influence of the imagination, become the victims
of the disease from the bite of rabid animals, and moreover, the
disease is often communicated from animal to animal in the same
way, a fact which proves beyond a doubt, that the imagination
has but little to do in generating the disease.

It has also been argued that the bite of a healthy animal can
induce the disease, and that it varies but little, if at all, from
traumatic tetanus. There is undoubtedly a resemblance between
these diseases, but they are not identical, and the fact must be ac-
knowledged, that a rabid animal is capable of communicating a
poison to men by inocculation, which induces a specific action
upon the nervous centres, and produces the disease which is
known under the name rabies or hydrophobia. *Andral* supposes
that the disease is communicated exclusively through a wound, or
a surface where the cuticle has been removed, but that it may be
communicated by placing the virus in contact with a mucus
membrane whose epithelium is entire, and *Chausier* says, the application to the nose of a handkerchief impregnated with the
saliva of a mad dog, has been known to produce the disease in
man.

Most writers have agreed, that the saliva, modified by some
morbific cause, is the agent by which the disease is induced in man,
yet some have believed that the hydrophobic virus is a secretion by
itself, mixed with the saliva, and with it applied to the wounded
part. The investigations of *Marochetti*, a Russian physician, led
him to take this view from the fact that from the third to the

ninth day of the disease, whitish pustules are perceptible near the frænum linguæ, which open spontaneously about the thirteenth day. The only confirmation of this learned gentleman's views has resulted from the dissection of numerous persons, who have died of hydrophobia, in whom were found considerable development, mostly inflammatory, of the mucous crypts at the base of the tongue, the pharynx and the upper aperture of the larynx. It would seem, also, from the analogy, that the hydrophobic poison was a secretion from the blood, from the fact that lambs have become affected from merely suckling ewes that had been bitten by a rabid dog.

Hydrophobia does not always result from the bites of animals known to be decidedly rabid. *Wagner* remarks that he has witnessed a number of instances of the kind, where the remedies employed were merely such as were superstitiously regardl effectual; and from this fact, he was led to infer that a predisposition to the disease rarely exists in man.

It is generally believed, that man laboring under the disease can communicate it to his fellow-man, but there are no facts to warrant the conclusion, yet the feeling is that he can. *Breschet* innoculated a dog with the saliva of a man suffering from hydrophobia, and in thirty-eight hours the animal became rabid, and bit several dogs, which also became rabid. How the hydrophobic virus placed thus eccentrically, affects the great nervous centres, is a mystery. The wound often heals entirely before the disease breaks out, and in some instances the recollection of the occurrence has been entirely obliterated.

TREATMENT.—Hydrophobia has uniformly been regarded a hopeless disease to attack, but cases have been cured under Homœopathic treatment. Doctor *Ramsbotham*, of Nova Scotia, has cited a case of cure of confirmed rabies in a man, and Doctor *Comstock*, of St. Louis, has also detailed the successful treatment of a case that came under his care. The most important part of the treatment to be employed, however, is that which obviates an attack of the disease, after a person has been bitten. There are judicious means to be employed at once for the purpose of extracting the virus when one has been bitten, and none will be more likely to prove successful than the use of the potential cautery, or red-hot iron, held so near the wound as to attract to the surface the poison that may have been communicated. Should the application of the cautery fail, but little advantage can be gained from excision of the part, or by disorganizing the entire surface of the wound, as absorption takes place so rapidly that the whole system may be under the influence of the virus before the knife could be successfully brought to bear in the case. A variety of means have been suggested to be employed, as prophylactics, that need not be detailed, as nearly all of them have failed, in cases where there was no want of evidence of the virus having been communicated.

In the Homœopathic treatment of this disease and its prevention, the following remedies may be employed, viz: *dry or radiating heat, Belladonna, Cantharides, Hyoscyamus, Lachesis* and *Stramonium.*

Hahnemann cites *Belladonna* as a certain preventative of hydrophobia, to be given every three or four days, but the application of radiating heat at the same time is commended. This may be done by means of a red-hot iron or live coal, placed as near the wound as possible without burning the skin or causing too intense pain; the heat should be continued for an hour, or until the patient begins to shiver and stretch himself.

Cantharides 6x dil., a useful preventative, as well as a curative, may be employed when there is great dryness and burning in the mouth and throat, much aggravated on attempting deglutition; or paroxysms of fury, alternating with convulsions, which are renewed by any pressure on the throat or abdomen, and also by the sight of water; fiery redness and sparkling of the eyes, which become prominent and frightfully convulsed; spasms in the throat, excited by pain produced by the action of the muscles of deglutition, when attempting to take fluids. *Belladonna* 6x is more available when there is drowsiness, with ineffectual efforts to sleep, in consequence of mental anguish and agitation, sense of burning in the throat, with accumulation of frothy saliva in the throat and mouth; frequent desire for drinks, which are spurned on being presented, and a suffocating or constrictive sensation in the throat on attempting to swallow; the muscles of deglutition spasmodically affected, so that the patient cannot swallow; glowing redness and bloated appearance of the face; pupils immovable and generally dilated; great dread; occasional desire to strike, spit at, or bite or tear anything the hands are laid upon; inclination to run away, continual tossing about, great physical activity, twitching in various muscles, especially those of the face, ungovernable fury, foaming at the mouth and tetanic spasms.

Along with *Belladonna*, or either before or after the use of this remedy, *Hyoscyamus* may be employed where the convulsions are severe and of long duration, and when the inclination to spit or bite is not so apparent, but a desire to injure those who attend in some way; dread of liquids on the account of the pain of swallowing and spitting out the *saliva* for the same reason; excessive convulsions, with loss of consciousness soon after an attempt to exercise the organs of deglutition.

When strong convulsions result from fixing the eye upon brilliant objects, or polished surfaces, or whatever reminds the patient of water, *Stramonium* may be employed, and especially when there are fits of laughter and singing; severe convulsions, alternating with ungovernable fury. *Lachesis*, when the convulsions take place, may prove a useful remedy.

Argentum nit., *Mercurius viv.* and *Veratrum*, are remedies that may also be consulted in the treatment of this distressing malady.

Delirium and Delirium Tremens.

By this term is meant a kind of incoherence so often associated with fever, a wandering or straying of the mind from strict rationality.

CAUSES.—These may be *centric* or *eccentric*, or those that are seated out of the encephalon, or those acting immediately upon it.

In persons highly impressible, the slightest pain in any locality by inducing modifications of the cerebral function, may cause it eccentrically, and it may be caused centrically, by cerebritis, hyperæmia, or from any cause acting immediately upon the cerebral hemispheres or their meninges; or it may occur from want of excitement in this nervous centre, which may be occasioned by loss of blood, or loss of vital power occasioned by the over-action of the nervous function, as in typhoid fevers. It may also be occasioned by exciting or intoxicating drinks and narcotics, or any thing that impairs the function of that part of the brain mmediately concerned as the seat of the mental faculties.

The only *pathological appearances* that have been disclosed by post-mortem examinations, where persons have died in a state of delirium, are traces of inflammation of the meninges, and of the convolutions and hyperæmia of the blood-vessels of the cerebrum

TREATMENT.—Delirium being for the most part a symptom attendant upon febrile diseases, it is to the peculiarity of the symptom, or rather to the kind of delirium manifest, that we are to direct the attention, in order to ascertain the remedy that may be indicated.

Against delirium in general, the following remedies may be employed: *Aconite, Arnica, Aurum, Belladonna, Bryonia, Hyoscyamus, Stramonium,* and *Sulphur.*

When the delirium appears marked with anxiety or fright, as if the patient were very solicitous about something, or is actually frightened on the account of something illusory, the remedies that have been found to answer the best are, *Belladonna, Hyoscyamus, Opium* and *Stramonium.* If the pulse appears to be full and bounding, or other signs of inflammatory action, *Aconite* may be employed. If there is gastric derangement, or constipation of the bowels, *Nux vomica,* or if at the age of puberty in young females, *Pulsatilla* and *Calcarea carb.* may prove useful.

When the delirium is characterized by the patient indulging in all kinds of fancies, Belladonna, Stramonium and Sulphur are three of the most prominent remedies to be employed. Hyoscyamus and Opium are sometimes useful, and so also may Chamomilla, Sepia, and Silicea be called for in certain temperaments.

For loquacious delirium, Belladonna, Rhus tox., Stramonium and Veratrum. When the patient is merry, Belladonna, or else, Aconite, Opium and Veratrum.

For a low muttering delirium, Arsenicum, Belladonna, Hyoscyamus and Stramonium are most frequently employed. Carbo vegetabilis, Nux vomica and Opium are also worthy of being consulted.

For furious delirium, Belladonna, Bryonia and Opium, are among the most prominent remedies. Aconite and Colocynthis are sometimes useful, to meet certain conditions. Plumbum and Veratrum are also indicated; the former, when there is obstinate constipation, as in cerebral inflammations, and the latter, when there is great prostration and tendency to diarrhœa.

For delirium characterized by singing, Belladonna is indicated. The symptom presents so many phases, as being mirthful, sad, melancholic, etc., that it is not unlikely that the polychrests may be the most reliable remedies to consult, but in prescribing for this single phenomenon, the fact must not be lost sight of, that the age, temperament, general features of the disease, in other respects, are severally to be taken into account.

Mental Alienation.

The apparent distinction between delirium and mental aliena-tion is that the former is attendant upon febrile conditions of the system and the latter is not; but the term " mental alienation" is not easily defined, although it is usually employed to denote a continued or intermittent derangement of the intellectual and moral faculties.   When the system is exalted by fever, the de-rangement of the mind varies as the fever rages in a greater or less degree, but in cases of pure mental alienation where no fever is present, the variable symptoms are attributed to other causes. Most writers have considered the following divisions of mental alienation advisable to be borne in mind in order to facilitate ac-curate statistical comparisons which are so desirable.

1st. Those cases of mental alienation which consist in a mere perversion of the mental and moral faculties, and

2nd. Those which consist in the impairment or loss of the same faculties.

Under the first may be recorded *mania*, in which the intellect is completely perverted upon all subjects; second, *monomania*, or partial insanity, in which the perversion is restricted to one sub-ject; and third, *moral insanity*, which consists in a morbid perver-sion of the natural feelings, affections, inclinations, temper, habits, moral disposition and natural impulses, without any remarkable disorder of the intellect, and particularly without any insane illusions.

Under the second may be reckoned, first, *dementia*, in which the intellect has been impaired or destroyed; and second *idiocy*, where the deficiency of the intellect is congenital.

The *symptoms of mental alienation consisting in perversion of the intellectual and moral faculties* are as follows, viz.:   some strange aberrations are first noticed in the tastes, habits and no-tions, differing entirely from those of a person of sound mind. These may continue for an uncertain period before the disease becomes fully formed, after which the strangest hallucinations are experienced, the patient sees objects that exist only in his own imagination; he hears unusual sounds, and the senses of taste and smell are also subject to equal illusions. He will often expose himself to the extremes of temperature, either to the cold until his limbs become stiffened, or to extreme heat sufficient to roast them, without uttering any complaint. It is thought by some that extreme cold has not the same effect upon the insane as the sane, but this is a mistake; the organs of perception being disordered the painful sensations may not be experienced, though the physical effects may be the same. The reason, at times, becomes entirely dethroned, and then there may be incessant and incoherent talking in the most excited manner. At other times the reason may seem all right upon all subjects but one, and when this cord is touched the insane delirium is excited.

Although the reasoning faculties may be perverted, the memory of past events may be perfectly retained, but the affections towards friends and associates may be perfectly transformed into unwarrantable suspicions and hatred. The feelings and actions are of the strangest character; some may be gay, timid, wild, frank and humble; others sober, dull, passionate, cunning, mischievous and haughty. Some are destructive and quarrelsome, and will do violence to persons and things that surround them, and some seem engrossed with melancholy and are full of religion. The expression of the countenance betrays the predominant emotion. When excited, the face is flushed, the eyes sparkling, the voice is clear and loud; when otherwise the face is usually pale, the expression tranquil, and the voice weak. Sleep is banished for the most part, or when indulged in it is generally disturbed, and by no means refreshing. Unlike the febrile delirium, the insane condition presents no derangement of the nutritive function; the appetite may be as good and the digestion as easy as in persons enjoying sound health.

In *mania* the mental perversion is generally excited; when its highest pitch is attained suddenly, it has been termed *acute mania*, or raving madness. When more tardy, and the disease seems protracted, it is termed *chronic*.

In *monomania*, or in cases where the insane delirium concerns but one idea, the patient, if ambitious, fancies himself a king, or some exalted personage; if religious, he is perpetually praying; if misanthropic, he indulges in hatred of his fellow men; and if despairing, he is in constant dread of his fate hereafter, etc.

Moral insanity consists in a morbid perversion of the sentiments, feelings and affections, and frequently without any derangement of the mental faculties; the patient is singular, eccentric, fickle, and capricious, and manifests a tendency to gloom or sadness or to preternatural excitement of angry and malicious feelings, and a propensity to steal or to commit other kinds of mischief, and, in short, the whole moral character of the patient is changed.

The symptoms of mental alienation which consist in the impairment or loss of the intellectual and moral faculties, are such as may result from dotage, and are characterized by total incoherence of ideas, absence of all faculty of reflection, and the sensorium seems to have lost all power of receiving impressions from without; the recollection of the past is lost, though sometimes what transpired in early life is recollected. In complete dementia, however, nothing is remembered, all intellectual and moral manifestation is gone, and the patient only lives as a helpless and deplorable character. Sometimes the animal feelings persist, and he cries or laughs, without any assignable cause.

This form of the disease usually takes place gradually, and sometimes after furious mania, and at others, the sinking is but a gradual subsidence of the faculties.

Idiocy differs from *dementia* or loss of the faculties, in being a congenital difficulty, usually dependent upon imperfect organization of the encephalon, and it may exist in various degrees.

The *symptoms* that are characteristic of fully developed idiocy cannot well be mistaken; a vacant stare of the eyes, slavering from the mouth, which is usually open. The cerebral convolutions for the most part appear to be undeveloped; the head is deformed, so as to attract the attention even of the unprofessional, and accompanying these deformities are usually found a faulty memory, and great difficulty of learning; an imperfect articulation, rendering it difficult to pronounce a single word; an absence of ideas, and in some instances a total want of comprehension. The degree to which the power of speech exists, has been regarded as a measure of the intelligence. The idiocy is extreme when the subject cannot appreciate words spoken to him so as to be able to repeat them, but less so, when the degree of comprehension is greater.

In consequence of this deficiency of intellect, the animal propensities, developed at the age of puberty, being uncontrolled by reason, are often offensively manifested, and the idiot requires constant attention to guard him against filth, and to prevent him from disgusting exhibitions.

In some rare cases, the memory is not much impaired or a talent for music, or something analogous, may be so great as to excite astonishment.

In advanced stages of insanity, a *general paralysis* has been observed, supposed by some to be dependent upon chronic inflammation of the circumference of the brain. This happens to men more frequently than women, and especially in cases that have already passed into dementia. Impaired action of the tongue, causing the articulation to become difficult, is usually the first sign of impaired action, after which the muscles of the inferior extremities partake of the difficulty, so that the gait becomes unsteady, and perhaps after an elapse of months, the patient is unable to preserve an erect posture, and he is compelled to remain seated, or in a horizontal posture all the time. The parts subjected to pressure under such circumstances, become irritated, and gangrenous blisters will form, establishing an irritation that may fatally implicate the vital organs. *Calmeil* has stated the mean duration of the paralysis to be thirteen months, and that it rarely happens that recovery takes place.

Causes of mental alienation.—There is no doubt but that a constitutional predisposition to insanity exists, either hereditary or original, from the fact that the application of the same exciting causes will induce it in some that will have no such effect upon others. It has been observed that persons born after insanity had been developed in their parents, are more subject to the disease than those born before, and that where such hereditary disposition exists, the disease is liable to appear in the different members of a family at a particular period of life.

Andral mentions the fact, that children have become affected from a powerful emotion experienced by the mother during utero-gestation, and in consequence have become predisposed to insanity at the age of puberty.

Mental imbecility is common before the age of puberty, but mental alienation seldom occurs till after. It has been observed, that insanity is most frequent between the ages of thirty and forty, and a greater proportion of females than males are thus afflicted.

The influence of previous attacks is one of the most powerful predisposing causes, and most commonly after one attack, the individual is more liable than before. There have been rare cases however, that after repeated attacks of insanity, the predisposition has been lost.

An elevation of temperature has an injurious effect upon insane persons, and the summer is more exciting to them than cold weather, and besides it is known that heat may operate as a cause of the disease. It has been observed that recruits predisposed to insanity, when drafted for service in the torrid region, are in most instances, subject to development of the disease. The number of admissions to the insane asylums, it has been observed, are much greater during the heat of summer than in winter.

The idea was formerly cherished, that the influence of the full moon was detrimental to the insane, and on this account they received the appellation of *lunatics*, and insanity became designated by the term *lunacy*, and light often proves exciting to the insane, and this is likely to be the case at the full of the moon and at the break of day. The stimulus of light frightens some, pleases others, and agitates all, and this will account for the insane being more agitated at the full of the moon than at other periods. *Coup de soleil*, or sunstroke, has been assigned as a cause of madness, but by no means common. Injuries of the head sometimes induce mania, but not suddenly. Misfortunes of the kind more frequently cause inflammation of the brain, as the immediate consequence; and when mental alienation does supervene, it is not usually until the lapse of considerable time after receiving the injury. Intemperance, it is thought, may prove an indirect cause of mental alienation, by inducing previous states that favor the development of the disease. The excessive use of prostrating drugs, may so tax the vital energies of the economy, as to shatter the nervous system and bring on insanity. Excessive venery has not only been reckoned among the causes of insanity, but, also, as one of the prominent causes of dementia. Sudden suppression of the catamenia, pregnancy, undue lactation, and even celibacy, have been included among the causes of mental alienation. Various diseases of the brain may have this deplorable result. Violent mental emotions, misery, and great calamities, are well known causes, and to these we may add, as occasional causes, care, anxiety, passions, apprehensions relative to salvation, indigestion and diseases of the intestinal canal, loss of blood and many other circumstances.

Idiocy is common in Norway and in the mountainous countries generally, owing, it is believed, to the absence of society, while on the contrary, mental perversion is the product of society and of intellectual and moral influences. In idiocy, causes have interfered to interrupt the development of the organs. In madness, the brain being over excited, has transcended the normal boundaries.

Locality may have some influence in the production of certain forms of insanity, as well as in the generation of other forms of disease, but it is doubtful whether a mountainous country is more favorable in this respect than one more level. It is said that in Wales, which is unusually mountainous, and Italy, which is traversed by ridges, the proportion of the insane is very small.

Cretinism is one of the most striking instances of idiocy induced by locality. This seems to be a species of fatuity connected with personal deformity, as known to exist in the mountains of Switzerland.

Almost any serious derangement, or even torpidity of the digestive tube, is likely to produce some form of insanity, but most commonly that of hypochondriasis.

Diseases of the pulmonary organs, on the contrary, may not give rise to cerebral disturbances, the intellect may continue unclouded until within a very limited period previous to dissolution.

The pathology of mental alienation, has enlisted the attention of the most critical observers. *Pinel,* and others, after many examinations of the dead, came to the conclusion, that no lesions were discovered, calculated to throw any steady light upon the true nature of the disease. More modern observers have maintained that the brain presents alterations which may be detected by pathologists—and these alterations differ according as the disease is acute or chronic, and with the nature of the symptoms, whether they pertain to the intellect or otherwise.

That insanity is a purely nervous disease upon which pathological investigations can throw but little light, is indeed probable. The vital forces of the brain may become deranged without the supervening of any alteration of structure that can be detected. It is known that both acute and chronic inflammations of the viscus may take place, and it seems probable that the latter may be the sequel of the former, and be the primary physical cause of insanity. Some writers have maintained that disease in some other locality may establish an irritation by metastasis in the cerebral convolutions. Post mortem disclosures have utterly failed of establishing the truth of these propositions and we are still left to conjecture as to the pathological condition of the cerebral hemispheres attendant on mental alienation.

There are, however, some appearances that have been described, worthy of attentive study; they may be regarded as letters in the alphabet that may ultimately come into use in throwing light upon the subject.

Foville and *Pinel* have each recorded the result of his observations on the vesicular matter, viz.: that it is injected of a deep red color and preternaturally soft; that the membranes are opaque and covered with serum, lymph or pus. The bones have been found, in some cases, unnaturaly indurated and thickened, and in other cases they have presented a kind of atrophy to which the diploe had disappeared, allowing the external plate to crowd upon the internal so as to present a manifest depression externally. But even if these appearances are confirmed, an interesting question might arise as to whether they are to be regarded the organic cause of insanity or the effect.

The *morbid appearance* of the brain, in cases where persons have died demented, are better confirmed. Paleness of the viscus, as if from the absence of blood, has been well confirmed; a collapsed condition of the convolutions has also been observed, sometimes indurated, at others softened.

In congenital idiocy, the convolutions are seldom developed, and some of the constituents of the brain in its healthy condition are believed to be wanting. The brain is classed among the albuminous tissues, and when normal, the fact that it contains a definite proportion of phosphorus and sulphur, would argue that its health would cease if either of these were wanting or deficient. *Vauquelin's* chemical analysis of the brain, in numerous instances, disclosed the interesting fact that the due proportion of phosphorus and sulphur was essentially wanting in the brains of idiots. And it is not improbable but that acute encephalitis, such as occurs in malignant cases of scarlatina, may diminish the quantity of these essential ingredients, and be one cause of the dementiæ that is sometimes witnessed in the cases that recover.

The researches of *Esquirol* present many interesting facts with regard to the shape of the skull as having some relation to the intellectual faculties; but though these researches have been great, they may not have accomplished, as yet, anything remarkable by way of elucidating the relations which these malformations may have to disordered intellects.

TREATMENT.—Insanity was regarded in the earlier ages an awful dispensation of the Almighty, entirely out of the province of medicine, but in more modern times it has been regarded a disease that may often prove curable under a proper course of treatment. Since the attention of philanthopists have been turned to the insane, much has been accomplished of a praiseworthy character in providing for the proper treatment of this unfortunate class.

Asylums have been provided in all Christian countries, that have been the means of exerting a beneficial influence, and in the United States the results have been very encouraging. A very great proportion of the *lunatics* admitted into these asylums have been cured, but whether by any therapeutical treatment that has been brought to bear, is exceedingly doubtful. But little opportunity as yet has been presented for testing Homœopathic treatment in these cases in asylums. In private practice, however, many cases have received Homœopathic treatment, and it is believed with salutary results. The moral treatment that has been provided in connection with asylums, has undoubtedly proved of the utmost advantage, for it must appear reasonable that insane patients surrounded by a combination of circumstances in every way calculated to favor the recuperation of the physical powers, and at the same time well adapted for the training of the moral and intellectual faculties, are placed in a better condition for receiving benefit than they otherwise would be if left unprotected and exposed.

The most reasonable course of treatment is that which may be divided into the *moral* and *medicinal*.

The *moral treatment* relates to the management of the insane by secluding them from such influences, as appear to be unfavorable to their mental condition, and this, it must be admitted, can better be accomplished by placing them in appropriate seclusion in some well regulated asylum, than by leaving them to the care of relations or servants at home.

There may be cases, however, in which patients are attached to their homes, and relations and associates, to a degree that secures to them sufficient reason to prevent them from violent outbreaks. Such cases may not be benefitted by forcibly taking them hence; great caution should be exercised in cases of the kind, and regard must be had to the manifestations in all cases, both of mania and monomania. But in a large majority of cases, the maniac detests his nearest and dearest relatives and friends, and it becomes essential, both for his protection and recovery, as well as to secure safety of others, that he should be placed in an asylum.

In every well regulated insane establishment, the patients are classified. The furious should be separated from the more peaceable, and those who are convalescent should be allowed a secluded quarter of their own. The very violent should be so secluded and restrained, as to subdue their turbulence, if possible without the strait jacket or chains, for these shackles too often prove baneful in their influences, and excite and infuriate the unfortunate victims. It is now a well settled principle, that the insane should never be harshly treated, firmness and the absence of everything like temper in the attendant, are absolutely indispensable, and this course, it has been found, rarely fails of tranquillizing the most furious and malevolent. In all cases, however, the maniac and monomaniac should be so well guarded, as to be continually under the observation of the keeper. The entire abolition of all personal restraint, in the management of the insane, has of late been found entirely effective. To accomplish this a most rigid system of constant superintendance is necessary—the attendants should be humane and mild, and always ready to speak a kind and soothing word, and moreover to seek for pleasing subjects to interest the minds of the insane, when practicable. The results of this course of treatment have been highly satisfactory in many of the most prominent insane institutions of this country, France and England.

In cases where corporeal restraint cannot be entirely dispensed with, it has been found useful to place the patient by himself under as favorable circumstances as possible, and in the best possible situation for him to receive all the kindness that can be bestowed upon him.

This kind of discipline for the insane, it is believed, has been salutary in many cases, without even a resort to medicinal treatment at all, and all systematic efforts to induce a mental occupation of any kind to prevent insane ideas from intruding, must favor the convalescence of the patient. By carefully studying the mental characteristics and inclinations of patients, it is probable, that nearly all may be provided with labor or amusement that will exert the most beneficial influence. Some may delight in agriculture, some in horticulture, some in work shop, some in music, some in reading pleasing stories, or narratives—all these classes should be provided with occupations in accordance with their tastes, for the very one provided requires the attention in such a way as to produce a moral revulsion, preventing the topics of hallucination from engrossing the mind. Statistical reports are sufficiently abundant to prove the salutary influence of this kind of training for the minds of the insane.

It has been found impossible to benefit monomaniacs by trying to reason them out of their peculiar notions; all arguing with them should be avoided. Whatever insane idea the monomaniac may possess should be indulged; as for instance, when one fancies that some live animal is in him a counter-impression may be made by pretending to submit him to a process for its removal. *Esquirol* mentions the case of one who fancied he could not void his urine on account of producing a second deluge, but was prevailed upon by being told that the town was on fire and that he could save it from destruction by allowing his urine to pass from him. Other interesting cases of the sort are recorded, showing the necessity of refraining from contradiction, while at the same time a judicious course, apparently favoring the insane idea, may prove effectual in curing the difficulty.

It is impossible to point out the precise course to be pursued in the moral treatment of the insane under all cases. Much must be left to the discretion of physicians.

The *moral treatment* of those suffering from *dementia* and idiots, has of late years attracted the atention of philanthropists.

That the mind can be improved by culture, is a fact universally admitted. A systematic method of training or cultivating any degree of mental endowment that may exist in the idiot, it is probable, may contribute to his improvement, if not to his entire restoration. Mr. Richards, in his school for idiots, has demonstrated that a vast amount can be accomplished by bringing into action in a methodical manner the most obscure minds of the idiotic class.

HOMŒOPATHIC TREATMENT.—After the most judicious moral treatment has been brought to bear upon the insane, a resort to remedial agents in the form of Homœopathic medicines may have a beneficial effect; but certain conditions of the physical system have to be noted, in precisely the same way as in persons of sound mind.

The remedies for the most part employed in the Homœopathic treatment of the insane, are Aconite, Agaricus, Antimonium, Argentum, Arnica, Arsenicum, Aurum, Belladonna, Calcarea, Camphor, Cannabis, Cantharis, Carbo animalis, Chamomilla, Cicuta, Cocculus, Conium, Crocus, Crotalus, Cuprum, Digitalis, Dulcamara, Hyoscyamus, Kali carb., Lachesis, Ledum palustre, Lycopodium, Mercurius, Mezereum, Moschus, Natrum muriaticum, Nux moschata, Nux vomica, Opium, Phosphorus, Phosphoric acid, Platina, Pulsatilla, Rhus tox., Silicea, Stramonium, Sulphur and Veratrum.

This may seem like a long list of remedies, but a little reflection will serve to render it probable in every one's mind, that many remedies will be required to meet the various deranged conditions of the insane.

Aconite, when there is fear of death, anguish with apprehensive and trembling state of mind, and bitter wailing; great tendency to start, sensitive and irritable mood, alternations of merry singing, or warbling and whining mood, raving and gesticulation, especially at night. The 30x dil. is the best form in which to give remedies to the insane, ten drops in a glass of water, dessert spoonful three times a day.

Agaricus, when there is no disposition to talk. Timorous craziness.

Antimonium c., when there is a loathing of life, with disposition to shoot or drown one's self.

Argentum, noisy mania and craziness, hypochondriasis, gloominess.

Arsenicum, excessive anxiety and restlessness driving one to and fro in the day time, and out of bed at night, especially in the evening, after lying down; dread of being alone, fear of death, or mania of suicide, crazy.

Arnica, hypochondriac anxiety, frivolity.

Aurum, melancholy, iresistible desire to weep, anguish increasing into suicide, despair of one's self and others, disposed to grumble and quarrel, vehement and disposed to fly into a passion.

Belladonna, raging mania, head-strong, hypochondriac lowness of spirits, anguish and restlessness, tremulous despondency, disposition to escape.

Calcarea, vehement and irascible, with disposition to censure and find fault, weeping mood, anxiety, tendency to start, out of humor, obstinate, aversion to others.

Camphor, whining anxiety, disposition to quarrel.

Cannabis, mania, at times merry, at others serious, and at others raging.

Cantharis, whining, and low spirited, great restlessness, rage with cries, barking, striking, hydrophobic mania.

Carbo animalis, full of fright in the evening, tendency to start.

Chamomilla, when there is great moaning and tossing about, vexed and whining mood with crying.

Cicuta, mania with dancing, laughing and foolish gesticulation.

Cocculus, melancholy, sad, reverie after being crossed, apprehensive anguish, fear of death, disposition to feel offended.

Conum, hysteric mania, characterized by anxiety, out of spirits, hypochondriac indifference, indolent and discouraged, vexed and irritable, confused thoughts with mania.

Crocus, merry, gesticulating mania with pale face, vehement, angry, alternate harshness and kindness of disposition, forgetful and absent minded.

Crotalus, when there is lowness of spirits, with indifference to every thing, anguish and restlessness, melancholy, quarrelsome.

Cuprum, for fits of craziness characterized by thoughts about some imaginary business, or by merry singing, or sullen and trickey disposition, generally accompanied by quick pulse, red inflamed eyes, wild look, and followed by sweat, rage, confusion of ideas.

Digitalis, when there is anguish, especially in the evening with whining mood, apprehensions for the future.

Dulcamara, when there is internal uneasiness and nightly delirium, impatience and disposition to dispute without being vexed.

Hyoscyamus, when there is distress and dread of men and disposition to escape during the night, inclination to laugh at everything, loquacious and given to jealousy.

Kali carb., when there is tendency to start, and an irritable mood.

Lachesis, for crazy jealousy, faultfinding, malicious, nightly delirium, mental alienation after chagrin, or after excessive studies, religious mania.

Ledum palustre, when there is misanthropy, peevishness and ill humor.

Lycopodium, when there is obstinacy and impeded activity of the mind.

Mercurius viv., when there is obstinacy, impatience and mania, illusions of the fancy, delirium, mental alienation of drunkards.

Mezereum, when there is ill humor, dullness of intellect, frequent vanishing of ideas.

Moschus, for hypochondriasis with palpitation of the heart; stupefaction as if intoxicated.

Natrum muriaticum, when there is apathy, vehemency, and alternations of good and ill humor.

Nux moschata, when there is disposition to laugh at every thing, alternations of seriousness and laughter.

Nux vomica, anguish and restlessness, frequently attended with palpitation of the heart, and mania of suicide, irritable, artful, malicious, and quarrelsome, mania from drunkenness.

Opium, tendency to start, illusions of fancy, mania with strange fancies, rage.

Phosphorus, anxious and uneasy when alone; hypochondriac, loss of shame, dread of labor, irritable.

Phos. acid, sad, anxious for the future, apathy.

Platina, mental derangement after fright or illness.

Pulsatilla, depression of spirits, dread of company, whimsical, especially suited to persons of mild disposition and females.

Rhus tox., when there is mania of suicide, illusions of fancy, and mental alienation.

Silicea, when there is want of cheerfulness, fixed ideas upon some unimportant point, gloominess, careworn countenance.

Stramonium, when there is melancholy, hurried movements, loud laughter, indomitable rage and mania, with an inexhaustible variety of fanciful visions, lascivious talk, conversation with spirits, affectation of proud and haughty manners, dancing, constant alternatives of ludicrous gesticulations and sad, serious gestures.

Sulphur, when the patient is obstinate, irritable, peevish, fretful, or full of fancies, philosophical and religious, and when the mania is such that the patient fancies himself in possession of all sorts of beautiful objects.

Veratrum, mental alienation with singing, moving about to and fro, having the appearance of much business, laughing, whistling; sometimes violent and ill-humored.

In the medical treatment of the insane, the general condition of the nutritive functions has to be noted as well as that of the animal functions, and the same rule may be observed in prescribing remedies for the insane, as for the sane in this respect. If there is fever, indigestion, disease of the kidneys, or any other functional derangement, the same remedies may be required, without regard to the mental alienation as in other cases.

DIET AND REGIMEN.—The diet of the insane should be plain, without excitants, such as stimulating condiments, malt liquors, wines or alcoholic beverages in general; coffee should be prohibited as well as tobacco, opium, and other agents that excite or depress the nervous system; freedom of exercise in the open air as well as judicious bathing, should be encouraged.

LOSS OF MIND, IMBECILITY.—The following remedies may be consulted.

TREATMENT.—Anacardium, Argentum n., Belladonna, Calcarea, Helleborus, Hyoscyamus, Lachesis, Opium, Sepia, Sulphur, China.

Anacardium, when there is an awkward and silly demeanor,

laughing at serious things, weakness of memory and mind, inability to collect the ideas.

Argentum nit., suitable for persons that have become imbecile from epilepsy, when there appears to be absence of thought, as if stupid, foolish demeanor, silly laughing and murmurs, with appearances of grimaces or closing the eyes in the day time.

Belladonna, when imbecility has supervened upon an attack of insanity, when there is forgetfulness, absence of thoughts, confusion of ideas.

Calcarea carb., when there is a loss of mental consciousness, obstinacy, thoughtlessness, and when the imbecility has resulted from intemperance, which has first produced *mania-a-potu*, and a talking about dogs, rats and mice.

Helleborus, dullness of the inner sense, dullness of sense, with thoughtless staring at one point, weak memory, imbecility after an acute attack of scarlatina, or attending a dropsical diathesis.

Hyoscyamus, congenital imbecility, or lascivious mania and ludicrous gesticulations, loss of memory, does not recollect any thing, no power to direct the thoughts, absence of ideas.

Lachesis, weak memory, forgets that which is just spoken, mistakes the time, mind worn out with study.

Opium, congenital idiocy, when there is complete stupefaction, loss of mind from intoxication.

China, when there is loss of mind, occasioned by loss of blood or debility.

Sulphur and *Sepia* are remedies that may have a beneficial effect in dotage attendant upon old age.

When the cause of mental imbecility is known, this may have some bearing in the selection of a remedy, as for instance, when arising from scarlatina, *Sulph.* and *Phos.*; when occasioned by a blow, or concussion of the brain, *Arnica.* All remedies to be used in the 12x dil.

The condition of the system has to be noted in the adaptation of a treatment, for, aside from the imbecility, the symptoms of diseased action may be precisely the same as in ordinary cases, and this fact would argue the propriety of resorting to the same kind of treatment, or rather to the same remedies as are ordinarily found serviceable in common deranged conditions.

For the treatment of that kind of imbecility common to old

age, nothing proves more advantageous to the patient than the utmost care and attention to his wants, when he suffers from an attack of a cold, administer for his relief, when from diarrhœa, pain in the head, or any local suffering whatever, administer such remedies as will prove most likely to relieve him.

DIET.—The diet and regimen for idiots and those suffering from imbecility, must be plain and nutritious, rich gravies and fat meats must be avoided, fruits may be allowed *ad libitum.* Ablutions at regular seasons are to be commended, as well as judicious bathing, when there is no physical infirmity that would render it improper.

Hypochondriasis.—Hypochondria.

This difficulty, for the most part, is classed among the neu roses as an affection separate and distinct from what we have been considering. But, in strict propriety, it cannot be separated from mental alienation. But without doubt it is a form of monomania—at least it has been so regarded by nearly all the modern writers upon the subject. There are, however, some who are still disposed to class it with dyspepsia, with which it is undoubtedly often associated.

In our former article, allusion was made to hypochondriacal monomania, where the subjects imagined they had some live animal within them. It is characteristic of monomaniacs to have the mind fixed upon some imaginary difficulty which they dread, and this being the ever present characteristic of hypochondriasis, would seem to argue the propriety of regarding the disease as being identical with that form of mental alienation termed monomania.

This kind of monomania, however, consists of a constant dread of diseases conjured up by the imagination, the most melancholy forebodings, as well as the most painful attention to real sufferings, which very frequently are of the most trifling character.

During the prevalence of some fearful endemic disease—such as cholera or yellow fever—it has been observed that a certain class of persons become fearfully alarmed, and they appear to be constantly anticipating an attack; and whatever ailment befalls them, however slight, they are apt to magnify it into that form of disease which they so much dread. Some become afflicted with a dread of hydrophobia, and become mad upon the subject; others really believe themselves in constant danger of some other fatal malady. Many singular examples of the *hydrophobic mania* have been recorded. The following has been recorded as a veritable fact: two brothers were bitten by a rabid dog at the same time in England. One of them set off for America soon afterwards, where he resided for twenty years. After this he returned to his native country, and on learning that his brother, who had been bitten at the same time with himself, had died with every symptom of hydrophobia his imagination became so wrought upon that he died soon afterwards with similar symptoms.

The symptoms of hypochondriasis are astonishingly diversified, and for the most part exist along with the healthy play of various functions. At other times there is considerable functional disease. There may be disordered digestion, a torpid action of the liver, or some derangement of the functions of some of the other organs, whereupon the fears of the patient overcome his reason, and he imagines the most trivial symptoms to be of the greatest moment. A slight flatulency, or distension of the stomach or abdomen may amount, in his imagination, to a positive inflammation of the most serious character, working great mischief in the abdominal viscera. The slightest irregularity in the movement of the bowels, or the slightest modification in the character of the evacuations may occasion him the greatest anxiety, and dread of some impending disease of a more formidable character, or perhaps death, which he imagines is staring him in the face. In this way he is made perpetually miserable.

Nothing has been elicited from morbid anatomy at all calculated to throw any light upon the nature of this malady, but from the phenomena that usually attend it, the conclusion has been arrived at that some inappreciable morbid change in the encephalon is the immediate cause of the disease.

TREATMENT.—This course must be based upon the same principles laid down under mental alienation. At the commencement the treatment must be moral, but it is to be borne in mind that it is not best to rudely contradict the patient's notion concerning his bodily diseases. It is believed to be better to fall in with them, and prescribe for their removal. Exercise in the open air, riding on horseback, and especially the exercise afforded by traveling, and coming in contact with different scenes that new impressions may be constantly engendered, are to be commended; gymnastic exercises are also advisable when the patient's general health is such as to admit of them. It is a well known fact that the hypochondriac is averse to all exertion, and if left to his own inclination he would dwell upon, and brood over his imaginary evils, and thus render his idea more decidedly confirmed, and, of course, more difficult to eradicate. But by efforts of a judicious character, he may be induced to move about, to go from home, or to engage in harmless amusements that give exercise to the body, and at the same time afford mental occupation of a buoyant character.

There is not much that can be offered concerning the moral treatment of this unfortunate class of patients; it is a question properly belonging to the physician, who will find it necessary to use his tact and his powers of perception so as to understand how to modify his proceedings so as to meet the different characters of those he has to treat; the physician is thrown wholly upon himself, and that, too, in a moment; when he comes into the presence of a hypochondriac he will be interrogated by the patient upon subjects of the most delicate nature. The physician must be philosophical in his treatment of such cases, or otherwise he may not have sufficient adroitness to gain an influence over a mind that is disturbed, suspicious and irritable, so as to have any beneficial effect. The really morbid phenomena that may manifest themselves in the hypochondriac may indicate the employment of remedial agents to meet each individual case. It is believed that Homœopathic remedies may be selected for given cases in accordance with the symptoms manifested.

For diseases of the stomach in hypochondriacs, Nux vomica, Cocculus.

FIXED NOTIONS.—Anacardium, Aurum, Belladonna, Cicuta, Cuprum, Hyoscyamus, Ignatia, Lachesis, Stramonium.

FOREBODING OF DEATH.—Belladonna, Lachesis, Nux vomica, Platina, Zincum.

FOR ILLUSORY NOTIONS IN GENERAL.—Aconitum, Arsenicum, Belladonna, Hyoscyamus, Lachesis, Mercurius, Moschus, Nux vomica, Pulsatilla, Stramonium, Sulphur and Veratrum.

If the patient fancies he is abandoned.—Carbo animalis, Stramonium.

If haunted with the idea of being a criminal.—Hyoscyamus.

If haunted with the idea of ghosts or demons.—Arsenicum, Belladonna.

If insane upon the condition of his stomach, imagining that it is ulcerated or corroded.—Ignatia, Sabadilla.

For melancholy in general.—Arsenicum, Aurum, Helleborus, Lycopodium, Pulsatilla, Silicea, Sepia, Sulphur and Veratrum.

For low spirits.—Bryonia, Calcarea, China, Natrum, Sulphur.

FOR RELIGIOUS MANIA.—Belladonna, Crocus, Hyoscyamus, Lachesis, Locopodium, Pulsatilla, Stramonium and Sulphur.

Hypochondriasis may be attended with so great a variety of symptoms that it would be impossible to enumerate all its phases and the remedies applicable to each. The mind may become fixed in any imaginable idea, and whatever its nature may be, the corresponding remedy may be suggested.

The diet for hypochondriacs should be carefully selected to meet the condition of the digestive organs. All stimulants should be prohibited, especially those that only afford a temporary exhilaration of the animal spirits, for a corresponding depression will invariably follow their use.

CHAPTER XLIX.

DISEASES OF THE NERVES.

The diseases that affect the nerves so as to produce sensible modification of structure, as well as of function, afford something more tangible than the neuroses that we have been considering.

Neuritis, Inflammation of the Nerves.

When the nerves are the subject of inflammation, the fact may be known by constant pain increased by pressure on the affected part; the pain may be augmented when the nerve is inflamed, but it does not occur in paroxysms, as it does in neuralgia. When any nerve is so situated that its course can be traced, the pain in case of inflammation may be aggravated by pressing along the affected nerve, and the parts to which the nerve may be distributed become variously affected; muscles may become convulsed or paralyzed. There may be loss of vision, and of the sense of hearing, if the optic and auditory nerves are the seat of inflammation. *Andral* says, that inflammation of the *pneumogastric nerve* gives rise to whooping cough, or acute gastritis. The disease may either be acute or chronic.

CAUSES.—Neuritis may be induced by external violence, as by bruises or puncture, sometimes it supervenes upon surgical operations; blood-letting has sometimes given rise to the difficulty, but at other times it makes its appearance from causes within the system, which cannot be explained.

TREATMENT.—When a nerve has been injured by puncture or bruise, the application of a dilute tincture of *Aconite* or *Hypericum* to the part may prove of service.

Aconite may be administered internally when the inflammation is violent, and when there is reason to believe that the nerve may be affected with hyperæmia; *Belladonna, Arnica* and *Hypericum* may be administered internally when the inflammation arises from a mechanical difficulty; but when it arises from causes within the economy, *Belladonna, Cicuta* or *Conium*, may be administered after *Aconite*, each in 3x dil., drop doses every hour.

Neuralgia, or Pain in the Nerves.

This disease, commonly termed *tic douloureux*, is one of the most painful to which humanity is subject. It consists essentially of a more or less acute, exacerbating, or intermittent pain, seated in the nerve, and shooting along its ramifications.

SYMPTOMS.—The pain in neuralgia, in a majority of instances, occurs suddenly, though sometimes there is a slight sensation of itching, or of heat, or creeping numbness in the part, which in a gradual manner becomes more and more intense.

Then again, the paroxysm of neuralgia is preceded by a feeling of coldness and numbness, the pain for the most part is exceedingly acute and lancinating, taking place instantaneously, and extending along the nerves like an electrical shock. When the pain is at its height, it seems as if burning needles were thrust into the effected parts; after a time the agony diminishes, and is alternately succeeded by a sense of numbness, which remains until the pain returns. Exacerbations and remissions of pain take place at intervals until, alternately, the suffering becomes so that it can be endured, which was hardly the case when it was at the height of the paroxysm.

When the affected nerves are distributed to muscles slight twitching will be observed in them, when the pain is protracted and severe, the heart and arteries may sympathize and beat with more force than usual, which is the result of suffering.

If the diseased nerve is distributed to secreting organs, their functions may become impaired, the permanent agitation of the muscles may give rise to involuntary catchings, which the French term *tics*, whence the name *tic douloureux*.

When the pain continues for a long time, it must inevitably give rise to constitutional disturbances, affecting the nutrition of the whole body, and the patient may become worn out and die of exhaustion. These extreme cases, however, are of rare occurrence.

It may be said of most cases, that a cure may be wrought by time and the employment of appropriate remedies; relapses are common until the habits of the body become such as to overcome all predisposition for them to return. During sleep, if the patient is fortunate enough to attain this state, his sufferings are usually suspended, the duration of the disease is uncertain, it may be ephemeral or it may last for months and years. Cases of cure are recorded where the patient has been afflicted for ten or twelve years.

Neuralgia has received several names, according to its locality. It is termed *facial neuralgia* when the pain is felt in the frontal or supra orbital region, infra orbital and maxillary regions. The *infra orbital* has received the name *tic douloureux*. It gives occasion at times to twitchings of the lower eyelid, cheeks and upper lip, and to agony almost beyond endurance.

Dental neuralgia is a form of *toothache*, but takes place when the teeth are apparently sound, with shooting along the jaw and along the nervous ramifications, so as to endure the extremest suffering.

Neuralgia sometimes affects the trunk, following the course of the intercostal nerve, and hence is termed *intercostal* neuralgia; at other times it is seated in the parieties of the thorax, and hence termed *thoracic* neuralgia. It occasionally attacks the female mamma, so as to induce the suspicion of the existence of cancer, this is termed *mammary* neuralgia. One of the severest forms affects the nerves of the spermatic cord and the testes, extending to the nates and thighs, implicating the bladder, so as to give rise to frequent micturition, the *ileo scrotal* neuralgia descends from the lumbar region along the psoas magnus to the scrotum.

The nerves of both the upper and lower extremities may be equally affected with this disease, but it is more frequently met with in the latter. The *sciatic* neuralgia extends from the sciatic notch along the back part of the thigh to the ham, and thence it sometimes extends to the foot. It is frequently met with in a slight degree during pregnancy.

These varieties, have, it will be seen, received special names, and without doubt many more might be enumerated.

There is a variety sometimes termed *false* neuralgia, occasioned by pressure upon a nerve, which will disappear when the pressure is removed.

Tumors in the pelvis may occasion pain along the sciatic nerve. Cases have been met with where syphilitic periostitis has produced the affection, as has been abundantly proved by relief being procured on the administration of mercury.

CAUSES.—The causes of this distressing malady are very obscure. There is, however, without doubt, a predisposition to the affection, of the precise nature of which we are altogether ignorant. Persons of a highly impressible nervous system are the most liable to the affection. The disease is altogether neuropathic, although some authors have regarded it an inflammation, or rather an inflammatory action going on in the nerve, but all the phenomena of the disease are adverse to the idea, and indicative of sufficient difference to discriminate between neuritis and neuralgia.

Neither very young nor very old persons are prone to suffer from the disease; some very curious differences with reference to age are observable, as respects the different forms of the disease. The infra-orbitar is most commonly met with in adults, but in the aged the femero-popliteal is more frequently observed.

Some authors have supposed that females are more susceptible to the disease than males, but this assertion fails of receiving that confirmation which is reliable, giving it the coloring of a fact. Both sexes appear to be equally subject to neuralgia of the face, while the sciatic neuralgia more frequently attacks men than women. When the system is very susceptible, as in some persons, the most trivial circumstances may bring on an attack, a cold, moist wind, and sometimes the slightest breath of air may develop facial neuralgia of the most excruciating character. Even the touch of the razor will sometimes excite the most tormenting pain. In a state of predisposition to other forms of neuralgia, damp and cold may oftener prove the exciting causes than other circumstances.   External injuries may cause neuralgia as well as neuritis, though some maintain that neuritis always results from external injuries.   The healing up of an old ulcer and leaving a cicatrice, it is said has occasioned neuralgia, and also when a patient has once suffered from the disease, and almost any exertion, bodily or mental, may bring it on, if indulged in to excess.

Some of the most distressing cases of neuralgia on record have been caused by wounds, and frequently the pain may be experienced in the sentient extremities of the nerves, at a considerable distance from the injured portion. And not unfrequently when we can find no cause near the seat of pain, we may find some source of irritation distinct in the trunk of the nerve. Severe losses may predispose the system to neuralgia, such as happen from miscarriage, or any other cause that detracts from the nutrition of the system.

Morbid anatomy throws no light upon this disease that is at all worthy of attention, as all that has ever been elicited from post mortem appearances is rather of a negative than of a decisive character; doubtless there is some molecular change in the substance of the nerve, but not such as to indicate anything with reference to treatment. All that serves as a guide in treatment are the symptoms of each individual case.

TREATMENT.—The Homœopathic treatment of neuralgia requires the following group of remedies: Aconite, Arsenicum, Aurum, Belladonna, Bryonia, Calc. carb., China, Colocynthis, Lycopodium, Pulsatilla, Platina, Sepia, Spigelia, Sulphur and some others, in 12x dil. for each.

Aconite, when there is redness and pain on one side of the face, or pain in the teeth or maxillary region without the presence of any decayed teeth.

Arsenicum, when there is apparently a periodicity in the attacks, and the pains are of a burning, pricking and rending character, and are experienced around the eyes, and occasionally in the temples, aggravated by cold, and temporarily relieved by heat.

Aurum, when the pains appear to be in the bones, and particularly when they occur after the excessive use of mercury or blue pills.

Belladonna, when there are darting pains in the cheek bones, jaws, nose or temples, or in the neck; twitches of the eyelids, and excruciating pain in the ball of the eye; for almost every form of faceache this remedy seems adapted.

China, when there is a tendency to periodicity in the attacks, and when there is extreme sensitiveness of the skin, and particularly when the disease has occurred after the system has become weakened by losses of blood, or acute disease.

Calc. carb., when there are twitchings of the lids, pressure in the eyes, tearing pains in the facial bones, pain in the teeth after taking a draught of cold water, or from exposure to a draught of cold air, digging pain like a sore, and beating.

Colocynthis, when there are violent, rending and darting

pains, which chiefly occupy the left side of the face, aggravated by the slightest touch, and extending to the head and temples.

Lycopodium, when the right side of the face seems to be the most affected, and also when there is a torpor and creeping pains extending towards the head and temples.

Pulsatilla, for facial neuralgia when there is a feeling of coldness, and torpor in the affected side of the face, with severe spasmodic pain in the cheek bone, with a sensation of crawling and aggravation or renewal of the suffering in the evening, and when in a state of rest; also when there is lacrymation, redness of the face, etc.

When neuralgia attends other difficulties, such as *prolapsus uteri*, *Sepia* and *Aurum* are worthy of attention. Neuralgia of the sciatic nerve may require the use of *Belladonna*, *Calcarea*, *Mercurius* or *Sulphur*. That which affects the lower extremities, *Bryonia*, *Rhus toxicodendron*, *Spigelia*, *Zincum*. *Spigelia* is also a useful remedy when the pain extends into the head, and is excruciating, aggravated by the slightest touch. For neuralgia of the skin, *Mercurius*. When there are acute and dragging pains in the hip joint, and a sensation of coldness in the part affected, and also when the pains appear to return periodically, *Arsenicum* is the remedy to be consulted. When the pains are aggravated at night, *Chamomilla*. When seated in the right hip, *Colocynthis*. When there are cutting pains on the slightest movement, *Ignatia*. When there is a sensation of stiffness of the limb, or sensation as if the limb were contracted, torpid or paralyzed, *Nux vomica*. *Rhus toxicodendron* is better suited when rest aggravates the suffering, and motion and warmth mitigates it. *Bryonia* is a good remedy when the neuralgia is in the right, upper and lower extremity.

DIET AND REGIMEN.—Patients suffering from neuralgia will often have an impaired appetite; the severity and duration of the pain may have produced some constitutional derangement. It is better under such circumstances to subsist upon a moderate diet, and one easy of digestion, and indeed one that will require hardly any labor of the digestive organs. All condiments must be avoided, such as vinegar, pepper, mustard, etc. When the patient's appetite remains, he may allow himself black tea, cocoa, and other non-medicinal drinks. When a warm room alleviates the suffering, it is best for the patient, but if heat aggravates his suffering, a moderately cold room is better. If rest relieves him, let him lie in bed, and if activity and motion contribute to his ease and comfort, let him enjoy them to the full extent.

Odontalgia, Toothache.

But little need be said by way of description of this malady, the affection is so common that but few have at all times been exempt from it.

The principal remedies employed to relieve aching teeth are Aconite, Arnica, Arsenicum, Belladonna, Chamomilla, Mercurius, Nux vomica, Pulsatilla and Sulphur, 12x dil. in water.

Aconite, when the toothache is accompanied by fever and heat about the head and when the toothache results from cold or from nervous excitement.

Arnica, when the pain is occasioned by a mechanical injury, as from extracting or plugging.

Arsenicum, when cold brings on a paroxysm, or aggravates the pain.

Belladonna, when from cold, there is severe pain in the teeth, involving the whole jaw, the pains extending off the side of the face and into the ear, and when the pain is aggravated by hot applications. When produced by coffee and *Chamomilla,* and also when attended by diarrhœa and flushed face, or swelling of one cheek, or when the pain extends into the ear, and worse when in the room than when out in the open air. *Mercurius viv.,* for pains in hollow teeth, worse in the morning; pain in the jaw bones. *Nux vomica,* when the toothache arises from cold, which at the same time affects the head and neck. *Pulsatilla,* suitable for persons of a mild, quiet, timid disposition, or for persons of a fretful temper, or when the toothache occurs in the spring, with earache and headache, and when it attends the menstrual period, and when the pains are of a jerking, tearing, or stinging character, or when cold air relieves the pain, or it is relieved by mastication.

Sulphur, suitable for jumping pains in hollow teeth, swelling and bleeding of the gums.

When the toothache occurs from pregnancy, Calc. carb., from nursing, China, from grief, Ignatia, etc. For ulceration of gums, Mercurius, Silicea, Hepar sulp., Calc., and Sulphur.

Persons suffering from toothache should avoid holding hot or acrid substances in the mouth, and refrain from the use of Kreasote, oil of cloves, or any agent that interferes with the action of the remedies. When it becomes apparent that any exciting cause will bring on the toothache, it is best to guard against it, as much as possible; when coffee or tea, wine, or other stimulants excite pain in decayed teeth, they should be prohibited.

Partial Paralysis, or Paralysis of Certain Muscles.

The paralysis that lesions of the nervous centres will produce, and especially that which arises from hæmorrhage in the nervous centres, has been already treated of. But there are cases where the muscle or muscles becomes paralyzed, without the possibility of tracing the cause to any morbid appearance on dissection, and yet when the effect has proceeded from some unappreciable cause or change that must have occurred in the nervous centres. We often find the paralysis confined to a small portion, and frequently it happens that only one muscle is implicated. When this is the case, and there are no signs whatever of any disturbance in the brain, the loss of power may be owing to pressure on the particular nerves that are distributed to the paralyzed muscle. Dislocation of the os humeri, by causing pressure on the circumflex nerve, has caused *paralysis of the deltoid*. In many cases, however, the paralysis of a single muscle is but the precursory sign that betokens the approach of some more serious difficulty; the falling down of the upper eyelid may. indicate the approach of apoplexy or of. hemiplegia, and the paralysis of one or more muscles of the fingers is at times a premonitory sign of the same difficulty.

The paralysis of one of the motor muscles produces *strabismus*, such as often occurs in advanced stages of encephalic disease. *Aphonia* appears to be produced in many cases by paralysis of the muscles whose office it is to stretch the vocal cords.

Paralysis of the tongue occurs as a symptom of general paralysis and ye t it may occur alone from pressure on the hypoglossal nerve.

Sometimes a morbid condition of the nerves distributed to the face will occasion *paralysis of the face*, although the same occurs in or accompanies hemiplegia.

Paralysis of the rectum produces a deplorable condition of the patient; a continual involuntary discharge of fæces. A paralysis of the sphincter of the bladder occasions involuntary discharge of urine.

The paralysis caused by lead, and also that attendant upon mental alienation may sometimes occur only in the partial form. Workers in mercury are liable to a form of partial paralysis that effects the muscles concerned in articulation and mastication and sometimes those of locomotion; arsenic when taken as a poison has been known to produce similar results.

CAUSES.—The ordinary causes of partial paralysis are the same of course that produce general paralysis; certain poisons are known to have produced the difficulty. Pressure upon the nervous centres or on that part from whence a nerve may arise that is distributed to a certain muscle may occasion its paralysis—contusions and concussions are among the exciting causes of the disease.

Partial Paralysis.

Partial paralysis may also be produced by cold acting upon the sentient extremities of nerves, occasioning loss of power in the nerves of any part. It may be brought on by intemperance, excessive sexual indulgence or self-abuse, and by whatever agency that may interrupt in any degree the function of the spinal nerves.

In regard to the prospect of affecting a cure of the various kinds of partial paralysis, much will depend upon the morbid condition. If there is complete destruction of the nerves proceeding to any single part, no cure can be effected; but if there be merely a compressing cause, such as may arise from a tumour, this may be removed by proper treatment. Those instances of paralysis that result from poison by lead or arsenic taken into the system, are, no doubt, curable. That which may result from teething may pass away when the cause subsides. The prognosis depends very much upon the morbific influence, and the length of time the patient has been afflicted. That which has continued for a long time, is liable to resist the effect of remedial means to a much greater extent than recent cases, and much doubt exists of effecting a perfect restoration when the cause is so obscure as not to be recognized.

The experience of the writer in the treatment of several cases

of local paralysis, leads him to believe that the effect of Homœopathic remedies is frequently successful. The higher attenuation
from the 12x to 30x, dil., for all cases. Doses repeated every
four hours.

For PARALYSIS OF THE BRAIN, which is denoted by loss of
mental and moral manifestation, and an absence of sensation in
the part, *Cuprum aceticum* 3x trit., three times a day.

For PARALYSIS OF THE ORGANS OF SPEECH, Belladonna 12x,
dil., has sometimes proved effectual. In a case occurring after
rush of blood to the head, in a gentleman about fifty years of age,
Belladonna 6th was given in daily doses for ten days without any
perceptible benefit. Sulphur was then given at night and Belladonna 12x, in the morning, for four days, which evidently produced a salutary effect; the power of speech was gradually recovered, and at length a complete restoration. In another case,
which seemed to occur from no definable cause, where there was
complete loss of speech, Graphites and Causticum 12x, dil., had a
good effect. In a child ten years of age, who had suffered from
an attack of inflammation of the brain and afterwards with loss
of speech, Causticum and China in the sixth dil. afforded a satisfactory result. The writer has used these remedies, however, in
another case without effect, where partial restoration was effected
by Belladonna.

Several cases of *paralysis of the tongue* have come under the
writer's observation, and in one in particular, where the patient
was very much prostrated, China, in the tincture, was given in
drop doses with good effect, although Belladonna, Causticum and
Dulcamara appeared to accomplish but little before. If paralysis
of the tongue occurs from acute hydrocephalus, Hyoscyamus
may prove of service; if from suppressed eruption, Graphites; if
after an attack of epilepsy, Belladonna or Stramonium. In some
cases of long standing paralysis of the organs of speech, and of the
tongue in particular, the effects of remedies did not become
apparent for some time. In such cases, however, Causticum and
Graphites may be employed. In case of paralysis of one arm,
Pulsatilla. Miss Mehetable Pancost, aged 39, after a severe attack of vomiting, suffered paralysis of the right arm and hand.
Pulsatilla given every twenty-four hours effected a cure in little
more than a week. In case of paralysis of the lower extremities,
Nux vomica may prove of essential service. When one side be-

comes paralyzed, Causticum, Cocculus and Lachesis are among the most prominent remedies. If partial paralysis occurs after rheumatism, China, Ferrum and Ruta may be regarded the most prominent remedies of the group to be consulted.

There is no resort but to internal remedies when any of the internal organs become the seat of paralysis, but friction may be resorted to with benefit when the local paralysis involves some of the external muscles of locomotion, as

PARALYSIS OF THE BLADDER requires the internal administration of Arsenicum 3x dil., Helleborus 3x dil., etc.

PARALYSIS OF THE NECK OF THE BLADDER requires Arsenicum, Bell. 3x dil., Cicuta 3x dil., Dulc. 3x dil., Hyoscy. 3x dil., Lach. 3x dil., etc., the Arsenicum 3x dil., Dulc., and Hyos., being the most prominent of the group.

PARALYSIS OF THE SPHINCTER ANI.—Acon., Bell., Hyosc., Laur.

PARALYSIS OF THE INTESTINAL CANAL.—Phosphorus.

PARALYSIS OF THE UPPER AND LOWER EXTREMITIES IN GENERAL.—Bell., Bry., Cocculus, Nux vom., Rhus. These several remedies may be applied externally as well as internally, in the following way: first, second, or third dilutions, five drops in a tumbler of water may be dermically applied over the region of the difficulty.

Friction over the region of the paralysis, by rubbing with the hand, may have a salutary effect, but counter-irritants seldom accomplish anything favorable for the patient. The very irritation they occasion may be thrown back upon the seat of the affection so as to aggravate rather than ameliorate the difficulty.

In regard to local paralysis affecting different parts of the organs of prehension, locomotion, etc.

IN THE TREATMENT OF PARALYSIS OF THE ARMS.—*Calcarea, Calc. phos., Cocculus, Nux vomica, Rhus, Sepia,* are the most prominent remedies. *China, Ferrum, Lycop., Belladonna* and *Veratrum* may be consulted for particular cases.

FOR RHEUMATIC PARALYSIS OF THE ARMS, *China* and *Cocculus, Ferrum* or *Tart. em.* have been employed.

FOR PARALYSIS OF THE ELBOW.—*Mezereum* and *Petroleum.*

FOR PARALYSIS OF THE FINGER JOINTS.—*Calcarea, Calc. phos., Magn. c.* and *Phos.*

FOR PARALYSIS OF THE THUMBS.—*Magn. c.*

FOR PARALYSIS OF THE LOWER EXTREMITIES.—*Belladonna, Cocculus, Nux vomica,* and *Rhus* are among the most decidedly useful remedies, and also *Bryonia, China., Jodatus* and *Veratrum.*

FOR PARALYSIS OF THE FEET, *Oleander* would seem to occupy the most prominent place, and *Ars., China* and *Plumb.* may be consulted.

FOR PARALYSIS OF THE KNEE AND KNEE JOINTS.—*Ambr., Ars., Baryt. c.*

FOR PARALYSIS OF LEGS.—*Aconite* and *Arsenicum.*

FOR PARALYSIS OF THE TARSAL JOINTS.—*Oleander,* or perhaps *China, Arsenicum* and *Plumbum.*

FOR PARALYSIS OF THE THIGHS.—*Aconite, Aurum, Chelidonum majus.*

FOR PARALYSIS OR THE LUNGS.—The most prominent remedies are *Arsenicum, Carbo. veg., Ipecacuanha, Lachesis,* and *Opium.* Those holding a subordinate relation, *Baryta, Graphites, Sambucus* or else *Aurum, Camphor, China, Pulsatilla* and *Tart. em.*

FOR PARALYSIS OF THE LUNGS FROM CONGESTION OF BLOOD.—*Aconite, Ipecac, Phosphorus* and *Sambucus,* or else *Bell., Bry.* and *China.* 12x dil.

FOR PARALYSIS OF THE LUNGS OF OLD PEOPLE.—*Lachesis* and *Opium* or else *Arsenicum, Aurum, Carbo. veg.* and *China,* 12x dil.

FOR PARALYSIS OF THE LUNGS AFTER A CATARRH.—*Arsenicum, Tart. em.* or else *China. Camphor, Ipecac.* For the same difficulty in children, *Aconite* and *Sambucus,* 12x dil.

During treatment the utmost care should be exercised in all cases to guard against agents that may interfere with the action of remedies. The patient should have the invigorating effects of a good atmosphere in well ventilated apartments.

There are numerous difficulties that affect the whole system that may implicate the nerves, or that the excitement of the nervous system is the chief agent in producing. Give the remedies in 5 to 10 drops of the dilution in half a glass of water. Dessert spoonful doses four times a day.

Palpitation of the Heart.—Palpitatio Cordis.

The beating of the heart may be caused by nervous irritation alone, as may be inferred from the effect of violent emotions, as fright or anxiety, upon the organ. Great debility of the nervous system may occasion the difficulty, and also severe pain may so act upon the nerves as to cause a violent beating of the heart. It is often the case that this affection is mistaken for organic disease of the heart, when well chosen remedies for nervous irritation will cure the affection. When the whole system suffers from debility, the weakened condition of the nerves may give rise to innumerable sufferings, and none more frequently than palpitation of the heart.

When this affection arises from debilitating losses, such as hæmorrhage or diarrhœa, *China* may exert a beneficial influence in promoting the recuperation of the system so as to obviate the difficulty.

When some violent emotion, as grief, produces palpitation of the heart, *Ignatia* will in all probability afford relief.

When produced from fright or fear, *Opium* may have a quieting effect so as to overcome the affection.

When connected with the menstrual function, *Pulsatilla* will relieve, and also when the nerves have become excited from having taken into the stomach a rich quality of food, as fat meats or gravy.

For the excitement of the nervous system produced by indigestion occasioning palpitation of the heart, and especially at night, Nux vomica 3x, trit., may procure relief for the patient, and also if the nerves have been excited from intoxicating drinks, producing palpitation, the same remedy in the 6x, dil. may be prescribed, ten drops in a gill of water, a dessert spoonful repeated every hour until relieved. When palpitation is connected with sick headache in females and especially those suffering from prolapsus uteri, *Sepia* in the 30x, dil., ten drops in a gill of water, given in spoonful doses will often cure. Arsenicum 30x, dil., will generally relieve palpitation, when accompanied by a paroxysm of nervous asthma. China 6x, dil., ten drops in a glass of water in spoonful doses every hour will relieve when the palpitation supervenes upon debility produced by fever, or the loss of blood.

When palpitation results from nervous debility alone,

Chamomilla 6x, dil., or Pulsatilla, Valerian and even Nux vom., each in the 6x, dil., prepared and administered as above.

Calcarea 6x, trit., and Ignatia 6x, trit., and Nux vom., Arsenicum and Pulsatilla each in the 6th dilution, may be given in small powders, or drop doses in water, to highly excitable nervous temperaments in case of anxiety and palpitation.

In all cases let the symptoms guide in the selection of the remedy. This totality will generally indicate a proper affiliation.

CHAPTER L.

The mucus membrane that lines the eyelids and the front part of the eye-ball is liable to become inflamed from exposure of the eyes to dust, smoke, cold winds, impure air, glare of light, etc. This affection is termed conjunctivitis, included in the general term opthalmia. Formerly all inflammatory affections of the eye were included under this term. But owing to the fact that there are several varieties of opthalmia, which require individual description and treatment, different terms may be necessary to express pathologically the nature of the affection and its precise locality. We will, therefore, deal with affections of the eye as we have found them.

Simple Ophthalmia.

This is known by a sensation of heat, or a sensation as if sand were under the lids. This imposes the necessity of an ocular inspection in order to ascertain if any foreign body is in the eye; if none can be found, the sensations are surely disease and afford indications for remedial treatment.

TREATMENT.—*Am.*, *Acon.* and *Bell.* in the 6x dil., may be used in drop doses internally, while a lotion of ten drops in two ounces of water may be applied externally.

Catarrhal Inflammation of the Eyes.

This consists of inflammation of the conjunctiva and mer-bornian glands, with a discharge of a mucus secretion, and by swelling and agglutination of the eyelids.

In this kind of ophthalmia there is a pricking pain felt on moving the eye, as if there were dust, sand or a small fly under the lids, a sense of stiffness on moving the lid, sensitiveness of the membrane to cold air; the eyes become watery and secrete a mucus which glues the lids together in the morning; the conjunctivæ exhibit a bright redness, which distinguishes their in-

flammation from that of the sclerotic coat. The iris is not
affected by this kind of inflammation. The discharge is sometimes abundant, but less so than in the purulent form. It is
nevertheless contagious, especially if the discharge is purulent.
The lids become sticky and difficult to open in the morning on
account of the dried secretion causing the lids to adhere together.
The lids are often swollen and red, and the discharge and pricking pains sometimes increase in severity, and both eyes become
affected at the same time. This part distinguishes the disease
from gonorrhœal opthalmia, which seldom affects more than one
eye at a time, especially at first. Catarrhal inflammation of the
eyes is sometimes epidemic, caused by exposure to extremes of
temperature, cold winds, and especially drafts of cold air. It
may spread through families, and even through neighborhoods, in
spite of all measures to prevent the contagion.

TREATMENT.—In Allopathic treatment various callyria are
recommended.

HOMŒOPATHIC TREATMENT. — *Euphrasia*, *Mercurius*, *Am.*
and *Bell.* in the 6x dil., drop doses every hour, are found to be
quite effectual.

Those afflicted with this kind of sore eyes should avoid exposure to damp, cold air, or to any stormy or inclement weather
during the attack, and should remain in a room of uniform temperature, and apply at night compresses of cold water; if the lids
are agglutinated in the morning, no attempt should be made to
open the lids without first moistening them with warm water, or
milk and water.

Purulent Ophthalmia.

This disease is an inflammation of the conjunctiva, accompanied by considerable secretion and pus, which mingle with the
tears. In the beginning of the attack, when it is yet mild, it
may be considered for catarrhal inflammation, but as it increases
in severity it appears to be similar to that which is gonorrhœal.
The symptoms are more violent, destructive and rapid in their
progress than those of the catarrhal or scrofulous. The tingling
sensations first experienced are soon followed by acute pains extending through the eyes to the temples and brain itself; the eyelids adhere; the flow of tears is soon changed into a profuse secretion of pus; the eyelids are inflamed, swollen and vascular,

and the vision is almost obscured; if the disease goes un-
checked, the cornea becomes cloudy, then ulcerates, or partly
sloughs away, portions of the iris may. protrude, and the eye is
destroyed. There are attendant on this condition headache,
nausea, quick pulse, hot skin, etc., sudden alternations from heat
to cold, the irritation of something foreign in the eyes, such as
sand in the eyes. *Metastasis* of measles, scarlatina, small-pox, etc.,
and also ill-ventilated, badly lighted and ill-drained dwellings
may be proximate causes of this formidable disease.

Among the causes of spreading this unfortunate disease, is
the carelessness of nurses in using towels and handkerchiefs, to
promote cleanliness, that have been used about patients suffering
from the disease. We were once in a family of several children,
who, after an attack of scarlatina, suffered from purulent
ophthalmia. The nurse in washing their faces, used towels which
had not been washed after having been used in other cases, and
from these towels the whole household became inoculated; and,
therefore, to prevent the spread of purulent ophthalmia, let it be
an established rule that no common use should be made of towels,
wash-basins or bed-clothing.

TREATMENT.—For purulent ophthalmia consists in the employment of *Arg. nit.*, *Hepar*, *Merc.*, *Nit. ac.*, *Phos.*, *Sulph.*,
each in the 6x dil., ten drops in a gill of water, to be used as a
lotion, and internally in teaspoonful doses every two hours, iced
water compresses on the eyes and the strictest cleanliness.

Purulent Ophthalmia of Infants.

It is true that this disease in the adult is nearly the same as
in infants, yet it becomes so modified in infants, by reason of
their rapid growth, that a different treatment is required.
This trouble commences soon after birth, and presents the common symptoms. Causes, inoculation at birth with gonorrhœal
or leucorrhœal discharges from the vagina. Contact of the
conjunctiva with these is too often prophetic of future misery
for the child.

Gonorrhœal Ophthalmia.

This formidable disease of the eyes is seldom cured of the
gonorrhœa, because the delicate and sensitive condition of the
eye, inoculated with the virus, is less liable to yield readily to

remedial measures. The same remedies, however, that act promptly in arresting gonorrhœa, are the ones to employ in this gonorrhœal sequel.

The cause of this affection in women is often the want of honesty in their husbands in not informing them of the danger of using the same towel and wash-bowl after coitus. This careless-ness often leads to an inoculation of the eyes, which inflame, suppurate and produce disorganization of the delicate tissues necessary for proper vision. An estimable lady, aged 37, gave birth to a daughter, and recovered well from the after illness. But as soon as her husband was permitted an embrace, she felt an uncomfortable itching and stinging on the labia. She used a towel for ablutions, and wiped her genitals and afterwards her face. Her eyes began to itch and smart and inflame, and became so red and swollen that she could not see. An oculist was called in, and after a critical examination found both eyes organically broken down, and all caused by an imprudent use of a towel impregnated with gonorrhœal matter unknown to her. These causes are more common than is imagined. During the war of the rebellion this species of ophthalmia prevailed exten-sively, not with gonorrhœal subjects, but with those whose eyes innocently came in contact with the infection. An eye and ear surgeon informed the writer that multitudes lost their sight in spite of medical treatment; but after Hildreth's method of placing a compress of 15 lbs. pressure over the eyes, excluding the light, the patient was placed in position for successful medical treatment. It will be perceived that the disease arises from the contact of gonorrhœal matter with the eye, and not from metastases of urinethretic gonorrhœa. As before stated, the mat-ter may be conveyed to the eye of a healthy person by or through the medium of clothes, towels, etc. Children are often con-taminated and lose their sight, at least of one eye.

TREATMENT. — The Allopathic treatment consists of as-tringents, *Collyria of Sulp.*, *Zinc.*, etc.

HOMŒOPATHIC TREATMENT, which has been most successful, is *Acon.*, 3x and 30x dil., *Arg.* n. 3x trit., *Merc.*, *Bell.*, *Sulph.*

Belladonna is suitable for pain, redness and swelling, throb-bing pains in the temples and eyes, intolerance of light. Twelve drops of the 1st dil. may be put in six teaspoonfuls of water; a teaspoonful may be given every hour.

Aconite is suitable for quick pulse arising from cold. The early administration of this remedy, while cold compresses are applied, will generally relieve the catarrhal ophthalmia; and *Dr. Angel* says the topical application of ice, and the same remedy is recommended in gonorrhœal ophthalmia.

Mercurius sol., 3x trit., may be given every hour in two-grain doses. *Merc. cor.*, 3x, may be given in like manner in the most violent forms of the disease.

Dr. Dudgeon recommends *Argentum nit.* as truly Homœopathic to gonorrhœal ophthalmia, two to four grains to an ounce of distilled water, a small quantity to be introduced by a camel's hair brush once or twice a day under the eyelids.

Phytolacca is suitable for the itching which gas-light aggravates. Diet should be spare and free from stimulants.

Iritis.

This peculiar affection of the eye is difficult of detection, on account of the situation of the iris, and the difficulty of characterizing the complaint by external symptoms; when this texture becomes inflamed there is considerable constitutional or febrile derangement of the external tunics. This is probably owing to the relaxed attachments of the conjunctiva to the eyes, and the more susceptible opportunity for effusions into the cellular tissue beneath.

Iritis commences with a dull, pressing, heavy, deep-seated pain in the orbit. The pupil is contracted. The natural color of the iris undergoes a change to a dark greenish or reddish hue. The conjunctiva presents a blush of a moderate rose-color. The eye is sensitive to the light, and the sight is somewhat obscured.

As the disease progresses, the pains become acute, and extend into the temples, and top of the head. The contraction is more apparent, flashes of light pass through the eyes, and the nervous system is greatly excited. The pulse becomes accelerated, the skin becomes hot and dry, the bowels are constipated, and there is a partial suppression of the urinary secretions, and there are other indications of constitutional derangement. After these acute sufferings have persisted for some time, the iris presents an irregular, angular, and thickened appearance covered with specks of yellow lymph. Minute abscesses now form on the iris, and ultimately burst into the anterior chamber, and afterwards commonly absorbed. If adhesions between the iris, and the capsule of the lens, or if the deep-seated or the comparatively deeper-seated parts have become involved in the trouble, it results usually in complete loss of sight.

The inflammation sometimes extends from the iris to the retina, the cornea, the choroides, finally the whole internal structure of the eye is implicated, and then the malady will present the characteristic symptoms of the inflammation of the different parts.

In such cases the symptoms are very violent, the pains greatly aggravated, and throbbing. There is a very rapid contraction of the pupil and speedy extinguishing of the sight. Then the constitutional signs become very alarming, and the condition of the patient shows an eminent danger of absolute loss of vision.

CAUSES.—The causes are somewhat variable. The most common cause is the abuse of mercury, and another nearly allied, is syphilis; these two agents are believed by many to exert a pernicious influence, but there are grave doubts about there being a genuine cause of iritis. Other causes are mechanical injuries, rheumatism, gout, and excessive study or use of the eyes over minute subjects.

TREATMENT.—For traumatic iritis Arn., both internally and externally. This should be prepared as follows: half an ounce of Arnica flowers should be put into a pint of cold water to macerate for twenty-four hours, and then filtered, and applied externally to the affected eye; let the decoction be heated to a temperature of 85° F., and compresses wet with it and applied to the affected eye or eyes, while Arn., 3x, dil., ten drops in a glass of water may be given in dessert spoonfuls, dose every two hours; Acon. 3x, dil., may be prepared and administered in the same manner, for febrile symptoms; Bell. 3x, dil., prepared as above when the pain shoots through the temples and produces a frontal headache.

Rheumatic Iritis.

Rheumatic Iritis,—accompanied by fever, also requires Acon. 3x, dil., administered as above, and for other symptoms *Spigelia* 3x, dil., Euphrasia 3x, dil., Merc. sol. 3x, trit., two grain doses, Clematis 3x, dil., Sulph. 3x, dil., Kali 3x., dil. In arthritic subjects, Ars. 3x, trit., in two-grain doses. In Syphilitic cases Merc. s., 3x, trit., Merc. jod., 3x, trit., Aurum met., 3x, trit., each in two grain doses, repeated at intervals of two hours. For iritis in scrofulous cases, Calc. carb., 3x, trit., Merc. corr., 3x, trit., each two grains. For *iritis* in gonorrhœal subjects Arg. nit., 6x., dil., internally and externally twice a day with application of dry warm wadding applied externally. Cold applications either of water or other resorts must be avoided. Atropium 6x, dil., may be given in drop doses to prevent the adhesion of the iris to the capsule of the lens and to avert permanent contraction of the pupil. Atropine is used to dilate the pupil, 3x, dil., applied externally. Belladonna 3x, dil., in drop doses, repeated every two hours, is especially useful in inflammation of the tissues of the eye.

Amblyopia.

This is simple weakness of sight, or morbid alteration thereof and includes all grades of the impairment of vision from mere dimness to absolute blindness.

CAUSES.—The causes are numerous, embracing various morbid conditions of the organism, gastric derangement, biliary diseases, over exertion of the eyes in executing fine work, etc.

TREATMENT.—For simple weakness of sight Anac., 3x, dil., Bell., 3x, dil., Hyos., 3x, dil., Caust., 3x, dil. Each of these remedies have a beneficial influence in protecting and strengthening the sight.

Other remedies for morbid weakness of sight are Aur., 3x, trit., Calc. carb., 3x, trit., Merc., 3x, trit. They may each be administered in two-grain doses repeated twice a day. China 3x, dil., Ver. vir., 2x, dil., Ruta 3x, dil. Each in drop doses repeated every hour when indicated will have a salutary influence in strengthening the sight.

Amaurosis.

This disease may be divided into two grades one of which is curable; and the other in spite of treatment is incurable.

CAUSES.—It is caused by fine work, suppression of habitual discharges, such as hæmorrhoids, menstruation, etc. It may also be caused by the suppression of measles and other exanthems. The metastasis of *gout* to the eyes; the abuse of mercury may also be included among the causes of *amaurosis;* it may also be caused by rheumatism, scrofula, intemperance, excessive use of tobacco, and sometimes by catching cold in the eyes and head, etc.

This disease is curable when the optic nerve is in a state of integrity, and suffers neither from paralysis or atrophy. For curable amaurosis the same remedies may be employed as in amblyopia.

TREATMENT.—The remedies must be employed in accordance with the symptoms attendant in the difficulty.

The congested amaurosis resulting from too great a flow of blood to the head and eyes requires Bell., 3x, dil., Cact., 3x, dil., Ver. vir., 3x, dil., Dig., 3x, dil. Each may be given in drop doses repeated every two hours when administered according to indications afforded by constitutional symptoms. If caused by biliary derangement, Nux vom., 3x, dil., Merc., 12x, dil. If caused by rheumatism Bry., 3x, dil., Puls., 3x, dil., Sulph., 3x, dil. The Bry. and Puls. may be given in drop doses, repeated at intervals of an hour, but the Sulphur at the same time may be given in 3rd trit., two grains every night. If caused by Dyspepsia, etc., Nux v., 3x, Merc., 3x, trit., Puls., 3x, dil., China 3x, dil. If caused from over use of the eyes, Ruta 3x, dil., and Arnica 3x, dil.

Muscæ Volitantes.

Spots before the eyes. This disease consists of an appearance of black motes before the vision, or of thin grey films, like the wings of a fly, or something like spider's webs, or if viewed on a white surface, there are appearances of luminous flashes or circles with a central aperture.

Various opinions have been entertained concerning the nature of these phenomena. Some suppose them to be debris of cells or corpuscles of the vitreous humor, and granules and fibres floating in the vitreous humor in and out of the field of vision.

CAUSES.—The exciting causes of these ocular spectus are excessive use of the eyes, in artificial light in badly ventilated rooms, or probably by insufficient sleep, or certain fevers, as enteric and typhus, or any morbid sensibility.

TREATMENT.—The prevailing treatment has been nerve tonics, such as Valerian virg., Snake-root, Sage tea, etc.

HOMŒOPATHIC TREATMENT consists of Hyos., 3x, dil., Conium 3x, Cocculus 3x, dil., three-drop doses daily. Rest from over labor with the eye is a *sine qua non*. A nourishing non-medicinal diet, out-door exercise in the country or by the sea-side, and frequently bathing the closed eyes with cold water, for two or three minutes, and according to our observation, the patient is likely to receive benefit.

Cataract.

It is well known that Homœopathy promises important results of treatment in this disease, although, strictly speaking, it belongs to the province of surgery. We nevertheless take the liberty of presenting a few words respecting the malady.

By the term cataract is understood an opacity of the crystalline lens, or capsule, which causes an obscuration or a total loss of vision. We have seen several varieties both of the lenticular and capsular. The firm or hard cataract occurs the most frequently to old people, and can be recognized by its density and hardness. It is of an amber color and small in size. Another kind has come under our observation; it is a fluid or milky cataract caused by a change of the lens into a white and semi-fluid mass of so large a size as to nearly obliterate the posterior chamber, impair the motions of the pupil and intercept the admission of the rays of light. There is yet another kind of soft or caseous cataract, somewhat like the last variety with enlargement of the lens, of a cheesy consistence, and of a light gray or sea-green color, destructive to the posterior chamber, interfering with the motion of the pupil and iris, resulting either in partial or total blindness, and there is yet another variety called the capsular cataract, and is an opacity of the capsule of the crystalline lens, beginning at the margin of the pupil in the form of distinct white shining points, specks or streaks, and of a light color, never altogether uniform even when the disease is completely formed. This kind of cataract occurs in children soon after birth, and it is styled congenital. Amaurosis and this kind of cataract are sometimes blended. The complication is difficult of detection, on account of a close resemblance of the symptoms of these two diseases. The first or primary indication of a forming cataract is a defect of sight when attempting to read fine print. All objects become indistinct at a distance. A strong light is required to read or write. A mist is constantly before the eye. Soon after this obscuration of vision a small speck begins just behind the center of the pupil, and continues to enlarge until the opacity is complete. A black ring encircles the edge of the pupil, and causes the sight to gradually disappear until blindness is complete. The cause of cataract in the various forms is frequent and long continued use of the eyes in reading and writing or looking at minute objects by a strong light, or by congestion of blood to the eyes, too much exercise in the sun, and where bright fires are kept, hereditary predisposition, mechanical injuries, etc. The prognosis of every form of cataract is by no means flattering. Primary obscuration of sight requires the strictest attention to remove the cause, careless indifference about the obscurity in which every thing seems to be involved should be met by strong mental effort to avoid all causes of aggravation. In the treatment of this disease Allopathy offers nothing except couching or extraction. We have but few remedies that present a chart of this difficulty in their pathogenesis, yet there has been successful results which have been observed from the use of remedies, and this renders it obligatory on us to avail ourselves of these.

TREATMENT.—Silicea 12x, trit., given in two-grain doses daily has operated satisfactorily in several cases, Graphites 12x, trit., has also been attended by favorable results. The local aplication of sulphuric ether vapor to the eye, has been beneficial in incipient cataracts. The internal remedies that have appeared to have the most salutary effect are Conium 3x, dil., Puls., 6x, dil., Magnesia carb., 6x, dil., and Sulphur 3x, dil. The sight may be improved when the cataract first impairs the vision by Phosphorus, Euphrasia, or Spigelia, each 6x, dil., in daily doses.

Sulphur is appropriate in those cases which seem to be connected with scrofulous or psoric diathesis; it has also been found curative in cataract complicated with amaurosis. Euphrasia or Spigelia may follow the use of Sulphur with benefit. They should be administered the same as directed in the same remedies in amblyopia. A lady, seventy-seven years of age, who had been blind four years, took Euphrasia 30x, dil. One month after she began to distinguish objects. Aug., 4th, objects began to look distorted. She continued the use of the Euphrasia for awhile and then changed to Cannabis 3x, dil. At the end of another month she could distinguish objects, could recognize the letters in a book, could resume her former occupation. Two months later she was able to thread a needle, and gave thanks for the benefit she had received.

Glaucoma.

This disease is an excessive infiltration of the eyeball, causing intra-ocular pressure characterized by morbid induration of the globe, restricting the field of vision, and fading sight, and ending, unless arrested by treatment, in total blindness.

This distressing malady affects pale, unhealthy persons, always beyond the middle age, in whom degeneration is apparent, affecting all the tissues of the body; it may be constitutional or idiopathic or it may be secondary to inflammation, or may be the result of an injury, in which event the disease becomes traumatic glaucoma, or it may arise from sudden disappointment or other mental shock, such as grief, loss or fright; women are more frequently the victims, and it is liable to be the sequel of physical and mental depression occasioned by fatigue in watching the sick, or grief for the loss of friends.

The primary symptoms of this disease are a rapid increase in the failure of vision, obliging the patient to provide for his comfort stronger glasses; another marked symptom is intermittent dimness of sight; objects in the afternoon appear to be enveloped in smoke, and also with slight redness and watering of the eyes, halos of various colors around the gas-light, lamp, or candle, great restriction of the field of vision, increased induration of the eyeball, the cornea exhibits a dullness like that of a glass that has been breathed on, and neuralgia in the nerves of the eye. It is a common occurrence for one of the eyes to be first implicated, but the other is liable to a similar affection soon afterwards. When acutely inflamed the eye exhibits signs of internal congestion, in the anterior chamber there is a distension of the vessels which contracts it. The pupil is dilated and sluggish. The sight disappears rapidly. The pain occasioned by the increased tension of the eye-ball is very severe and almost maddening; it is often mistaken for neuralgia; aching around the orbit and at the side and back of the head is intense. These sufferings often produce a sympathetic effect upon the stomach, resulting in severe vomiting, causing the sufferer to imagine himself the victim of a bilious attack. These severe symptoms may pass away and be succeeded by a partial restoration of sight, nevertheless the vision is still impaired and the severe symptoms are liable to return. If several attacks occur successively the glaucoma becomes established, and the eyeball acquires a stony hardness, the pupil becomes pushed out and appears of a sea-green color, and the pain is so great as to unsettle and break down the constitution. In simple and chronic cases there is less pain, but the disease gradually increases. The ophthalmoscope reveals the organic changes better than they can be described.

TREATMENT.—Kali hyd., 6x dil.; Ars., 6x dil.; Ipec., 3x dil., may be administered in drop doses to mitigate the congestion and inflammation of the choroid; for hepatic or syphilitic, Merc. 3x trit., in two-grain powders; for hæmorrhoidal complications, Nux vom., 3x dil.; Ham., 3x dil.; Colin., 3x dil., may be given in drop doses frequently repeated. For rheumatic and arthritic complications, Bry., 6x dil. and Colch., 3x dil. For neuralgic suffering, Mac., 6x dil.; Cham., 3x dil.; Sant., 2x trit., in two-grain doses is serviceable, applicable in the treatment of idiopathic cases. Rest is essential for the comfort of the patient. Hot water fomentations, medicated with Bell. or Opium, will often mitigate the pain. The only criterion by which to judge of the usefulness of the treatment, is the apparent effect in reducing the tension of the eye-ball in glaucoma. In some cases the disease has yielded to treatment, but in a majority of cases it ends in blindness.

The diet of the patient should be simple, nutritious, non-stimulant and non-medicinal. A practiced oculist should have charge of these cases.

Strabismus, or Squinting.

Squinting is a want of concord in the movement of the axes of the eyes, or when that of one eye is not parallel with that of the other; a loss of harmonious movement of the eyes; the closing of one of the eyes may enable the other to look straight. If the squint is directed towards the nose, it is called convergent; if outwards, it is divergent; if confined to one eye, it is monocular. If the squint alternates first with one eye, and then the other, it is binocular. This obliquity of vision commends itself to the careful manipulation of the surgeon, and a critical knowledge of the recti muscles, which control the movements of the eye.

The cause of congenital squinting is obscure. Its occurrence during childhood may be caused from an unequal use of the eyes, as from imitating those who squint, or trying to look at spots on the nose or face; or from the habit of turning the eye inward; or from cerebral irritation during an attack of measles or scarlatina; or from worms, from anger, and from general ill health. In adults, or aged persons, it is due to the partial paralysis of the inner muscle of the eye. Certain remedies carefully administered in accordance with the constitutional symptoms may remove the difficulty.

TREATMENT.—If the squinting occurs after an attack of scarlatina or measles, attended by cerebral irritation, Bell., 3x dil.; Hyos., 3x dil.; Gels., 3x dil., may be affiliated according to symptoms, and repeated in drop doses until there is a change. If from invermination, Cina., 3x dil.; Spig., 3x dil. Given in the same way when no cause can be assigned, Phos., 3x dil.; Sulph., 3x dil., may be employed. The careless use of the eye should be guarded against. An attempt may also be made to correct the deformity by fixing the vision, by closing the unaffected eye for several minutes at a time repeatedly through the day. When caused by dentition, worms, whooping cough, or gastric disturbances, the removal of the primary disease is generally sufficient to restore the normal position of the eyes.

Congenital strabismus can only be cured by surgical operation.

Inflammation of the Eyelids.

The symptoms are obvious, redness, soreness and swelling along the margin of the eye-lids, spreading over the whole lid.

TREATMENT.—When this affection has arisen from exposure to cold, with febrile symptoms, Acon 3x dil., ten drops in half a glass of water, teaspoonful doses each hour during a single day, will be sufficient to effect a cure. When there is bright redness of the lid, dread of light, Bell., 3x dil., prepared and given as above, may be sufficient. When there is much swelling and infiltration into the cellular tissue, Apis. mel., 3x dil., will afford prompt relief. For erysipelatous appearance of the lids, and the formation of small vesicles, Rhus tox., 3x dil., in drop doses, repeated frequently, may soon afford relief. Neglected cases with suppuration can be cured with Hepar sulph., 30x trit., a small powder twice a day. For chronic inflammation of the lids, Conium, 3x dil., is usually an effective remedy. Bathing the eye-lids with warm milk and water, or the early use of cold compresses, avoiding exposure to cold draughts of air, is commendable accessory treatment.

Sty on the Eyelids.

This is a small painful boil with slight inflammatory symptoms, projecting from the margin of the eyelids; debilitated persons or those having a scrofulous diathesis are subject to this kind of tumor.

TREATMENT.—The principal remedy and one that should first be administered alone or in alternation with Acon., is Puls., 3x, dil. If given early, a few drops applied externally often disperses the sty. When there is inflammation and restlessness give Acon., in alternation with Puls. A dose of Sulph., given morning and evening for a few days may prevent the recurrence of styes. Staph., is also useful for the same purpose. In persons of scrofulous constitution Calc., and Sulph., should be administered for a week each in succession, the former to be given morning and evening for a week, and after waiting a few days give Sulph. in the same manner, repeating the course if neccessary.

Inversion and Eversion of the Eyelids.

Inversion of the eyelid is termed entropium, is a growing inward of the eyelid and lashes so as to create great disfigurement and constant irritation of the globe of the eye, and is often caused by the employment of caustics used by ignorant persons to cure purulent ophthalmia in the lower ranks of society, and eversion of the eyelid termed ectropium may be caused by burns on the face or from the thickening of the conjunctiva from tarsal ophthalmia.

TREATMENT.—The treatment for this trouble is the same that we have before recommended for scrofulous sore eyes. Great benefit is often derived from bathing the eyes with cold or tepid water, and the local use of Calendular lotion, ten drops to a gill of water.

Tarsal Ophthalmia, Granular Eyelids, Eczema.

Palpebrarum and inflamed thickened condition of the conjunctiva and the enlargement of its cilia with disordered secretion of the meibomian glands, the conjunctiva and the skin itself causing irritation as from foreign bodies. Eczema in the eyelid occurs chiefly in the young, and is a chronic affection which may remain for years, and even for life. The granulations are rough and uneven. They can be detected by the touch. The secretion of pus may be so abundant that the eyelids stick together during sleep, encrusted with dried mucus chiefly from the meibomian se-.cretion. The tarsal border becomes thickened and rounded and a constant overflow of tears excoriating and irritating the edge of the lids greatly deranging the lachrymal secretion. The causes of this difficulty may be found in struma or hereditary taint, enlarged lymphatic glands, swollen upper lip, sore ears, digestive derangements, etc.

The disease sometimes occurs as the sequel of the eruptive fevers. Impure air, smoky and uncleanly dwellings, and especially overuse of the eyes in an unhealthy atmosphere.

TREATMENT.—The chief remedies are Merc., 6x, dil., Hep. sulph., 6x, dil., Calc., 6x, dil., Sulph., 6x, dil., Clematis, 6x dil., each when indicated may be administered, ten drops in a gill of water, spoonful doses three times a day. For chronic inflammation of the borders of the eyelids, with soreness and swelling of the glands, such as often occurs in scrofulous patients, Clematis, 3x dil., may be given three times a day, and during the remedial treatment the eyes should have rest, frequent bathing with tepid milk and water and avoidance of impure atmosphere, cold winds, etc. Other accessory treatment may suggest itself for individual cases as they occur.

46

CHAPTER LI.

DISEASES OF THE EARS AND NOSE.

Inflammation of the external ear, especially in the primary stages, may exist as an independent affection. But it is frequently connected with disease of the internal ear. It has a tendency to spread inwards, if neglected. A fetid discharge indicates disease within the tympanum.

SYMPTOMS.—The symptoms are dull, aching pain, increased by motion of the jaw; the external meatus is red, tender and swollen, the cervical glands often swell and become sensitive to the touch. The hearing in most cases is not interrupted. There is a general febrile disturbance and disorder of the nutritive function.

This affection is generally caused by exposure to cold when the ears are unprotected. A frost-bitten ear often takes on inflammation. The ears of children often inflame from the effects of teething, and both children and adults are liable to this trouble from mechanical injuries.

TREATMENT.—When there is excessive pain and soreness, and general disturbance of health, saline purgatives have been recommended.

HOMŒOPATHIC TREAMENT is to be preferred. For the feverishness, excessive pain, soreness, ten drops of the 3x dil. of Aconite, in half a glass of water, may be given in teaspoonful doses every half hour, until relieved. For red, shining swelling of the meatus, and for the throbbing in the ears and sensitiveness to noise, Belladonna, 3x dil., prepared and administered the same as directed for the Aconite. Belladonna, 3x dil. is indicated when there is violent pain in the head arising from inflammation of the helix and external meatus.

In less acute and more persistent forms of the disease, Pulsatilla 3x, dil., should be given, ten drops in half a glass of water; a teaspoonful should be given every two hours, and continued for some days, after the pain has ceased. For chronic inflammation, and when the disease is very apt to recur, and in scrofulous patients, Sulphur 3x, dil., in drop doses, should be given for four or five days, morning and evening. Bell., 3x, dil., may be given in the same way for several days after the Sulphur; Mercurius 3x, trit., may also be consulted. During the administration of remedies, careful application of fomentations will be found soothing. When the fomentations or poultices are removed, a little cotton wool in the ear is necessary to prevent a cold.

Abscesses.

Sometimes boils form in the outer part of the meatus, in persons of middle age, which are acutely painful, and require appropriate treatment in order to relieve the pain. They are nevertheless not prophetic of any serious consequences. Many little abscesses are the product of inflammation of the sebaceous glands, and correspond with the appearance of boils in other parts, and with styes on the eye lids. They invariably produce acute throbbing pains, darting into the ear.

TREATMENT.—Bell., 3x, dil., ten drops in half a glass of water, will probably relieve the pain, when administered hourly in spoonful doses. If the Bell. fails, give Arnica in the same manner. To arrest the appearance of these abscesses, give Silicea 30x, dil., in two-drop doses, and continue for three days. To facilitate the suppuration, Hepar sulph., 30x, dil., may be given in drop doses every two hours, until such change occurs. After the resolution is perfected, Sulphur 6x, dil., may be given twice a day in drop doses to prevent a reformation and suppuration of these abscesses. A free use of tepid water compresses may hasten a cure. Ham. ext., may be usefully applied to these abscesses.

Accumulation of Wax.

This occurs in consequence of an increased secretion of the ceruminous gland, and it may be a cause of deafness. It is therefore important to effect a change in the secreting gland as early as possible.

TREATMENT.—The accumulation of the wax should be removed if possible by repeated syringing with tepid water. The syringing should be discontinued if it causes pain. After the wax is carefully removed, Sulphur 3x, dil., may be given in drop doses once or twice a day, in order to establish the integrity and normal condition of the gland. Graphites 6x, trit., and Spongia 6x, dil., will be found remedial.

Diseases of the Membrana Tympani.

This membrane may be subject to inflammation, either acute or chronic. The symptoms first manifest are a slight uneasiness and buzzing inside the ear. On examination large red vessels may be seen on the membrane, which is opaque, swollen, and frequently attended by a secretion of viscid mucus. The hearing is somewhat impaired. In the chronic form, the membrane presents a leaden appearance, flattened, dense and rigid. The vessels are congested without perceptible pain, though tinnitis is often observed, and the hearing is greatly impaired.

CAUSES.—Exposure to cold, or a damp atmosphere. It may occur as a sequel of eruptive fevers, or the application of cold or irritating substances to the ear, or it may occur as co-incident with affections of the skin, or mucous membrane in the other parts of the body. Such cases are of frequent occurrence with children of scrofulous constitution, when weak or neglected.

TREATMENT.—Acon. 3x dil., may be given in drop doses, hourly, in the early stage of inflammation. When the vessels are congested, and attended by cerebral symptoms, Bell. 3x dil., may be given instead of the Acon. For the inflammation following measles, and attended by darting, tearing pains, Puls. 3x dil., may be given in drop doses until the pain is subdued. When the pain extends to the teeth, and is aggravated by warmth, or in a warm bed, Merc. cor. 3x trit., in two grain doses, repeated every two hours, may result in a favorable change. Sulph. 3x dil., is an excellent remedy to favor convalescence. Scrupulous cleanliness may be observed in the use of fomentations and poultices. When the ear is washed it must be thoroughly dried in order to guard against the inflammation. Sponging and friction must be habitually practiced.

Perforated Membrana Tympani.

The membrana tympani may be slightly perforated without much detriment to the hearing, only a trifling amount of deafness is apparent, and healthy appearance of the ear is generally noticed. If the perforation leaves a large aperture, and the membrane is torn with a ragged edge, the hearing is greatly impaired, and not likely to be cured. The symptoms of perforation, after the meatus has been thoroughly cleansed with warm water, and the aperture clearly seen by a speculum, or if it be minute, its position is marked by a peculiar pulsation, if there is no obstruction of eustachian tube, the patient can blow air into the tympanum; if there be perforation the air will escape through it into the meatus, with a whistling sound. The cause of perforation may be an ulcerated condition of the membrane itself, or mucus may accumulate in the tympanum, and find its way into the meatus by morbid destruction of the membrane.

TREATMENT.—The treatment should consist, first, in washing out the cavity by means of alkaline solutions passed from the meatus through the eustachian tube into the fauces. This is a simple process, unattended by danger. There are many other methods of cleansing the cavity than by this way, yet no injury other than a temporary giddiness takes place. Chronic perforations of the membrana tympani, should receive constant washing out of the cavity daily, until as many applications are made as necessity requires, and the ear should be well cleansed and dried each time. Calcarea carb., one dose a day of the the 3x trit., is of service during the tedious processes of washing.

Inflammation of the Mucous Membrane of the Tympanum.

In mild cases there is aching in the ears, tinnitus, dullness of hearing, which becomes more serious with subsequent attacks, leading finally to deafness. In more severe cases, intense throbbing, darting, burning pains extend over the side of the head, which are aggravated by swallowing; distressing noises, fever, delirium, congestion of the membrana tympani, are also manifest. Inflammation of the throat, and deafness, increasing in intensity. Sometimes the disorder may rapidly subside, and yet be the occasion of some of the severest and most dangerous diseases that afflict the ear, and lead to permanent and incurable deafness. Many months may elapse before complete restoration can take place.

TREATMENT.—Aconite 3x dil., as in the preceding article, in drop doses repeated every hour, will soon remove the feverishness. Bell. 3x dil., given in the same manner, will remove the brain

symptoms. Mercurius 6x dil., Sulphur 3x dil., ten drops each
in half a glass of water, may be given three times a day when
indicated.

Accessory treatment the same as in the preceding article.

Accumulation of Mucous within the Tympanum—Otorrhœa— Running from the Ears.

This disagreeable and offensive disease of the ear is quite
frequent, and is one of the most obvious and incurable causes of
deafness. When children complain of earache, it is frequently
followed by purulent discharge, caused by the disease. It is not
unlikely to be the cause of convulsions in children, who suffer
from other affections of the mucous membrane, and particularly
that of the bronchia and lungs.

When the child puts his hands to his ears and rubs them or cries
when they are roughly washed, and is unwilling to be towed
about or harshly handled, it is not unlikely that the child is suffering from otorrhœa. And also, when blowing the nose or
swallowing produces a continuous uneasiness, pain, tinnitus,
headache, sensation of ripening abscess about to burst and afford
relief, various degrees of deafness may be the result of ottorrhœa.

An ordinary cold affecting scrofulous children is a fruitful
source of tympanitic disease and running from the ears. Whooping cough and eruptive fevers are also causes of the disease. Any
deteriorating or exhausting illness, such as croup or diphtheria.
It is necessary to frequently examine the tympanum in order to
detect the first symptoms of the disease.

TREATMENT.—In case of thick, bloody and fetid discharge,
attended by rending pains in the affected side of the head and face,
and swelling and tenderness of the glands about the ears, or
when the affection has followed small-pox, Mercurius 3x trit.,
in two-grain powders may be given every four hours until there
is a mitigation or necessity for a change, Hepar sulph. 3x trit. is
indicated when there is a discharge of pus and blood, or when
the patient has been dosed with Mercury, two-grain doses three
times a day. When the discharge is of a thin, watery or purulent
character, and when it is the sequel of measles or mumps, Pulsatilla 3x. dil., and Kali bich. 3x. dil. may be given in drop
doses three or four times a day. Arsenicum 3x, trit., Mur. ac.

6x, dil., Causticum 6x, dil., may each be prescribed when indicated. Arsenicum when the discharge is excoriating, 2 grains morning and evening. For tedious cases Calcarea carb. 6x, trit., and Sulphur 6x, trit., are effective remedies in scrofulous patients.

Other measures are required, such as absolute cleanliness of the ears; neglect of this precaution may allow an accumulation within the meatus that undergoes changes that work mischief in the deeper structures. The careless use of the syringe by unskilled hands should be discouraged. A Carbolic acid lotion is of great value in otorrhœa. Further surgical treatment may be necessary.

Deafness.

This inconvenient affection may be congenital, or it may arise from constitutional debility. All causes of depression to the muscular and nervous system act injuriously on the ear. Functional deafness is painless and depends on an impaired digestion, low spirits and dull weather. This kind of deafness requires China 3x, dil., Petroleum 3x, dil., and Nux 3x, dil., the remedy selected to be given in drop doses, four doses daily. Deafness may be caused by brain diseases, excessive mental excitement, obstruction of the external and internal ear, and by the diseases considered in the preceding article, and by paralysis of the accoustic nerve and the poison of blood diseases, such as measles, mumps, scarlet and typhus, rheumatic and arthritic fevers. It is sometimes caused by mal-treatment of intermittents from massive doses of Sulph. of Quinine, from apoplexy, epilepsy, and from blows or the noise of sudden explosions, producing loud detonations, as from a clap of thunder. It may occur from a cold and catarrh, and is but an aggravation of pre-existing deafness.

The prognosis in all cases of deafness must be made with reference to age of the patient, hereditary proclivity to the disease, or the relation sustained to constitutional disease. A favorable result from treatment can scarcely be anticipated in these cases if caused by syphilis, or any of the chronic constitutional maladies, when deafness comes on gradually, and is not dependant on obstructions in the auditory apparatus, it is generally incurable. There are however many cases of deafness of an ephemeral kind allied to causes which can be removed.

TREATMENT.—The treatment of deafness, in order to be successful depends on the removal of the cause; in many cases this is impracticable and yet in some cases it is possible. It is in recent cases when the cause is obvious that skillful treatment is most successful. In those of long standing the capacity for hearing may be decidedly increased to a greater or less extent, our experience and observation leads us to predict favorable results from rightly chosen Homœopathic remedies, after the removable causes have been attended to. The remedies to be consulted for nervous deafness are Phos. China, in debilitated constitution and for periodic deafness. Phos. ac., and jod., when sounds at a distance cannot be heard. Cactus g. for deafness with palpitation and also Ars. and Spong. Each of these remedies may be employed in the 6x, dil., when indicated, in drop doses in water, four or five times a day.

When deafness arises from a cold, Arsen., Bell., Puls., Dulc., and Bry., may be consulted and affiliated in the 6x, dil., ten drops in half a glass of water and a dessert spoonful dose, repeated every two or three hours.

If deafness follows fevers, etc., with loss of power in the acoustic nerves, Bell., Puls., Sil., China. If after cerebrospinal meningitis, Phos. ac.

We had a case of this kind which recovered with loss of hearing, and after a few months treatment with daily doses of Phos., and Phos ac., the hearing was restored. When deafness arises from suppressed eruption or discharge from the ears, Hep. sulph., Aur. mur., each in the 6x, trit., may be given daily, morning and evening; Calc. carb., and Sulphur, may likewise be consulted. When deafness arises from enlarged tonsils, Baryta carb., 3x, trit., may be given twice a day until a change. There are many other phases of the disease associated with many abnormalities which we find it difficult to specify. But there is a wide range of therapeutic agents from which to select, according to their pathogeneses.

General Remarks Concerning the Ears.

In the course of many years' practice we have observed much to condemn in nurses and mothers in not being careful in washing the face and ears of children, and not taking pains to wipe the head and ears dry after the proceeding. This is particularly enjoined to guard against the danger of deafness when there is any discharge from the ears. Care should be taken in drying the ears without inflicting a mechanical injury by crowding portions of the towel into the ears, and giving a twist, for this irritates the passage. Blows on the head, or boxing the ears of children should be avoided. All mechanical injuries of the kind may have a dangerous effect on the delicate and sensitive structure of the ear, and bring on deafness.

TREATMENT.—For the slightest injury to the ears from blows, a few doses of *Arnica* 3x dil., taken internally will not be amiss.

Diseases of the Nose.

When treating the diseases of the respirative system, we described several distinct affections of the nares and their membraneous lining. Ozæna is an ulceration of the mucous membrane of the nose, from which a fetid, purulent discharge, or that of saneous matter occurs. The nasal cartilages are sometimes destroyed, and the sense of smell and taste become equally depraved. The causes; neglected catarrh, syphilis or scrofula.

TREATMENT.—If there are no organic lesions, Aurum met. The 30x trit., in two grain powders taken night and morning, cured a case of ozæna when there was a pain above the nose, with redness and swelling, heat and soreness of the nostrils, yellowish-green or yellow discharge, partially dry and watery fetid pus. For further information concerning catarrhal obstruction of the nares, see article on coryza and catarrh, under the head of diseases of the respiratory organs.

There is an obstruction of the nares known under the name of polypus. There appears to be two kinds of polypi; one is merely mucus, and the other is a fibrinous appendage to the schneiderean membrane; both are pear-shaped; the former is cured by Pulsatilla 3x dil., two doses a day; the latter is often cured by Calc. c. 3x trit., a powder every night. If this does not succeed in time, give Sanguinaria 3x dil., two-drop doses in water, three times a day.

Inflammation of the Nose, Nasitis.

A very severe catarrhal inflammation affects the schneiderean membrane. The intensity of this inflammation may result in ulceration. The treatment does not differ essentially from that recommended for common catarrh, or cold in the head. The same remedies may be consulted.

Bleeding from the Nose, Epistaxis.

This is generally a trifling affection, but it may require some discrimination to decide when to interfere, and when to let it alone, for it may be a symptom that points to serious constitutional derangement. No treatment is necessary for simple cases, when there is but a trifling flow of blood, but when the discharge is excessive, and continuous, or oft recurring, arising from debilitated conditions, under such circumstances the loss may be serious, and indicative of something of a more serious character.

For ordinary cases, the symptoms which precede the hæmorrhage are giddiness, weight or oppression in the forehead. The bleeding may come from only one nostril, and not always from the front; it may pass through the posterior nares, and thence into the stomach or larynx, and be mistaken for hæmatemesis or hæmoptesis.

The cause of *nose bleed* has always to be taken into account. It often arises from a blow on the nose or head. It may be brought on by overexertion, or from violent coughing, as in whooping cough, or from a fit of passion, or rush of blood to the head, or it may attend the hæmorrhagic diathesis, or apoplexy in old age. It may arise from suppression of bleeding piles, difficult menstruation. The predisposing cause is the extreme vascularity of the schneiderean membrane, the capillaries distended and favor hæmorrhage as vicarious menstruation in women, or the check of hæmorrhoidal flow in general.

TREATMENT.—For venous hæmorrhage in every form, Hamamelis extract is indicated. Aconite 3x, dil., from arterial excitement, Belladonna 3x, dil., when nose-bleed proceeds from cerebral congestion. For epistaxis in old persons, Carbo veg., 3x, trit., for other conditions Nux 3x, dil., Phos., 3x, dil., Arnica 3x, dil., China 3x, dil., etc. When the affection is vicarious, Puls., 3x. dil., or Podoph. 3x, dil.

The accessory treatment consists of the application of cold water or ice to the nose, forehead and feet, and by the use of styptics or styptic cotton for plugging the nostrils.

NOTE.—Any of the remedies selected to meet given cases may be administered in cold water, ten drops of the dilutions to half a glass of water, and ten-grains of any trituation, spoonful doses, may be repeated every hour until there is a change.

Perversion of the Sense of Smell.

This affection generally attends chronic catarrh and requires the same remedial agents, as required in the treatment of that disease. (See Chapter on nervous diseases.)

CHAPTER LII.

Urethritis.

This disease has been quite common and may be distinguished into that which is virulent and non-virulent. The former being by far the most familiar to physicians, while the latter is so vague and indefinite and of such rare occurrence that but little mention may be made concerning it.

The non-virulent urethritis is caused by irritation produced by foreign bodies in the urethra, calculi, etc., or it may be the result of excessive sexual intercourse or intercourse during menstruation. It may arise from irritating drugs such as Copaiva, etc. It may originate from cold or be a mere symptom of other inflammation. It may result from irritation of the bladder or prostate gland, without a shadow of suspicion of it being the result of impure coitus.

Gonorrhœa is quite a different thing, and almost invariably an infectious blenorrhœa of the urethra, occasioned by contact. That impure coition is the cause of the disease hardly admits of a doubt. Yet it is possible that it may result without sexual intercourse, but not without contact with gonorrhœal matter. It is not probable that patients always give reliable statements concerning the origin of the trouble. As a rule the disease is caused by impure sexual intercourse.

It is not necessary in this place to discuss the nature of gonorrhœal poison. Such discussion is fruitless. As many opinions have been entertained of the contagion as there have been treatises on the subject. Some assert one thing, and some another concerning its specific character, instead of having the moral courage to say they know nothing beyond the fact of a gonorrhœal disease. It is a useless waste of time to indulge in theorizing on a doubtful subject, we will therefore proceed to note the description and causes of the disease.

The first symptoms of the presence of gonorrhœa become apparent about eight days after exposure. In some cases they are manifest in from three to five days; it is difficult to learn

the precise time owing to the proneness of the victims to claim
that a much longer time has elapsed. This undoubtedly is a
deception, or at least an error. It sometimes commences so mild-
ly that some time may pass before cognizance is taken of the
difficulty. It is manifestly true that the degree of infection may
modify the length of time. The manifestation of the commencement is a painless titillation in the urethra, and often with a vo-
luptuous sensation, and a thin slimy secretion is discharged,
gluing the orifice together in the morning. The urethral mucus
membrane so far as visible reddens at this stage with considerable
tumefaction. The peculiar titillation is followed by frequent
inclination to urinate, and also by troublesome erections and nocturnal emissions. Pain ensues upon the titillation with a constant
urging to urinate frequently, creating severe pain in the urethra,
with intolerable smarting and burning. The urine, of which only
a few drops are voided at a time, is scalding hot, so that it becomes
like fire. The freer and more copious the stream when urinating,
the less will be the pain at the time; but soon after the pains return more violently. The more urine in the bladder in the morning the more distressing it is to urinate. The orifice of the urethra
begins to swell and participate in the affection—the lips look very
red. The secretion still is scanty, looks yellow or greenish-yellow,
is thick. Stiffens the linen with yellow or greenish stains, and
in the morning the secretion can be squeezed from the urethra in
abundance. The sensitiveness of the urethra to pressure now
reaches to the fossa navicularis. The erections at night become
more frequent and continuous, causing the patient much pain in
consequence of the stretching of the urethra, which is very sensitive. Emissions at this stage very rarely occur, if ever. The
purulent secretion in quantity, increases greatly, still preserving
its greenish-yellow color. The parts are stained by the discharge.
The glands and prepuce swell, sometimes enormously. An old
gentleman called on the writer for advice on account of severe
swelling of prepuce which was nearly as large as the head of a
newly born infant, and his suffering from urethral inflammation
was great, and yet he thought it unaccountable, for he had indulged in but one intercourse with a young girl who peddled
trinkets. So far as could be learned the disease with him had
made rapid progress. Aconite 3x, dil. in hourly doses soon
relieved him of pain. Cannabis 3x, dil. followed Aconite, given

in the same way, effected a cure in eight days. After the disease
has progressed to the stage here described, excoriations take
place and small superficial ulcers show themselves. The inflammatory irritation of the prepuce easily results in phymosis. The
further progress of the disease becomes apparent by the soreness
and tenderness that extends the entire length of the urethra.
The disease seldom remains confined to the anterior portion of
the urethra, except in a few cases. What is usually denominated
the inflammatory stage continues about a week or two weeks.
There appears to be but little general fever, but often there is
much mental excitement and intense pain.

The discharge becomes very copious toward the termination
of the first stages, but its color changes more and more to that of
a whitish mucus, and assumes a more fluid consistence. The pains
at urinating almost entirely disappear, the erections become le s
frequent and painful, the nocturnal emissions are inclined to
greater frequency, the white secretion leaves gray and stiff stains
on the linen, with a yellow point in the center. If no unfavorable
complications are present the whole disease may terminate in
about six weeks. If complications exist a much longer time may
elapse before the patient is well. The inflammatory stage may
be protracted with distinct febrile characteristics. Inflammation
of the prostate gland is attended with danger of obstructing the
urethra. Orchitis, or swelling of the testes is another complication. Gonorrhœal buboes in the inguinal glands constitutes a
serious complication. And another painful complication is called
chordee and is specially noted. It is a painful curving of the
penis downwards during an erection. It is caused when corpora
cavernosa have become involved in the inflammation. This
trouble is serious, and treated in a faulty manner may result in
permanent disorganization.

A chronic urethritis may supervene upon an acute attack of
gonorrhœa, which becomes apparent in the form of a gleet or a
secondary siege of the affection. This is so common that it may
pass for a common rule. This gleet sometimes continues for
years. There is no positive evidence of its being infectious, yet
it is a source of anxiety to those so afflicted.

The sequellæ of gonorrhœa may involve the bladder, prostate
gland, etc. Strictures are by far too common a result and require
careful treatment. It is always advisable to use a well oiled bougie,

this may be the only resort capable of affording relief; we could add much more by way of describing attendant ailments but from what we have stated no one need mistake the trouble.

TREATMENT.—During the inflammatory stage when there is considerable pain, Aconite 12x, dil., 10 drops in half a glass of water, a table spoonful three times a day. After Aconite, Gels., 3x, dil., may be prepared and given in the same manner. *Cannabis sat.* 3x, dil., given in drop doses in a spoonful of water repeated every three hours. This remedy is applicable in all the stages and its use should be continued for weeks if necessary, in the following order: 3x, dil. for four days, 6x, dil. for the same length of time, 12x, dil. for the same length of time also, and if the disease is not cured let the next trial be made with 30x, dil. To ensure a favorable action of the remedy and a speedy cure the patient must keep quiet and abstain from heating and stimulating drinks and the women. For violent inflammation, suppression of urine, priapism, painful erections, and chordee, give *Cantharis* from 3x, dil. to 30x, dil., as directed for *Cannabis sat.* It is better to remain quiet during any attack of gonnorrhœa. The violent pains are somewhat mitigated by Gels. 3x, dil., in drop doses frequently repeated. When Cannabis does not fully cure the patient in two or three weeks, Merc. sol. 3x, trit., a two-grain powder to be given morning and evening, until the cure is effected.

For gonorrhœa and chancre combined, Merc. jod., 3x, trit., a powder morning and evening; if not cured in ten days change to Kali hyd., 6x, dil., two drops three times a day.

For figwarts give three drops of Thuja 3x, dil., three times daily; if not removed or cured in two weeks, change to Nit. ac., 6x, dil., to be used in the same way.

For orchitis, Clematis 3x, dil., bowels to be moved by tepid enemas, and three drops of the remedy, three times during the day at intervals of four hours each.

When the disease has been mismanaged with doses of Copaiva or Cubebs, give a dose of the 3x, trit., of Sulphur every night, and three drop doses of Phytolacca 3x, dil., in a spoonful of water every morning. For severe inflammatory symptoms, Acon. 3x, dil., Cann., 3x, dil., each in drop doses in water, or ten drops in ten teaspoonfuls of water, and a teaspoonful every two hours alternately.

For yellowish green discharge, Cannabis 3x, dil., and Mercurius 6x, trit., in alternation at intervals of six hours.

For strangury and difficult urination Cantharis 3x, dil., ten drops in half a glass of water, and a spoonful every hour until relieved. For milky discharges give Capsicum 3x, trit., every morning and evening. For *prostatitis* Nit. ac., 6x, dil., Puls 3x, dil., Thuja 3x, dil. Rest and quiet, and abstinence from stimulating drinks is recommended.

Syphilis.

This venereal disease is a specific ulcer or chancre produced only by contagion, produced through an abrasion from sexual intercourse with an infected person, the peculiar action of the poison in the blood being marked by a sequel of symptoms, which make their appearance twenty days after the absorption of the virus, that may result in affecting various tissues of the body for a longer or shorter period. It is in consequence of the duration and severity of the syphilitic poison, that this disease demands critical attention.

The disease is undoubtedly contracted, sometimes from accident, from soiled clothing, or water-closets, or from patient to the nurse, and it is difficult to eradicate this poison from the system. It often remains latent, long after an apparent cure. The taint, by reason of this persistency, is often transmitted from parents to offspring, as its manifestation may be seen in infantile diseases of the genitals; associated with wasting of the limbs, distortion and crookedness of the bones, ulceration of the tonsils, throat, and general feebleness in succeeding generations. This and much more can be predicated as the result of mercurial syphilis which has existed on the part of parents or ancestors still more remote.

It is difficult to define the limits of constitutional syphilis, and yet the extinguishment of the virus is within the range of possibilities. Syphilitic disease, ranges from the simple chancre which is specifically termed *primary* while limited to the part innoculated or lymphatic glands connected with it. It is termed secondary or constitutional syphilis when it affects parts not directly inoculated, such as the mouth, throat, tonsil, eyes and skin from the effects of the virus in the blood. It is termed *tertiary* when symptoms arise later in the disease, after a lapse of time in which there is an apparent freedom from the disease. Changes of tissue resulting in tainted blood. According to some pathologists the secondary evils are due to changes in the blood, and the *tertiary* to changes in the tissue. These changes include bone affections, cachetic ulcers,—fibro-plastic deposit nodes, etc. The nodes may form in various parts of the body, in the bones, brain, heart and lungs, liver, muscles and areolar tissue. A vast number of diseases are but outstanding effects of this virulent poison in the blood.

Syphilis in the three stages is contagious, and too great care cannot be exercised in preventing contact with other persons.

Hereditary syphilis is constitutional when the fœtus becomes impregnated from one of its parents. The infant may be healthy when born, or apparently so, but its skin is of a dull color, attended by an expression of age.

There are two kinds of chancre, one is infectious, and the other is not. The infectious chancre does not commence till three or four weeks after coitus. It first appears as a pimple, abrasion or crack, and develops slowly. Unless the sore is irritated the discharge is but slight. It soon becomes circumscribed, and seldom becomes phagedenic. The sore remains alone after glandular enlargement and infection of the system, and it is apt to be followed by indurated buboes.

Those chancres which are not infectious, begin within a period of three days. It first appears as a red spot, and soon becomes a pustule, and then a suppurating sore, which develops rapidly and suppurates profusely. It becomes phagedenic. It can be transplanted to other parts of the body, and often multiplies into clusters, a single suppurating bubo. A careful, discriminating observation of the two kinds of chancre, may prove to be eminently practical.

The primary syphilis is more tedious than any of the other specific fevers. The poison possesses the power of reproduction in the patient's body. The smallest possible quantity of virus is self-propagating, and suffices in time to inoculate all the solids and fluids of the body. The time required is much more protracted than for other constitutional dyscrasias, and the stages are prolonged indefinitely. We may count the time by weeks, and even months. The disease may last years without causing the patient to abandon social life, or refrain from matrimony, or becom-

47

ing parents, whose progeny cannot escape from the taint of syphilitic poison. This circumstance stamps the whole subject with an importance which attaches to the physician and surgeon the greatest responsibility. It behooves him not to sanction a matrimonial alliance, where there is a probability of this taint being in the constitution of one or both of the parties.

In order to better understand the nature of the disease, with reference to treatment, we will explicitly state the symptoms and diagnosis of the different stages.

The period of incubation varies from three days to seven or nine weeks. First there appears a red spot, which rapidly develops, becomes transparent, breaks, and forms a sore, which spreads with a peculiarity not common to other sores. Its form is circular with hard edges, cut clean, with a base which is grayish, or lardaceous, and irregular as if worm eaten. This is the ordinary form of the *primary* disease, which frequently gives rise to secondary symptoms. The second form is the *soft* or superficial sore from which, as before stated, no *secondary* symptoms arise. The margins of the ulcer are elevated, and the base is a reddish color and discharges copiously.

The phagedenic chancre is developed in persons of a scrofulous diathesis. Its edges are dark colored, irregular and thin, and a fetid thin secretion. It commonly increases in size and becomes rapidly disorganizing.

It is the primary or hard chancre which for the part claims our attention, for this is the kind that causes enlargement of the lymphatic glands in all parts, which become indurated, and especially those of the groin, which become hard and in some cases suppurate.

The secondary symptoms may arise after awhile and give the appearance of copper colored eruptions and ulceration of the throat and soft palate, with loss of the hair and pain in the bones and joints, with general febrile disturbance. In the *tertiary* form ulcerations of the mouth and throat which are inclined to spread, ulceration of the skin, diseases of the periosteum, cellular tissues, muscles, etc. The *diagnosis* of constitutional syphilis is important. It is just manifest on the skin because this tissue is the most superficial and when accompanied by deeper seated affections and we take into account the antecedant symptoms, peculiarities, color and form, the diagnosis is not difficult, and especially if the inguinal glands are enlarged. The case is made quite certain with these symptoms without further .enumeration of symptoms.

TREATMENT.—Mercurius sol., 3x, trit., given in two-grain powders every three hours is believed to be an antidote to the venereal poison in the system. It is specially indicated in chancre with red margins, cheesy or lardaceous bottom, painful, and inclined to bleed.

Nitric acid 6x, dil. is an effective remedy in constitutional syphilitic ulcerations, especially those inherited by children, and when the Mercurial cachexia has been engrafted upon inherited syphilis. Nitric acid 6x, dil. is also useful in primary chancre with spongy, elevated margins, not painful but readily bleeding profusely. After administering the remedy in the 6x, dil. in water, ten drops to a gill of water, and a spoonful of the solution three or four times a day, the 30x, dil. is recommended, to be prepared and administered in the same way. Kali hyd. 6x, dil., twenty drops in half a glass of water and given in tablespoonful doses three or four times a day is one of the surest antidotes to syphilitic poison in the secondary and especially in the tertiary form of the disease, with all its varied manifestations, nodes, tubercular skin eruptions, ulcers on the tonsils and throat, etc. Merc. corr. 6x, trit., in two grain powders, given every four hours, will cure a chancre with ichor adhering to the bottom and discharging thin pus which stains the linen.

The same remedy prepared in the same way will cure that miserable combination of chancre and gonorrhœa, buboes and skin affections; the symptoms being worse in bed.

When similar symptoms show themselves in scrofulous persons, *Cinnabaris* 6x, trit., may be prepared and given as above.

Arsen., 3x, and Kreasote 3x, dil., twenty drops in a glass of water given in spoonful doses three or four times a day, will cure gangrenous ulcers with florid unhealthy granulations, which bleed on the slightest touch, and are otherwise painful and burning.

Ars. iod., in 2x and 3x, trit., will cure a venereal bubo the most rapidly; it eclipses all other remedies, says *Dr. H. Noah Martin,* of Philadelphia.

Merc. jod 3x, trit., in two-grain powders given twice a day cured an inveterate case of syphilis, which had been under treat-

ment two years. The patient was obliged to keep his bed, and
the first time we saw him, his throat was terribly ulcerated,
implicating the tonsils, and palate, his breath so foul as to assault my olfactories unmercifully, his skin was studded with
tubercles, and offensive scaly sores, great ulcers on his legs and
thighs. He had spent hundreds of dollars with specialists and
was not benefited. We prescribed the Merc. jod. 3x, trit., to be
taken as above stated, we also ordered the sores washed with clean
warm water without soap, an application of 2x, trit. Merc., jod.
to each ulcer, while we had his mouth washed with a solution of
Chloride of Soda. We called the second time twenty-four hours
after and found no reason for changing the prescription as he
was comparatively easier.

We made our third visit the next day and found the throat
somewhat improved and the skin more emollient; the ulcers presenting a better appearance. Continued the same remedy internally, and on the fourth day there was a visible improvement.
Continued the external dressing, and prescribed, Merc. jod., 6x,
trit., two-grain doses a day. This treatment was continued for
twenty days, the patient improving all the time. As long as the
patient did well we made no change, at the end of six weeks we
discharged the patient so nearly cured that further attendance
was unnecessary.

CASE II. Was a young woman of the town, full of loathsome sores, with her mouth and tongue ulcerated, the labia
enormously swollen from inflammation. We prescribed nearly
the same treatment in this case for a week with no effect. We
then changed to Merc. jod. rubrum 6x, trit., a powder three
times a day, and she soon began to improve. The swelling and
ulceration of the labia was entirely gone in two weeks and she
was able to stand on her feet, and walk without pain. We continued this remedy until the loathsome sores healed and her
mouth and tongue appeared to be well, have not seen her since.

We cured a case of sore throat in a syphilis patient who had
been mercuralized with Phytolacca.

We have used Bell., 3x, dil., in cases of great pain, redness
and erysipelatous appearance. We have prescribed Aurum mur.
3x, trit., but for ulcerations of the mouth and nose, ozæna, bone
d seases and sarcocele, this remedy is invaluable when the sys-

tem has been broken down by combined action of syphilis and Mercury.

For orchitis, Clematis erecta excels all other remedies; 3x, dil., in drop doses every one or two hours, will speedily effect a favorable change, and also when there are excrescences, scabies and tetters, discharging bloody matter; and pain and irritation worse at night. Accessory treatment to meet each case is left to the physician.

Spermatorrhœa.

The meaning of this term is an abnormal and involuntary discharge of the semen. It may be caused by masturbation, excessive venery, or it may occur spontaneously as well as involuntarily during the night.

Any unnatural excitement which augments such a vitalized secretion as semen, which constitutes the sole contribution of the male in behalf of the propagation of the species, never fails, when of long standing, to result in nervous exhaustion, or other disorders of the nervous and digestive system.

SYMPTOMS.—A marked depression of the nervous system, and a manifest impairment of the mental faculties, inability to concentrate the mind either on study or business, the memory becomes treacherous, the physical powers are weakened, cowardice and want of energy are generally apparent; the patient is languid, debilitated, hypochondriac and misanthropic, and is apt to indulge in fearful forebodings and distrust of his abilities. He becomes dyspeptic, emaciated, without any evidence of real organic disorder.

TREATMENT.—The treatment of this trouble is by local means and remedies. In the treatment of spermatorrhœa, which occurs without erections, and is attendant on the stools, a warm hip bath in which the patient must sit five minutes three times a day, and the cauterization of the verumontanum has effectually cured some bad cases. Self compulsion against any indulgence in masturbation is an absolute condition, as the habit may result in insanity or dementia. Cheerful associations and good society are indispensable.

We have found best the 3x, trit. of Digitaline, 3 grain doses night and morning. If but little benefit results in the first ten days, change to Digitaline 6x. trit., and then to 30x, trit. By perseverance with this remedy in the manner prescribed, great benefit may be expected.

A gentleman was for five years afflicted with involuntary emissions and subject to great bodily and mental weakness, and emaciation; was on the point of abandoning all treatment as useless; was induced to take Aurum 3x, trit., in three grain doses, repeated daily; soon began to improve rapidly, gaining flesh. After five weeks Aurum 6x, trit. was substituted; the improvement continued and a cure was the result. Mercurius, 3x, trit. had been given in the case without benefit.

Nux vom. cured a case of habitual masturbation in a woman who contracted the habit when a child from itching of the pudenda. At 25 she gave birth to a child, after which she suffered from gastralgia, three or four times in 24 hours, great pressure in the stomach and head, great weakness of the knees and want of memory. Her habit was followed by spinal irritation and great sensitiveness to the touch. Many other derangements were the result of this secret vice and no effort had been made to induce her to abandon it. She took Nux 3x, trit., 3 grains twice a day, eight doses, and then one dose a day. With this treatment she was cured in four weeks, but after a few months she relapsed. Nux 3x, trit., after ten doses, restored her; she continued well.

Cuprum aceticum, 6x, dil. cured a case of impotence of two years standing in a robust young man aged 38 years. China, 3x, dil. will cure nocturnal emissions, provided the patient avoids self abuse and attends regularly to the evacuation of the bladder. Nux 3x.

Impotence of males can often be cured provided the cause becomes known. If it arises from debility, which may first manifest itself in loss of sexual power, *Agnus castus* in the tincture may be given in drop doses, four times a day for a week. Agn. c. 1x dil. may then be given in the same way, and 3x, dil. may follow for a week, and then the 12x, dil. and soon the 30x, dil. By persevering with this remedy in anticipation of the best results, in nine cases out of ten a cure will be effected. The loss of sexual power in some cases has been restored by Nux mosch. 3x, trit., a three grain powder every night. Baryta 3x, trit., has been found exceedingly useful for early loss of sexual power, in married life. Petroleum 6x, dil., for persons of bilious temperaments, who from fickleness and loss of sexual power become hypochondriacs. Ten drops may be put in a cup of water and given in spoonful doses night and morning. We have witnessed the good effect of this remedy in quite a number of cases.

When spinal irritation is caused by this debility, *Conium m ac.*, 3x, dil., ten drops in a glass of water, and a spoonful three times a day; *Cicuta vir.*, when a patient complains of weak back, and greater or less weakness in the lower extremities and finds him *non passum* in family matters, the 3x, dil., in half a glass of water, and take a tablespoonful morning and evening.

For priapism or erections from unnatural excitement *Cantharis* 3x dil, 10 drops in a glass of water, a tablespoonful every night, half an hour before retiring. If this trouble is caused by hæmorrhoids, Æsculus, 3x, dil., Nux vom., 3x dil., each ten drops in half a glass of water, spoonful doses every night. Camphor solution is a good remedy for this phenomenon. For further information on this subject see work *Decline of Manhood* published by Duncan Brothers.

CHAPTER LIII.

Metritis.

Uterine inflammation is attended by great pain, tenderness and swelling of the womb, and frequently arises from miscarriage, from tampering with instruments, and drastic medicines to procure one.

TREATMENT.—When from unavoidable miscarriage followed by fever, and caused by fright, and there is hot skin, hard and rapid pulse, intense thirst, Aconite, 3x, dil., 10 drops in half a glass of water, may be given in teaspoonful doses every hour until the fever subsides. *Belladonna* is the proper remedy for metritis when it occurs during confinement and attended by pains in the hips, joints, and small of the back, as if bruised or broken, and great sensitiveness on pressure. Bryonia, 3x, dil., when the least motion aggravates the suffering, she cannot sit up because of nausea.

In nine cases out of ten of metritis or its complication, peritonitis, Acon. given in the form above described and followed by Belladonna, will effect a cure. We have had considerable experience that will confirm this statement.

Macrotin in the 12th dilution is regarded an excellent remedy for uterine inflammation, but it must not be given in any low attenuation because of its tendency to produce aggravation if the uterus is sensitive in consequence of any active irritation. The late *Dr. Douglas* relates an interesting cure of chronic metritis, which was treated with Merc. sol., 3x, trit., one grain morning and evening and then with Sepia 6x, dil., three drops three times a day. After 24 days treatment of the two remedies, a resort to Macrotin, 3x, trit., one grain morning and evening, effected a permanent cure. *Dr. D.* regarded this case an inflammation of the lining of the mucus membrane of the womb, secreting pus with probable ulceration.

CANTHARIS.—When violent tenesmus of the bladder attends metritis, and there is a constant urging to urinate, this remed may be given in 3x, dil., 2 drops in a teaspoonful of water once in two hours. In very bad cases of metritis, when the patients lie in unconsciousness, with their arms stretched out along the sides of the body, interrupted by sudden starting up, screaming, throwing the arms about, and then signs of the affection of internal organs, this medicine in the 6x, dil., ten drops in half a glass of water and a tablespoonful every three hours. When the disease is caused by a fit of anger or chagrin after confinement, Chamomilla, 3x, dil., ten drops in half a glass of water, may be given in teaspoonful doses every half hour until relieved. When sudden joy comes over a woman after parturition and she in consequence suffers from sensitiveness, and cannot bear to be touched, a few doses of Coffea cones, disks or pellets, will generally give relief.

If inflammation of the womb be developed by emotional disturbances, and attended by spasmodic symptoms, jerks of the extremities, face, and eyelids, Hyoscyamus, 3x, dil., 10 drops in half a glass of water; teaspoonful doses may be repeated every half hour. In those cases in which typhoid symptoms supervene with delirium and restlessness, throwing about the limbs, pushing off the bed clothes and baring the body, this remedy given as above will be of service.

When metritis is attended by acute pain in the mamma, which also gets sore, especially in a low cachectic state of the system, and feeble pulse, Iodium, 3x, dil., may be prepared and administered, the same as directed for Hyoscyamus.

When no pressure whatever can be borne upon the uterine region, not even from the bed clothing, and the patient wishes frequently to lift them up, not on account of extreme tenderness of the abdomen, but because she is uneasy and feels as if the pains were ascending toward the chest, Lachesis 12x, dil., prepared in the same way as directed for Hyoscyamus, and given every two hours.

This remedy prepared as above is the most remarkable in its effects when given for metritis at the critical age, when there is great aggravation after sleep, and an amelioration of the pains by a flow of blood from the vagina, and alternate chilliness and heat of the skin, distended abdomen; or when metritis is attended by the discharge of thin ichorous lochia.

If metritis gives rise to stitching, aching or boring pains

with an indifferent amount of heat, moist tongue, chills and sweats, and worse the entire night, Mercurius sol., 6x, trit., if given in two-grain powders and repeated every two hours, will probably effect a speedy cure.

In many cases of this disease attended by general derangement of the system, such as violent aching in the hypogastrium, aggravated by pressure or contact, violent pains in the back and loins, constipation, nausea, frequent desire to urinate with scalding, and burning pain, and a feeling as if bruised, all the symptoms worse towards morning, Nux vomica 6x, trit., is indespensable, if given in small powders, two-grains, one every three hours, relief will almost certainly follow.

When suppression of the lochia causes metritis and there is a dark or sanious discharge from the womb which seems to have a strong tendency to become putrescent, Secale 3x, dil., ten drops in a glass of water and given in spoonful doses, every two hours until a favorable change occurs.

When during inflammation of the neck of the womb the patient feels that she must cross her limbs to prevent a protrusion, Sepia 6x, dil., may be prepared and given the same as Secale.

When inflammation of the womb is attended by stinging, thrusting pains, similar to such as arise from the sting of a bee, with entire absence of thirst, and scanty urine, Apis mel., 3x, trit., in grain powders, may be given and repeated every hour until a change occurs.

Arsenicum 3x, trit., in grain powders, may be given three times a day ,for burning, throbbing, lancinating pains, with restlessness and anguish, and fear of death; great thirst and cold drinks aggravate the trouble.

Cantharides 6x, dil., drop doses in water every hour, will be a source of relief to that violent tenesmus of the bladder that sometimes attends metritis.

Should severe, colicky pains attend metritis, causing the patient to bend double, with great restlessness, and distension of the bowels, diarrhœa, great thirst, and peritoneal tenderness, Colocynth 3x, dil., ten drops in ten teaspoonfuls of water may be given in teaspoonful doses every hour, at the same time, water as hot as the patient can drink it should be taken in small draughts every hour, in alternation with the remedy.

PULSATILLA 3x, dil., twenty drops in a glass of water, should be given every hour, in teaspoonful doses, when the patient complains of tension and contraction in the abdomen, as if the menses would appear, with nausea and vomiting of mucus, semi-lateral headache, bad taste in the mouth, no thirst, nightly diarrhœa and scanty menstruation.

DIET.—That which is exceedingly nutritious, easy of digestion in the form of gruel, broth, with crumbs of bread, chicken broth, rice, black tea, etc.

Amenorrhœa.

This affection of young and old women may be considered under separate heads, viz., *Retention* and *Suppression*. Retention of the menses beyond the natural period, from constitutional causes or mechanical obstruction. The period at which young girls change is called puberty, which in our climate and in the temperate regions generally takes place with girls at an age varying from twelve to fifteen years. In very warm or hot climates, menstruation occurs at an earlier period, *i.e.*, from the age of eight to eleven years. Whatever age is disclosed by observation to be the standard, enables the physician to form an idea of the abnormality of the retention if any exists.

CAUSES.—There are many causes that may provoke a delay that creates more or less anxiety on the part of mothers. After allowing for variation of time in individual cases, a change is expected, and the regular periods of menstruation are expected. If this change does not take place without too great a deviation from what is anticipated it is natural to inquire into the probable cause.

From many year's experience and observation I have come to the conclusion that retention may be prolonged from a natural delicacy of the constitution, a highly impressible nervous system, and a lymphatic temperament. There are general conditions which have more or less influence in opposition of the change.

TREATMENT.—Therefore a subject of naturally delicate constitution should not escape the attention of the physician. He should take cognizance of the natural struggles, if any, to merge into womanhood, and seek means or remedies to strengthen these struggles until the anticipated physiological change takes place. How shall this be done? First note the condition of the organic functions, and try to ascertain if the digestion and assimilation of food properly take place, or if there is palpitation, or nervous irritability. *Pulsatilla* will remove all these symptoms, and in a majority of cases be a successful aid to nature's efforts. The dose and administration should be stated so plainly that mistakes may not be possible. Drop into a glass of water ten or fifteen drops of Pulsatilla and direct a table spoonful to be given the patient three times a day. If this mixture does not prove to be successful in ten days, try the first decimal dilution in the same way and then after a trial with 1x, dil., change to 3x dil., and pursue the same course, and allow me to say, I have rarely known a failure of bringing about the desirable result. A single dose of the 3x, trit. of Sulphur, given first, may render the system more impressible to the action of the Pulsatilla.

The timid, nervous constitution should receive the same critical attention. The girl may suffer from pain in the back and loins, and from general uneasiness and twitching, without courage sufficient to make formal complaints. She has headache and sometimes derangement of the stomach. These symptoms are not uncommon as the period of puberty draws near; nature is struggling for a normal manifestation in this constitution and temperament, and I am satisfied from experience that Senecio aurens 3x, dil., fifteen drops in a glass of water, in morning and evening doses of a tablespoonful, will prove a valuable aid. Should this remedy fail, follow with *Calcarea carb.*, 3x, trit., a grain dose morning and evening, and if still further remedial measures are needed, Sepia may be prepared and given the same as Calcarea.

When amenorrhœa occurs in the most robust females, or rather when retention takes place and the delay appears anomalous, Nux vom., 3x, trit., a grain dose, morning, noon and night. From the 3x, trit., change to 6x, trit., to be employed in the same way, and also *Aconite* 3x, dil.; *Bell.*, 3x, dil., might in some cases be given; *Bryonia* when there is violent headache owing to congestion of blood to the head and chest, and when every motion is painful, and a flow of blood from the nose, with dry lips and thirst.

When a young girl near puberty, exhibits a pale face with blue margins around the eyes, fulness and distension of the abdomen, etc., give *China* 3x, dil., fifteen drops in a glass of water, spoonful doses three times a day.

Singular phenomena are more or less rarely observed at the age of puberty which require specific treatment. Instead of normal periodical evacuation, hæmorrhages occur from different parts in the place of the usual flow from the womb. In some very rare cases, *vicarious* menstruation has taken place from the top of the head, the ends of the fingers, the soles of the feet, the stomach, the intestines, the nose, the lungs, and other parts of the body, apparently assuming the place of the monthly discharges; of course they must be vicarious.

The treatment of this must accord with the symptoms and their locality. If the flow is from the top of the head, with headache and dimness of vision, we should prescribe *Glonoine*, 3x, dil., first, for immediate relief, and then we would recommend a two grain dose of the 30x, trit., of Calc. carb., to be taken every night for the ensuing three weeks, and then we should follow with Macrotin, 3x, trit., until the period occurs. When the vicarious discharge takes place from the fingers, we should prescribe *Caulophyllum*, 3x, dil., to be taken in drop doses, every three hours till the period passes off, and then we would recommend anti-psoric treatment for 20 days, and Caulophyllum again. We would recommend the same treatment for the flow of blood from the foot. When it flows from the stomach, *Ipecac* 3x, dil. When from the nose, *Aconite*, 3x, dil., and Belladonna. It is well to precede specific remedies indicated in all cases with anti-psorics.

The revolution which nature causes at the age of puberty ought always to be manifest in the menstrual flux, but the causes of derangement are numerous, and the departure from the normal standard diversified.

Suppression of the Menses.

The affection is common and from a variety of causes. After menstruation becomes once established and takes place at regular monthly periods, great care is required of all such persons not to expose themselves to extremes of temperature, or to the chill of autumn or winter evenings. Wet feet may cause suppression, so may sitting in a cold room; intense anxiety, mental emotion, fright or sudden shocks cause suppression. Sickness, pregnancy, and want of reconciliation to unavoidable misfortunes, whatever be the cause of suppression, must be taken into account.

Amenorrhœa is often followed by disturbing maladies, and more frequently from suppression than from the delay of the menses previous to puberty. A sudden suppression of the menstrual flow is sometimes followed by congestion of the lungs and the head, causing fainting and convulsions.

TREATMENT.—If caused by a cold bath, Dulcamara, 3x, dil., in drop doses, may soon procure relief; the doses should be repeated every hour, and a free use of the flesh brush should be accessory.

Caulophyllum, 3x, dil., is a salutary remedy for suppression caused by a cold; administer as follows: Drop 5 drops of the dil. in as many tablespoonfuls of water and give a tablespoonful at a time every 12 hours.

When suppression is caused by grief or trouble or suppressed grief, Ignatia, 3x, dil., ten drops in ten teaspoonfuls of water may be given in teaspoonful doses every two hours.

Am·norrhœa in young girls who lead a sedentary life, and suffer from a tendency of blood to the head or chest, and particularly if the menstrual flow has become suppressed by sitting in a cold room; and if on rising up they suffer from vertigo, nose bleed, or if the suppression is caused by fright or chagrin, Aconite 6x, dil., ten drops in as many tablespoonfuls of water, may be given in teaspoonful doses every two hours; at the same time they should go out when pleasant and exercise in the open air.

In case of suppression caused by indigestion, or other causes, characterized by violent contracting pain in the abdomen, and bearing down sensation, with inclination to support the bowels with the hand; leucorrhœa not copious but transparent, and passing imperceptibly from the relaxed parts, spotting the linen yellow; and nausea as from eating fat food; hysteria with maniacal lasciviousness, Agnus castus, 3x, dil., twenty drops in a glass of water may be given in teaspoonful doses every hour. If the 3x, dil. fails, 6x, dil. may be substituted, prepared and administered in the same manner; and when suppression is caused by working in water and is attended by dropsical symptoms, Calc. carb., 3x, trit., may be given in grain doses morning and evening. This same remedy, prepared in the same way, may be given when there is frequent rush of blood to the head, with dizziness and buzzing in the ears constricted feeling around the waist, quick and irregular beating of the heart increased by motion.

Graphites 6x, trit., in grain doses, may be called into requisition when there is dryness of the vagina, burning and itching of the labia during the scanty flow of the menses, which, when they are not suppressed, are pale and attended by pains in the abdomen and limbs, swelling of the hands and feet, itching blotches here and there on the skin, from which oozes a gelatinous fluid. The remedy may be given every 24 hours, in the morning. This remedy is in the menopausial period, what *Pulsatilla* is in youth.

Chlorosis.

Young unmarried ladies of delicate, lymphatic constitutions, slight figures, and highly impressible nervous systems, are by far most liable to attacks of this disease.

DIAGNOSIS.—The symptoms commonly observed during the incipient stage of chlorosis are gastric derangement, with more or less affection of the bowels, manifested by a pale and bloated appearance of the tongue, foul breath, partial or total loss of appetite, morbid craving for certain indigestible articles, like chalk, slate pencils, coal, clay, pickles, etc., torpid state of the bowels, tympanitic distension of the abdomen, and occasionally griping pain. What passes from the bowels is composed of crude and imperfectly digested aliments, unnatural in color and consistence.

Chlorosis occurs chiefly between the ages of 13 and 24 years, seldom at a later period. If it does occur it is not difficult to trace it to secondary disturbances, such as rapid succession of confinements of young women and especially if they nurse their own children.

The disease is evidently connected with the sexual sphere; as an entirely primary disease it only assails unmarried women. It sometimes occurs previous to the first appearance of the menses, but more frequently after several menstrual periods.

There is reason for believing it to be hereditary; females of pale complexion are more likely to become the victims of this disease, but no constitution appears to be exempt from it; and yet delicate persons with irritable nerves are more impressible.

Among a variety of causes we may mention sedentary habits, insufficient exercise, mental exertions without corresponding muscular activity, excitement of the imagination or fancy from persistent novel reading, excitement of the sexual feelings by self abuse and improper relations to the opposite sex, any interference with the free expansion of the chest, the deprivation of open air, and moreover by tight lacing. This latter cause, if kept up, will surely drag the patient down into confirmed tuberculosis. Close attention is therefore necessary to note every symptom, especially in the case of robust young girls who exchange a country life and plenty of fresh air, for the restrictions which surround a residence in the city.

We must be the more careful in fortifying the system against chlorosis because it is an idiopathic disease, occuring exclusively among women, and difficult to account for by any precise and logical reasoning.

The disease is more common in cold than in warm climates, and when it is taken into consideration that in cold climates, children, a large portion of the time are kept in closed rooms, at a temperature of 75° or 80° Fahrenheit, thus preventing that free development of the body which would result from pure air and abundant exercise. That this pernicious custom prevails during a large part of the year, at the north, accounts unmistakably for the frequent instances of chlorosis in families composed of young ladies.

It is manifestly true that persons and especially females of frail, nervous and lymphatic constitutions cannot withstand the severities of the temperate latitudes, without suffering more or less from glandular and membranous disorders. Men even, of studious and sedentary habits, who have refrained from taking much exercise have occasionally suffered from chlorosis.

Some of the symptoms of chlorosis frequently assume a serious local aspect as the disease progresses, and thus pave the way for exceeding dangerous complaints.

These are enumerated by MARSHALL HALL as follows: "First, pain in the back; second, cough and dyspnœa, third, palpitation of the heart; fourth, pain and tenderness of the side; fifth, pain and tenderness of the abdomen; sixth, constipation, seventh, diarrhœa; eighth, anæmia; ninth, menorrhagia; thirteenth, hysteric affections; fourteenth, œdema, anasarca erythema nodosum."

These complications are nothing more than symptoms of the original disease, and must receive a corresponding treatment. It is well to impress this fact on the mind, because when any of the symptoms here enumerated, are taken for the disease itself, any one of these symptoms may become so prominent, as to lead to an erroneous opinion respecting the importance of the case. As for example, frequent pains in the chest, violent palpitation of the heart, on the slightest exertion, and an irregular and intermittent pulse, have often misled attending physicians, and caused them to fear the gravest organic lesions of the heart. When this impression or conclusion gives place to true ideas of the case that chlorosis is a constitutional disease, and should be treated the same as other constitutional maladies. That it is formidable and requires the most critical attention to all the features of the disease. The practitioner who encounters a case of this chlorosis sees before him a case of great debility, with prominent symptoms which serve as a guide for the employment of remedial measures. In a veritable case of "green sickness" the patient in the process of time becomes, listless, irritable, fond of being alone, with no inclination to engage in any physical or mental exertion; the menses become irregular, the face pale and tumid, the lips lose their color, the eyelids are swollen and surrounded by a dark greenish or yellowish color, and now the function of nutrition fails, emaciation begins, and a variety of symptoms follow, such as lassitude, hysteria, dyspnœa and palpitation of the heart, or a fluttering about the region thereof, which becomes signally apparent in ascending stairs, or while rapidly walking, or from sudden emotions of the mind. A train of illusory, or real troubles, tend to derange and depress the spirits. The patient is subject to vertigo, ringing in the ears and head, and disturbed by unpleasant dreams.

As the disease progresses all these symptoms become more strongly marked. The whole surface of the body assumes a smooth and puffy appearance, the skin is sallowish or lead-colored, the muscles soft and flabby, the lower extremities become œdematous, particularly the feet and ankles. If no barrier is interposed to arrest the progress of the disease, the entire organism is subject

48

to its influence, and universal derangement of the organs and functions entering into the economy of human life.

Now what are the predisposing and exciting causes of this derangement? Why should young girls, just blossoming into womanhood, have such a dreary life before them? What are the proximate causes of all these troubles? These queries are important in a pathological and therapeutic point of view. Let us trace then, the natural history of the malady. It is a well settled fact that chlorosis manifests itself in rare instances, in young girls at the early age of three or four years; and the *first* indication, or rather first abnormality in the system noted, is the prominent gastric and intestinal derangement. This invariably attends the first commencement of chlorosis. This alone is sufficient to lay the foundation for an indescribable number of derangements that develop the disease.

It therefore seems probable that a *therapeusis* capable of reaching all the phases of the disease, must call into requisition a large portion of our materia medica. But the pathological condition of the patient may be likened to the branches of a tree which are too numerous to count and yet with this root there is only a single tree. The gastric and intestinal derangement first seen in chlorosis, is capable of exhibiting an amount of phenomena equal to what has been described as characteristic of the disease.

TREATMENT.—Ferrum, 3x, trit., in one grain powders every three hours, in the cachexia will gradually produce a favorable change. *Ferrum pyrophos.* 3x, trit., is a valuable remedy because it is soluble in the blood. The commencement of chlorosis treated faithfully with Ferruginous tonics will do much toward obviating the early symptoms, and here I will venture the remark, that the .ferrated elixir of Calisaya has apparently changed the cachectic condition of anæmic debility of chlorotic girls. This accords with our experience.

Alumina, 3x, trit., a grain powder night and morning will be suitable for those who complain of constant chilliness, craving chalk or clay, and are subject to scanty menstruation of pale blood, and also when hysteric symptoms, such as spasmodic laughter and jerks, and anxiety enter into the group, and moreover when the sight of a knife suggests suicide, and when low spirited on waking.

Arsenicum and *Arsenate of Iron*, 3x, trit., are desirable remedies when chlorotic girls exhibit a high degree of debility with excessive irritability, œdematous paleness, cardial disturbances even when at rest, *pernicious anæmia*, fever with dropsy and petechial effusion. A small powder of either preparation may be given three times a day, half an hour after each meal.

CALC. CARB., 30x, dil., twenty drops in a glass of water, a tablespoonful, night and morning, and given persistently, has cured inveterate cases in strumous subjects. Anorexia, chronic acidity; pallor of the countenance, leucorrhœa and defective assimilation, are symptoms which call for this remedy.

In uncomplicated cases of chlorosis, with scanty menses or amenia, loss of appetite or taste, tendency to relaxed bowels, and with inclination to weep, Pulsatilla 3x, dil., drop doses for a week, morning, noon and night, then 12x, dil., drop doses, three times a day, for the succeeding week, and then follow with the 30x, dil., the third week. In this practice I have the greatest confidence, having seen the most desirable results.

CASE I. Miss A. C. P., aged twenty-three, came under my care. A long siege of treatment for chlorotic amenorrhœa, of sixteen months standing, her stomach was greatly deranged, and accompanied by a tedious diarrhœa. She had little appetite, her face was pale, with discoloration of the infra-orbital region. Her parents had no confidence in Homœopathy; her uncle was a highly respected physician of the regular school. She had been under his treatment nearly up to the time when we were called in and during the entire period she had gradually lost flesh and strength; as a dernier resort they concluded to try Homœopathic treatment.

After making critical inquiry into the antecedents of the case, we prescribed drop doses of the tincture of *Sulphur* at night and the same of the tincture of *Pulsatilla* in the morning. She took the remedies as prescribed and derived benefit. After a week 3x, dil., of each was substituted, and the result was eagerly watched by her parents, and their hopes were so much revived in her case, that they immediately sought for a physician of our school whose reputation would entirely eclipse ours. To him they stated her case, and then he requested them to inquire of us what remedies she had been taking. The desired information was given, and our successor informed. He recommended a perseverance with the same. Under the salutary effects of these two remedies she recovered, married, and for several years, she has been comparatively a healthy woman, and a mother of four children.

CASE II. A girl aged sixteen; hereditarily scrofulous, had not menstruated, was sorely troubled with gastric derangement and occasional diarrhœa, pain in the back and general debility, pale countenance with greenish blue circles around the orbits, was placed under our care. We found some difficulty in deciding between amenorrhœa and chlorosis; finally we recognized both and commenced our treatment. We ordered bathing in warm salt and water and the free use of the flesh brush, and then we gave *Macrotin* 6x, dil., drop doses every three hours, for several days, with no apparent benefit; we then reconsidered her case, and decided to give *Calc. carb.*, 6x, trit., a grain dose, night and morning. At the same time we tempted her appetite with nutritious broths or essence of beef. After one week's treatment with *Calcarea* alone we prescribed *Senecio aureus* 3x, dil., three drop doses, to be taken in alternation every six hours. Under this treatment changes began to take place. The gastric symptoms passed away, and there was little or no diarrhœa, and her appetite began to crave substantial food. In ten days her first menstrual period occurred, but with little pain, and was pale and scanty. The dropsy which before had been noticed passed away and we felt quite sanguine of conquering the chlorotic symptoms by the time her next period came round, and we were not disappointed. We recommended a daily perseverance with the remedies until the premonitory signs of another period. This direction was followed, at the same time she was able to eat beef broiled and roasted and without any gastric disturbance. The second menstruation was five weeks after the first, and was decidedly healthy. She flowed four days bright red blood, and felt well and strong. All the chlorotic symptoms were for a time effaced. This case convinced me of the utility of alternating an antipsoric with a psoric remedy in such cases.

CASE III. A married lady suffering from chlorosis during pregnancy, and being anæmic and debilitated, and liable to suffer from difficult digestion and flatulence, was very greatly benefited by *Aletris far.*, 3x, dil., 10 drops in a glass of water and spoonful doses every morning, noon and night.

CASE IV. A lady who had been in trouble induced by mental emotions, caused by fright, and who was superlatively sensitive and inclined to hysteria and other complaints, derived great benefit from *Ignatia*, 3x, dil., 5 drops on a lump of sugar, night and morning. She had for some time suffered from chlorosis, which was palpably manifest in her countenance.

CASE V. M. J. C., aged 18 years, dark complexion and black hair and eyes, had her menstrual periods at the age of 11 years, and at each period she flowed profusely, until a change arising from gastric irritation caused a cessation. She then began to suffer from headache, peevishness, loss of appetite, derangement of the bowels, excessive malaise and weakness; she must lie down for hours with no disposition to exercise in the open air; pale, cachectic, and a veritable victim of green sickness; was cured by the persistent use of the 3x, trit. of *Antim. crud.*, 2 grains night and morning.

CASE VI. A case of a lady aged 35, of nervous temperament. She suffered from irregular and scanty menstruation, leucorrhœa, sick headache and constipation; her face was pale and tumefied, dark greenish blue circles around the orbits, no appetite, melancholy, fever spots on the skin, and great debility; was so far benefited by the employment of Sepia, 30x, dil., 5 drops in a spoonful of water, night and morning, that she was able to resume her millinery business.

We might further show the benefit of treatment by citing examples, but let it be understood that a faithful and judicious treatment of chlorosis may save many estimable young ladies from an untimely grave.

Cancer of the Mammary Gland.

The distressing symptoms of a malignant growth in the mammary glands lead at once to an inquiry into its nature. It is an induration of the gland, caused in many instances by mechanical injuries. Morbid changes take place in this indurated nucleus and the growth of a fibroid structure formed of meshes, enclosing non-united and non-uniform granules, nuclei and cells, whose tendency is to spread indefinitely into the contiguous structures, and in the course of the lymphatics of the parts affected to produce itself in remote parts of the body, and to proceed to ulceration and ultimate exhaustion.

There are non-malignant tumors that affect the mammary gland. They are usually unattended by pain. These are sometimes curable, but malignant cancer is a constitutional disease and if excised is liable to be reproduced.

The non-malignant can be effectually removed if not cured. We have had several ladies who supposed themselves doomed by reason of having a mammary cancer. We could find evidence of constitutional diathesis and we have called on skillful surgeons to remove them.

TREATMENT.—In other cases where the entire gland became indurated, we have been successful in the employment of remedies. *Carbo. animalis*, 3x, trit., *Ars.*, 3x, trit., *Hydrastis*, 3x, trit., are remedies that we have used with success.

There is much testimony in favor of the use of *phenic acid*, administered hypodermically or by the mouth. Our experience is limited, but we unhesitatingly favor the treatment. We would suggest that all indurations of the mammæ should receive the earliest attention, and in this way a malignant growth may be prevented.

Cancer of the Womb.

Cancer or scirrhus or carcinoma of the womb. The specific character of these tumors is the same in any locality of the body, and the remedies that will exert a favorable effect in one locality, in all probability will act well in another. Our definition of induration and cancer of the mammary gland is apropos to the same trouble in the uterus. What is malignant and constitutional is the most dangerous, because there are greater obstacles in the way of a cure.

TREATMENT.—*Carb. an.* will cure indurations of the womb in many cases, 3x, trit., a two grain powder twice a day. For real carcinoma of the uterus there is no remedy that promises the success as that of the *phenic acid*, used after the manner prescribed by the late *Dr. N. F. Cooke*, and his preceptor, *Dr. De Clat.* Graphites, 3x, trit., has been used in grain doses daily. Kreosote, 2x, dil., has also been employed with at least a palliative effect.

Hydrastis is recommended for all varieties of cancer, but it will only act as a regulator of nutrition when it is faulty, and thus acts favorably on cancers. It is used in the 1x, 2x, and 3x, dilutions, in drop doses several times a day. The *phagedenic* ulcers of the womb can be greatly benefited by *Nit. ac.*, 6x, dil., drop doses, repeated every two hours during the day. There are other remedies that can be usefully employed in the treatment of these painful affections of the uterus.

We once called the late *Dr. H. K. Boardman* in consultation in a case of cancer of the mammæ, and after preparing the patient by daily doses of appropriate remedies, he removed the *cancer* with the knife. Its weight was more than a pound. The lady recovered and is alive and well at this time of writing.

Dysmenorrhœa.

The meaning of the word is difficult and painful menstruation, with severe pains in the back, loins and region of the ovarry. It does not always appear in the same form, because it originates from various causes. It may be connected with derangement of the stomach, and difficult digestion. It occurs in connection with the rheumatic diathesis, and probably more frequently in gouty constitutions. It is frequently associated with hysteria and neuralgia. In connection with uterine inflammation, implicating the os and cervix, dysmenorrhœa frequently occurs, and moreover it arises from ovarian irritation.

DIAGNOSIS.—Painful menstruation occurs more frequently with plethoric and robust ladies of ardent, sanguinous and animated temperaments. There is no irregularity in the monthly sickness; it comes on at the regular time, but generally in small quantity, if there is any show at all, and then it may be entirely suppressed for some hours, and then it returns again, and this may be repeated. Women troubled with dysmenorrhœa, as a rule, suffer from constipation and frequent headaches from rush of blood to the head during the intervals between the menstrual periods. The most marked symptom attending nearly every case of dysmenorrhœa is bearing down pains in the region of the womb, very much like labor pains, coming on in paroxysms; constant aching in the small of the back, loins and hips, pelvis and the lower extremities. Accelerated action of the heart and arteries, flushed cheeks, cutting and pressing pains in the abdomen, flatulence, eructations, oppression of the chest, anxiety, scanty discharge of non-coagulable blood and lymph and shreds of membranous structures or clots of blood. So great has been the desire to cure this suffering in women, that a frequent resort to local treatment has been an injury instead of a benefit. Too free a use of catheters has caused local ulceration, more tedious to endure than the real disease.

Dysmenorrhœa presents itself in different forms which becomes necessary to recognize. First, the *neuralgic form*. Unmarried ladies or those who have never borne children, are liable to suffer from this form. In cases such as these, both the sterility and painful menstruation are undoubtedly the product of ovarian disease. Second, *congestiv form*. Congestive dysmenorrhœa is not uncommon with unmarried young ladies. It is sometimes cured by marriage, though it often occurs with those who have had children, especially with those of healthy robust constitutions, and of plethoric sanguine temperament.

CAUSES.—The causes that operate in the production of amenorrhœa and further derange the health in rheumatic, nervous, scrofulous constitutions, are the same that produce dysmenorrhœa. The severe and excessive pain depends on *ovaralgia*. It is deep-seated, and neuralgic in character, amounting in severe cases to inflammation of the ovaries, and neuritis. As civilization progresses, this distressing trouble among women seems to be more common. It is entirely unknown in savage life, and in that state of society which forbids such unreasonable resorts to genteelly shape the body as have been practiced. When we reflect upon the habits and modes of life which the customs of refined society impose upon young females, we need not wonder that the important function of the uterus so often becomes disturbed. The demands of *fashion* are unreasonable, and the foolish mother is anxious that her daughter should grow up according to the laws of a false elegance, with a shape of body moulded to suit the *code of fashion*, rather than to leave the physical system to develop itself according to the proportions marked out by infinite wisdom. From many years' observation in practice, we are convinced that more constitutions are ruined, more suffering has been provoked by interfering with nature's endowment than otherwise exists, from unavoidable causes. Mechanical devices to shape the female form into the artificial thing recognized and known as a specimen of gentility, with deranged functions, productive of chlorosis, *dysmenorrhœa*, consumption and organic affections of the heart, are in the present age more disastrous to health, then the lethal influences wafted on the wings of the winds, in the malarious districts. Another cause of *dysmenorrhœu* is the want of out-door exercise, and too close confinement to study. Another is the accumulation of indurated fæces in the colon, rectum, etc.

TREATMENT.—Much depends on good hygienic treatment in this disease. An active exercise in the open air, several times a day, a plain regimen and abstinence from green tea, coffee and wine, and a temperature not exceeding 68° Fahrenheit within

doors are prime conditions to the successful treatment of dysmenorrhœa.

When the disease arises from an inflammatory condition of
the uterus, attended with fever, rapid pulse, hot skin, thirst and
hurried respiration, headache and general restlessness, Aconite
3x, dil., ten drops in a glass of water, may be given in spoonful
doses every hour.

If the menses are scanty, and attended by cutting pains in the
uterine region, abdomen, back and loins, vertigo, loss of appetite,
chilliness, nausea and discharge of thick black blood, alternating
with short discharges of bright red blood, Pulsatilla 3x, dil.,
prepared and administered the same as directed for the Aconite.

Agnus castus 3x, dil., given as directed for Aconite for
dysmenorrhœa with *ovarian neuralgia*, menses profuse, coitus
painful and abhorrent.

Belladonna, 3x, dil,, 10 drops in half a glass of water, given
in teaspoonful doses every hour, is an admirable remedy for dysmenorrhœa, when the patient is of a plethoric habit and sanguine temperament, and the disorder has originated from some
violent emotion, and is attended by serious determination to the
brain. It is well to proceed with this remedy after Aconite has
been administered.

Prof. Ludlam made a statement in his report to the World's
Convention of Homœopathic physicians held in Philadelphia in
1876, that repelled eruptions, in many instances, were the source
of membranous dysmenorrhœa, and that a successful treatment
of this painful disorder consists in employing such remedies as
are suitable for the eruptive disease, from whence the trouble
has originated. As for instance, *Urtica urens*, when from nettle-
rash; scarlatina, Belladonna; from erysipelas, Rhus, 10x; from
measles, Bry. (See vol. 1st, p. 969, Transactions of the World's
Convention, held in Philadelphia in 1876.

Prof. Ludlam, was the first, we believe, who observed this
connection between eruptive fevers and this menstrual difficulty.
His observation has been abundantly confirmed since. And we
venture the opinion that the skin and mucous membrane are so
intimately related, that a repelled eruption of any kind would
naturally exhibit its effect on that portion of the mucus membrane
immediately implicated during the catamenia.

Guaiacum tincture, in drop doses has been much lauded as a remedy in dysmenorrhœa. *Dr. Dewes*, formerly professor of obstetrics and diseases of women made a favorable mention thereof.

Mercurius corr.—In complications of dysentery and dysmenorrhœa, this remedy in 3x, trit., may be given in grain doses every two hours. The symptoms indicating it are severe and burning pains of a forcing character, as if there was a struggle to force an obstacle from the neck of the womb. Tenesmus as in dysentery, burning, straining.

Borax, 3x, trit., may be given in grain doses every two hours in an attack of membranous dysmenorrhœa, which occurs when the menses comes on too early and too profuse, attended with colic and nausea. We will give a few examples that have come under our observation:

CASE I. Young lady aged 19, suffered intensely at every menstrual period. She was invariably in the greatest agony for two or three days, clenching her fists and throwing herself about in the bed and groaning with pain; after this agonizing pain she flowed profusely, suffering from colicky pains. It became necessary to resort to palliatives to lessen the suffering. She had tried Anastesia, the recommendation of her previous medical attendant, and to no good result. We tried to lessen her sufferings by warm hip baths, and warm fomentations applied over the uterine region, which for brief intervals afforded some relief. We then tried the 3x, trit., of *Borax*, a grain powder on her tongue, repeated every two hours; after the third dose she experienced some relief. 6x, trit., was then recommended, grain doses to be repeated as before, and in 12 hours she was entirely relieved, and soon recovered her normal health, and in order to protect her from such agony in the future, grain doses of 3x, trit. was prescribed, to be taken every night until the succeeding menstrual period, and to her great joy the period returned and she experienced a healthy flow, and apparently free from pain. A continuance of the same preparation in like doses was prescribed, to be taken every three days during the succeeding interim; and the next period was entirely normal, and she and her mother considered her cured. This was a veritable case of membranous dysmenorrhœa, and confirmed our opinion of the utility of Borax in such cases.

CASE II. A married lady aged forty-four; had suffered intensely at her menstrual periods with membranous dysmenorrhœa, she had submitted to several operations with bougies and other dilators of the cervix uteri, and always without beneficial results. She rather thought herself the victim of injury from these attempts to relieve her mechanically. The irritation which the instruments had produced independent of the difficult menstruation, added to her suffering. She suffered at each period violent contractive spasms which lasted from six to twelve hours, leaving the entire uterine region very sore; at every return of the catamenia it was too early and too profuse, of bright red blood, and the interims between the periods, was very far from being a season of comfortable health; she felt exhausted, and particularly after shreds of a membranous character had been passed off, after which audible emissions of flatus passed from the vagina. During the interim she was depressed in spirits and gave up to melancholy foreboding and just before her periods, she suffered from fullness of the head and chest, and difficult respiration, headache and an abnormal sensation all over the body. We have thus been particular in describing this case because we verily believed its protracted character was greatly due to the abortive attempts to give relief by unreasonable mechanical measures to dilate the os uteri. She was at the acme of the suffering, when I was called to prescribe, unable to leave her bed or stir without fainting. Our first prescription was *Caulophyllum* 1x, dil., in drop doses every hour; after six doses and no relief, on further consideration we decided to give *Bromium*, which in a brief period was followed by marked relief; we prescribed the 6x, dil., ten drops in half a glass of water, and a teaspoonful every hour, and continued for twenty-four hours. We then gave the 12x, dil., and continued its use until the end of the period which she claimed was more tolerable than she had experienced for years. This remedy was followed by such good results it was continued over several periods; each succeeding one was less painful and finally, it being near the critical age, we changed to *Lachesis* 12x, dil., prepared and given in water, one drop to a teaspoonful, three times a day. Under this treatment she gained strength and suffered but little pain, although her system had been so worn down by previous suffering and mal-practice she never resumed a robust constitution. She never had borne any children.

CASE III. Mrs. E. S., a full, plethoric lady, suffered at each menstrual period so greatly, that she seemingly craved death as a relief. She always suffered from extreme languor before the menses; intense colic at the time, with loss of appetite, attended with nausea, vomiting, headache, pain in the back and limbs, and a continual pressing down in the abdomen, and constipation. After casting about for remedies, and prescribing many unsuccessful, we determined to give her Belladonna in repeated drop doses of the 3x, dil., from which she obtained some relief. We then substituted *Atropine* 3x trit., in grain doses; with this remedy we have been enabled to obviate her suffering from dysmenorrhœa for years.

We might detail the characteristic features of a multitude of cases which we have treated within the last thirty years. One case we relieved and cured with Hyos., and Puls., in hourly alternation, ten drops of the 3x, dil., each in a gill of water, a spoonful at a dose. Perseverance with these remedies, over two periods, proved to be sufficient. Some we have greatly benefited with Causticum, some with Arnica, some with Platina, Sepia and Calc. In most all cases we begin with the 3x, dil., or 3x, trit., and advance to higher attenuations of the same remedy. We have utterly failed to cure in many cases, which we have attributed in part to our faulty selection of a remedy. Our accessory treatment has been mainly confined to tepid or hot water compresses, with well ventilated apartments, kept reasonably warm. My experience warrants me in commending the use of critically affiliated remedies at reasonably short intervals, between the periods.

Menorrhagia.

This disease consists in profuse uterine hæmorrhage, which may take place at any time from puberty to extreme old age, without regard to any particular constitutions. But the most common which commands the attention of physicians, happens at the monthly periods, from congestion or relaxation of the uterine vessels. The natural secretion of the menstrual fluid each month, may vary somewhat in quantity, according to temperament, constitution and habits of life. Robust and plethoric women who live generously, may suffer considerable loss of blood at each period, and suffer no inconvenience from it; while individuals of delicate frame and relaxed tissues, would immediately become sensible of ill effects of so profuse a flow. When the natural monthly flow becomes morbidly affected and increased, the designation of uterine hæmorrhage is applied, because it is an abnormal condition that requires medical treatment.

Dangerous uterine hæmorrhages frequently occur during pregnancies, from rupture or disturbance of the placental membrane, and also from falls, mechanical injuries or blows, violent exercise, fright, anger, miscarriages, or cathartics and emenagogues.

The symptoms which precede menorrhagia which occurs at the menstrual period, are general uneasiness and dissatisfaction, petulancy, sense of dullness and oppression of the head, lassitude, weariness, and wandering pains in the back, and loins, and lower extremities, sense of weight and pressure in the pelvis, chilliness, deranged circulation, loss of appetite, cold feet, etc.

In light cases of menorrhagia, such as may occur at the regular catamenial period, there is generally a sense of lassitude and debility, with faintness and weariness, uneasy sensations in the back and limbs, with absolute inclination to rest, and no disposition to exercise, a death-like feeling at the pit of the stomach, paleness of the face, cold extremities, feeble and unsatisfactory respiration.

In more serious cases the patient becomes almost entirely void of blood; the face, lips, and cheeks become blanched, the muscular strength almost gone; every attempt to move or converse induces faintness. There is an evident determination of blood to the head, as there are sharp pains, delirium, ringing in the ears, and throbbings of the carotid and temporal arteries; the sight becomes obscured, sparks or spots float before the eyes; the breathing is labored, and the most moderate movement or exercise causes palpitation of the heart; rapid pulse and feeble; general coldness of the surface; great uneasiness and nervous irritation. The blood gushes upon every exertion to move or change posture, and on coughing, sneezing, or vomiting. Frequent and protracted syncopy comes on after the patient has lost sufficient to come into a very low state. Respiration and circulation can hardly be detected; they appear to be almost suspended. The blood clots at the mouth of the uterine vessels, and this causes a temporary arrest of the flowing. After a reaction takes place in the general organism, the clots are liable to be expelled, and a return of the hæmorrhage takes place. There may be alternations of the conditions for several months, or until a condition of the system ensues from which there is no reaction, and there is no expulsion of the clots. And now time is allowed for the uterine vessels to recover themselves sufficiently to sustain themselves, and to resist any further morbid secretion. Cases of this description have occurred under our own observation, and we have witnessed the kind offices of nature in bringing about a physical condition from which recuperation could commence.

Among the symptoms of this complaint we have enumerated determination of blood to the head, and inflammation of the brain. These symptoms have been so frequently observed in connection with profuse hæmorrhages, that the question of *bloodletting*, as a Homœopathic resort for cerebral inflammation consequent on menorrhagia, has been raised.

When menorrhagia originates from organic derangements of the womb, such as indurations, cancers, fibroid tumors, and ulcers, symptoms peculiar to these morbid productions will present themselves, in addition to the ordinary signs.

Cases of this kind will require careful attention, both in a diagnostic and a therapeutic point of view. As for instance, were the disease to depend on a scrofulous diathesis, or syphilitic taint, our remedies must be directed as well to their original and general causes as to those which are more immediate and local. By pursuing this course we may strike an enemy in ambush while subduing those already apparent to the senses.

The causes of menorrhagia are both *remote* and *proximate*. We include under the former head, neglect of proper physical and moral education, excesses in eating and drinking, and low diet, hereditary taints, pressure of the abdominal viscera downwards upon the womb by mechanical contrivances, etc. Under the latter head we include irritation and congestion or inflammation of the secretory vessels of the uterus; to disturbances and injuries that may occur during pregnancy, and from *accouchment*, tumors of different kinds, etc.

The *prognosis* is favorable when no organic affection exists; nevertheless, the uterine hæmorrhages which occur from miscarriage, or confinement, or those which take place during pregnancy, must receive critical attention, and proper measures of relief must be brought to bear, or the victims may bleed to death. But no woman need bleed to death under any of these circumstances, if there is proper knowledge and decision on the part of the attending physician.

The circumstances which oblige us to make an unfavorable prognosis are chronic induration and softening of the uterus, cancerous and other organic derangements, known to be incurable. But even in these apparently hopeless cases we should never despair, for the resources of Homœopathy often surpass our most sanguine expectations.

TREATMENT consists in removing as far as possible all disturbing causes, and then the critical affiliation of suitable remedies to aid the recuperative efforts of nature. From the following a selection can be made that will probably obviate all functional derangements: Belladonna, Ipecac, Sabina, Crocus, China, Sepia, Erigeron, Causticum, Pulsatilla, Macrotin, Platina, and other remedies. Our best remedy in superabundant menstruation proceeding from irritation and active congestion, or determination of blood to the head, is *Belladonna*, 3x, dil., 10 drops in half a glass of water, and teaspoonful doses repeated every hour. The patient should try to be quiet and free from anxiety as much as possible.

CASE I. A lady 30 years of age, of full habit, suffered from profuse discharge of bright red blood, which felt hot as it escaped from the vulva, was cured by a few doses of Belladonna, prepared and given as above directed. She had experienced these hæmorrhages at every menstrual period, and sometimes between the periods for several months.

CASE II. Mrs. S., after confinement, flowed profusely and continuously until her case became alarming to her father, who was a physician of the regular school. He resorted to such measures as appeared to him reasonable, without success; he called in counsel one of the same school, who suggested various remedies, and still the flow was not lessened. The use of the tampon and astringents had only a temporary effect. She was suffering from nausea that proceeded from the stomach, without a moment's relief, even after vomiting. The flow of blood increased with every effort to vomit; she began to gasp for breath and faint, and her medical attendants thought her case hopeless. The nurse begged of the father for permission to call in a Homœopathic physician as a dernier resort, which was granted. The Homœopath came at once and soon decided to give *Ipecacuanha*, in the form of saturated globules, and before the third hourly dose the hæmorrhage was arrested. The effect was witnessed by the father and his counsel, who at once asked why the saturated globules of Ipecac were followed by such happy results; and the reply was, "because the remedy was Homœopatic to the case." The lady was soon relieved of the nausea, and the sense of pressure over the uterus, and she began to recuperate gradually and felt that she had made a happy escape.

CASE III. A young married lady miscarried at three months. She had for a time felt uncomfortable sensations extending between the sacrum and pubis; when she miscarried, the embryo and placenta seemed to pass from her spontaneously; she continued to flow profusely, with clots of bright red blood, aggravated by the slightest movement. *Sabina*, 3x, dil. was given, two drops at a time in a spoonful of water, and repeated every hour; and though she had been flowing for forty-two hours, and was much enfeebled by the loss of blood, the remedy acted promptly in procuring relief and she soon recovered.

CASE IV. We had a lady patient, recently married, who

at her menstrual period, flowed for a week dark, stringy blood, resembling worms intermingling in a knot. We found it difficult to arrest the flow at once, after an unsuccessful trial with several remedies. She was cured with two-drop doses of *Crocus sat.*, administered in dessert spoonfuls of water, repeated hourly, for one day.

CASE V. Was a middle aged lady suffering from profuse hæmorrhage, from no definable cause, except debility and atony of the womb. She had seasons of discharging clots of dark blood, with uterine spasms, and colic. Her employment was dress-making, and she was interrupted by painful distention of the abdomen, coldness and blueness of the skin, and great weakness from the loss of blood. This trouble was a monthly occurrence. She was cured and permanently fortified against a return of the symptoms by the employment of *China*, 3x, dil., two-drop doses in a spoonful of water, repeated every two hours, without interfering with sleep, for ten days.

CASE VI. Was the wife of an attorney, aged 35, of nervous temperament, who had been brought to the verge of the grave by persistent uterine hæmorrhage, attended by sick headache and a painful sense of emptiness at the pit of the stomach, and yellow maculæ on the face and nose. She suffered from inveterate constipation and escape of flatus from the bowels. She was permanently cured by taking *Sepia suc.*, 3x, trit., a two-grain power morning, noon and night, for six days.

CASE VII. A woman who had long resided in the south was afflicted with painless flooding. She was cachectic, and suffered from general coldness at times, and at other seasons she complained of being too warm, and did not wish to be covered. She had a feverish pulse, and suffered from a passive hæmorrhage of dark colored blood, seldom in clots, but perpetually annoying. *Secale*, 1x, trit., was given for three days without effect. The 3x, trit., was then given in two-grain doses every three hours for a week, with very slight improvement. Being satisfied that Secale was the remedy, we gave 30x, trit., for another week, and she rejoiced in finding herself much better. We continued the same remedy in a still higher attenuation, 60x, trit., under which she recovered as fully as her feeble constitution would permit.

We have employed *Erigeron*, 3x. dil., in profuse and alarming hæmorrhages; and also Causticum, Pulsatilla, Macrotin, and Platina, all in 3x to 6x attenuation, with satisfactory results. As soon as menorrhagia or metrorrhagia patients can take food, feed them lightly at first, and gradually more generously, until the normal strength is regained.

Metrorrhagia.

We have treated of menorrhagia as a profuse menstrual flow that may occur any time after puberty, and varies in the amount of flow from that which is normal in quantity to a profuseness somewhat alarming and threatening in its character. Metrorrhagia also signifies a uterine hæmorrhage, but that which takes place at or anteriorly near the change of life. To distinguish menorrhagia and metrorrhagia is quite difficult unless we affirm one to be hæmorrhage, which takes place at every menstrual period, in the commencement after puberty; and the other takes place at or near the menopausial period, and is attended with more or less danger.

TREATMENT.—Hæmorrhages at the critical age, *Pulsatilla*, 3x, dil., 10 drops in a gill of water, and teaspoonful doses. When there is a cessation of the menstrual discharge for a time, and then returns with great force, the blood black and mixed with coagulated lumps, and when the metrorrhagia is most profuse with women given to reveries, or at the critical period, patient is always better in the open air, Belladonna, 3x, dil., prepared the same as Pulsatilla, teaspoonful doses every hour until relieved. When the face is flushed, and the head aches with a pulsating tremor all over the body, and when there is a painful pressure over the sexual organs, as if all would escape from the vulva. Lachesis, 6x, dil., given in the same way when there is pain in the right ovarian region, extending towards the womb, increasing in severity till relieved by a discharge of blood. *Platina*, 3x, trit., two-grain powder night and morning, for metrorrhagia, with blood dark and thick, like tar, and pain in the back, penetrating into both groins, with excessive sensitiveness of the genital organs.

Secale, 3x, trit., for painless flooding of the feeble, two-grain powder night and morning. *Laurocerasus*, 3x, dil., Trillium, 3x, dil., Calc., 3x, trit., may be consulted.

Metrorrhagia is identical with menorrhagia.

Leucorrhœa.

This disease consists in a discharge from the womb and vagina, of a muco-purulent character, sometimes white, yellow, or greenish; either thin and watery or the consistence of starch pre-

49

pared for use, or gelatine. The disease arises from a benignant
morbid action, and, unlike gonorrhœa, it is non-contagious. Those
authorities which maintain the identity of leucorrhœa and gonorrhœa, are evidently in an error. The former originates from an
unhealthy or impaired condition of the mucus membrane. The
latter from a small quantity of gonorrhœal matter coming in
contact with the most sound and healthy membrane. An ordinary inflammation analagous to that of catarrh or chronic bronchitis, may result from the former. The latter results from the
application of a specific infection, the result of contact with a purulent secretion.

When the *cervix uteri* is inflamed, a white discharge called
fluor albus generally results. If the inflammation be severe the
discharge may be tinged with blood.

A purulent leucorrhœa is apt to follow a vaginal or urethral
inflammation, and if acute, the discharge is yellowish or greenish
and often tinged with blood. The chronic form of this malady
presents a thinner, more glairy and muco-purulent secretion. A
uterine cancer causes an ichorous, bloody and fetid discharge.

In light cases of leucorrhœa the discharge is usually thin,
glairy, transparent, and starchy. A patient of delicate or cachectic habit, with confirmed leucorrhœa, the fluid may be muco-purulent, serous, sanious, and of a white, greenish, or yellow color.
The discharge is generally worse about the period of the catamenia,
probably owing to the determination of blood to the parts during
their natural appearance.

CAUSES.—Taking cold from sitting on a damp seat or cold
ground, or exposure of the neck and shoulders, over excitement
of the sexual organs, and too frequent submission to sexual intercourse, tight lacing, hæmorrhoids, miscarriages and abortions,
prolapsus uteri, purgatives, etc., etc.

SYMPTOMS attending the disease, heat and soreness of the
parts, general debility, face pale or sallow, eyes surrounded by dark
or leaden colored circles, irritable stomach and bowels, a weary
dragging sensation in the left side, dull pains in back and loins,
and abdomen, cold extremities, nausea, palpitation and dyspnœa
after exercising. Mental and physical energy, depression. Sexual
propensity sometimes exalted, at other times diminished. The
protracted and severe forms of the trouble generally give rise to
these symptoms. But a mild form of the difficulty may last for

years, with little inconvenience. The rich, indolent, luxurious and dissipated are much more liable to suffer from the disease than those in more active life. The disease is more common in cities, than in the country. This very common and prevalent weakness, accounts for unfruitfulness of many married women, and for the frequent miscarriages which occur in large towns. Leucorrhœa occurs at all periods of life, but more common after puberty and previous to the change of life, when so many influences induce a free determination of blood to the utero-genitals.

Leucorrhœa, often accompanies *prolapsus uteri*, not however as a sequence, but rather as a cause; for the former has often existed for years as a drain upon, before the signs of prolapsus manifest themselves, and owing to this debilitating flux, impairing the tone of the uterus, its muscles and ligaments lose strength and contractility.

There appears to be no period of life, exempt from this trouble; it is the most common after puberty, and just previous to the change of life.

When we take into consideration the great variety of causes productive of leucorrhœa in cities, it is not strange that so great a degeneracy in the offspring of enfeebled women should be apparent in the puny and sickly growth which follow.

It is incumbent on physicians to suggest the removal of all avoidable causes of this weakness, whether they relate to corsets and lacing, or want of exercise in the open air, or too close confinement in illy ventilated appartments, too frequent attendance on balls, concerts, or theatricals, irregular hours of pleasure, including late hours at night.

HYGIENIC TREATMENT.—Abundant exercise in the open air, and an avoidance of all sexual excess, and the pleasures of the table, a withdrawal of the thoughts and affections from exciting spectacles, from crowded halls and parties; from lascivious imaginary romances and intrigues, and a careful attention to personal cleanliness of the utero-genital organs. Frequent daily ablutions are a *sine qua non*, in order to ensure the removal from the mucus membrane a morbid secretion which, if left to accumulate breeds evil to the delicate sensitive structures. It is liable to undergo partial decomposition and become fetid and highly pernicious in its effects. On this account the thorough use of tepid, or cold water should be locally employed as circumstances may require.

TREATMENT.—There are many remedies which may be usefully employed in this complaint, but we need enumerate those only known to act therapeutically from the most extensive observation.

Calc. carb. is positively an excellent remedy in chronic leucorrhœa, affecting debilitated and scrofulous females, when the menses are too frequent and too profuse; when the leucorrhœa consists of a milky discharge, transparent, mucilaginous, starchy, unirritating, and accompanied by itching of the parts, lassitude, depression of spirits, etc., etc. The remedy is recommended in the 3x, trit., 6x, trit. and 30x, trit. First give a grain dose night and morning of the 3x, trit., for a week; then the same of 6x, trit., for the second week, and then the same of 30x, trit., for the third week, and wait under the regulation of hygienic treatment for the result, which without doubt will be favorable.

In all persons of a scrofulous or psoric diathesis, anti-psoric remedies, such as *Sulphur, Stannum* and *Iodium*, will be required and must be used as directed for Calc. carb., in the 3x, trit., 6x, trit., and 30x, trit. The discharge in these cases is thin or yellowish, and irritating to the parts with which it comes in contact. There is much debility and many signs of tuberculosis, hectic fever and emaciation.

Sepia, in 3x, trit., 6x, trit., and 30x, trit., given as directed for Calcarea, will be suitable for females naturally delicate and sensitive, with clear, transparent complexions. The discharge is mucus, white, yellowish, or watery, mild or acrid in its nature, most abundant just previous and just after the menses, and attended by falling of the womb, itching and stitching pains in the genital organs.

Pulsatilla, 3x, 6x, and 30x, dil., is a desirable remedy for leucorrhœa attendant on pregnancy, and also when it becomes profuse about the period of the monthly sickness. The discharge is thick, white, burning, and tenacious. Drop doses may be given three or four times a day.

Alumina has proved successful in several varieties of whites, particularly indicated when the discharge is acrid and profuse during the day, when walking and immediately antecedent to the menstrual periods, attended with itching and burning of the genital organs and rectum, 3x, trit., 6x, trit., and 30x, trit., to be used in the same manner as directed for Calc. carb.

Lycopodium, Phosphorus and Cocculus 3x, 6x, 30x, trit., in grain doses, day by day persistently, when the "Whites" are brought on by self abuse, and occuring at intervals with milky, serous, ichorous or reddish discharge. The remedies are suitable for lymphatic temperaments and those highly sensitive to cold, and subject to catarrhal affections, and of a morbidly excitable nervous system.

Sabina is suitable in the 3x, dil., for whites dependent on weakness of the womb and vagina, when arising from suppression of the menses, miscarriage, or severe, protracted labors. Polypi and prolapsion of the womb, ten drops in ten teaspoonfuls of water, a teaspoonful every two hours. *Secale cornutum* 3x, trit., in daily doses of two grains, is also suitable.

China 3x, dil., in drop doses every hour, when the whites originate from excessive losses of blood, or other animal fluids, extreme weakness from febrile diseases and malaria.

Arnica 3x, dil., is a suitable remedy for the traumatism described by *Prof. Ludlam* arising from difficult labor and mechanical injuries during accouchments, and especially for the subsequent leucorrhœa. In plethoric females of full, bounding pulse, suffering from whites, Aconite 3x, dil., may be given three or four times a day with a probable certainty of cure, fifteen drops in half a tumbler of water may be administered in spoonful doses every four hours.

Many other remedies may be consulted and affiliated according to the guiding symptoms.

CHAPTER LV

CLINICAL NOTES AND OBSERVATIONS.

Arsenicum in Brights Disease.

A gentleman aged 40, a confirmed dyspeptic, found himself rapidly declining and passing large quantities of albumen daily, was cured by the persistent use of Ars., 30x and 200x, dil.

Apis Mellifica in Intermittent Fever.

Several cases of intermittent fever of a stubborn character have been broken up by this remedy, after other remedies had failed. The late *Dr. Hering*, of Philadelphia, regarded this remedy of great value in many forms of ague.

Baryta Carb. in Whooping Cough.

When whooping cough assails aged people this remedy has been found of great use, especially when they complain of roughness of the throat and a tickling sensation in the epigastrium.

Eucalyptus in Hay Fever.

Mrs. C——, aged 50, had suffered for years with this annoyance, which commenced annually about the 15th of August, and lasting about six weeks, obliging her to seek a more dense atmosphere for relief, has latterly experienced perfect relief, from Eucalyptus, administered by olfaction, 2x, dil.

Eucalyptus in Erysipelas.

A case of gangrenous erysipelas of the leg was cured with drop doses of the tincture taken internally three times a day, and a compress wet with a solution of the same remedy, in the proportion of 60 drops to half a glass of water, applied to the surface, after being washed and cleaned as far as possible. Eucalyptus also cured a case of hæmaturia. It was given in five-drop doses on a lump of sugar once in three hours.

Gelsemium in Hay Fever.

A gentleman aged 44 years, cured himself of an annual attack of hay fever by taking 3 or 4 drops of the tincture in a spoonful of water, morning, noon and night before meals, and before retiring. Duration of the attack, eight days.

Naphthalin in Hay Fever.

We have had some delightful experience in the use of this remedy in hay asthma the present season; several cases were relieved or cured in the course of one week, with the 2x trit.

Alcohol in Chronic Ottorrhœa.

Pure, undiluted alcohol has cured a number of cases of chronic otitis. The application of undiluted alcohol does not produce intense pain; for a few moments there is a smarting, slightly burning feeling, which gives rise to a sensation described by patients as that of an "agreeable warmth." This latter lasts for considerable time. (*Dr. A. W. Calhoun.*)

Aconite in Arachnitis.

A child of C. S. D., Esq., aged two and a half years, was taken ill after exposure to cold and damp surroundings. The face was flushed, the eyes were fiery, the head was intensely hot, the anterior fontanel exhibited a convexity and heat in an aggravated form, and truly alarming, the pulse was greatly accelerated, the thirst for cold water was immeasurably great, vomiting was incessant, and the child's shrill screeches were sufficient to alarm a neighborhood. From the heat of the cerebrum, and inflammatory convexity from the anterior fontanel, we recognized a case of acute *arachnitis.* Arsenicum, 3x, dil., 20 drops in a tumbler of water, was first prescribed. We found no change six hours after, and the case looked dubious. Instead of gratifying the thirst by supplying all the cold water the child could wish, we prepared a tumbler of water with 20 drops of the 3x, dil., of Aconite, and ordered the nurse to swab his mouth with it continuously, hoping to allay thirst. This was followed for several days, and then the heat of the head disappeared, the vomiting ceased, and the child's thirst was better. It lay quiet for a few days in a comatose sleep; the swollen fontanel was better. The child recovered.

Zizia Aurea in Epileptiform Diseases.

We have observed the salutary effect of the 3x, dil., of this remedy in the convulsions of children, and must confess that we have great confidence in its therapeutic power. *Epilepsy* in its incipiency is susceptible of being cured by this remedy.

The following notes and observations are taken from those furnished by the author to the last four vols. of the U. S. M. & S. Journal and recent observations.

Gambogia in Dysentery.

This remedy, in the 3d trituration, has been found of great use in dysentery attended with burning tenesmus and prolapsion of the anus; and also when the stools are watery and attended with colic, or green mixed with mucus, accompanied with tenesmus. Many cases of dysentery characterized by chill and pain in the back, bitter taste in the mouth, burning of the tongue, and soreness all over, that will not yield to Mercurius cor., are readily cured by this remedy.

Helleborus Niger in Dropsies.

This remedy, in the 6th attenuation, has cured hydrothorax supervening upon measles, in a child six years old. It cured a case of hydrocele in a youth who had just recovered from scarlatina. In anasarca after scarlatina, it has proved eminently successful. It cured a child 16 months old of acute hydrocephalus after his case has been abandoned as hopeless by his previous medical attendant. This remedy should always be preceded by a dose of the 3d trituration of Calc. carb., in scrofulous subjects.

Hypericum Perforatum for Injury and Laceration of the Nerves.

A young woman, aged twenty, fell and injured her spine, in the region of the lower dorsal vertebræ. She lost the use of the lower extremities immediately after, and suffered greatly from heaviness in the head, derangement of the stomach, torpidity of the bowels, and tympanitic distention thereof. Gave Arnica, the 3d decimal attenuation, and had her back bathed with a strong dilution of the tincture. But it afforded no relief. The surface of the lower extremities was cold as ice; there was spasmodic twitching of the muscles of the face and upper extremities. The 3d decimal attenuation of Hypericum was given, and repeated at intervals of two hours. Her back in the meantime was bathed in the tincture, and a compress wet with the same was applied to the injured region of the spine. In twenty-four hours the twitching ceased; the pulse, which had been depressed, became more active, and the lower extremities began to assume a natural warmth. The remedy and application to the surface were continued for several days; the heavy, dull pressure of the head disappeared; the digestive function became established, and she was able to move the lower extremities, with considerable effort of the will. The treatment was continued for a week or more. There was, however, great soreness of the surface, and a constant inclination to spasms, but less and less until they disappeared. When she had recovered sufficiently to express her feelings, she remarked that the Hypericum made her feel better every time she took it, or had a fresh compress applied to the spine, and under the use of it she fully recovered, and no unpleasant sequel was entailed.

This remedy appears to be particularly adapted to injury of the nerves and nervous centers, resulting in trismus or tetanus.

Ignatia Amara in Quotidian Fever.

In a case of intermittent fever, attended with great pain and thirst during the chill and no thirst during the fever and heat which followed, Ignatia, the 3d decimal was prescribed. The succeeding paroxysm was lighter; the next was lighter still, and no others occurred. This patient had suffered from daily paroxysms for more than a week.

Ignatia in Chorea.

A little girl of 11 years, of delicate constitution, and exceedingly sensitive, was unable by volition to control the movement of the upper and lower extremities and muscles of the face. She had thus suffered without any acute pains, for more than a year. Gave her a dose of Calc. carb., 3d trituration, and followed it six hours after with the third dilution of Ignatia. She soon began to improve, and at the end of the first month's treatment she had quite recovered.

Ignatia in Affections of the Heart.

Was called to see a distinguished lady, who for six or eight years had been stricken with grief. I found her in bed suffering from great pain and anguish in the region of the heart. In making a critical examination with the stethoscope, found no evidence of organic heart disease. Ten drops of the 2d dilution of Ignatia was dropped in half a goblet of water, and a dessert-spoonful was directed to be given every four hours. The first dose gave much relief, and in less than a week she felt quite well. This was the lady's first resort to Homœopathic treatment.

Iodine in Goitre.

Miss H., of slender form and lymphatic temperament, presented her case for consideration. The difficulty was bronchocele, or goitre. She had been treated by external applications of the officinal tincture of Iodine, and strong Iodine ointment, and without relief. Having considered the subject thoroughly, the conclusion was reached that Iodine in some form was the remedy. A half ounce of globules was saturated with the 2d decimal dilution, and she was directed to take the remedy persistently, three globules morning and evening, and take no other remedy until she had exhausted these. She obeyed the directions to the letter. For three months but little change was noticed. But afterwards the swelling began to diminish gradually, and had wholly disappeared at the end of the year.

Iodine in Croup.

A case of croup, which came on with hoarseness and dryness of the throat, and afterwards with tenacious mucus in the larynx and trachea, was relieved promptly by the administration of the 6th attenuation of Iodine. The medicine was prepared by putting ten drops of the dilution in water, and then a teaspoonful was directed every thirty minutes until relieved, or there was necessity for a change of remedy.

Iodine in Indurated Swelling of the Glands.

I have given Iodine, the 3d decimal, with good effect in swelling and induration of the inguinal glands, and also in swelling and induration of the cervical and salivary glands, and also for the swelling of the glands in general. One or two doses a day have proved sufficient.

Iris Versicolor in Sick Headache.

Have found this remedy beneficial in several cases of semi-lateral headache, attended with gastric derangement and vomiting of watery mucus, and where the paroxysm came on at irregular periods, with aching through the temples and the eyes, more marked in the right side. The 2d or 3d attenuation has usually been employed.

Iris Versicolor in Choleroid Affections.

When the cholera was raging in Chicago in 1866, this remedy proved very efficacious in the colliquative diarrhœas, which often proved the incipient stage of cholera. When looseness of the bowels first showed itself, with more or less pain in the bowels, and near the region of the liver, I gave the remedy in the tincture and 1st attenuation, and repeated frequently.

Kali Bichromicum in Diphtheritic Croup.

I have found the 3d attenuation of this remedy of the greatest value in diphtheritic croup when administered early after the manifestation of the difficulty. I have given it when the following symptoms were present: Hoarse, croupy cough; sore throat; the appearance of livid patches, indicative of false membrane at the posterior of the fauces, great prostration and laborious breathing. The mode of administration is to drop ten drops of the dilution into a goblet, fill it half full of water, and then mix it well. The liquid should be turned back and forth from one glass to another many times. A teaspoonful may then be given every thirty minutes.

Kali Bichromicum in Membranous Croup.

Have found this remedy of the greatest use in arresting the progress of membranous croup when the attack came on in the morning with hoarseness and accumulation of mucus in the larynx, tending to pseudo-membranous formation. After a few doses of Aconite, the 3d decimal, to allay the arterial excitement, Kali bichromicum the 3d decimal, in water, administered at short intervals, has produced a speedy cure. This remedy has also had the happiest effect in croupy pneumonia, prepared and administered as above.

Kali Carbonicum in Asthma.

This remedy in the 6th decimal attenuation cured a case of asthma in a gentleman 59 years old. He was inclined to rheumatism and cough, with expectorations of tenacious, ropy mucus. Until he was relieved by this remedy, he had been unable to lie down for many weeks, but subsequently his breathing improved so greatly that he could lie down and take regular rest.

Kali Hydriodicum in Rheumatism.

A gentleman, aged 46 years, had a severe attack of acute rheumatism, which was characterized by painful swelling of the joints, involving both the upper and lower extremities. After the employment of Aconite, Bryonia, Nux vomica, and Rhus tox., the acute stage passed off, leaving great soreness, weakness and stiffness of the joints, together with a severe asthmatic cough at night. Various remedies were employed to remove the suffering, with no perceptible advantage. At the recommendation of one who had suffered from a similar difficulty for six months, and had been cured by a solution of one drachm of pure Kali hydriodicum in a quart of water, taken in tablespoonful doses three times a day, he took the same and was cured in a few days.

Lachesis in Chronic Sore Throat.

Mrs. D., aged 33 years, had been suffering with a sore throat for two years. She had a painful dryness of the fauces and a sensation of something being lodged in the larynx. She had the advice of several eminent physicians, and took their prescriptions without obtaining relief. She stated her case to me and was radically cured by a single prescription of Lachesis 30th, *Hering's* preparation. She knew of another lady affected in some respects as she had been, and procured the same preparation for her, and it had a like effect.

Lachesis in Quinsy.

A well known lady of P., had been subject to attacks of quinsy, which had occurred many times during an elapse of five years after her first and only confinement. During each attack she suffered all the while with great soreness and sensitiveness of the pharynx and tonsils, and a sensation as if she had a plug in her throat. So sensitive was the exterior of the throat, that she was unable to endure the slightest touch or pressure upon the surface. Lachesis the 30th was prescribed, to be taken in globules upon the tongue every two hours. The effect of the first day's treatment was to relieve the great sensitiveness externally and internally. The second day she was unable to swallow fluids, and yet the tumor in the throat was less painful. The third day she was able to swallow food in the form of a custard. The fourth day she felt the tumor to be less, and each succeeding day it gradually diminished, until the whole disappeared, it having terminated by resolution, and never after had she an attack of the disease.

Lachesis in Bronchitis and Pneumonia.

Mrs. N., 63 years of age, of delicate constitution and spare habit, has been afflicted more or less for several years with cough and expectoration of mucus, that would require more than one effort of coughing to dislodge, after which she experienced a smarting sensation in the throat and stitches in the left side. She had taken a variety of remedies, some of which had given temporary relief; but on every exposure to cold, or to the intensely hot weather of the summer, the disease would return. Finally Lachesis the 30th was prescribed, and apparently with the greatest advantage. She took two doses a day for several weeks and fully recovered, and has remained well, with the exception of one or two attacks of ordinary cold, during the last two and a half years.

Lachesis in Heart Disease.

Have treated several cases of alleged heart disease with Lachesis 30th where there was deep sighing every few minutes, and occasionally fits of suffocation and fainting, weak pulse, often intermittent, and stitches in the left side of the chest.

Laurocerasus in Phthisis Pulmonalis.

Mrs. S., a victim of phthisis, an irregular pulse, hectic fever, characterized by alternations of chilliness and heat, and night sweats. She was much emaciated, and, at times, very hoarse, with great accumulation of mucus in the throat. Her breathing was difficult, and she had frequent paroxysms of coughing and raising a thick, bloody mucus. Laurocerasus the 6th attenuation in water (ten drops in four tablespoonfuls,) was given in teaspoonful doses every three hours. She was relieved of her fever and night sweats; her cough was much better; her appetite became restored, and she became quite comfortable, and remained so for some time, after which she relapsed and died.

Lobelia Inflata in Asthma.

The third decimal attenuation of Lobelia cured a case of asthma of long standing in a lady, aged 37. She complained of waterbrash and cardialgia. Sensation as if something was lodged in the throat, difficult and asthmatic respiration. She had frequent attacks of vomiting, which invariably were succeeded by a paroxysm of asthma. The daily administration of this remedy for a few weeks affected a radical cure.

Lycopodium in Pneumonia.

A young boy, nine years of age, complained of chilliness, followed by pain in the head and chest, which soon developed into a latent typhoid pneumonia. He suffered from extreme prostration, a feeble and rapid pulse, together with a troublesome cough and expectoration of rusty sputa. His bowels were very torpid; his countenance seemed sunken and pinched, and his appetite entirely gone. He was quiet, motionless and comatose for several days. A dose of the 30th of Lycopodium in globules was given him three or four times a day. This apparently wrought a favorable change. His bowels moved normally; the expectoration became favorable; the cough less violent; a natural secretion manifested itself upon the margin of the tongue; the coma disappeared and he convalesced rapidly. This remedy has generally proved salutary in incipient phthisis when symptoms of pneumonia or deep seated bronchial inflammation were present.

Mercurius Vivus for Cough.

I have found no remedy that acts so promptly and satisfactorily in removing a hoarse cough, with much tickling in the larynx. It is also an excellent remedy in a dry, racking cough, especially if it occurs at night, with a distressing distension of the chest. Have found it useful in cough with putrid, sweetish or saltish expectoration. The potency the most used is the 3d trituration.

Mercurius Corrosivus for Sore Mouth.

Mrs. M., a lady of 35, and mother of four children, became afflicted with nursing sore mouth, when her infant was only two months old. The sores upon her tongue were inclined to inflame very much, and to dip deep below the surface. She had quite a number of these deep fissures or ulcers. Her tongue and mouth were so sore and painful that the effort to swallow fluids even was very much dreaded. After trying various remedies without much relief, gave Mercurius corrosivus in the 3d decimal trituration, after which she experienced relief.

Mercurius Corrosivus in Dysentery.

In those dysenteries preceded by chilliness with colic, cold sweat and distension of the abdomen, and thence by bilious diarrhœa, running into discharges of bloody mucus, attended with burning colic, straining and tenesmus, Mercurius corrosivus in the 3d decimal trituration has generally proved effectual.

Mercurius Iodatus for Nasal Catarrh.

A case of nasal catarrh of long standing, characterized by dull headache on waking in the morning, and great accumulation of mucus in the posterior nares, was cured by daily doses of the 3d trituration of this remedy taken persistently for two weeks.

Mercurius Dulcis in Cholera Infantum.

This remedy, in the 3d decimal trituration, has often produced the most favorable change in those cases of cholera infantum where there was great thirst and frequent discharges of white watery stools, with straining, and particularly when there was some nausea and disinclination to take nourishment.

Moschus in Nervous Prostration.

In the case of a lady, aged 33, of feeble pulse and coldness of the extremities, and given to melancholy, Moschus the 6th attenuation, produced great relief, and was followed by a great flow of spirits and warmth of the surface of the body.

Moschus in Hysteria.

Have found this remedy effectual in removing hysterical headache, fainting spasms and sense of constriction of the chest, and chilliness over the entire surface of the body, and particularly where there was inclination to involuntary stools, and a copious flow of colorless urine, and great restlessness of the lower extremities. Have generally employed the 3d decimal attenuation, ten drops in half a tumbler of water, and have given a teaspoonful every two hours.

Natrum Muriaticum in Herpes.

In a case of herpes in the bend of the joints of a lady 40 years of age. She had an eruption first in the bend of the elbow, which became so inflamed, that the skin became rough and painful, and the itching and smarting extremely annoying. Gave Natrum muriaticum, 30th centesimal attenuation, and the eruption began gradually to diminish, after which a slight eruption of the kind manifested itself upon the face, the knee joints became painful, and the skin in the bend of the joint became red and inflamed. Continued the use of the remedy until the whole disappeared.

Sulphate of Nickel in Headache.

A lady was subject to periodical attacks of headache, which lasted three or four days every two weeks. The pain seemed to be the most acute at the root of the nose, extending to the vertex and through the temples. She had some nausea, but no vomiting. She was unable to raise her head from the pillow when the attack was upon her. The distress was so great during the paroxysms that she lay and groaned in anguish. After administering Cuprum, Ignatia, Sepia, Calcarea, Sulphur, and other remedies without effect, gave a two-grain dose of the 3d trituration of the Sulphate of Nickel, and the succeeding paroxysm was lighter. Repeated the remedy every day during the period. The next attack was comparatively light, and after this there was no return for four months—a respite which she had not enjoyed for ten years.

Nux Juglans in Noli-me-tangere.

A young man had been afflicted with this dyscrasia for more than two years. His nose and mouth were the seat of sores which often became aggravated and painful. He was cured by drinking the cold infusion of the leaves of the tree, gathered in June, a wine-glass full three times a day.

Nux Juglans in Scrofulous Consumption.

Was called upon to prescribe for a woman who had been confined to her bed for months, with what her medical attendant pronounced an incurable consumption. She was of a scrofulous constitution and extremely emaciated. Having but little hope of benefiting her, and yet to gratify her with a prescription, she was directed to pluck some leaves from an English walnut tree, and pour cold water upon them, and after twelve hours to commence taking a wine-glass full three times a day. Six months after this prescription the lady was met in the street quite recovered. She said she drank the infusion as directed and found decided relief. Her appetite returned. Nutrition became established. She regained her normal amount of flesh and strength, and considered herself quite well.

[NOTE.—This cold infusion has been used with great advantage in scrofula and scrofulous swelling of the glands, and may be considered a useful remedy in these complaints.]

50

Nux Moschata for Headache.

A middle-aged lady had suffered much from headache and drowsiness for many months, with great debility and slight pains in the præcordial region. She suffered also more or less from indigestion, and complained of a saltish taste in the mouth. Three or four grain doses of the 3d decimal trituration of Nux moschata cured her.

Nux Vomica in Sleeplessness.

In several cases of sleeplessness in hypochondriacal persons known to have been irritable and in haste, and somewhat troubled with vertigo, and easily fatigued with mental exercise, and wakeful at night, Nux vomica in a grain dose of the 3d trituration has sufficed to quiet the nerves and to produce sleep. Nux vomica given in the same form has remedied the sleeplessness of inebriates, and is the best remedy known for procuring sleep in victims to mania-a-potu.

Oleum Jecoris in Rheumatism.

The gentleman had been suffering from chronic rheumatism for more than a year, and frequent cramps in his feet. He was greatly emaciated; had dryness of the mouth; was hoarse and suffered more or less from cough. Cod liver oil was directed in teaspoonful doses three times a day, from the use of which he was greatly benefited, and marvellously relieved from the disease.

Opium in Coma.

This symptom frequently follows pain in the head and marks the development of typhoid. When the coma is light, Belladonna is a useful remedy. When it amounts to sopor, and great difficulty has been apparent in arousing the patient, a single dose of one drop of the 3d dilution in a spoonful of water has been found efficient.

Petroleum in Hypochondria.

Mrs. M., of bilious temperament, greatly depressed in spirits and given up to fearful forebodings—fancying herself friendless—

and hopelessly demented, was cured by a few doses of this remedy in the 6th attenuation.

Sulphate of Zinc in Dysentery.

A case of chronic dysentery, which had baffled treatment for more than a year, and which presented the appearance of being an organic trouble, was cured by a single prescription of Sulphate of Zinc, 3d trituration. The symptoms most complained of by this patient were thin, pale, bloody stools, several times a day, with painful tenesmus, great desire for food, which apparently failed of supplying nutrition to the system. The patient was extremely emaciated at the time Sulphate of Zinc was prescribed, since which the appetite has become normal, the stomach free from irritability. In a word, all the functions are carried on harmoniously; the recuperation of strength and regaining of the flesh are palpably manifest.

Sulphur in Chronic Dysentery.

A case of chronic dysentery, characterized by difficult respiration, violent tenesmus at night, and blood-streaked stools, and occasionally some pus mixed with the mucus and blood in them. The patient was a lady, whose figure was tall and slender, whose hair and eyes were black, and she had been suffering for seven months. A few doses of Sulphur, the 6th attenuation, cured her. Her diet, while under treatment, was mutton broth and boiled milk, with one-fourth of an ounce of Russia Isinglass to a quart.

Plumbum in Dysentery.

A case of dysentery, presenting the following symptoms, was cured by Plumbum, 6th attenuation: Constant tenesmus through the day, with continual but ineffectual efforts to evacuate the bowels, cutting pains, almost unbearable, and retraction of the abdomen.

Hamamelis in Dysentery.

I have witnessed the rapid recovery of several cases of protracted dysentery, where the stools were composed mostly of dark-colored blood, and so frequent as almost to amount to a hæmorrhage; under the use of Hamamelis tincture, ten drops in half a tumbler of water, and a dessert-spoonful administered every hour until convalescence was evident. I have known some of these cases to relapse from the nurse allowing them chicken soup, which is always a pernicious diet in dysentery. Mutton broth or beef tea is preferable. Barley water or gruel is the best for drink.

Cantharis in Dysentery.

A dysentery presenting the following symptoms was cured by Cantharis, 6th attenuation: Cold hands and feet, with burning like fire in the arms, with an occasional discharge of matter that resembled the scrapings of intestines, sore throat and mouth, small pulse, and great thirst during the tenesmus and pain.

Colchicum and Iris in Dysentery.

When dysentery is accompanied by cramps in the calves of the legs and prolapsus ani, discharges of jelly-like mucus, great swelling of the lower abdomen, and frequent shuddering down the back, Colchicum has proved an efficient remedy. In a case of bilious dysentery, when the patient complained of feeling cold, and when the skin was blue, and also when he manifested great prostration and complained of griping in the umbilical region and much rumbling, Iris versicolor in the 3d attenuation, was given with good effect, and the patient soon recovered.

Merc. viv. in Dysentery.

In the case of a little girl, aged seven years, who complained of severe burning, tenesmus and excrutiating discharges, and griping in the lower abdomen, aggravated by walking, putrid taste in the mouth, nausea, and offensive perspiration, and great pain previous to stool, Merc. viv. gave prompt relief.

Merc. cor. in Tenesmus.

A gentleman, aged forty-four years, complained of severe pains in the rectum. He had cold hands and face, and could not move without increasing his suffering, and after every stool the severe and painful tenesmus continued; was cured by Merc. corrosivus, 3d trituration. The first dose gave partial relief; the second, given three hours after, was followed by relief from suffering, and in two days he was quite well.

China in Dysentery.

China, 3d attenuation, in dysenteries that occur in marshy districts with intermittent symptoms, has cured promptly in many cases, when Arsenicum, Mercurius, and other remedies, had failed to give relief. In one case of a young gentleman of sanguine temperament, who had discharges of a cadaverous odor, worse at night, and of chocolate color, China the 3d was the remedy required to remove the unpleasant symptoms, and after it was administered the patient rapidly recovered.

Iris Versicolor in Bilious Diarrhœa.

A married lady, aged 33, of sedentary habits, was affected with bilious diarrhœa and frequent discharges of dark bilious matter from the rectum. Resorted to various remedies, which totally failed of affording any relief. She applied to a physician of the older school, who treated her for several weeks, and all the while her diarrhœa gradually grew worse. She became very much prostrated and emaciated, and it was feared on the part of her friends that she had consumption of the bowels. When first called upon to treat her she complained of great thirst and nausea, severe griping in the abdomen, and general nervous restlessness. A fever of a low order began to show itself, and she had more or less pain in the right temporal region and over the right eye. Arsenicum, 6th, was given at intervals of two hours for a whole day and night, and no relief was experienced. Iris versicolor, 3d decimal, was then prescribed, and, to use her own words, the first dose reached the right place and gave temporary relief. The second was given two hours after, and still but little change for the better was apparent. The remedy was continued for twenty-four hours, and a perceptible change for the better was the result. The medicine was discontinued for several hours, and all the while she continued to improve; the medicine was repeated at intervals of six hours for two days, and she was evidently cured of the malady. She gained strength, her appetite returned, normal stools became established, and she gradually regained all that she had lost, and found herself quite well.

Phosphoric Acid in a case of Chronic Diarrhœa.

Mr. H. M., aged 56, suffered for a long time with dull pain in the head, with considerable gastric derangement, and four or five stools every day of a grayish, thin character, and at times almost involuntary. Phos. ac., the 3d decimal, was prescribed to be given at intervals of three hours. In twenty-four hours the head was relieved, the gastric irritability allayed, and the diarrhœa ceased; recuperation followed rapidly, and the patient fully recovered.

Phosphorus in Chronic Diarrhœa.

Was called to treat a case of chronic diarrhœa. A gentleman somewhat advanced in life, who complained of great tenderness, on pressure, in the region of the umbilicus, both above and below, and every morning he was subject to copious discharges of watery fæces, which poured from him profusely. He experienced a sense of great weakness in the abdomen and of general debility. After three or four evacuations of this kind his bowels remained quiet for the most part through the day, although at night there was considerable rumbling and uneasiness, interfering with rest. When this gentleman first became affected he was erect and robust and weighed 180 lbs. But he gradually lost strength and vivacity until he was unable to leave his room. His pulse was small and quick, the coating upon his tongue was a grayish white, and his appetite indifferent. His respiration was somewhat feeble, his skin dry and hard. He had been treated for more than six months, and had derived but little benefit. After studying his case faithfully, and consulting with an eminent German practitioner in Philadelphia, it was concluded to give him Phosphorus 30th, and repeat the dose every four hours. No other remedy was required, as from the moment he took the first dose he greatly improved until he quite regained his health.

Iris Versicolor in Chronic Diarrhœa.

Mrs. D., of rather slender form, pale face and clear skin, was subject daily to one or two evacuations from the bowels, which came on after much uneasiness and pain in the lower abdomen, and was followed by burning in the rectum and anus. At first she regarded the disease as of trivial character, and gave it little attention. But it became so persistent, and each day about the same, she became alarmed, and called in a physician of the older school, who gave her a brisk purgative of Calomel and Rhubarb, and although exceedingly prostrated after the operation of this dose, she fancied herself better. But she soon found that the difficulty remained the same, after the medicine had done operating. Through the persuasion of friends she called on me to prescribe in her case. After giving Arsenicum, Veratrum and Mercurius, I found but little improvement. I then prescribed Iris versicolor of the 3d decimal attenuation. A few doses cured her, and she remains well to the present hour.

Rheum in the treatment of Diarrhœa in Teething Children.

I have had many cases of persistent diarrhœa in teething children, which proved stubborn under the use of Chamomilla, Pulsatilla, Ipecac, etc., that have yielded kindly upon the administration of Rheum, 6th attenuation. The symptoms indicating the use of this remedy are, acid stools with colicky pains and slimy evacuations, great restlessness when sleeping, tossing about, frequently crying out with pain, frequent straining when awake to evacuate the bowels. Rheum in the 6th decimal attenuation has generally proved in nearly all such a well chosen remedy, and in the heat of the summer, when diarrhœas are common among teething children, this remedy is prominent in the group which the successful treatment of children requires.

Dulcamara in Diarrhœa.

From many years' observation I have found this remedy adapted to such patients as contract diarrhœa from lying on cold ground, or whenever it is the result of a chill. Diarrhœa from a cold determining towards the bowels is usually attended with prostration, and the stools are slimy, varying in color from green, yellow and white. In camp diarrhœa, during the late war of the rebellion, Dulcamara was found one of the most useful remedies. A distinguished officer at the battle of Pittsburg Landing informed me that a bottle of Dulcamara carried by his quartermaster did more essential service in camp than the surgeon upon his staff. When, according to a common phrase, "a cold settles on the bowels," whether in camp or out, this is a valuable remedy. Mrs. G——, a frail constitution physically, was accustomed to suffer from nightly evacuations for many years, always worse in cold weather. She had more or less colic, prostration and restlessness. She took Dulcamara 3d by the advice of her physician, persistently, in daily doses, until she found, to her great satisfaction, a change in the condition of her system. She was completely relieved and cured, and since then her constitution is able to resist the effects of cold in a much greater degree than ever before since her marriage, a period of twenty-five years.

Colocynth in Diarrhœa.

Mrs. J——, of nervous temperament, and subject to hysteria, was for a long time a victim to severe attacks of colic, attended by bilious or watery diarrhœa, retching, etc. She evidently was a dyspeptic, and suffered mostly with these attacks after eating. The only relief she had sought was from taking Morphine, or some preparation of Opium. Her mind was exercised to get relief from suffering, not to remove the cause and thus prevent the paroxysms from returning. Being called upon to prescribe in one of these attacks, I became convinced that she might be permanently relieved from this periodical suffering. After administering one or two doses of Calc., I gave her Colocynth, sixth decimal, and continued it daily until she ceased to have the colicky paroxysms, and her health was altogether improved. The diarrhœa continued for some time, and gradually disappeared. The digestion was better, her appetite returned, and she soon regained her normal health.

Veratrum in Diarrhœa.

When cholera was prevailing epidemically a few years since, I encountered many cases of exhausting diarrhœa where there was great weakness after each stool, and cold sweat on the forehead and all over the body. The discharges were brownish or greenish, watery or papescent, and sometimes the patients complained of coldness of the abdomen, and sometimes of nausea. I found Veratrum album uniformly an effectual remedy.

Pulsatilla in Diarrhœa.

I have had uniform success with this remedy in the treatment of diarrhœa of a watery, slimy or bilious character, and particularly when it came on at night unconsciously, and also when there was a disagreeable taste in the mouth that rendered every article of diet unpleasant, and when there was unpleasant eructations or bitter vomitings. The 6th dilution has generally been employed—fifteen drops in a half tumbler of water, and a teaspoonful given every two hours until a change.

This remedy has also been effectual in diarrhœa when there was much pain *before* each evacuation of watery matter, and when there was much rumbling in the bowels, but very little or no thirst. The same dilution, prepared as above, may be given in the same way.

China in Cholera Infantum.

During the heat of summer it is of daily occurrence to meet with young children, and even infants, suffering with this disorder. When the diarrhœa comes on gradually, assuming more and more a watery character, apparently colored with blood, so as to give the discharges a pale pinkish appearance, and when the little sufferers emaciate rapidly, and seem completely exhausted, China, third dilution, has proved a valuable remedy, and given every two hours, in water, it often has a salutary effect in staying the progress of the disease and effecting a cure.

Chamomilla in Cholera Infantum.

I have seen the grandest results from the use of this remedy in cholera infantum in teething children. When the irritative fever is palpably manifest, with flushed cheeks, slight heat of the head, and copious perspiration about the chest, and when the stools are watery, profuse and frequent, and particularly when the child cries out frequently with colicky pains, twenty drops of the third or sixth dilution in half a tumbler of water may be administered, a teaspoonful at a time, every two hours. In the meantime let the child be carried into the open air by the side of the water, or in a steamboat upon the water, for the purpose of inhaling an invigorating atmosphere, and in a majority of cases this excellent remedy will prove sufficiently curative without resorting to other means.

Chamomilla in a case of Protracted Colic.

Col. A——, aged 50, had a severe attack of colic, which obliged him to take his bed and send for his physician, a member of the "regular" school in good standing. When the physician came he found the Colonel in the greatest agony, from colic, which seemed to be located in the epigastric region. He gave him Camphor, Peppermint, and a carminative, without effect. He then gave two drachms of the Camphorated Tincture of Opium and still the suffering seemed aggravated rather than diminished; and for six weeks this physician administered opiate after opiate, in some form or other, and still there was no let up to the colic. Being exhausted and discouraged, he was induced to believe that a chronic inflammation had all the time been gaining ground in the stomach. A consulting physician was called, and a new formula of opiates was substituted for the old, but all to no purpose. The Colonel gave up in despair, and said he could not live much longer. At this juncture his daughter interfered, and insisted, much against his will, that he should see a Homœopathic physician. Without faith, and with violent protestations against such a course, he let his daughter call one, and addressed him as follows: "Well, Doctor, what can you do? I have had the benefit of the best talent in the profession, and here I am, with one foot in the grave and one foot out; and I have no confidence in you, but to please my daughter I will let you prescribe." On examining the case it was ascertained that there was great pressure and fullness in the pit of the stomach, tearing and drawing pains, that kept him tossing and turning in bed. He complained of a sensation as if the bowels were drawn up in a ball—leaving the whole abdomen empty—and that he had nightly aggravations of the suffering. Seeing in these symptoms an indication for the use of Chamomilla, it was prescribed in drop doses of the third dilution, or, in other words, twenty drops were mixed in twenty teaspoonfuls of water, and a teaspoonful was directed to be given every half hour. When the first teaspoonful was administered he simply remarked that "it was ridiculous;" but before the half hour had expired he fancied that he felt the effects of the remedy all over him, and that he was relieved from pain—the first respite he had felt for six weeks. The second dose was given, and he then declared it was the most powerful medicine,

and he feared to take any more. On being reassured that the
medicine could not poison him, but that it only relieved his pain
and would permanently cure him, he replied. "Then I want a
gallon of it." Convalescence became at once established, and he
soon recovered, a thorough convert to Homœopathy.

Pneumonia.

Cases of inflammation of the lungs are more frequently met
with during seasons of dry and cold weather. The exciting cause
may be a cold north, north-east or north-west wind acting upon
predisposed victims. When the system is heated abnormally, a
drink of ice water may provoke a chill, so may violent emotions,
or loud talking against the wind, or excessive fatigue, first inducing a copious perspiration and then a subsequent chill. In most
cases pneumonia sets in with a chill, and yet observation discloses
the fact that in nearly all cases of pneumonia the subject has
been sensible of weariness, inappetency and sensitiveness to cold
air several days before anything like a distinct chill occurs; but
when it does come it is followed by a continuous dry heat upon the
surface, more or less pain in the chest, tending somewhat to the
left side. There is at the same time a sense of oppression or
weight in one or both lungs, which gradually gives way to a
stinging, aching pain, causing great anxiety, with short and hurried respiration. The breath is hot and feverish, the face flushed,
and the carotids distended. When both lungs are inflamed, and
the intercostal muscles are somewhat implicated, inspiration is
effected by the abdominal muscles and diaphragm, without raising
the thorax or ribs, and this renders it more tolerable for the patient. If only one lung is inflamed, the pain will be severe only
in that lung and in the side that is implicated. When both lungs
are inflamed, and heat and pain are felt in the whole cavity of the
chest, the patient is in great danger, unable to indulge in a full
inspiration because of the violent stitches it produces. At this
stage a dry cough adds to the distress of the patient. After a while
a transparent, tenacious and frequently reddish mucus is expectorated. The bowels are usually constipated, the urine is hot and
reddish in color. The pulse is usually full and tense. This is what
is termed the first stage of the disease, and requires, according to
the symptoms, Aconite. I have known a few drops of the 3d dilution of Aconite, put in half a tumbler of water, and administered

in teaspoonful doses every hour, to be followed by moisture upon
the skin, a reduction of the pulse, a mitigation of the pain in the
lungs, and a general relief to the whole system. In most cases,
Aconite must be continued until the fever is considerably moderated, and a copious, warm perspiration appears.

The second stage of pneumonia takes place when the inflammation becomes extended so as to interfere with the function of
respiration; and in order to detect the severity and extent of the
inflammation, a physical examination becomes necessary. This
may consist of auscultation and percussion. When the tissue of
the lungs is filled with air only, as in a condition of health, the
normal sounds of respiration can be heard by placing the ear to
the chest, or by the aid of a stethoscope, and the sound elicited
on percussion is resonant, clear and distinct. If this is not the
case, the lungs are either filled or partially filled with blood or
serum, as in hepatization, or with pus, as in tuberculosis.

It is better to select the back part of the patient's chest for
percussion, because it has been observed that infiltration of the
tissues naturally gravitates towards the posterior wall of the thorax, and is therefore more easily detected by percussion in this
region, which yields a dull sound, and more so in proportion to
the degree of infiltration. The normal respiratory murmur, when
infiltration occurs, gradually disappears, and what is usually
termed the bronchial murmur takes its place. When these physical signs exist there is considerable dyspnœa and a constant desire to draw a long breath; the stitches become more and more
violent, and there is a short, hacking cough, with bloody expectoration. When this second stage sets in, Bryonia 3d attenuation, may be given every hour. When this condition has
presented itself in females, I have seen beneficial results from
the use of the 3d of Pulsatilla in alternation every hour with
Aconite.

When the expectoration becomes rusty, Phosphorus 3d, has
generally acted favorably—five drops of the 3d dilution in half a
tumbler of water may be given hourly in spoonful doses, or every
two hours as the symptoms improve.

When there is excessive accumulation of mucus in the air
passages, and much rattling, and threatening of suffocation, and
some dyspnœa, Tartar emetic may take the place of Phosphorus.
In a case of pneumonia in a child six years old, when there was

severe pain in the head and chest, a few doses of Belladonna 6th, given at intervals of an hour, relieved the pain in the head and lungs, but an excessive accumulation of mucus in the respiratory passages, ensued, which three or four doses of Tartar emetic, given at intervals of an hour, cured.

I have observed that in most cases, pneumonia will yield in the first stage, sometimes, to Aconite alone; and when there is a palpable indication of capillary congestion of the bronchia, and chilliness, with headache, Belladonna after the Aconite will complete the cure; and when the cough causes pain in the head, as if it would split, Bryonia, after Aconite, will bring about recovery.

For the pneumonia that sometimes supervenes upon measles, Aconite 3d may be given frequently at first, and afterwards Bryonia 3d and Sulphur; the two remedies first named may be given in water, a spoonful every hour or two hours as the case may be more or less severe, and the latter may be given in the 3d decimal trituration once a day. I have also employed the higher potencies with success, when the fever has been active and pain in the chest was very severe.

I have noticed that patients sometimes recover from this disease, and, when able to leave the bed, still complain of oppression and weakness of the lungs. In such cases a dose or two of the 200th of Lycopodium or Phosphorus given daily will soon cure them; and also when the fever is intense and the patient suffers from delirium I have seen the whole difficulty yield to a few doses of Belladonna 30th given at intervals of an hour. And here let me note that in a majority of cases of pneumonia in children, Aconite 30th may be given every hour until the arterial excitement ceases, and then Belladonna 30th, continued for a brief period, will result favorably.

When typhoid symptoms supervene, Rhus tox. 30th will operate favorably. In a case of ten days' sickness, the patient having been in a state of coma most of the time, Rhus rad. 6th produced a favorable change in a few hours; and the patient's cough, which before had been dry and painful, became looser and less painful, and recovery soon followed.

A case of pneumonia in a gentleman aged 30, of sanguine temperament, who had been bled profusely, but who nevertheless still suffered from high fever and great debility, dry

cough and rusty expectoration, was cured in the space of a
week by the use of Aconite 30th and China 30th in alternation
every hour.

In asthmatic subjects it has been observed that Arsenicum
and Ipecac are valuable remedies to consult. An aged gentleman
who had suffered from asthma most of his life was exposed to the
extremes of temperature, which resulted in an attack of pneumonia. He complained of chilliness and hot flashes and thirst, his
tongue was coated with a thick, white coating. His cough was
exceedingly painful, and his respiration difficult. His skin was
dry and hard. Aconite 30th was first given, with little effect.
Arsenicum 30th removed the fever and chilliness gradually; the
remedy was continued for two days. But after the chilliness and
hot flushes subsided the pain in the chest, cough, and difficult
breathing remained. Ipecac 30th was given in water, a spoonful
every hour, with good effect. He finally recovered from the attack, and remained quite free from the asthma, that had frequently troubled him before, ever afterwards. It has been customary
to describe two forms of pneumonia, one of which is termed
spurious or pneumonia notha, which is characterized by an accelerated, soft pulse, slight stinging pains in the sides of the chest,
felt only when drawing a long breath; anxiety and oppression,
or a sense of weight in the lungs, with expectoration of blood
from day to day; faint sound of the voice, and interruption of
speech by frequent attacks of coughing—usually attend this form
of the disease. In the commencement, Aconite is required; a few
drops of the 6th attenuation dissolved in a cup of water, and
thoroughly mixed may be given, a dessert spoonful at a time,
and repeated every hour when the symptoms become aggravated.
Mercurius solubilis, the 6th, may be prepared in the same manner, and administered as directed for the Aconite. These two
remedies have generally proved sufficient; in some cases, however
Mercurius vivus may have the preference, especially in those of
sallow complexion and subject to biliary derangement. When
the cough is dry and hacking, with more or less constriction in
the chest, Chamomilla 6th prepared in the same way may be given,
with advantageous result. If there is hurried and anxious respiration, Ipecac 6th should be called into requisition. When the
constriction of the chest is accompanied with great anxiety, and
coldness of the extremities, Veratrum album. 6th must be given

as above. I have also found Arsenicum 6th a valuable remedy when there is great prostration.

In the more malignant forms of pneumonia, when several days elapse before the disease actually manifests itself, and the patient begins to complain of an inexplicable sense of suffering, and a chill sets in, followed by shortness of breath and pressure in the chest, and these symptoms are accompanied by heat, cold, and clammy sweats, dry and blackish tongue, muttering when asleep, and the urine and fæces are passed involuntarily, Bryonia 1st attenuation may be given in water every hour. If this remedy does not change the condition of the patient in a few hours, I have found Rhus tox. a valuable remedy to follow. If the patient manifests considerable stupor, Opium 3d is indicated. If the disease has been brought on by excessive fatigue, Arnica 3d in water may be given after the Opium; and if the prostration and coldness remain, Ars. and Veratrum may be called into requisition.

One of the most favorable signs of a change for the better in these severe cases, is a copious and vaporous perspiration; also when the pulse becomes calm, and the respiration free and easy, with signs of returning moisture at the nostrils, and copious deposits of urates in the urine, and free expectoration. The absence of fever is not always a sign that the danger is over.

When the inflammation extends to both lungs, and there is great anxiety and distress for breath, and the pulse becomes rapid and small and finally compressible, and also when the breathing is laborious and rattling and performed exclusively by the abdominal muscles, and particularly when the countenance is pale and sunken and the patient settles down in bed unable to help himself, the indications are altogether unfavorable.

Before giving practical illustrations by citing numerous cases that have come under my personal observation, I will append the symptoms in general that call into requisition each particular remedy.

Aconite is indicated when there is a chill, followed by dry heat and burning of the skin and violent thirst, anxious breathing, stitches in the chest, dry cough, hurried and full pulse, vertigo on raising the head, and a reddish sediment in the urine, which is hot and scalding.

Arnica is indicated where the pneumonia is occasioned by a mechanical injury, and when the stitches in the chest are very much aggravated by coughing.

Belladonna.—When there is evidence of congestion of blood to the head and lungs, with flushed and bloated countenance, obscure vision, severe pain in the head, and delirium, burning heat over the entire body, rapid and full pulse, short and laborious breathing, cough with expectoration, lancinating stitches in the chest, expectoration of bloody mucus, dark or brown urine. This remedy is suitable to follow Aconite, and especially if Aconite has failed to produce the desired result.

Bryonia.—When the skin is dry and there is violent thirst, rapid pulse, subdued and anxious breathing, with desire to make deep and full inspirations, stitches in both lungs, made worse by coughing, and when a sudden pain in the head is produced by the cough, attended with expectoration streaked with blood or of a rusty color, and hot urine, which deposits a reddish or brown sediment.

Pulsatilla.—When the pneumonia sets in after menstrual suppression. It may follow the use of Aconite, and when the patient moans and feels anxious and listless, the pulse rapid, and soft, rattling respiration, stitches in the chest, cough and expectoration of coagulated mucus and blood, with rheumatic pains in the limbs.

Tartar emetic.—When there is a copious catarrh in the air passages, and expectoration of mucus, producing suffocation and distress, incipient œdema of the lungs, great dyspnœa and paralytic weakness of the chest.

China.—In case of loss of blood, by being bled, or from the rupture of some vessel, which sometimes occurs from coughing, when the pulse is soft and there is a general debility, and also when the respiration is short and hurried, and there is much rattling of mucus in the air passages.

Phosphorus is indicated when there is heat with anxiety, rapid pulse, tense and wiry, oppression of the chest as from a load, and anxious breathing, stitches in the lungs, cough with rusty sputa, urine dark, becomes turbid in a short time.

Mercury.—When there is heat in the whole body, thirst and desire for cold drinks, fetid night-sweats, stitches in the chest, made worse by sneezing, rapid motion or breathing, cough with bloody expectoration, dark red or brown urine.

Nux vomica is generally indicated for pneumonia in inebriates, or after sudden suppression of piles, and particularly when there is obstinate constipation.

Rhus tox., and *Rhus radicans* are indicated when there is great prostration and inclination to coma and other indications of a typhoid fever.

Lycopodium is indicated when during convalescence there still remains deep-seated pain in one or both lungs, and also if the bowels are seriously constipated, and particularly when the pneumonia has passed off, and a deep-seated bronchial irritation remains. It is also indicated in hepatization and tuberculous degeneration.

Carbo veg., is indicated in chronic inflammation of the lungs when there is coldness of the hands and feet, and pains in the lumbar region, and dull pains in the head.

Sulphur.—When pneumonia occurs after some eruption has been suppressed, and when the disease is imperfectly developed.

Calcarea carb., is also indicated when pneumonia supervenes upon any of the exanthematous diseases.

Other remedies may be called into requisition in the treatment of this painful disease, such as Gelsemium, Sanguinaria, Macrotin, Veratrum viride, and Carbo animalis, when the condition and symptoms indicate their use.

From this group of remedies, selections can be made that will meet almost all cases of pneumonia, from the mildest to the severest form of the disease, and it will be our aim to cite from experience, examples and cases illustrative of the practical application of these various remedies.

Phosphorus in Pneumonia.

A lady aged 61 years, after an exposure to a cold, damp wind, was seized with a chill, which was followed by a violent fever and pain in the head and chest; her pulse was somewhat accelerated, full and bounding; her tongue was coated with a thick white fur; she complained of dryness of the throat and mouth; severe pain in the right lung; short hacking cough with a trifling expectoration of mucus; her skin was hot and dry; her urine

51

highly colored and deposited a brownish sediment; she had no appetite and was quite debilitated. Aconite 3d was given in water, five drops in half a tumbler, and a spoonful once an hour. In twelve hours a warm perspiration broke out, and the arterial excitement was much less. After waiting several hours from the time the perspiration commenced, the following symptoms were noted: The pain had continued in the right lung, and the cough was more severe, and the expectoration was slightly tinged with blood, and every time she coughed, she suffered from pain in the head, and rheumatic pains about the chest. Gave Bryonia 6th, prepared in water, a spoonful every hour for twelve hours; found at the expiration of time but a slight improvement. The pain in the right lung was slightly better, but the cough remains about the same; the expectoration was slightly rusty, and the fever somewhat worse. Gave Aconite again for three successive hours. The skin being moist, a change was then made to Phosphorus. Five drops were put in half a tumbler of water, and a spoonful was administered every hour. In less than a day, the pain subsided. In the lungs the cough became looser, and the rusty sputa was no longer expectorated, but simply a dark colored thick mucus was thrown off by the cough. The nostrils became moist, and the nose began to discharge freely. Towards evening there was an aggravation of the fever, and a copious secretion of mucus was heard to settle in the air-passages. Tartar emetic was given, the 6th attenuation, in water; a spoonful every hour during the night. except when the patient was asleep. The next morning there was scarcely any fever; the respiration was free; the coating had disappeared from the tongue, and the appetite was decidedly improved, and altogether the signs seemed favorable for convalescence. The Tartar emetic was continued at longer intervals, until the cough was better. The patient gradually improved until her usual health returned.

Carbo Animalis in Pneumonia.

A lady aged 37; the wife of a master mechanic; complained for several days of feeling dull and weary. She had no appetite; her tongue was furred and her breath offensive. About the 5th day she experienced a slight chill and rigors extending down the spine, followed by considerable fever, full pulse, pain in the upper portion of the chest that greatly interferes with inspiration.

She suffered from dryness of the fauces and throat, skin and palms. She complains of pain in the back and over the thorax, a dry, racking cough and expectoration of tough, ropy mucus. Five drops of the 3d dilution of Aconite in half a tumbler of water was prepared, and a spoonful directed to be given every hour until the pulse became soft and the skin moist. Bryonia was then prepared in water, and spoonful doses were substituted for the Aconite. A few hours after, the fever returned with great violence, and the inflammation of the lungs seemed greatly aggravated, and every time the patient coughed, she screamed with pain. Five drops of the 3d of Belladonna were put in half a glass of water, and given every half hour. The patient, after taking four or five doses, was greatly relieved of the intensity of the pain in the lungs, but her head commenced paining her, and the pain became more and more intense, until she became quite delirious. Bell. 30th, was substituted, which had a wonderful effect in relieving the head and delirium, and there was much less pain in the chest, and yet there was considerable dyspnœa, and a manifest certainty that hepatization had taken place. There was dullness on percussion in the inter-scapular region, and a short and laborious respiration, that gave evidence of the derangement. As the fever and arterial excitement seemed great, Aconite in water was again prescribed, and after a few doses, a copious perspiration set in; at the same time the cough was intensely severe, and the respiration more seriously impaired. At this stage, an eminent practitioner of our school from New York City was invited to counsel with me in the case. A physical examination by him, confirmed the conclusions I had come to concerning the location of the difficulty, and the extent of its interference with the function of respiration. He expressed himself frankly, that an abcess of a fatal character must result from so formidable a hepatization. He suggested that Bryonia should be given in alternation with Aconite, and kept up for a day, which was done. We met at the bedside of the patient 24 hours after, and found no satisfactory improvement. At his suggestion, the violent and vapory perspiration, which through the night had been extremely copious, indicated the use of Carbo animalis. Concurring in the use of this remedy, it was administered in the 3d centesimal trituration, about one grain every two hours. A marked improvement in respiration, cough and fever followed at once. The expectoration became exceedingly copious but contained no pus. The remedy was continued for 24 hours more, and the improvement in the patient's condition was obvious to all. The tongue exhibited a moist and normal condition; the respiration was not so rapid, and the hepatized portion of the right lung gave signs of passing away without suppuration. The remedy was still continued at intervals of six hours. The patient improved gradually, and no other remedy was employed. Recovery in about two weeks was the result of treatment in this case.

Aconite in Pneumonia.

In all cases of this disease where the pulse is accelerated and full, the skin dry, the urine highly colored and depositing a brick-dust sediment, Aconite 6th, given every hour, or two hours in mild cases, may prove sufficient.

A lad six years of age, on coming from a warm school-room into a cold north-east wind on his way home, had a violent chill immediately after entering the house, which lasted for an entire hour. As it began to subside and the fever set in, the respiration became hurried; the skin dry and hot; the thirst violent and the urine hot and of a bright red color. A dry cough commenced, attended with painful stitches in the chest. Aconite, 3d dilution, a few drops in half a tumbler of water, was given in teaspoonful doses every hour until the fever subsided and the heat of the skin disappeared. About six hours after the chill the patient fell into a disturbed sleep, moaning at every breath; the cough continued to appear every few minutes, and was dry and distressing; the Aconite was continued through the night. In the morning he seemed better in some respects; at 10 A. M. he complained of aching in his limbs and feeling cold; his head commenced to ache, and every time he coughed he cried out with pain. The fever, during the afternoon, was considerable, but less than the previous day; about 10 P. M. he fell asleep, and awoke in delirium in about one hour. Belladonna 6th was then substituted for the Aconite, and one or two doses produced quietness, and he went to sleep and did not awake till morning. At 9 A. M. he seemed dull and inclined to a comatose sleep; he was aroused, however, by the nurse, and he took a little nourishment and sunk off to sleep again. He now complained of little pain, but his breathing was difficult, and the cough still dry. Gave Bryonia 6th, a few drops in half a tumbler of water, a teaspoonful every hour; after four doses, he began to expectorate a small quantity of dark-colored mucus; at night again he had considerable fever, but was dull and sleepy. The following morning his cough was loose and he seemed quite free from fever, and the coma had disappeared, and in all respects he seemed better. At noon his cough and expectoration had been considerable; his skin was moist and he had none of those stitches in his chest. At night the catarrhal symptoms seemed most prominent, the expectoration was greatly increased, and the cough gave him but little pain. Gave a dose of Stibium 3d, to be repeated in two hours. About midnight he had some return of fever, but the next morning he was greatly improved, called for something to eat. There was no burning thirst or dryness of the skin afterwards. He continued to cough and expectorate for several days, and then there was a mitigation; he soon regained his normal strength, and was well.

A little girl, daughter of Mr. B., played out in the cold on the first day of May, and became so chilled that the blood settled under the finger nails, and it was difficult to get up a warmth over the surface of the body; the pulse was 150 a minute; the respiration about 50. She suffered from intense thirst, dry cough, but no pain. She lay in a sunken, comatose condition for several days. She had previously had whooping cough and measles. She took Aconite with no perceptible effect, and also Bryonia and Rhus radicans. The strength was entirely gone, but when she laid still and motionless she complained of no suffering except from thirst. Arsenicum, 6th and 30th, were given without effect. Carbo veg., and other remedies that were evidently indicated had no effect whatever, and in spite of all the remedies, she gradually sank and died on the 22d day. There was something mysterious about the case. No remedy that seemed indicated had the slightest beneficial effect. She had the most persistent and critical treatment, and the best nursing that was possible, and yet there was no vital reaction from the time she was taken sick until she died. Was this the sudden result of the incipient sequel of measles and whooping cough? She appeared to be in good health when she was out at play. This case is reported on account of the failure of any remedies to produce the slightest mitigation, though prescribed by the concurrent skill of three experienced members of the profession.

A lad ten years old, of nervous sanguine temperament, taken sick about the middle of March; he first complained of feeling cold, and afterwards he complained of a severe pain in the head over the eyes, and shooting pains through the temples. His countenance was pale, tongue coated white, and considerable thirst. The pulse was more rapid than normal; the skin was hot and the urine highly colored. Gave a dose of Aconite 6th, and repeated it in two hours, after which he became dull and sleepy; so much so that it was difficult to arouse him; as yet there was no cough, and no indication of pneumonia. Gave Belladonna 6th, in water, and repeated several times at intervals of one hour, and still he remained dull and in a stupor. Cerebral disease was feared, as his forehead felt hot and moist. He remained in this condition for three days, and then the coma ceased and a circumscribed redness of the cheeks appearing in marked contrast with his otherwise white and clear complexion, which led to the suspicion that his lungs were implicated. Gave Belladonna 30th, five drops of the dilution in a cup of water, a teaspoonful every hour; after taking a few doses, his head seemed clear and free from pain, but a cough ensued, short, dry and painful; considerable fever attended the cough, and the act of coughing caused the head to ache again. Gave Bryonia 6th, five drops in a cup of water, a teaspoonful every hour. Expectoration of a rusty appearance followed, and the redness of the cheeks was more apparent. Every paroxysm of coughing caused the patient to cry out with pain in the chest. The respiration was short and hurried, the pulse quick. Aconite 6th, was substituted for the Bryonia, and a warm perspiration soon followed, and for twenty-four hours there appeared to be considerable improvement; but the fever returned, the cough increased, the expectoration was still rusty, and the flush of the cheeks was greatly increased. Every time the patient coughed there was a moan, indicating great distress. Phosphorus 6th, five drops in a cup of water, was directed to be given in teaspoonful doses, every hour. After three or four doses, the severity of the cough ceased, the fever subsided, the appearance of the sputa changed, and for the next twenty-four hours the signs of recovery were satisfactory. The fever returned with less severity, as did the accompanying symptoms. Phosphorus 6th, was continued,—the expectoration became more copious and catarrhal, the cough was unattended with pain. The improvement during the next 24 hours was very marked. There was no return of fever or pain; the cough continued with considerable mucus expectoration for several days, and gradually disappeared. Recovery soon followed.

A gentleman aged 39, naturally robust, contracted a severe cold from exposure to a heated and then to a chilly atmosphere, from which he experienced severe pain in both lungs, accompanied by considerable arterial excitement. He was very thirsty, and his breathing hurried and painful; he had a hot, dry skin, and passed but a moderate quantity of urine having a reddish sediment. Aconite, 3d attenuation, was prepared in water and administered every hour until his fever subsided; the skin became moist, and the pain in the lungs was gone; after which his recovery was rapid, being able to return to his business in seven days from the time he was taken.

Stibium in Pneumonia.

A young lady aged twenty-three, of fair complexion and light hair, was cured of pneumonia of several days' standing by Stibium 3d. She complanied of considerable pain in the right lung, accompanied by cough and copious expectoration of mucus. She also had a dull pain in the head, and coryza. The remedy was given in powders of the 3d trituration and repeated at inter vals of three hours. She was speedily relieved and her recovery was rapid.

Sulphur in Typhoid Pneumonia.

Typhoid pneumonia in a male patient of adult age, characterized by sunken countenance, coma and stertorous respiration, a rapid wiry pulse, and great prostration. *Opium* 6th was given at intervals of three hours for a day and night, followed by Ars., 6th, in doses of four pellets every three hours; but little change occurred for two or three days. There was considerable rattling in the chest, for which Bryonia 6th was prescribed with apparently good effect; but after two days the debility and difficult respiration increased; gave one dose of Sulphur, four pellets, and after four hours gave *Rhus tox.*, after which convalescence became evident, and a gradual improvement from day to day resulted, in recovery. There was in this case some degree of hepatization in the right lung which the *Sulphur* removed, as indicated by an expectoration of pus, after its administration.

Aconite in Chills.

A young man, an accountant, was seized with a chill on the 10th of February, which was followed by pain in the chest and fever; his countenance soon became sallow; he complained of severe pain under the right shoulder-blade, and there was a marked irregularity of the heart's action. Aconite 3d was first given at intervals of an hour for an entire day. This was followed by moist perspiration over the chest, but no alleviation of the pain. Chelidonium was then administered in drop doses of the 3d attenuation. This was followed by relief of the pain under the right shoulder-blade, and the heart symptoms also disappeared. The patient rapidly recovered, and no other remedies were given.

Lachesis in Tuberculous Deposits.

In a feeble, cachectic subject, evidently suffering from tuberculous deposits, after having been treated for acute inflammation, Lachesis 9th afforded great relief. In this case there was invariably a paroxysm of coughing after sleeping. This patient did not recover, but was greatly relieved by the remedy.

Lycopodium in Pneumonia.

A son of a well-known merchant was observed to be failing, losing flesh, and becoming greatly debilitated; a deep, hollow cough and a low fever betokened a formidable case. Bryonia 6th was given without relief. Other remedies were tried with like effect. Lycopodium 6th was then given, and the result was favorable. This remedy was continued, and the young man fully recovered after a protracted illness of five weeks.

Tartar Emetic in Pneumonia.

A lady advanced to the seventh month in pregnancy took a severe cold, which resulted in catarrhal inflammation of the lungs. She suffered from a severe and painful cough of an extremely suffocating form. She had considerable fever, dry and hot skin,

and more or less aching in the head and back. Aconite simply
allayed the fever. This remedy was followed by Ipecac 6th with
very little effect. Tart. emetic, 6th dilution, was then given in
drop doses at intervals of an hour, and all the formidable symptoms yielded. She fully recovered after an illness of eight
days.

In the delicate condition of this patient we often find it
difficult to subdue the cough when attended with catarrhal inflammation, and after considerable experience and observation, I am
inclined to give Stibium the preference over many other remedies.
It possesses the power of relieving the air passages, allaying the
fever and cough in many cases, and particularly when the
paroxysms of coughing are so suffocating as to almost arrest the
breathing, and also when there is considerable rattling of
mucus and a hollow cough, and anxious oppression of the
chest.

Bituminous Coal in Pneumonia.

A real estate dealer, aged 54, of bilious temperament,
after being exposed to a storm of snow and rain, became
very cold, and found it difficult to get warm for several days; he felt chilly even in a warm room; he found
himself yawning and very much prostrated. From morning till
evening he suffered intensely from aching in the limbs and from
coldness of the extremities. A dry, hollow cough, and considerable pain in the chest were constantly troubling; he was thirsty,
and his tongue was considerably coated; he had no appetite, and
grew weaker every day; his bowels were constipated, the urine
was not profuse but reddish, and deposited a pale, brick-dust sediment in the chamber. He finally was obliged to keep his bed, and
resort to bottles of warm water to keep him comfortable. He
continued in this cold and sunken state for more than a week,
neither external warmth nor internal stimulants had the effect to
warm up his system. The pulse was feeble, and the cough indicated considerable capillary congestion. At last his head began to
ache, and a febrile reaction began to take place and continued to
increase until he began to complain of feeling excessively hot;
the pulse beat more strongly, the respiration began to be effected,
and he complained of severe pain in both lungs, and when he
coughed the suffering was great. That there was decided inflam-

mation of the lungs could not be doubted. Aconite, 3d dilution,
a few drops in a goblet of water was directed, in teaspoonful
doses, to be given every hour. This remedy was continued for
twenty-four hours, and still the pain did not abate either in his
head or chest. The dry and shriveled appearance of the skin remained the same. Belladonna 3d, prepared in the same way, was
then given in dessert-spoonful doses for another twenty-four
hours; his head was somewhat relieved, and the cough became
less painful, but when he turned or moved, the pain was greatly
increased; the countenance was pale and sunken, and the thirst
was great. Arsenicum, 6th, was given, four or five doses in succession, at intervals of two hours. This removed in some degree
the dryness of his mouth, and he was less inclined to call for
drink. Still he had no appetite for food, and was becoming
weaker. He expectorated a white, frothy mucus, and could not
be moved without extreme pain. Bryonia was given the following morning, in the way directed for Aconite, and yet it made
but little impression until evening, when for the first time there
was a slight moisture upon the head and chest. During the night
he had a copious perspiration; the following morning he had
less pain, and the respiration was less difficult. The same remedy
was continued the following day, and at night he had clammy
perspiration which lasted for several hours; in the morning he
seemed a little better, the fever was continuous, he was unable to
take any food but oatmeal gruel, and this in limited quantities.
He began to expectorate a dark-colored mucus. Bryonia was
continued for another day, and at night he had a copious sweat;
the next morning he coughed up a quantity of rusty sputa. Phosphorus 6th, was given every two hours during the day, and at
night he had a more copious sweat, which lasted till morning;
there was also a fetid odor from his breath. Carbo animalis, in
the 3d trituration, was given every three hours until evening, and
he seemed less restless and inclined to sleep in short naps; towards
morning he felt chilly, and complained of a dead ache in the
lumbar region; the urine was scanty and thick, and altogether he
seemed no better; cold hands and feet led to some fears of an additional recurrence of fever. A very carefully prepared trituration of bituminous coal was being proved by *Dr. W. H. Burt;*
he had prepared the 3d centesimal, which was administered in
grain doses, at intervals of four hours. The effect of this remedy

was somewhat remarkable; the patient, after taking the third dose, had a gentle moisture upon the skin, less thirst and less pain. The tongue became moist, and the taste became so improved that an orange afforded some delight as he sucked it. At night he seemed quiet, and fell to sleep and rested well between the paroxysms of coughing. The same remedy was continued the following day, and at evening the patient was evidently stronger and better, and from this time he gradually gained in strength, and fully recovered after a siege of six weeks' illness. When he first sat up his feet became much swollen, and it was some days before he could use them to advantage. Arsenicum and China were usefully employed in the restoration of the strength.

Chelidonium in Pneumonia.

A less formidable case of inflammation of the lungs, with pain in the right side and under the right shoulder-blade, sal low countenance and painful inspirations, was cured by Chelidonium alone. Complete recovery took place after one week's illness.

Gelsemium in Pneumonia.

A German girl, who went from hot steam where she was washing into a cold atmosphere to relieve herself from the perspiration the hot steam had occasioned, received a sudden check of perspiration, which resulted in congestive pneumonia, very threatening to her life. For some days she complained of severe pains in the chest, and there was considerable coldness on the surface of her body. She coughed up mucus streaked with blood. Gelsemium the 3d, was given in this case, and continued for nearly two days. As the remedy gave decided relief; no other was employed. The girl soon recovered. Gelsemium is invariably applicable to these cases, where the most suffering is found under the scapulæ of both sides, caused by sudden check of perspiration from cold. The remedy breaks up the disease by producing copious perspiration.

Phytolacca Decandra in Diphtheria.

In the group of remedies known to have a beneficial effect in diphtheritic sore throat, Phytolacca deservedly occupies a prominent place. Having had occasion to try its virtues in quite a number of cases, I have always found satisfactory results when the patient complained of feeling cold in the evening and during the night, with dryness of the throat and soreness in the morning. In several cases where evening chilliness was followed by soreness of the throat in the morning, I have found livid exudations upon the tonsils and fauces, difficult deglutition and extreme sensitiveness of the amygdalæ, and also considerable fever and arterial excitement. Phytolacca 3d attenuation, has generally operated satisfactorily, removing these diphtheritic symptoms.

When my patients complain of a choking sensation in the throat, caused by swelling of the soft palate and tonsils, and when there is a fiery redness of the velum palati, I take the alarm and give Phytolacca in the 3d decimal attenuation, and rarely without satisfactory results; and also when my patients complain of roughness or rawness of the throat, which is so sensitive as to forbid the mechanical contact of any solid food, while they are made nearly frantic by attempting to swallow fluids, I have found Phytolacca in the 3d decimal attenuation an effectual remedy. In short, let it be said that in cold weather, when diphtheritic inflammations are liable to prevail, Phytolacca in the 3d or 6th attenuation may be recommended in almost every case of incipient dryness or soreness of the throat that may result in diphtheria.

Phytolacca in Rheumatism.

There is truth in the common saying that coming events cast their shadows before them. It has been a tradition among the Indians and yeomanry of America from time immemorial, that Phytolacca may be made into a tea, drank for the cure of rheumatism. It has undoubtedly proved a salutary remedy for many forms of the disease, when administered in this way. But in modern times the provings of this remedy have confirmed its use in these affections.

Mrs. S——, aged forty-three years, had suffered for many weeks with rheumatism in the small of her back, so that she could not assume the erect position without great pain. She had no perceptible fever or thirst; her appetite was not much impaired. She suffered no pain except in the lumbar region, and this was so excruciating that fears were entertained that renal inflammation was the cause; and yet, from the fact that the usual quantity of urine was passed daily without difficulty, this idea could not be entertained. Rheumatism of the muscles of the back was evidently the difficulty, and in accordance with this conviction, the 6th of Phytolacca was prescribed, in drop doses, to be repeated every three hours until relieved. She took the remedy for two days, found herself much relieved, and ceased taking it; in a few days after she found herself perfectly well, and free from the suffering. This remedy has been useful in cases of chronic rheumatism, when other remedial measures seemed to fail, as follows: Rev. Mr. W——, who had suffered for many months with rheumatism of the back and hip-joint, was cured by a few doses of Phytolacca, 3d dil., and he was past fifty years of age. So conscious was he of this remedy being sure relief for him, he never traveled without it; and moreover, I have heard him say that he has recommended it with satisfactory success in many cases of sciatica and rheumatism of the arms and shoulders. Rheumatic patients have frequently complained of a sensation of dryness and swelling, as if something was in the throat, while taking this remedy.

Phytolacca in Swelling, Induration, and Abscess of Mammary Gland.

Mrs. T——, a stout, fleshy lady, on the third week after her confinement, began to complain of heat and swelling in the right breast. The nurse was directed to rub the same with lard and to keep the milk drawn out, in hopes of escaping the painful ordeal of a mammary abscess. But all efforts to prevent the caking seemed to fail, and the gland was hot, painful and swollen. Drop doses of the 1st dilution of Phytolacca were directed to be given every hour, and by the time the lady had taken the sixth dose, the gland was evidently relieved of the heat and distension. She discontinued the medicine, convalescence went on, and in two days her breast was restored to its normal condition. I have likewise found the external application of the tincture of Phytolacca, while taking a dilution, as an internal remedy, to be exceedingly effective in these mammary difficulties. Thirty drops of the tincture to an ounce vial of water, will form a lotion of sufficient strength, while ten drops of the 1st dilution in half a pint of water will be sufficiently strong for internal administration. I have generally found Phytolacca a useful remedy in the early stages of mammary inflammation and not unfrequently in those more advanced, when suppuration has commenced. In the mother tincture it may be applied to excoriated or cracked nipples with the certain prospect of relief. The use of this remedy cannot be too highly commended.

Pulsatilla Nuttiliana in Irregular Menstruation.

In a case of irregular and painful menstruation, the subject being a young lady, aged 20, Pulsatilla nut., wrought a wonderful change. Her menstrual periods commenced when she was 17 years of age. At her first change she suffered intensely from colic and restlessness, severe pain in head and back; after two days this suffering passed off, and she seemed to recover her usual health. Her next period occurred in seven weeks, and was ushered in with great agony and restlessness, her head, back and stomach all seemed severely affected. She took stimulants without relief, and the period of suffering was worn out in a few days as before. The next period occurred at a shorter interval, but with the suffering unmitigated, and in this way she went on for two years or more, sometimes four, sometimes five, or even six or seven weeks would elapse between her periods. She had the last year been subject to Homœopathic treatment, but with very little benefit. She had taken the Anemone Pulsatilla, Sulphur and other remedies, such as Hyoscyamus, Ignatia and Belladonna, etc. During one of her late periods she took twenty drops of the Puls. nut., in half a tumbler of water, a teaspoonful every hour, and a few doses relieved her suffering, and the period passed off more pleasantly than ever before. The following period occurred at the regular time and with little suffering, and for the last year she has been regular, and subject to no greater suffering than in ordinary cases.

A lady approaching the climacteric period, who had not menstruated for three months, and had suffered greatly with her head and distension of the abdomen, was speedily relieved by a few drop doses of the 2d dilution of this remedy.

A case of amenorrhœa was cured after taking this remedy four or five days, three times a day, ten drops of the 2d dilution in half a tumbler of water, a teaspoonful at a dose

The clinical use of this remedy up to this time has been either in the tincture or lower dilutions, but it is believed that much of the headache, nausea or diarrhœa that follows the administration of larger doses, even when it is designed to correct derangements of the menstrual functions, may be obviated without lessening the curative action, by higher attenuations.

Polygonum Hydropiper in Amenorrhœa.

I have known a decoction of smartweed to be called into requisition in domestic practice, to overcome the amenia in young girls, but it was hardly possible to get at all the facts attendant upon its use under such circumstances. We have received however the impression that " *smartweed tea* " has rendered some useful service. This impression has been confirmed by the provings of *Dr. W. E. Payne*, and the late *B. F. Joslin, M. D.*, but now from its clinical use we can state that Miss C. C——, nervo-bilious temperament, suffered at every period several day's delay, during which time she was hardly able to keep about. She had taken many remedies to overcome this habit, but without effect; finally a resort was had to the tincture of Polygonum hydropiper, in five-drop doses, and the habit was corrected. In several other cases of amenorrhœa this remedy has been used with more than ordinary good results.

Polygonum Hydropiper in the Treatment of Ulcers.

In some females at the climacteric period there is a proneness to suffer from superficial ulcers and sores upon the lower extremities. I have found no remedy more efficacious in removing them. Twenty drops of the tincture in half a tumbler of water, in doses of a tablespoonful three times a day internally, while the sores are dressed with a compress wet with a lotion of one part of tincture to four of water, will effect a cure in a short time. Sometimes a decoction of the herb is used for a wash with like effect. I recollect of hearing an experienced nurse remark, that she had never failed of healing these sores with simple Cerate, after having poulticed them with *smartweed* mixed up with *corn meal*.

Rhus Glabrum in Syphilitic Ulceration.

A gentleman, aged 50 years, of nervo-sanguine temperament, who had suffered from syphilis, and often, as he supposed, had been cured, suffered from ulceration of the mouth—the ul-

cers took the form of deep fissures in the tongue, gums and sides
of the mouth—so severe and painful as to render it difficult to
masticate his food or swallow liquids. The nutrition of the system
was so obstructed that great emaciation was the consequence.
He was treated with nitric acid, nitrate of silver, and other local
applications, without effect. A number of remedies prescribed
Homœopathically afforded no relief. At last a wash prepared from
the sumach berries was used with a swab, while the 2d dilution
of the tincture was administered in five-drop doses several times a
day. Immediately after a resort to this treatment, the inflammation and soreness of the ulcers disappeared and they began to heal.
His recovery was rapid—complete, since which he has remained
in sound health. After the use of mercurials in the treatment of
syphilis, I have several times found a tincture of the berries effectual in removing soreness of the gums, throat, and ulcerated mucus surfaces generally, and there can be but little doubt of this
remedy being Homœopathic to all such cases.

Rhus Venenata in Erysipelas.

Was called to treat a lady, aged 38, of lymphatic temper-
ment, who had been suffering from a vesicular eruption upon the
face and hands. Her face was much swollen, as were her hands,
arms, and lower extremities. She complained of intolerable itching and burning. The arterial excitement was marked, the pulse
was full and bounding. Gave Aconite, 3d dilution; first, ten
drops in half a tumbler of water, teaspoonful every hour, till perspiration became somewhat profuse, then gave the 3d decimal attenuation of Rhus tox., with little effect. After this gave the 3d
decimal of Rhus venenata, and after a few doses the itching and
burning ceased, the tumefaction disappeared, and the patient soon
recovered.

Pepsin for Dyspepsia.

Although we have no elaborate proving of this remedy, there
is a limited amount of clinical experience recorded of its use sufficient to justify a favorable consideration of its merits. Mrs. S——,
aged 51 years, had suffered much from indigestion for a long time.
Her stomach was in that condition which forbids indulgence in
an ordinarily nutritious diet without causing great pain. She no
sooner swallowed her food than the stomach would become dis-

tended and painful. Some kinds of aliment caused greater distress than others, but even the most simple and digestible would excite pain, attended with regurgitation of wind and retching. This had been so uniformly the case that she suffered daily for years, in spite of all the measures she had resorted to for relief. She was first treated with tonics and alteratives, acids, alkalies and stimulants, which neither mitigated her suffering nor caused her even a temporary relief. Afterwards she placed herself under the care of a Homœopathic physician, who prescribed faithfully various remedies which did not reach the case, and the conclusion was that she suffered from some organic lesion that remedies would not reach, and she gave up treatment for some time. Finally she applied to another practitioner of the Homœopathic school, who prescribed the 1st decimal trituration of Pepsin, to be taken in doses of two or three grains immediately after each meal. She had taken the remedy but the brief period of two weeks, when she found herself much improved. She continued the same for another two weeks and then discontinued it because her health was fully restored. Previous to this last trial she was emaciated and greatly depressed in spirits, but afterwards she gained in flesh, and exhibited a cheerfulness that betokened ease in body and mind.

Lycopersicum Esculatum in Tetter.

We know but little of the medicinal virtue of the common tomato plant, and therefore we call attention to the following case, hoping that something valuable may come out of it. *Dr. Whiteside*, formerly of Harrisburgh, Pa., and later of Philadelphia, related his own case, as follows: "I suffered for many years from an inveterate tetter on the palmer surface of both hands, and resorted to every remedial measure that seemed available to get rid of it, but derived no benefit either from external applications or internal remedies, but after the bearing season of a tomato patch in the garden was over, in using the hands to pull up the stalks while they were yet green, they became painfully inflamed, but in a few days the inflammation subsided, and with it the tetter disappeared, and never was there a sign of its reappearance afterwards." The expressed juice of the plant has been tried in similar cases with beneficial results.

52

Rumex Crispus in Diarrhœa.

In the case of a lad troubled with diarrhœa, which uniformly came on after a night's sleep, and was characterized by a succession of stools in the forenoon, attended with but little pain, Rumex 6th affected a speedy cure. And also in the case of a lady subject to cough and diarrhœa past midnight. She was frequently awakened about two or three o'clock in the morning by a tickling cough, which was followed by several profuse, offensive, and watery evacuations. After trying several remedies which failed to cure her, Rumex 6th was given with good effect. I have found this remedy useful in the treatment of children suffering from diarrhœa worse in the morning, when no cough was present, and when the stools were of a dark and colliquative character.

Rumex C. in Cough.

During the prevalence of an epidemic catarrh which prevailed in Chicago in November, 1864, which appeared to implicate both the Schneiderian and mucous membrane of the larynx and bronchiæ, characterized by tickling and constant inclination to cough, *Rumex crispus* in the 30th attenuation was found generally useful and curative. And here it may be remarked, that this remedy will prove effectual in most cases of catarrh that are worse in the morning, when there is an inclination to sneeze and cough from a sense of titilation in the nares, trachea or bronchial tubes, and particularly when there is simultaneously a diarrhœa, as from a cold, causing thin and brownish evacuations.

Spigelia in Neuralgia of the Face.

Mrs. H——, aged thirty-five, had been suffering, during a cold, damp spell of weather, with severe neuralgic headache and pain in the face. Atropine 3d relieved the pain in the head, but the pain in the face became excruciating, affecting the left eye, which exhibited a red and inflamed appearance, attended with extreme pain, extending deep into the socket, and was very sensitive to the light. The slightest motion aggravated the suffering. Spigelia, the 3d decimal, afforded prompt relief. This remedy seems appropriate for general use in neuralgia of the trigemini *in cold, damp weather*, and it is seldom prescribed under such circumstances without beneficial results.

Spigelia in Disease of the Heart.

Miss E——, aged twenty-three, was subject at times to syncope, accompanied by pain in the left shoulder, hurried respiration and quick pulse. Her face exhibited a bluish paleness, and the heart's action was violent and oppressive. In listening to the sounds of the heart, a wheezing, short and quick, resembling somewhat the sound produced by a hand bellows, could be distinctly heard. The young lady suffered much from a sense of fullness in the head, and at times with headache extending to the vertex. Gave Veratrum viride and Digitalis with scarcely any effect, after which Spigelia the 3d was given in drop doses, and repeated every two hours. After taking the remedy a few times, the heart's action became less violent and the pain in the shoulder disappeared. The remedy was continued at intervals of three hours, and under its use the patient became stronger and felt much better in every respect. The remedy was discontinued; after a day or two the sense of fullness of the head returned, accompanied by a pain in the upper portions of the left breast. Spigelia in the 200th attenuation was prescribed, a mitigation of the symptoms followed, and the patient was more comfortable than she had been for many weeks previous, and the improvement seemed to be permanent.

Urtica Urens in Burns.

Having had several cases of severe burns to treat, I have witnessed the effect of this remedy as being salutary in allaying the febrile symptoms when administered in the 6th attenuation internally. I have also seen the best results from its external use as a lotion when there are no abrasions of the skin or destruction of the tissues.

Veratrum Viride in Convulsions.

This remedy has been employed with the most salutary results in the treatment of convulsions in children. When they occur during dentition and follow in rapid succession, apparently jeopardizing the life of the child, a few doses of the 6th decimal attenuation have sufficed to bring about a permanent cure. *Dr. W. H. Burt*, who was one of the most prominent provers of this remedy, has found it uniformly useful in convulsions arising from emotional excitement, and particularly in those of a puerperal character. In convulsions that occur during labor, he has found that a few drop doses of the tincture will very generally control the abnormal action; and in cases where they occur after the delivery, he has found it absolutely curative.

Stannum in Chronic Bronchitis.

In the personal observations which we have made concerning the treatment of this very common disease of the temperate regions of the globe, reference has been had to the recent pathology of the subject. It is only within the present century that the pathology of chronic bronchitis has been clearly understood. In 1808 *Badlam* wrote a treatise on acute bronchitis, and soon after *Hastings* wrote on the chronic forms of the disease. Since, the mucous lining of the bronchial tubes has received the general attention of pathologists.

Acute bronchitis may terminate in the chronic form, but in very many instances the latter exists where there is no evidence of its supervening on the former. The symptoms vary materially, but in every case there is a cough, differing in character and intensity, but generally more marked than in other diseases of the respiratory organs. The expectoration varies—sometimes it is clear and transparent, and at other times frothy—viscid, adhesive, and containing small white grains, which adhere to the vessel. Some authors have regarded these particles as indicative of tubercular disease; but to relieve the doubt, place some of them on a piece of paper and expose them to heat. If the matter is from mucus follicles, a greasy stain will be left on the paper, which will not be the case with tuberculous matter. In some cases the sputum is yellow-greenish or purulent, and generally inodorous. We have seen many cases of this kind which under our care have recovered. Great and exhaustive quantities of matter are sometimes coughed up from the lower tubes, and at other times the quantity is trifling, and the cough quite dry. In mild cases the respiration is not much affected, though sometimes it is complicated with a humid asthma, and paroxysms of difficult breathing.

The greatest suffering in chronic bronchitis is from the severity of the cough. Scarcely any signs of fever are noticed in many cases, and yet in others of a sub-acute form there is a febrile reaction, which affects the nutritive function, and results in emaciation, and ultimately in a regular heated fever.

The severe forms of the disease present symptoms like those of pulmonary consumption, and may soon wear out the life of the patient. In milder cases, individuals may be affected for years with chronic cough and expectoration without material injury to the physical health. It almost always disappears in the summer and returns in the winter. This fact has given to the disease the name of "winter cough." The prognosis of these cases accompanied by heated fever, is by no means favorable, neither is bronchitis in old people liable to pass off without making them its victims. And when the disease is complicated with pleuritis or cardiac troubles, the prognosis is not greatly in favor of the patient's recovery. The physical signs are similar to those of the acute form. The chest may be resonant throughout. The different ronchi may be heard. The vesicular murmur may be heard, as well as that peculiar rattling which has been compared to the clacking of small valves.

A married lady, aged thirty years, experienced a tickling sensation in the bronchial tubes, which she believed to be the result of inhaling some irritating vapor from the atmosphere. The tickling caused a cough which, at first, was unattended with expectoration, but the tickling and inclination to cough did not subside as she anticipated, and the irritation of the mucous membrane increased until it settled into a chronic inflammation. She then began to expectorate a white, frothy mucus, attended with no pain except from severe paroxysms of coughing. At this stage the case came under our treatment. Our first prescription was *Hepar sulph.*, 6th attenuation, in water, a table-spoonful twice a day. After two days there was a change in the expectoration, but the cough remained about the same, and she expectorated a yellowish, tough phlegm. *Phosphorus* 6th, a few drops in half a glass of water, a dessert-spoonful three times a day, was prescribed. She took this remedy for three days, and derived apparently considerable benefit. The cough was less severe, and the expectoration free, but unchanged in color. She coughed mostly in the morning. Continued *Phosphorus* 30th, after the same manner, for several days, and there was considerable mitigation. The cough and expectoration were less, and for several days she continued to improve. But, it being late in the fall, and much changeable weather, she contracted a slight cold, and had a relapse, and now the cough changed from the morning to the evening and night, and came on in paroxysms. The expectoration also changed color, and she complained of an indistinct, deep-seated pain in the bronchial tubes. *Lycopodium*, 6th attenuation, was given in water in the same way, and during the next 24 hours there was a slight improvement. The indistinct pain was removed, and the paroxysms of coughing were less exhausting and frequent, and the expectoration, though the same in character, was less. *Lycopodium* 30th continued. During the next four days she continued to improve. The cough had mostly disappeared, and the signs of complete recovery were quite satisfactory. The appetite was fair, and the strength but little impaired. She continued better for some weeks, and then had a relapse; coughed much during the night, and with little expectoration. *Hyoscyamus* 6th was given in water, as the remedies before mentioned, and the cough at night ceased altogether, and she rested well.

She had frequent relapses during the winter, and each seemed to be of a different character, and called for a corresponding remedy. At the menstrual periods, she coughed much at nights, and the expectoration was of a greenish color. PULSATILLA 6th invariably relieved the cough at these times.

When the winter was far advanced, and the March winds set in she was attacked acutely with the cough again, and was much prostrated under its influence. The expectoration was of a muco-purulent character, and very copious, and her appetite was somewhat impaired. Gave *Stannum*, 6th dilution, at first, and afterwards the 30th, two doses daily. Under this treatment, she improved rapidly until the warm weather set in, after which recovery was complete, with the exception of the predisponent left in the system, and she remained quite well until the cold and changeable weather late in the fall, when there was a palpable indication of the return of the disease. Looking forward to a winter of severe suffering, she, with her husband, spent the winter in Florida, and by this means she escaped the severe relapses which were sure to be her lot in the frigid climate of the

North. In the spring after the weather became warm, she returned home and remained well ever after for several years. This case presents an argument in favor of the influence of protracted warm weather in effecting the cure of chronic bronchitis.

Sulphur in Chronic Bronchitis.

A preacher of the Society of Friends took a severe cold, which greatly affected the mucous lining of the bronchial tubes, and it terminated in a stubborn case of chronic bronchitis, which persisted in spite of treatment from early fall till the warm weather of the succeeding spring. For two successive winters he had been treated Allopathically with cough syrups and expectorants, which only palliated the severity of the disease. Not deeming it practicable to repair to a warmer climate, he concluded to hazard another winter at his home in Eastern Pennsylvania. He was much better during the summer, and until the fall, when a recurrence of his disease was inevitable. Being called upon to take charge of his case, we found him, Sept. 10th, suffering greatly from a suffocative cough and copious expectoration of tough, white, viscid mucus; quite weak and emaciated, with swollen feet. *Sambucus* 3d was our first prescription, to be given in drop doses, in water, every three hours. He felt better after taking the remedy twenty-four hours, and continued in about the same way until Sept. 25th, not improving under the *Sambucus* beyond a certain point; and having at times considerable suffocation from the accumulation of mucus and cough, *Phosphorus* 6th was given in drop doses, repeated every three hours, for several days. The improvement was very marked under this remedy up to a certain point, and here he remained stationary. The cough was somewhat troublesome and the difficulty of sneezing was extreme. His appetite was indifferent. *Tart. emetic* 6th was given in drop doses, in water, for twenty-four hours, after which expectoration was effected without difficulty and there was a return of appetite and the cough became different. It was a short, hacking cough, without suffocation, but exceedingly annoying both day and night. *Sulphur* in the 3d trituration was given daily for a week, at the close of which he was in all respects better, with improved strength and a good appetite; and with exercise in the open air, and great care to keep himself well clothed, he passed the cold season with but little cough, in comparative ease and comfort, and the following season he was able to attend to business. By the employment of Homœopathic remedies to ward off approaching attacks, he passed the succeeding winter in the same comfortable way. This man was an esteemed member of the Society of Friends, and in all respects a model of temperance. For four years he braved the storms of winter, and ultimately regained his health so perfectly that he went out in all weathers without experiencing the slightest injury; and he maintained that the *Sulphur* was the curative remedy in his case.

Baryta Carb. in Asthma.

A widow, aged 65 years, had been troubled with what she termed the "winter cough," for ten years, and during the entire time she had received only palliative relief from expectorants and cough mixtures. The constitution appeared to be good and her appetite but little impaired. She finally concluded to try Homœopathic treatment, and she came under our care. She had the following symptoms when I first saw her: A suffocating paroxysmal cough and difficult expectoration. She had no fever, but every paroxysm of coughing nearly exhausted her strength. She appeared pale, thin and emaciated, and somewhat asthmatic. *Arsenicum* 6th, was directed in drop doses, in water, to be repeated every two hours. This gave her some relief, the paroxysms of coughing were less severe, her respiration was improved and she felt less prostration than she had experienced for weeks. After *Arsenicum* had exhausted its effects we gave *Ipecac*, which still further removed the suffocative and asthmatic symptoms. We then gave *Baryta carb.*, which seemed to agree with her case, and under the use of which she bore up against the vicissitudes of the weather better than she had done during her ten years' sickness. She took no other remedies during the attack, and she remained quite well during the entire year.

Ferrum Met. in Bronchial Cough.

A clergyman of the Unitarian denomination was the victim of a congenital bronchial cough, with little or no expectoration until he had reached adult age. Coughing apparently was so fixed in his constitution that it made a part of it. Whether this

cough depended on a chronic congenital inflammation or not, we
are unable to say; but one thing was evident, that the cough
was a necessity, and with this gentleman was a standard of health.
So often did this cough excite the sympathy of friends, that
from week to week anodyne cough preparations were pressed
upon him to repress it. But whenever a measure of the kind was
brought to bear to suspend the cough, he invariably became sick,
and suffered much until his cough returned. After he attained
the age of 21 years, and while yet a pupil at the university, he
for the first time coughed up some mucus streaked with blood,
but this was after violent exercise in the gymnasium. We prescribed *Arnica* for his relief, and were not disappointed. After
taking the remedy one or two days he was cured of the expectoration, but the cough was what it had been up to that event.
The cough could be temporarily suppressed by an effort of the
will. At the age of 23 he left the university and was trained
for the pulpit; at the age of 25 he was installed as pastor of
the first Unitarian Society of S——, and preached regularly
every Sunday for seven years. By an effort of the will he could,
in the main, control his cough when speaking, but he was compelled to indulge in a complete paroxysm a short time after each
effort.

At the conclusion of the seven years it was found that
his health remained about the same, and he neither grew
better nor worse from the exercise of his voice in elocution, and
every time an attempt was made to smother his cough or suspend
it by the action of a sedative, he was made sick, and remained so
until his cough returned, and then he invariably found himself in
a normal state of health for him. From the age of thirty-two,
he began to expectorate freely. At first, mucus from the membranous lining of the bronchial tubes; and this pre-expectora-
tion attended every effort of coughing. *Phosphorus* 3rd was
given in drop doses, several times a day. This remedy, like those
taken by him before, did not palliate his cough, but it seemed to
diminish the expectoration for a time, and then it returned in
another form. The sputum was tinged and streaked with blood,
and appeared to be a mixture of mucus and blood. He at the
same time looked pale, and was exceedingly debilitated. *China*
was now given in the 3rd dilution in water, ten drops to a gill,
and a dessertspoonful every two hours, which gave temporary re-

lief to all the symptoms except the cough. After taking the *China* his cough seemed to assume an asthmatic character, for which *Ipecac* was prescribed, and relief of the asthma was followed by the same old cough, purulent expectoration, which was very copious and exhausting to vitality. He rallied again under the use of *Calcarea*, and afterwards *Ferrum met.*, and was able to labor quite regularly until 37 years of age, coughing and expectorating moderately all of the time, when a sudden development of worse features of the disease, in the form of quick consumption, terminated his life. The interesting features of this case are the imperative necessity for the cough, and the action of remedies in changing the character of the expectoration.

Dioscorea in Chronic Bronchitis.

A cure of chronic bronchitis after an attack of measles: The subject was 17 years of age when she was attacked with measles of a severe type, with excessively severe cough, which manifested itself several days before the eruption appeared. The cough, in a great measure, subsided when the eruption was the most marked. It is worthy of mention, however, that the eruption was unusually tardy in making its appearance. After recovery from the measles, a bronchial cough remained as a sequel. She coughed most when lying down, and expectorated considerable; complained of chilliness, and rigors down the back, and also pain in the head, with more or less fever every day. *Belladonna* 6th was prescribed with satisfactory results; the pain in the head ceased, the chilliness and rigors disappeared, and the cough was less painful; expectoration of mucus continued. Observing that the cough was aggravated on lying, and better when sitting up, gave *Hyoscyamus* 6th, at intervals of two hours, and continued the remedy for several days, but with little benefit. Changed to *Ipecac*, and afterwards to *Pulsatilla*, but little change for the better. Gave *Phosphorus* 6th and 30th for several days, and the cough changed from its humid character to a racking cough, and considerable soreness of the chest. After this change gave *Dioscorea* 6th, in drop doses in water, repeated at intervals of two hours, and she began immediately to improve from day to day until the cough disappeared entirely, and she was able to lie down with ease. She soon recovered her normal health and strength.

Hamamelis in Pneumonia.

A gentleman aged 31, had a severe attack of pneumonia, and was treated by an Allopathic physician. A cough remained after the pneumonia passed off, which settled into a chronic form, and for six months he was treated with cough mixtures and expectorants, from which but little benefit was derived. A temporary palliation, at best, was all that could be claimed for this resort. Not deriving any permanent benefit from this treatment, he was induced to try Homœopathy. The case presented the following symptoms: A dry bronchial cough, which for most of the time was quiet during the night, but came on in the morning in paroxysms, and continued at frequent intervals through the day. Every time a paroxysm occurred, the head would ache as if it would split. The coughing each time was attended with soreness, and heat of the chest, but seldom with perceptible fever. *Bryonia* 3rd, ten drops in half a glass of water, was given in teaspoonful doses, and repeated immediately after each paroxysm. The result of this prescription was decidedly favorable. The cough became less painful, and was unattended with the pain in the head, and more or less expectoration followed, which at first was frothy and white. *Bryonia* 30th was then given for three or four days, at intervals of two hours. The patient continued to cough and expectorate mucus somewhat frothy and white, without further mitigation. *Lycopodium* was substituted for the *Bryonia*, a dose three times a day. After four days the expectoration changed to a thick yellow sputum, while the cough, not painful, continued, and evinced no sign of disappearing. *Stannum* 30th was substituted for the *Lycopodium*, and a drop to a dessertspoonful of water was given half an hour before each meal. The cough became better under the use of this remedy, but there was a tendency to chilliness, and fever, and night sweats, for which *Carbo vegetabilis* was prescribed, and to be administered in the same form as directed for *Stannum*. The patient found great relief from this remedy, and seemed to be rapidly improving until a fresh cold aggravated the cough to a degree that brought on hæmorrhage, from the rupture of a small vessel, and for this *Hamamelis virginica* was prescribed with salutary effects; the hæmorrhage ceased, the abrasion healed, and the consequent soreness was no longer felt. There was a gradual improvement from this time, and final recovery was the result.

Without citing other cases illustrative of the possibility of curing permanently these chronic bronchial inflammations, we would suggest that much depends upon the hygienic treatment that should accompany the medicine. When the patient is able to go about, or away from home, it is necessary to be well protected with suitable clothing, and especially over the chest. The Scotch chest protector, which consists of a felt covering for the chest, attached to an elastic band to fit around the neck, is useful. Fresh air, or out-door exercise is to be commended, but in cold weather it is of the utmost importance to avoid sitting in a cold room, or standing in a cold, damp place.

Belladonna in Chronic Laryngitis.

We seldom meet with this disease in very young children, unless it supervenes upon some acute malady, such as scarlatina, measles, diphtheria, or croup. It is mostly confined to persons of middle age, and more frequently it affects men, and less frequently women. According to our observation, chronic inflammation of the larynx is a secondary affection. It is usually preceded by some acute form of the disorder, or a cold. It may proceed from talking, singing, or other causes, and is sometimes perfectly curable, while at others it is accompanied by an irritative fever, and gradually increases in severity until the patient dies. I have found the following remedies of service in treating the disease:

Causticum acts favorably in allaying a chronic inflammation of the larynx, when there is a racking cough and chronic hoarseness. A case of chronic hoarseness and pain in the larynx, of six months standing, was radically cured by this remedy.

Belladonna.—In treating chronic laryngitis, I have often observed that slight exposures would provoke acute aggravations, such as stitches in the larynx, with much inflammation and soreness; and, also in sudden attacks of hoarseness, feeble, low voice, hollow, dry cough, and sometimes with paroxysms of suffocation, or croupy cough, *Belladonna* has afforded great relief, and for these acute aggravations we need a remedy that will act promptly in subduing capillary congestion. Nothing is more likely to have this effect than *Belladonna*, and, although the chronic form of the malady remains, the cough is not so painful. According to my observation, other remedies should follow *Belladonna*. If there is an irritative fever, and there is all the appearance of

laryngeal phthisis, *Carbo vegetabilis* should follow *Belladonna*.
I have found *Carbo animalis* an excellent remedy when there was
a cough with greenish expectoration and pneumonia of the right
lung, degenerating into suppuration, while at the same time the
larynx seemed to be chronically inflamed.

Hepar sulph. calc. is one of the remedies which I have found
indispensable in mitigating the severer forms of chronic laryngitis. It will generally remove, or mitigate, a racking or painful cough. It will cure a croupy cough; more or less soreness
of the throat. I have observed that soreness of the throat, implicating the larynx, and sometimes quite painful in subjects
that have become victims of the mercurial cachexia, is speedily
relieved by Hepar sulph. In laryngeal consumption, when
the cough is rough and the expectoration of muco-purulent
matter is considerable, *Hepar sulph.* gives great palliative relief.

Iodine, in scrofulous subjects, and where there is more or less
hectic fever, I have found serviceable in chronic laryngitis, and especially when the trachea is also implicated, and there has been
long standing hoarseness and croupy symptoms.

Kali bichromicum, in chronic laryngitis, where there is pain
and titillation in the larynx, with dry cough day and night, or
cough, with expectoration of tenacious phlegm, is a valuable
remedy.

Drosera.—In some cases of chronic laryngitis after measles,
where there has been considerable hoarseness with spasmodic
cough, I have known this remedy to effect a cure.

Mercurius vivus, and *M. solubilis*, in chronic laryngitis of
those who suffer from dry, racking cough, stiffness of the neck,
and occasional expectoration of blood, have been found useful.
When chronic laryngitis is the sequel of intermittent fever, and
there is cough caused by tickling in the throat, that sometimes
induces retching or vomiting, I have found *Natrum muriaticum* a
curative remedy.

Phosphorus cured a case of chronic hoarseness and aphonia
in a gentleman, aged 32 years, who had for many months been
suffering from the disease.

Sepia, *Sulphur* and *Spongia* are also valuable remedies that
have been employed against chronic laryngitis.

It must be borne in mind, however, that the treatment of
this malady under the most favorable surroundings, with remedies,

does not always promise a cure. They often mitigate and relieve the most distressing symptoms after an irritative fever sets in. In constitutions free from hereditary taint, they often effect a radical cure.

Hepar Sulph. in Acute Laryngitis.

A young man, 24 years of age, contracted a cold, which first affected the Schneiderian membrane and afterwards the mucous lining of the larynx. There was some fever and a peculiar tickling, a slight degree of soreness and burning in the throat, which coughing and talking aggravated. The voice was altered and hoarse, every articulation was characterized by a deep, metallic sound. The patient complained of pricking and heat, and a sense of constriction, quite severe after speaking or coughing, or when pressure was made upon the larynx. There was scarcely any expectoration. The cough dry and hard. Aconite 6th was given, four globules dry on the tongue, and the dose was repeated every hour during the evening.

At 9 A. M. the next morning the patient began to expectorate mucus tinged with blood. Belladonna 6th was given hourly, in doses of four globules; previous to the administration of this remedy the fever had become more apparent and a gentle perspiration had occurred, and the pain in the larynx was violent and stinging. After several doses of the remedy had been given, the severity of the symptoms was less, and the expectoration of mucus was increased, but the cough was painful and distressing. Belladonna 6th was continued until the following morning. All the symptoms except the cough were considerably mitigated. The appearance of the sputa was somewhat changed and was of a greenish color. Belladonna 12th was given through the day, and towards evening the hoarseness increased almost to complete aphonia, but there was less soreness and more rattling of mucus in the larynx. Hepar sul., 6th attenuation, was given every two hours during the night; this was followed by a partial relief of the hoarseness and rattling of mucus; at 10 A. M. the cough was less painful; talking did not increase the distress of the patient. The expectoration was difficult on account of the tenacity of the mucus. Tartar emetic, 6th, was given and repeated in two hours, and that removed the difficulty and the patient expectorated more freely and continued quite comfortable through the day; at night

the cough increased, and was allayed by a single dose of Hyoscya-
·mus 3d, in water, after which the patient passed a better night
and in the morning was much improved. A slight soreness of
the throat returned, which was promptly relieved by Belladonna.
Deglutition from the first was more or less difficult and the patient
could take no food except that which was entirely divested of
roughness, such as custard, etc.

When the convalescence of this patient became fairly established, he sometimes complained of chilliness and great sensitiveness to cold. Mercurius sol. gave relief in this respect and also
removed the remaining soreness of the throat. The patient now
progressed rapidly toward health, which was fully regained in a
brief period.

It has been observed that acute laryngitis is much more
common in males than females, and in adults between the age
of 21 and 40 years, nevertheless we have met several interesting
cases in females, and we here append this description and treatment.

Moschus in Laryngitis.

Miss F. E., aged 35, was constantly impressed that her throat
was too sensitive to allow any cold air to come in contact with it,
and consequently she kept it wrapped with several layers of flannel during the cold season. She rode in an open buggy for several hours, in a cold wind, and after which she complained of
soreness of the throat, with pricking sensation in the larynx,
which was so sore she could not bear any pressure upon it. She
felt languid and chilly, her pulse considerably accelerated, and at
times she complained of headache, and considerable heat and fever.
The voice at first sounded rough and hoarse, soon became extinct
and complete aphonia and constriction of the larynx lasted for
several weeks. There was much of the time a complete prostration, the patient being unable to sit up. It was exceedingly distressing for her to speak in a whisper, and coughing almost suffocated her. Deglutition was rendered difficult by reason of the
pharynx being somewhat implicated. She constantly held her
hand to the throat and looked wild and anxious. The mucous
membrane of the larynx was so completely coated with a tenacious
sputa, coughing could not dislodge it, and its persistency excited
some fears that hæmatosis might be interrupted. Finding consid-

erable arterial excitement and dry, hot skin, my first prescription
was Aconite 6th, in water, given every hour. After the sixth
dose the skin became soft and moist, but there was no mitigation
of the pain in the larynx or improvement of the voice. Gave
Mercurius jod. 3x trit., in small powders every two hours during
the day without any perceptible relief. All the symptoms, except the moisture upon the surface, remaining the same, I gave
Kali bich. 3x trit., in water, teaspoonful every hour. The pain
and soreness of the larynx was some better, but the aphonia remained the same, and the patient was unable to sit up, or take
much nourishment. Continued the remedy for several days, and
changed to Hepar sul. 6th, and then to Hepar sul. 3d, and then
to Hepar sul. 200th, but derived but little advantage. Followed
Hepar sul. with Causticum 3d, 30th and 200th, with beneficial
results. The expectoration became free and the sense of constriction was greatly relieved, but still an effort to talk was attended by great distress and fatigue. Continued Causticum 200th
as long as the patient seemed to improve, which was for an entire
week. The patient had now been in bed four weeks, and was
but very little improved, and it was greatly feared that her disease would become chronic. Gave Jodium in different attenuations, and also Spong., and still the hoarseness remained persistent.
The patient complained of a pain in the back of the neck and was
exceedingly wakeful. She scarcely closed her eyes in sleep for
several days and nights. Gave Moschus 3d in water, a teaspoonful every two hours. She very soon felt better, the appetite returned, deglutition was performed without difficulty, the hoarseness began to mitigate and the cough dislodged chunks of mucus,
yellowish and thick. The voice showed signs of returning and
some words were audibly spoken, much to the joy of her friends.
When the dryness and tenseness of the mucous membrane became
lubricated and expectoration became profuse almost to suffocation
Tartar emetic was given with decided benefit. The patient began
to improve in strength, as the laryngitis left and she fully recov
ered.

This lady unquestionably predisposed herself to the protracted illness from which she suffered, by keeping too much
warmth around the neck. It is known from observation that
those who expose the neck in cold weather are less liable to
laryngitis than those who act upon the mistaken idea that it is
necessary to keep the neck warmly clothed.

Causticum in Laryngitis.

Miss R——, aged 20, had attended a meeting of the church choir, exposed to a snow storm, and indulged for some hours in vocal exercise. On returning home she experienced a slight tickling and pricking in the larynx, accompanied by cough and expectoration. During the night there was dryness and soreness of the throat and some fever. Hoarseness, and a deep cough set in, having a croupy sound. Articulation became difficult as the hoarseness increased. The voice became extinct, and the patient could not speak above a whisper. All the while she had complained of soreness of the throat and pricking in the larynx. Aconite 6th was first administered for an entire day, five drops in half a tumbler of water, a teaspoonful every hour, after which there was less fever. Hepar sul. 6th was given after the Aconite, and before the termination of another twenty-four hours the character of the cough was changed, and the dryness gave place to a whitish mucus expectoration in which there were no streaks of blood. Hepar sul. was continued, and during the next twenty-four hours the soreness and pricking in the larynx nearly disappeared, and the cough was less severe. The patient remained much the same for one or two days, expectorating considerable tough, greenish mucus. The cough was worse at night. Gave Hyoscyamus 6th, two or three doses at intervals of two hours. The expectoration increased in quantity, and quite a number of lumps of thick, heavy mucus was thrown off, and yet there was no restoration of the voice. Causticum 30th and 200th were given with good effect, and the hoarseness gave way, and the patient was able to speak aloud. Observing the caution not to indulge in conversation, she gradually recovered her normal health.

Hepar Sul. in Laryngitis.

Caused by speaking for a long time in the open air. The patient was very hoarse and complained of great soreness in the larynx, and fever. Aconite 6th was given first, and afterwards Hepar sul. 6th; recovery took place readily under the use of these remedies.

We have also seen many cases of acute laryngitis in singers —caused by excessive use of the voice, and Hepar sul. in most cases will cure. The slightest catarrhal inflammation of the

53

larynx will bring on hoarseness, but seldom aphonia. Hepar sul. has usually proved an excellent remedy.

Acute laryngitis in adults, if properly treated at first, generally terminates favorably, but if neglected it may become so formidable as to jeopardize the life of the patient. We have known several cases to terminate fatally from an accumulation of mucus in the larynx and trachea, interrupting the process of hæmatosis.

Acute laryngitis in children is generally complicated with tracheitis, and assumes the form of croup, which is an inflammation of the larynx and trachea, resulting in a copious exudation upon the mucous membrane. The causes that operate in the production of the disease are obscure, and as attacks often occur in warm weather, it is by no means certain that exposure to cold, or the extremes of temperature can be classed among the causes; so far as observation can be relied upon, the frequent attacks of croup occur in children from two to seven years of age, who may be suspected of some hereditary scrofulous taint.

Kali Bich. in Laryngitis.

A child aged three years, whose mother had died of consumption, was observed to be dull and languid for several days, was suddenly seized at midnight with a paroxysm of acute fever, hoarse, rough cough, and a filling up of the larynx and trachea, rendering respiration laborious and difficult. The symptoms were so alarming that prompt measures were required, and Aconite 3d was given in drop doses every twenty minutes; after an hour and forty minutes, drop doses of the 3d of Spongia were given every fifteen minutes. This gave temporary relief, and the child fell asleep; after an hour it awoke with coughing peculiar to the disease, with increased difficulty of breathing. The 3d trit. of Hepar, dissolved in water, was given every twenty minutes by the teaspoonful, until the respiration became less difficult, and the choking was relieved. The child fell asleep again, and awoke in the morning quite free from all croupy symptoms. Another attack occurred in the afternoon more formidable than the previous. Kali bich. 3d trit., dissolved in water, was given in teaspoonful doses every twenty minutes. The child threw off a large quantity of mucus and lymph, and seemed effectually relieved, and the next morning seemed bright and playful. The remedy was continued at intervals of an hour, until it was evident that the disease was conquered. Care was taken afterwards, to avoid exciting causes, and the child escaped further trouble from the disease.

Tartar Em. in Croup.

A little son of C. P. K., Esq., aged two years, became hoarse and croupy from almost any exciting cause. His father was an asthmatic subject, and his mother was feeble and cachectic, and their little son was, on the whole, far from being strong and vigorous. His nurse had observed for some days that he was indifferent about his playthings, and wanted to be held in her arms, and yet he ate and slept as usual. Without any previous exposure, a severe attack of croup came on in the middle of the night; all at once he became hoarse, and coughed frequently. Being called immediately, I observed that his breathing was very labored, and that a profuse perspiration was standing upon the face, and that the trachea and larynx were rapidly contracting. Gave Tart. emetic, 3d trit., about five grains in a half a tumbler of water, and a teaspoonful every ten or fifteen minutes. The effect was almost magical, as the disease seemed to be arrested at once. The medicine was continued for more than an hour, when the little fellow went to sleep. He breathed better and better, until he awoke quite relieved. He had attacks subsequently which the same remedy promptly removed.

Bromine in Membranous Croup.

Child of S. L. S., aged one year. Although lively and playful till within four or five days of its extreme illness, was observed to droop and appear languid and feverish. A slight hoarseness was perceptible, and a short, dry cough. The nurse gave a few pellets of Aconite, and afterwards the child refused its food and had great difficulty in swallowing. The cough became rough and caused the child to cry out with pain at each paroxysm. From this it was concluded that the child had a sore throat, and probably inflammation of the larynx. Belladonna was given, 3d centesimal, and still the child grew worse. On the fourth day the disease suddenly developed into membranous croup, which threatened to be speedily fatal. The child's breathing was so difficult and laborious that its face and head were constantly dripping with perspiration from the exertion. Tartar emetic, 3d trit., dissolved in water, was given—a teaspoonful of the solution every fifteen minutes. After a few doses the breathing was slightly improved, and remained so for several hours. At midnight there was an alarming struggle for breath, the throat having filled again; every respiratory act was heard distinctly all over the house, varying from a loud rattling to a whistling sound. The countenance was pale and evinced extreme distress. A very copious perspiration stood upon the child's face and head, and its strength seemed to be failing. Gave Spongia, 3d dilution, ten drops in half a tumbler of water, a teaspoonful every fifteen minutes for awhile, and then gave the higher attenuation in the same way, and there was apparently no relief, and a change was made to Kali bich. 3d, ten drops in half a tumbler of water, and given in the same way. A perceptible amelioration followed. The crude Kali bich. was put in boiling water and the vapors allowed to impregnate the air of the room. Under this treatment the child grew better very gradually, and in the morning discharged several portions of false membrane, and continued better for most of the day. At evening the throat partially filled again and the distressing symptoms, though less violent, returned. The same measures and remedy were repeated, and evidently to some advantage. The night was more favorable than the preceding, and the child's countenance wore a lively expression in the morning. It coughed up additional portions of membrane, which the nurse took from its mouth in strings, and yet the respiration was loud and rattling. The improvement through the day was not much. At night another change of remedy was made. Bromine 3d, ten drops in half a tumbler of water, was given in teaspoonful doses of the solution every twenty minutes, with satisfactory results. The breathing was relieved, the cough became loose, and the child's skin became warm and moist, and he was playful in the morning, though exceedingly weak and inclined to sleep. There was no aggravation of symptoms the following evening, and the night was passed with no return of alarming symptoms. The child continued to improve from day to day until he was entirely well.

Bromine in Catarrhal Croup.

A child two years and a half old, son of S. R., was observed to be fretful and languid for many days, and frequently would drop off to sleep, surrounded by his playthings. On the 6th of February, in the afternoon, he coughed some, and acted as if his throat was sore. In the evening he commenced with a deep, croupy cough and a physician was called. The child was quite feverish, his pulse rapid, and the skin hot and dry. He gave three globules of Aconite, and repeated the dose several times, at intervals of thirty minutes. There was no mitigation of the alarming symptoms; on the contrary, they grew worse. He then gave Spongia, and remained with the child during the night, and the symptoms seemed to be worse in the morning. February 7th, 9 A. M., Hepar sul. 6th, was given frequently, and without producing any improvement. The child remained about the same until the next morning. After due consideration he gave Iodine 6th, and though the child grew no worse, there was no perceptible improvement. On the 9th of February he gave Tartar emetic, and still there was no change, except that the child's breathing became harsh and severely asthmatic. On the 10th and 11th, Kali bich., 6th, was persistently given, prepared in water, and administered every half hour, and yet the symptoms remained about the same. At the request of the parents, I was called as counsel. I thought the remedies had been well chosen and faithfully administered. I found, on critical examination, that a pseudo-membranous deposit was evident, which I feared would prove fatal, as the remedies which had been given had failed of affording relief. I suggested Bromine, 3d dilution, ten drops in a gill of water, to be given in teaspoonful doses every twenty minutes. This remedy acted like magic. A perfect absolution from all the alarming symptoms followed at once, and the child soon recovered. Two years after, when the little boy was four and a half years old, he had another attack. He was treated by another physician, whose prescriptions were made with admirable judgment. Being called upon to assist him also, I arrived just in time to witness a fatal termination of the case.

In most cases of catarrhal croup, I have found Aconite and Hepar sul. all the remedies required. When spasmodic and suffocating, Belladonna has proved useful. Let me remark here, that the higher potencies in my hands, have proved, for the most part, efficient in the treatment of the various forms of croup, if well-chosen. In the most violent cases of membranous croup, I have relied more upon the low attenuations, and perhaps from a morbid fear that the high would not have a sufficiently speedy effect in relieving the respiration.

Argentum in Chronic Laryngitis.

A gentleman of 35, a professor of elocution, became the victim of chronic inflammation of the larynx, which disabled him for nearly two years, and most of the time he had been under medical treatment. After duly studying his case I gave him Argentum met. 30th, which gave partial relief. I followed it with Argentum 200th, and he improved until the inflammation left and he felt quite well.

Causticum in Chronic Hoarseness.

A case of chronic hoarseness after an attack of acute laryngitis was entirely cured by Causticum 30th.

Hepar Sul. in Laryngitis.

A lady accustomed to exercise her voice in singing, first experienced a slight soreness of the larynx, afterwards it increased in severity until she found it impossible to sing or converse long without becoming hoarse, while at the same time she suffered from pain in the throat, which was continuous. For more than two years she suffered in this way. She was finally cured by Hepar sul. 30th.

According to my observation, au acute attack of laryngitis, even if the patient fully recovers, leaves behind a predisposition to the chronic form which must be carefully watched. All exciting causes should be studiously avoided. When talking fatigues, it is time to desist, and the same is true with regard to singing, while at the same time too much clothing around the neck is a detriment. We have occasionally, though rarely, met with cases of chronic laryngitis in persons of feeble constitution, where spasm of the glottis would occur after contracting a fresh cold. This would be noted by great difficulty of inspiration, and a hissing sound when the air is drawn in by the act, while at the same time expiration would be attended with but little difficulty. To remove the acute suffering attendant on this condition, Ignatia, Moschus and Sambucus, in the 3d attenuation, are useful remedies. We have also observed that this difficulty is not uncommon in feeble children inclined to croup. With such the attack comes on suddenly, awaking the victim from sleep about midnight. They have to sit up in order to catch breath, as they can only make short, hissing inspirations. Ipecacuanha, Sambucus and Arsenicum are remedies found to afford relief.

Belladonna in Acute Bronchitis.

A boy eleven years old had been experiencing a feeling of malaise for several days; began to complain of a succession of creeping chills, and afterwards a dryness of the nose and throat. A dry, spasmodic cough attended with a raw or sore feeling of the chest; his breathing was somewhat oppressed and for several days there was no expectoration. He complained of pain in the head, which the cough aggravated. Bryonia 3d, was given in drop doses every two hours, and after the fourth dose he began to expectorate a yellowish, tenacious mucus, still, complaining of the chills creeping down his back. Belladonna 3d was then given in the same way, and after two days the expectoration became more copious, white and lumpy. The chills ceased, the soreness of the chest disappeared, the cough gradually subsided, and the boy recovered.

Belladonna in Cough.

A plethoric gentleman, aged forty-six, was exposed for several hours to a damp snow-storm, from which at the time he felt no particular inconvenience. Before retiring at night he felt dull and heavy, with some aching of the limbs, and without any other indications a violent chill suddenly came upon him. This chill was followed by a comparatively moderate febrile reaction and a slight acceleration of the pulse, a severe headache, and some rheumatic pains in the back and lower extremities, and motion was generally followed by chilliness, a sense of great weariness, and inability to remain out of bed. The next development of the difficulty was a sore, burning pain in the chest, under the sternum, that rendered full or normal inspiration quite painful. At the same time a cough set in which greatly aggravated the suffering.

It was dry and not attended with hoarseness or any expectoration at first. The pulse became more accelerated, the skin hot and dry, and the breathing greatly oppressed. Aconite 6th was given in drop doses every hour during the dry stage of the cough, and until there was some moisture upon the skin and some expectoration of a greenish yellow mucus. The pain and soreness of the chest remained and was worse towards evening, and the head ached as if it would split at every paroxysm of coughing. Gave Bryonia 6th, in drop doses, every hour, and the next day the pain and soreness of the chest was much better and the cough occasioned less pain in the head. Continued the remedy every two hours. The appetite was entirely gone, the tongue was coated, and there was at times a sense of constriction across the chest. Belladonna 6th was given in drop doses in water, at intervals of an hour. A few doses produced a very beneficial result, and the patient afterwards coughed and raised without soreness or pain. He continued to improve, and found himself quite recovered after an illness of nine days.

Nux Vom. in Acute Articular Rheumatism.

A young gentleman aged 30, of sanguine temperament, became greatly fatigued from a protracted struggle to reach home by travelling on foot through a deep snow, and while in a state of general perspiration from the exercise, allowed himself to cool off in a northeast wind, at the termination of his journey. For several days a vague feeling of general malaise and slight catarrhal symptoms came over him, attended with dry skin and considerable fever, and this was followed by pain and swelling of the knee and ankle joints. For some days the arterial excitement increased, and his suffering became more and more intense. His bowels were constipated, his tongue coated with a thick, white coating. He was frequently covered with a copious acrid perspiration, and the slightest movement caused him to cry out with pain. His pulse full and hard, and the action of the heart somewhat violent. His first prescription, Aconite 30th, to be taken at intervals of three hours, was evidently of great service in eliminating *materies morbi* from the blood, as it promoted a warm perspiration for twenty-four hours, and a perceptible diminution of the pain in the swollen joints. The Aconite was continued until the warm perspiration ceased, and the pains were superceded by stiffness of the joints and some of the muscles. Nux vom. 30th was then prescribed, and given at intervals of three hours. Rapid convalescence followed the use of this remedy.

Arnica in Rheumatic Fever.

A robust gentleman, aged 44 years, had indulged in several glasses of hot whiskey punch, and became much heated in a warm room, and perspired freely. In order to cool himself, he went into the street when the thermometer stood several degrees below the freezing point. The result was a sudden check of perspiration, followed by an acute attack of articular rheumatism. For several days after this exposure to the extremes of temperature, he suffered from chilliness and pains in the larger joints, and particularly in the knees. He had considerable fever, and was inclined to sleep at first, but after a day or two his sufferings became so acute, that to sleep was impossible, and he spent a succession of days and nights in morbid wakefulness; much of the time his fever was so intense, and the pain in his joints so great, that the bed clothing was kept wet with perspiration of a strong acid odor, while mentally he was much bewildered, and often quite delirious. Aconite was administered quite frequently to subdue the arterial excitement; it had a good effect. He complained of severe pain in the back, his urine was highly colored, yielding a thick, reddish sediment; his joints, at first so excruciatingly painful, had now become enormously swollen and less painful; his appetite was quite impaired, and his bowels constipated. Pulsatilla 6th was given at intervals of two hours after the Aconite, from which he derived much benefit for a while, and then the pain and swelling would recur again. In this way the patient lingered along for six weeks—better and worse—with a greater or less amount of fever every day, and so sensitive to touch that he would cry out with pain when the bed was touched, or when the floor was shaken by any one walking in the room. The fever finally passed off, and the perspiration ceased, leaving great soreness and stiffness of the joints, and accessory muscles. Rhus tox. 6th was now given for two days, at intervals of three hours. The stiffness passed off, but the soreness remained. The knee joints ceased to be painful, but were so weakened and relaxed that the patient could not stand without assistance. The least exertion seemed to quicken the action of the heart and produce laborious respiration. Arsenicum 30th was given, and recuperation followed, but there still remained a dull, sore pain in the renal region, which was cured by a few doses of Arnica 3d. So severe had this case of rheumatic fever been, that even after all obstacles had been removed to a return to health, much time elapsed before the patient fully regained his health, or all appearance of soreness was banished from the joints.

In these cases we find evidence which goes to confirm the views of *Liebig*, that a sudden check of perspiration from cold when the body is fatigued, throws back upon the system the lactic acid and lactate of ammonia which otherwise might have been eliminated. This view of the case, together with the group of symptoms that ensue, naturally suggests the employment of eliminating remedies, and where there is a full and bounding pulse, dry skin, and pain in the joints, Aconite from the 3d to the 30th, may be employed with advantage, because it promotes perspiration. But when there is much renal suffering, and a soreness as if bruised, Arnica will have a curative action, and in cases of nephritis supervening upon rheumatism, and particularly where minute renal calculi are supposed to produce some mechanical injury in the ureters, producing the most excruciating pains, Arnica has afforded speedy relief.

Sulphur in Chronic Rheumatism.

Chronic rheumatism, in an adult, aged 55 years, characterized by stiffness of the joints and pain in the lumbar region, that interfered greatly with the exercise of rising up or sitting down, was cured by Sulphur 30th.

Kali Hyd. in Acute Muscular Rheumatism.

A gentleman exposed to hard manual labor, after a severe cold, suffered from an attack of acute muscular rheumatism which affected the muscles of the upper and lower extremities, as well as those of the neck and back. He was unable to move without great pain; his tongue was considerably coated, his appetite impaired, and his skin was hot and sensitive. His pulse was full and rapid, his urine was highly colored and deposited a brownish sediment; his bowels were constipated, and his head ached considerably, the pain being of a dull, heavy character. Aconite 3d was given first to subdue the fever; its effect was satisfactory in producing a copious acid perspiration and in changing the character of the pulse. Bryonia 3d was then administered at intervals of two hours for a day and night, but he still was unable to move without some pain. Nux vom. 3d was then given in the same way for twenty-four hours. In the meantime his bowels were moved and his suffering was less when turned from side to side in bed. But he still complained of great pain and stiffness of the muscles of the neck and back. China 3d was given with no good result. Macrotin 3d was also prescribed, as was Phytolacca, without producing beneficial results. Belladonna 3d relieved the pain in the head, neck and back, but failed to relieve the upper and lower extremities. Kali hydriodicum 3d was then given, after which the patient was generally better. This remedy was continued for several days and he continued to improve to a certain point and then remain stationary. Caulophyllin 3d was given with good effect, after which the suffering subsided, leaving the patient very weak. China 3d was given again for a day, at intervals of two hours, and the strength began to return; the appetite was restored, and there was a gradual improvement until completely restored.

Nux Vom. in Chronic Rheumatism.

A laboring man, aged 27, of sanguine temperament, had been several years a victim of chronic rheumatism in the back that interfered with stooping or sitting. A single dose of Sulphur 3d, was given, and no improvement for forty-eight hours. Nux vomica 3d was then given, every four hours, for several days, and there was a perceptible improvement. The Nux was continued at longer intervals and the patient still improved. No other remedy was employed and the patient fully recovered in twenty-five days.

It would seem that when the skin fails to excrete, an increased task is thrown upon the kidneys, materially deranging the function of these organs, and if these organs fail, the lactic acid accumulates in the blood, and probably acts as a ferment in producing more of this, or its kindred lithic acid, and its compounds and products. In inflammatory subjects they excite rheumatic fever. In cachectic persons they have a different effect, producing miliary fever, erysipelas, or pemphigus, and in more torpid frames,

they produce local rheumatism or gout. All these cases are remarkable for the acid character of the cutaneous and renal excretions. In the low forms of rheumatism, oxalic acid is supposed
to constitute the *materies morbi* in the blood, especially those of
a neuralgic kind. It would seem, therefore, that such remedies
should be employed as will carry on the work of eliminating these
poisons from the blood, which has to be accomplished through
the kidneys and skin. But in order to select the proper remedies,
we must understand the pathogenesis of those that are known
to excite the action of these organs in healthy persons. Of these
we may name Aconite, Arnica, Bryonia, Calc. carb., China, Hyoscyamus, Hellebore, Ignatia, Kali hydriodicum, Nux vomica,
Pulsatilla, Rhus tox. and Sulphur.

Bryonia in Pemphigus.

A lady aged 30, rode under the scorching rays of the sun on
a hot summer's day for several miles, was much fatigued and
perspired freely, laid herself on the ground in the shade to get
relief, and being of a scrofulous habit, she contracted a cold,
which checked the perspiration, and for twenty-four hours she
suffered the most excruciating pains all over her body, and violent chills running down the back. A violent febrile reaction
occurred, which brought out large blisters on her face and neck,
and on some unexposed parts of her body. This was a case of
pemphigus. Bryonia 6th was given every two hours. She commenced perspiring, and the secretion was of an offensive acid
odor, and so was the urinary secretion. No other remedy was directed, and she fully recovered in four or five days.

Belladonna in Erysipelas.

A lady, unmarried, walked several miles in the heat of the
sun, and when thus fatigued and perspiring, she went into a
spring-house and took cold; a chill followed with a violent headache, fever and rheumatic pains. These were followed by erysipelas of the face, which became enormously swollen. The skin
was dry and hot; her pulse greatly accelerated and weak. Gave
Bell. 6th every three hours continuously until the headache and
chills ceased and convalescence became established.

Belladonna in Chills.

A little boy aged 12, of scrofulous parents, after a hard play with his schoolmates, went into an ice-house, and had a chill, which was followed by a distressing headache and vomiting of greenish biliary matter. A violent fever set in, and brought out a miliary eruption all over the body. Aconite 6th was given, and repeated at intervals of three hours, until he began to perspire. The same acid odor characterized the secretion of the kidneys and skin. Bell. 6th was then prescribed, and this was followed by general relief; the headache passed off, and he recovered rapidly.

Bryonia in Acute Rheumatism.

A cachectic child, three years old, always at play, while fatigued threw himself down to rest upon a cold floor and fell asleep. On awakening the little fellow had a violent chill, and cried bitterly with pain. His head was hot, his face began to swell, his limbs were painful and swollen. He vomited several times, and his fever was so intense that alarming cerebral symptoms began to show themselves. He was quite delirious. His skin was hot and dry. The swelling of his face continued until both eyes were closed, and a few blisters began to show themselves on his cheeks; Aconite 6th was given every hour, and still his skin remained parched and dry, and he passed but little urine, which was strongly tinctured with an acid odor. Gave Calc. carb., a dose, and in two hours after gave Bryonia, after which he broke out in a warm perspiration, decidedly acid. No other remedy was required; the Bryonia gave prompt relief from suffering, and the little boy recovered.

From the cases cited it would seem evident that cold is the most common exciting cause of rheumatism, acute and chronic, of erysipelas, exanthemata and gout, where the system is rendered impressible by fatigue and perspiration; and, moreover, that the various characteristics of these maladies are mainly attributable to the difference in the constitutions assailed, as matter in the blood may proclaim its presence in the form of rheumatism in some, of urticaria in some, of eczema in some, of psoriasis in some, and in some it may take the form of gout. Both the exciting and predisposing causes are precisely the same.

Change of Climate for Asthma.

A young gentleman, aged 20, who had been a sufferer from frequent and repeated attacks since the age of puberty, at his home in Kentucky, found complete absolution by removing to Illinois.

A lady, aged 60, who passed the menopausial period at 40, was a victim to frequent attacks of asthma from this period so long as she resided in Philadelphia; but upon a change of residence to Brooklyn, L. I., her asthma left her and she has remained quite free from it since.

A young unmarried lady suffered intensely from successive attacks of asthma when residing upon the shore of Lake Michigan. Her sufferings were never completely relieved, but only mitigated by remedies. She finally married and removed to one of the cities upon the Atlantic coast, and soon after recovered entirely, and permanently.

A gentleman, now past 60, has nearly all his life suffered from distressing paroxysms of asthma, with brief intervals of rest; has removed from place to place, a score or more of times, hoping to find some climate or atmosphere that might exempt him from the suffering, but as yet he has found but little in the way of relief. He has tried almost all kinds of asthmatic remedies with a like result. He has tried electricity and magnetism. He has smoked saltpetre cigarettes and stramonium leaves. Vomited himself with Ipecacuanha and Lobelia, but all to no purpose. He now remains the disconsolate victim of the disease, proof-hardened against all manner of remedies. This case shows that even change of climite does not always prove salutary.

A young lady who had been a sufferer from a child with frequently recurring paroxysms of asthma, was sent by her parents to the hot springs of Arkansas, hoping that the change of climate and the influence of bathing would effect a favorable change in her condition, and these efforts were so far crowned with success that her paroxysms became lighter and less frequent. But on returning to her home in Chicago there appeared to be an augmentation rather than a diminution of her attacks. A trip to Lake Superior in midsummer was recommended, and the bracing atmosphere of that region afforded unmistakable relief.

Inasmuch as we have no satisfactory ætiology of this disease, we can make no generalization respecting the cause. Yet we are safe in making the following prognosis: In the early stages but. little impression is made upon the general health, but if left to go on without being in some measure controlled, oft-repeated struggles to bear up against the paroxysms wear so heavily upon the vital forces that other complications set in, such as dropsy or heart-disease, and a fatal termination is the frequent result. But are there no remedies that can be affiliated to mitigate, if not cure, these distressing cases, wherever they may be found? We think there are, and a brief account of beneficial results from well-chosen Homœopathic remedies may prove of practical benefit.

Kali Hyd. in Asthma.

A stout, plethoric gentleman, who for years was in the habit of flying to stimulants to afford him temporary relief at night, without which he declared his inability to assume the recumbent posture during an attack, which usually lasted from four days to two weeks. He had resorted to many remedies without effect. He had swallowed Lobelia emetics, Tartar emetic, Ipecacuanha and Sulphated zinc, until he was disgusted with the mention of them, and still they made no favorable impression upon the disease. He had been nearly smothered in vapor baths, and had passed through a purgatory of perspiration and rubbing under the skillful administration of the Turkish bath, time after time. He had smoked stramonium leaves and tobacco, until disgusted with this fog of his own creating. He had tried the effects of galvanism and other forms of electricity, and all to no purpose. A solution of the crude Kali hydriodicum, sixty grains to a pint of rain water, was prescribed to be taken persistently in dessert-spoonful doses four times a day. He had not taken up the first pint before he found benefit. Sixty grains were then ordered to be dissolved in a quart of rain water, to be taken, four doses daily, as before. He persevered in taking this solution for fifty or sixty days, and found to his satisfaction that he could breathe easier, and that his respiration was free from that wheezing which had annoyed him constantly before. He found that ascending stairs, or rapid walking, did not provoke a return of the suffering, as had been the case before. A third sixty grains was ordered in a quart and a half of water, and he was recommended to persevere· in taking four doses daily as before. Under the use of this last prescription he fully regained his health, and for more than five years has had no return of the malady.

Kali Hyd. in Asthma.

A lady who had not enjoyed a respite from asthmatic suffering for a longer period than two weeks for years, although her attacks had been mitigated by Arsenicum and some other remedies. Being still a sufferer to some extent, at our urgent request she entered perseveringly upon the use of Kali hydriodicum. She was directed to take a teaspoonful of a solution of twenty grains in half a pint of water, every three hours, except when it interfered with sleeping or eating. The relief which she gradually obtained induced her to adhere to the directions for several months, and though she was not absolutely cured, her relief was great, beyond her anticipations, and for the last two years she has had comparatively little suffering from the disease. And here it may be remarked that no other remedy, Homœopathically indicated, seemed to have a beneficial effect.

Kali Hyd. in Asthma.

A gentleman aged 50, a victim of inflammatory rheumatism and frequent attacks of asthma, went to Europe for his health. When in England, he was advised to take the 3d trituration of Kali hydriodicum, three times a day, in grain doses. He did so, and after a time his rheumatism and asthma both left him; and though in damp weather, or when laboring under the effect of cold, he experiences some slight return, he nevertheless has been comparatively well for the last seven years.

Kali Hyd. in Congenital Asthma.

A young infant afflicted with congenital asthma, was cured with the 6th attenuation of Arsenicum, given in daily doses of two globules. When a year and two months old, it had an attack of asthmatic croup, which proved very obstinate. Ipecac, 6th, was first given, and then Tart. emetic, 6th, but without much effect. Spongia 6th, and Kali bichrom. 6th, seemed to be followed by no encouraging result. Kali hydriodicum 6th was followed by partial relief, and the child remained to all appearances in a stationary condition. The 30th attenuation of the same remedy was given, without material change. The 3d attenuation was given, and the child began to improve, and soon recovered.

In the cases cited above, except the last, the patients had all suffered in some degree from inflammatory rheumatism, and this may be the reason why Kali hydriodicum proved so signally useful. Another class of asthmatic patients, treated with this remedy, have derived no advantage. In those cases which seem to be void of any humid characteristics, I have found Arsenicum useful, and sometimes curative. In a few cases complicated with hydrothorax, Apis mellifica, 3d attenuation, has afforded great relief; and in those cases characterized by increased action of the heart, Digitalis, either the 3d or 6th, has palliated the suffering and rendered the respiration less difficult.

In several cases of asthma, in weak, cachectic constitutions, subject to sudden attacks of laborious respiration from cold, I have found Belladonna essentially beneficial, and in all cases where the asthma is accompanied by fever and an indication of capillary congestion in the bronchial tubes, I have found the 3d or 6th of Aconite, followed in an hour by the 3d or 6th of Belladonna, to have a beneficial and satisfactory effect.

In those cases preceded by paroxysms of coughing at night which end in paroxysms of asthma, Hyoscyamus 6th will generally afford relief. In persons affected with chronic bronchitis, and subject to attacks of humid asthma, no remedy acts more promptly in giving temporary relief than Tartar emetic, and especially when the patient is suffering from impotency and feebleness, for the want of proper nourishment. Arsenicum and Ipecacuanha, of the 6th attenuation, given alternately, will generally palliate the sufferings of an acute paroxysm of asthma, even if they do not cure. There is a satisfaction to be gained in this respect, even when remedies fail of radically curing the patient.

Rhus in Typhoid Fever.

In the latter part of June last, we were called upon to treat the case of a merchant aged 40 years, of nervous sanguine temperament, who was taken with severe pain in the occiput and lumbar region, with constant thirst, and tongue furred with thick, yellowish-brown coating, entire loss of appetite, and extreme
54

wakefulness. The urine was highly colored, and deposited a thick, brown sediment of nearly the color of coffee grounds.

Under the use of Belladonna and Rhus tox., the pain in the head and back ceased about the ninth day; the coating upon the tongue remained; the patient continued wakeful and restless; very much prostrated, but complained of no pain. The coating upon the tongue, intense thirst and severe prostration seemed to indicate the use of Arsenicum, which was given in the 3d attenuation until the thirst abated, and a copious warm perspiration followed, after which the patient was somewhat relieved, and experienced a slight return of appetite.

In the meantime an adult patient in the adjoining room, taken sick about the same time, and as near as we could learn, with very similar symptoms, and who had been placed under heroic treatment, died. The event operated to depress our patient very much; his spirits became depressed, his countenance sunken and pallid; he became emaciated and unable to eat or sleep. The coating upon his tongue had nearly disappeared, although it was red with a dry streak through the center, exhibiting an inflamed and cracked appearance. Under the use of Calc. carb. 6th, administered every three hours, this condition disappeared; all the while the patient was unconscious of having slept. The bowels having remained constipated and unmoved, an enema of soap and water was ordered, which moved them freely.

For several succeeding days the patient appeared more comfortable, although he had fever every afternoon, and a slight perspiration at night. For this condition Merc. 6th was given every six hours, for three or four days, without perceptible change, except that the patient felt a little stronger. Four weeks had now elapsed, and the patient had continued to lose flesh, and there was no evidence of a decided break up of the fever. During the whole time he declared he had not slept. There being a slight tendency to diarrhœa, and a little bleeding at the nose, Rhus 6th was given every three hours, until the tongue became moist and there were no further indications of diarrhœa and nosebleed. The patient remained apparently in this state for nearly two weeks, when all traces of fever appeared to be gone, the appetite returned, unmistakable signs of convalescence ensued; in a few days after, the patient left his room, relieved of thirty-six pounds of his accustomed weight, which under the auspices of a good appetite and renovated powers of nutrition, he soon regained with more than legal interest. From the commencement of this case there was but a slight acceleration of the pulse.

Bry. and Rhus in Typhoid Fever.

A young lady of 14 years, of nervous temperament, in the same house, was taken with severe pain in the sinciput and sickness at the stomach; thick white coating upon the tongue; not much thirst; the pulse was somewhat rapid but feeble; under the use of Aconite, followed by Belladonna, she was relieved of the pain in her head about the fifth day, until which time she had not slept. On the sixth and seventh days she slept continuously. The center of the tongue became dry and of a brownish color. There was considerable tendency to diarrhœa and epistaxis. She sunk into a kind of torpor and prostration, which continued for nearly a week, during which time she had Bry. 2d and Rhus 6th in alternation at intervals of three hours. She took but very little nourishment during the time. Then ensued a more marked degree of fever in the afternoon, and a copious perspiration at night, after which her tongue became dry and moist at intervals, until her fever abated entirely, after which her appetite returned and she soon regained her usual health.

Aconite in Typhoid Fever.

A little girl, aged 8 years, was taken with a chill, which lasted about four hours, after which a fever ensued, which was attended with intense thirst; a dry red tongue, slightly coated; constipation of the bowels, and at times severe pain in the abdomen, which was distended and tympanitic. The fever continued for nearly a week without intermission, and only a slight mitigation early in the morning of each day. She had several attacks of bleeding at the nose, and frequent seasons of comatose sleep; under the use of Aconite 6th her fever somewhat abated. About the ninth day she broke out into warm perspiration, and her bowels moved. From this time she rapidly recovered. Aconite, Bryonia and Phos. having been employed in bringing about the change, and China after the fever had subsided.

Arsenicum in Typhoid Fever.

A young gentleman from Providence, R. I., had been traveling in the Valley of the Mississippi, and contracted a diarrhœa
which continued until he arrived in Chicago—a period of sixteen
days. Enfeebled and overcome by exertion, a fever began to
manifest itself as soon as he took lodgings. We were called upon
to prescribe in his case the 4th of August. Our first prescription
was Phosphorus 6th. He then complained of dull pain in the
region of the umbilicus, which was accompanied by dark watery
discharges from the bowels, exceedingly offensive. The Phos. appeared to relieve the pain in the bowels, and the stools became
less frequent. The fever increased, the pulse became weak and
fluttering; great thirst; cold moisture at times made its appearance upon the skin. Under the use of Arsenicum 3d, these symptoms disappeared, and he complained of being starved. He was
so weak that he could not lift his hand to his head. His face was
flushed with fever, his thirst could not be satisfied, and at the
same time he begged for the strongest kind of food, declaring
that he would starve unless he had it. Believing this appetite to
be morbid entirely, we endeavored to satisfy him with rice, mutton
broth and toast, which he would devour after the manner of
a beast of prey, and then mutter starvation. We continued the
use of Arsenicum 3d every two hours until satisfied that a change
was indicated, then we substituted China in the place of Arsenicum. Under the use of this remedy the morbid appetite disappeared, as did also the diarrhœa. But for four hours each
morning for several days, he would lie as cold and motionless as
if dead, and then a reaction would take place, and his skin would
become warm; during the night he would have little or no perspiration till near morning, and then a cold clammy sweat would
remain for some time upon the surface of his body. In view of
his great prostration, and apparently increasing fever, his case
appeared to be desperate. We increased the dose of Arsenicum,
followed by China, 3d decimal of the former, and the tincture of
the latter, and he began to rally. His pulse began to acquire
volume, his bowels became regular, and after a period of thirty-
five days he was able to help himself out of bed, and in a few days
more he began to walk out. In addition to the remedies prescribed in his case we directed vigorous friction over the surface

of body and extremities with a coarse towel, which had a beneficial effect. We may mention, however, of this case, that he had been under powerful medication under what is sometimes called the thorough treatment before he came under our care. This, added to the naturally torpid condition of his biliary system, and the palpable indications of an ulcerated condition of the mucous coat of the bowels, rendered the case altogether a difficult one to treat.

Phosphorus in Asthma.

A middle aged gentleman, subject to asthmatic difficulties, had been troubled with looseness of the bowels for several months, and every afternoon and evening a perceptible degree of fever. Much of the time he had experienced a dull pain in the region of the umbilicus—to the right. When called on to prescribe for his case, the following symptoms were present: Flushed face, laborious respiration, dry tongue, a dark streak in the center, coating otherwise thick, of a greyish color, a dry, racking cough, dull pain in the head, very much aggravated when coughing, an inclination to drowsiness, though frequently aroused by the cough. He complained of burning in the palms of the hands. His bowels became constipated after a dose of the 6th of Phosphorus, and the fever and drowsiness at first increased. A second dose of the remedy was given twelve hours after, and this was followed by a mitigation of the cough and fever, the tongue became moist, and the greenish coating began to disappear from the tongue. A third dose was given in twenty-four hours, and the patient continued to improve. No other remedy was given. A complete change in his system was apparent and he soon attained his accustomed health.

Merc. Viv. in Typhoid Fever.

A gentleman, aged 49, contracted a severe cold in a damp cellar. This cold soon ripened into a settled fever of considerable violence. A physician was called and he ordered a brisk cathartic, and the patient sunk into a low typhoid, which alarmed his family, and the first physician was superseded by two others of the same school, who resorted to an equally prostrating treatment. The right side of the patient became paralyzed, his speech was interrupted, and he gave indications of great prostration otherwise. He lay in a semi-conscious state, eyes half closed, his respiration was labored and difficult. His physicians expressed the belief that he could not survive twenty-four hours, and that his case was hopeless. His family, anxious to try other skill, again superseded his medical attendants by physicians of the Homœopathic school. After learning the history of the case, and in view of the extremely prostrated and unconscious condition of the patient, they gave but little encouragement to hope for any beneficial result from their treatment, but expressed a willingness to try. He had been ill twenty-eight days, and when the treatment was changed he exhibited the following symptoms: Hemiplegia, involuntary discharges from the bowels and bladder, apparently unconscious, pulse 100 per minute, tongue thickly furred, difficult deglutition, sunken appearance of the countenance, incoherent utterances, offensive breath and aphthous condition of the mouth. Sulph. 6th was given in the evening, and the following morning he was more conscious, and was able to take a little nourishment. In view of the aphthous condition of his tongue, Mercurius viv. 6th was given at 10 A. M. At 7 P. M. his tongue and mouth seemed to be in a better condition; his bowels had not moved, and there was evidently less prostration: Merc. viv. 6th continued. At 10 A. M. next morning, was informed by his nurse that he had slept considerable, and had taken beef tea, and the signs of recuperation were quite satisfactory. He had acquired sufficient strength to express his wants distinctly. He continued to improve for more than a week, and gave encouraging signs of recovery. On the thirty-seventh day of his illness he was unable to evacuate the bladder, which was considerably distended. A single dose of Hyoscyamus 3d removed this difficulty. There was an aggravation of the aphthous condition of the mouth that interfered greatly with his taking food. The dry and cracked appearance of his tongue suggested the employment of Nitric ac. 3d, which acted kindly; and for another week he barely held his own. During this time he had but little fever, and was greatly prostrated. China 6th was first administered, without effect, for two days, and then China 30th, and still no beneficial result. Arsenicum 6th and 30th, were given with like result. His bowels remained constipated, his skin was moist, but he was restless and wakeful. Sulph. ac. 3d was given, and this was followed by temporary relief, but he soon relapsed, and a troublesome and ominous hiccough set in. He had now been three weeks under Homœopathic treatment, which, at times, gave promise of ultimately promoting recovery. The paralysis, which his return to consciousness gave favorable indications of disappearing, now seemed aggravated, and this, with the incessant and violent hiccough, did not promise anything favorable. After studying his case thoroughly, and trying several remedies without effect, it was decided to give him Moschus 3d, and repeat the dose every two hours until the remedy was fairly tried. After the second dose the hiccough mitigated, and he had a respite of some hours, at the termination of which he signified his wish for the bed pan, and he had a copious evacuation from the bowels. After which he was at first much prostrated; his hiccough did not return, and for ten days he seemed much better, and his case seemed in some respects hopeful. At this period he complained of feeling cold and soon he began to shudder. A violent febrile reaction soon brought his sufferings to a close, forty days after his former physicians gave their opinion that he could not live twenty-four hours. This case is related to show the salutary effect of certain remedies in removing painful symptoms even in fatal sickness.

Arsenicum in Typhoid Fever.

Was that of an actor, age 25, who had a protracted chill, which was followed by intense fever and thirst, violent pain in the head, soreness of the muscles, pains in the bones, copious diarrhœa, and great prostration. A physician was called in who prescribed 20 grs. of Quinine, and this was followed by a temporary cessation of the diarrhœa but in other respects the patient was worse off. He sank into a col l, lifeless condition, characterized by cold, clammy perspiration, a pinched expression of the countenance, and a return of the diarrhœa after a respite of one day. All the while he had intense thirst, violent headache, entire loss of appetite and intense weakness. His physicians dealt out to him several crude drugs in a vain attempt to change his condition. A coma came over him and he lay for several days in a stupor, at times breaking out in a wild delirium. His bowels continued to move frequently, with profuse watery discharges of an exceedingly offensive odor. The sordes began to collect about his teeth, and the corners of his mouth became sore. The friends not being

satisfied with the progress, called in a physician of the Homœopathic
school, who inquired particularly into the history of the case,
and noting the symptoms present when called in, prescribed
Arsenicum 3d, to be repeated every two hours. In twelve
hours it was quite evident that the diarrhœa was lessening
and the character of the stools changed. This remedy was
continued, and in twelve hours more there was a moisture
upon the tongue, and the comatose condition was also disappearing. Ars. 6th was then given and repeated as before.
The patient gradually returned to full consciousness, his diarrhœa
diminishing until his bowels were moved none too frequently, and
his stools of a normal character. The remedy was discontinued
after the fifth day, as the patient complained of no thirst, and there
was less prostration and less fever, with all the signs of convalescence established. He was directed after the fever had disappeared, to take two doses of China each day until he was able to
leave his bed and room, which occurred on the fourth week of his
illness.

Phosphorus in Typhoid Fever.

A child, aged 5 years, was seized with a chill which lasted
all the morning, and was followed in the afternoon by a high
fever, great restlessness, pain in the head and chest, and general
perspiration. A second paroxysm of the kind occurred in a few
hours, and even a third after this, all within thirty-six hours, and
then a continued fever set in characterized by pains through the
temples and over the orbits, considerable nausea, tongue coated
white, and occasional rigors passing down the spine. Belladonna
3d was prescribed during the first paroxysm, Gelsemium 3d the
second, Atropine 3d afterwards. But when the fever became
continued, and there was severe pain in the head, and at times a
tendency to vomit, which was invariably preceded by drowsiness,
the Belladonna was prescribed to be followed by Ipecac, and this
prescription relieved the head and nausea; but a short, hacking
cough, and pain in the chest, a hot breath, quick, full pulse and
labored respiration, told too decidedly that the case was ripening
into acute pneumonia. Every time she coughed her head would
ache as if it would split open, and she would place her hands to
her chest and cry out with pain. Between the spells of coughing
she would be drowsy and unconscious, and sometimes awake just

before coughing, quite delirious. Bryonia was given and continued for two days. The remedy removed the heat from the chest, mitigated the pain in the head, and changed the character of the cough. The skin became moist, the expectoration from a rusty sputa became more free and less colored. The cough, though frequent, was not so painful. Phos. 6th was then given every hour, except when she was asleep. In twenty-four hours she was free from fever, sat up in bed and called for her playthings. The Phosphorus was discontinued for twenty-four hours, and still she continued to improve; her appetite returned, and her cough gradually disappeared and finally left her. She soon regained her normal health and strength.

Tartar Em. in Typhoid Fever.

A little boy, aged 5 years, son of an eminent lawyer, was seized suddenly with a pain in his head while at school, and on being brought home a violent and protracted chill ensued; this was followed by an intense fever and deep sopor, which lasted for thirty-six hours. At the commencement of the fever his skin was dry and hot, his pulse 150 a minute, and during the continuance of the sopor his arms and lower extremities would frequently twitch. Aconite 3d repeated every hour was given to allay the arterial excitement. After the first twenty-four hours, his skin over the region of the entire body became moist, although there was no profuse perspiration. His head seemed quite free from heat except in the frontal region over the eyes. Belladonna 3d was then prescribed, and continued in hourly doses from morning to evening, when he awoke, with a restless moan and cry, quite delirious, and shortly fell into a deep sleep again. The Belladonna was continued, and about every hour, until 11 p. m., he would arouse and cry out. About midnight he became very restless, and showed some indications of pain in his chest, and yet there was apparently but little inclination to cough. In view of his restlessness, and inquietude and delirium on waking, Hyoscyamus 6th was given at intervals of an hour the remainder of the night. In the morning he had a lucid interval, and a slight hacking cough. At 10 p. m. his face became flushed with fever, and he complained of pain in his left side. Aconite was substituted for the Hyoscyamus during the continuance of the febrile paroxysm. At 10 p. m. being very restless, and his eyes having a fiery expression, Belladonna was prescribed again. After two doses, one hour apart, he quieted off to rest and was quiet until 5:30 A. M. He awoke perfectly rational, with a dry, hacking cough. At 10 A. M., Tart. emetic 3d was given, and until 1 P. M. his fever raged considerably, but when it subsided, his cough was quite loose and he complained of no pain either in his head or chest. He continued quite comfortable during the afternoon and through the night. His bowels moved quite naturally in the morning. Tart. emetic was continued at intervals of two hours. He called for something to eat, and his tongue, pulse and skin all seemed to be in good order on the seventh day of this violent sickness, which had deprived him of strength so that he could not stand upon his feet. He looked cheerful and happy, and was quite playful. He had no medicine after the ninth day, as he was free from disease, with a good appetite, and only required a little time to regain his strength.

Nux. Vom. in Antecedent Heart Disease.

The frequent occurrence of death from heart disease, so sudden and unexpected, begets an inquiry into the nature of the proximate causes of so painful and startling an occurrence. Cases are not infrequent where a man or a woman, apparently lively and in good health, evincing no concern about any physical ill that may be ripening, arrests the social enjoyment of the family circle and society, by suddenly falling prostrate in death. Every occurrence of the kind shocks the community for a time, while many suppose there may have been no antecedent cause for the abrupt flight of the vital spark.

On the first of January, 1866, Mrs. S., while receiving New Year's calls, and while in the midst of a smiling compliment of the season, or at the close of a half uttered wish of " Happy New Year " to a gentleman friend, fell to the floor in a dead and breathless faint—pulseless and cold. She had been unusually vivacious and cheerful during the early morning hours, not effacing from her pleasant countenance the gracious smile even after the spirit had fled. Nine years previous to this shocking occurrence, she was the victim of wandering rheumatic pains, or fugitive drawing pains, from muscular rheumatism which she had experienced after a protracted exposure to cold and damp surroundings. Her sufferings at that time were greatly aggravated when reposing in a cold, damp air, or when any cold, damp application to her person was made. Warm applications either wet or dry, afforded

some relief. She also suffered from pains in the left shoulder and
right hip. She was of a nervo-sanguine temperament, red hair.
She suffered for many weeks. Was finally relieved and apparently cured by careful nursing, and the third trituration of Nux
moschata. For four years she experienced no return. She even
passed through the painful ordeal of parturition five years after,
and for a year or more previous to her sudden demise, she apparently suffered but little, not sufficient to keep her in the house,
though she had occasionally rheumatic pains. These, associated
with the previous attack, lead to the conclusion that rheumatism
was the primary trouble, which probably ended in embolism and
sudden death.

Another case was that of a lad, who for some time had suffered from rheumatic pains in the lower extremities, and stiffness
of the muscles to a degree that deprived him of locomotion.
At the same time he had palpitation, and occasional syncope.
His case was diagnosed rheumatism with evident tendency by
metastasis to affect the heart. Remedies were prescribed in accordance with the symptoms, but not salutary. He died after
four days' severe suffering. An autopsy revealed a valvular
trouble of the heart. Mitral regurgitation in this case had resulted in hypertrophy.

What might have been done to avert the calamity in one so
young, cannot be told. The earliest manifestation of any disease known, in many cases, to be followed by cardiac lesions,
should at once receive the most careful and judicious medical attention. The vantage-ground is often lost by waiting for full
development of symptoms before remedies are properly affiliated.
The diseases to which cardiac suffering is secondary, must receive
early attention if eliminated before they spend their force on the
central vital organs.

So common has it been for cardiac diseases to become secondary to some form of rheumatism, that in a tabular statement
of seventy-seven cases in which a precise early history had been
obtained, thirty-four had suffered from one or more attacks of
rheumatic fever, and thirteen from rheumatic pains. Forty-seven
out of seven-seven cases would indicate the necessity of the most
skillful treatment of the antecedents of heart disease, in order
to protect the heart against their invasion.

Several cases of prostration from heart troubles have been
observed, where the victims had complained from time to time of
rheumatic lameness, but not sufficient to deprive them from attending to business. It is the manifest duty of physicians to take
charge of such cases in earnest, for this is the veritable battle-

ground. Such cases if neglected will soon gain a complete victory over medical skill, and end in fatal cardiac lesions.

W. M., aged forty years, not very temperate in his habits, had experienced more or less discomfort from rheumatic lameness, which cared but little for, was suddenly seized with severe pain in the heart, which caused him to faint, pant for breath, etc. The nearest physician was called, and from one to two dozen leeches were promptly applied to the præcordial region. These hungry and blood-thirsty worms soon gave temporary relief from the cardiac congestion. The rheumatic pains had fled as soon as the cardiac pain occurred. This case shows the intimate relation between rheumatic and cardiac diseases. The subject was under Allopathic treatment, and died soon after the palliative relief furnished by the leeches. Had this patient taken heed to the hints which his lameness gave, and subjected himself to a proper regimen and medical treatment, his life might have been prolonged.

Many fatal cases of heart disease might be cited where the victims had suffered for months, and even years, with what they regarded trifling rheumatic pains. The autopsy of Mrs. P., who fell dead in the middle of a cheerful word in taking leave of one of her friends, made by the late *Dr. Boardman*, elicited the fact that embolism lay at the bottom of the fatal result. This lady had also neglected to give herself the requisite care and treatment for more or less rheumatic suffering during the latter years of her life.

Though rheumatism is the more common antecedent of heart disease, fourteen of the seventy-seven cases before cited had not suffered from this disorder, but from indigestion or gastritis.

The late President of the Academy of Sciences, for many months previous to his decease, was subject to indescribable suffering, and during the time his pulse now and then would become so accelerated that it was difficult to count. We have been at his bedside when the pulse was beating two hundred times a minute. Such rapid diastolic and systolic motion of the heart must have had its disastrous effect. He was subject to chronic gastritis, and this was antecedent to any heart trouble, for he had suffered intensely for many months from indigestion, and ultimately from inflammation and ulceration of the coats of the stomach. Autopsy revealed the organic changes that must have taken place gradually from indigestion, and its final effect on the heart, which was greatly enlarged above the normal size.

In order to prevent a disastrous effect from dyspepsia which may fall on the circulatory organs, Nux vomica and its analogies should be consulted, and especially when complicated with hepatic derangement or obstruction in the portal system that is liable to be followed by hypertrophy of the heart.

Morbus Brightii, especially of the chronic form, is followed by cardiac lesions. The connection between renal and cardiac lesions is especially important. When structural disease affects the kidneys, elimination of the urinary solids is imperfect, and their retention results in vaso-motor irritation and obstruction to the passage of the blood through the arteries, and a demand is made on the heart for increased propulsive power, and hypertrophy is the result.

When severe forms of scarlatina are badly treated, the sequel is usually albuminuria, which is apt to become chronic and thus pave the way to cardiac lesion.

Diphtheria is a disease that requires careful management in protecting the *vis nervosa*, which too frequently becomes so diminished that nervous prostration is the general result, in which partial or general paralysis occurs, and sooner or later the heart becomes fatally implicated. When this disease first made its appearance in this country, it is said that a celebrated physician lost ninety per cent. of the cases which he treated. Afterward it is said by the same authority that ninety per cent. recovered under a continued stimulating treatment during the attacks of the disease. Inasmuch, therefore, as both scarlet fever and diphtheria may be classed among the antecedents of cardiac disease, it follows that a correct therapeusis in their earliest stages is all-important.

In all blood diseases, and particularly in the exanthems, inflammation of the arteries is liable to occur, and thence atheroma or embolism obstructing the arterial circulation, and finally ending in valvular regurgitations or hypertrophy. In some cases venous thrombosis, or coagulation of the blood in the veins, takes place in a certain class of subjects, and thence putrefaction, septicæmia and death.

It is therefore evident that nearly all the above diseases, including the zymotic, if improperly treated, may be included among the antecedents of heart disease. And here let it be remarked, that a critical study of the therapeutics required for each and every disease that may be classed with the antecedents of cardiac troubles, while yet in the periphery of the vital domain, as well as careful affiliation of remedies indicated by symptoms in accordance with the only known law of cure, it is presumed that the defensive warfare against the lethal dregs of diseases that assault the heart would, in many instances, be a triumphant success.

As prolonged study, mental emotions, anxieties and disappointments are apt to impose severe labor, and often violent palpitation of the heart, resulting in dilation of its cavities or hypertrophy, it would seem necessary to affiliate remedies for the sentient and emotive spheres, while pouring the soothing oil of religious consolation to still the troubled waters.

Diseases Which Generate Cardiac Lesions.

About ten per cent. of the cases of heart disease may be congenital or idiopathic. It is impossible to arrive at a definite conclusion concerning the condition of the heart in these cases, except by the physical signs. One of the earliest signs is cyanosis. It is known by the color of the skin, which is blue, caused by the stagnation of blood in the cutaneous capillaries and by heart disease. The therapeusis of *cyanosis cardiaca* must necessarily be palliative, even if guided by the characteristic symptoms, because when rightly interpreted they show a congenital organic defect; nevertheless pains can be somewhat alleviated by treatment.

When a child cannot be turned in bed, or suddenly moved without the appearance of being faint and sick at the stomach; or if with chilliness or cold hands and feet, with blue lips, tongue, nails and a manifestly irregular pulse, give Digitalis. If it has suffocating attacks on touching the larynx or moving the chest Lachesis may afford some relief. In older children which have a slow and feeble pulse, and whose breathing is almost imperceptible, with slight moaning, give Laurocerasus.

Non-congenital heart disease seldom commences in the heart; the *materies morbi* appear to be generated from localities remote from the heart, and if not eliminated perfectly, by imbibition they are liable to reach the heart, and be productive of cardiac lesions. Cardiac lesions in a majority of instances originate from diseases which begin in the periphery of the body. Rheumatic fever when it accompanies acute rheumatism is usually very marked, with temperature ranging from 102°, 104·, 104.9° F. in exceptional cases, but generally the temperature rarely exceeds 100° or 101° F. during the fever. The pulse in some instances becomes accelerated to 100 beats a minute, but more frequently its rapidity is not much above the normal. The heart palpitates and the respiration is often accelerated. The skin takes on an additional degree of heat and transpires profusely without producing amelioration. Acute rheumatism may attack the synovial membranes of the joints, which generally become inflamed and swollen. From the acute the chronic form may originate. *Acute muscular* rheumatism has its seat in the muscles.

It is well known that the synovial membranes of the joints are composed of the same anatomical elements that enter into the structure of the pericardium and endocardium. This consideration renders it probable that a metastasis or transfer of the inflammation to a similar structure to that of its primary location might occur, and therefore to successfully defend and protect the heart and its surroundings, arthritic rheumatism and synovitis should receive prompt medical and hygienic treatment as soon as the primary symptoms and fever become apparent. A gentleman of sanguineous temperament, aged forty-five, complained of debility and malaise and occasional chilliness, succeeded by fever, accompanied by pain in one or several joints, which soon began to swell and redden. The swelling relieved the pain partially. The disease did not remain stationary in the joint first attacked. It traveled from one to another until nearly every joint in the upper and lower extremities became implicated and even the cervical and spinal articulations were beset with pain of an excruciating character and almost unendurable from the slightest motion; and yet, being tortured by restlessness, he was compelled to move even if it caused the greatest suffering. The fever in this case ran very high, and the temperature was several degrees above the normal; the pulse was full and tense, but not rapid; murmurs were heard in the cardiac region, together with an audible palpitation. The respiration was considerably accelerated. A profuse, warm, acid perspiration was eliminated from the skin, which afforded no relief. The urine was scanty, and loaded with urea and uric acid, which after cooling presented a thick deposit. We have thus been particular in presenting a record of this case, because, under the influence of rightly chosen remedies, the patient recovered from the attack in less than twenty days, and has remained in perfect health for several years. The chief remedies employed in the treatment of this case were Aconite and Bryonia. The Aconite, 3d dilution, in water, was given in teaspoonful doses every two hours, in the first onset of the fever, and Bryonia, 3d dilution, a few drops in half a tumbler of water, was given every hour or two, or three after, until the disease had finished its course. And here let it be stated that the Bryonia quelled the palpitation and murmurs, and the accelerated respiration. Judging from what we have observed in other cases, the Bryonia stayed the progress of the disease before it reached the pericardium, or brought the endocardium or its valves into its range. Up to the stage depicted in the case cited above, acute rheumatism is curable with properly affiliated remedies. When improperly treated, it may linger in the system until cardiac lesions become a secondary result.

Several years ago our esteemed colleague, Prof. T. S. Hoyne, had a painful attack of acute rheumatism, generally implicating his joints, with severe pain and swelling. After weeks of excruciating pain, he was relieved and radically cured by the frequent administration of Bryonia. Every vestige of the disease appeared to be eliminated, and for the last ten years he has not been conscious of any predisposition to another attack. This case adds to the proof that rheumatism previous to, and not complicated with any organic change can be cured.

Acute muscular rheumatism which has its seat in the muscles, tendons and other fibrous tissues is attended with burning, shooting and stinging pains in the affected muscles, sometimes worse, and at other times relieved by motion. This kind of rheumatism, under some circumstances, by injudicious treatment, and faulty medication, may extend to the muscular fibres of the heart. It may occur in the muscles of the upper and lower extremities, in those of the neck, back and chest, or any other portion of the muscles, but in whatever locality, let therapeutics do its work at once. If in the lower extremities, attended with a sense of lameness, worse when at rest, and better during motion, Rhus tox. is in the center of the group of remedies to be consulted. Rheumatism in any of the muscles attended with synochal fever must be first treated with Aconite. If rheumatism has its seat in the muscles of the shoulder, Lycopodium; in the fingers, Caulophyllin. When muscular rheumatism has located itself, search for a remedy suited to the locality and symptoms.

A gentleman aged 50, who had suffered from repeated attacks of muscular rheumatism with cardiac complications, and always recovered under Homœopathic treatment, was suddenly taken off his feet by a "kink in the back," and wishing to be relieved at once he called on an old school physician, who treated him to hypodermic injections of morphine. After two weeks' confinement with this kink he sent for his Homœopathic physician, who gave him a dose of Belladonna, and the next 'day he was a sterling advocate of Homœopathic practice, and remains so to the present time. Phytolacca, Nux vom., Pulsatilla, Calcarea carb., and many other remedies are applicable in the cure of lumbago. The characteristic symptoms in each individual case, whether the pain be in the pectoral, intercostal, femoral, humeral, or muscles of any other locality, must guide in the selection of remedies.

With regard to the origin of heart disease from rheumatism, says *Peacock*, "Out of 100 cases in which a precise early history could be obtained, sixty-one occurred from rheumatism, either acute or chronic, implicating the joints or muscles, seventeen cases were secondary to indigestion without any previous rheumatic pains, four from rheumatic gout, six from scarlet fever, six from typhoid fever, five from renal disease, and in five cases the disease was evidently congenital." The estimate of *Samson* is similar, varying but slightly.

In a minority of instances endocarditis is secondary to pleuritis, pneumonia and morbus. Brightii pericarditis is more frequently secondary to arthritic inflammation. Hypertrophy of the heart generally results from valvular lesions, which result from Bright's disease. The connection between the renal lesion and the heart is obvious; for where structural disease affects the kidney the elimination of urinary solids is so greatly obstructed that their retention results in vaso-motor irritation that interrupts the passage of the blood through the capillaries, and subjects the heart to a great increase of propulsive power, and hypertrophy ensues.

Cardiac degeneration is intimately associated with hypertrophy consequent upon valvular lesions or chronic Bright's disease,

inasmuch as these processes induce degenerative changes in the
aorta, which lessen the activity of the circulation, and develop the
same difficulty in the coronary arteries. The fact of this pathological condition being so formidable as to resist the curative effect
of remedies simply argues that the antecedents did not receive
early and efficient attention. It is well known that the intemperate use of intoxicating liquors causes renal lesions and albuminuria.
Then let alcoholism receive due attention—enjoin abstinence when
the degeneracy first seizes the patient. Let Nux vom. have its
remedial effect sufficiently early to successfully protect both the
heart and arteries.

We find occasionally the initiation of heart disease from
scarlet fever. An error in the treatment of this formidable
disease may be the cause of sequellæ, which ripen into dropsy
and Bright's disease, and are liable to operate insidiously in
producing cardiac degeneration. Simple albuminuria, anasarca
and local dropsies in their incipiency often yield to remedial
treatment, with Apis mel., Apocynum, Asclepias and their analogues.

Any disease dependent on some morbific principle, whether
epidemic, endemic, sporadic or contagious, which acts disastrously
in the circulatory system, if not carefully eliminated may result
in atheroma or thrombosis, and thence in cardiac lesions. Diphtheria and other zymotic diseases, the major exanthems, typhoid
fever and pyelitis have in many instances been the antecedents
of heart disease. It will be seen that idiopathic affections of the
heart are rare compared with those generated by disease, at first
remote from the center of the circulation. So varied are the diseases that directly or indirectly end in organic heart troubles,
either from negligence or maltreatment, it would seem requisite
to affiliate a correct treatment for each in the earliest stage of its
manifestation. When cardiac lesions are known to be secondary
to certain specific diseases, and if these diseases are not aborted
or cured prior to their extreme development, this fact alone would
indicate the necessity for the most critical therapeusis in the onset
of such as are liable to inaugurate a series of disturbances in the
circulatory system which have a direct or indirect action on the
heart. And inasmuch as any invasion of disease is expressed by
symptoms which indicate the efforts of nature to eliminate from
the system the *materies morbi* that have invaded and deranged the

vital forces, it is manifestly plain that no other aid than the selection of remedies whose pathogenetic symptoms are similar to those presented by the disease is acceptable assistance to nature in her struggles. The reason is the similarity existing between the pathogenesis and the symptoms of the disease, showing that the medicinal action will be in the direction of nature's struggles, and thus a positive aid to her eliminating efforts. It is impossible to estimate the good that can be accomplished by a critical adherence to that law of cure expressed in the formula, *similia similibus curantur*. Such a course would undoubtedly prevent many diseases in the periphery of the body from encroaching on the vital domain, and ultimately with disastrous and fatal effects.

INDEX.

A

Abscesses, 723.
Abdominal typhus, 553.
Acute bronchitis, 341.
Acute cystitis, 495.
Acute rheumatism, 503.
Accumulation of serous fluid in the nervous centres, 614.
Acne, 513.
Aconite in arachnitis, 795.
Aconite in pneumonia, 804.
Aconite in chills, 808.
Aconite in typhoid fever, 851.
Accumulation of wax in the ears, 723.
Adipous diarrhœa, 230.
Adults, spasm of the glottis in, 334.
Affections, dropsical, 323.
Affections of the heart, Ignatia in, 778.
Affections, choleroid, Iris versicolor in, 779.
A general view of the structure of the body, 87.
A general view of health and disease, 45.
A general view of physiology, 97.
Agents cognizable in causing disease, 49.
Agents non-cognizable in causing disease, 57.

Ague, irregular, 541.
Ague, dumb, or marked, 540
Air in the pleura, 431.
Alcohol in chronic ottorhœa, 775.
Albuminuria, 485.
Alienation, mental, 674.
Amaurosis, 713.
Amenorrhœa, 747.
Amblyopia, 713.
Aneurism, 452.
Ani, prolapsus of, 209.
Anginæ, the, 323.
Anginose, scarlatina, 324.
Angina, pectoris, 448.
Anginosa, scarlatina, 525.
Anæsthesia, asphyxia from, 435.
Anæmia of the nervous centres, 604.
Anthrax, 522.
Apoplexy, 606.
Apoplexy, nervous, 614.
Apis mellifica in intermittents, 775.
Arteries, diseases of the, 461.
Arteries, inflammation of the, 461.
Arteries, ossification of the, 462.
Arsenicum in Bright's disease, 774.
Argentum in chronic laryngitis, 838.
Arnica in rheumatic fever, 841.

Arsenicum in typhoid fever, 852.
Arsenicum in typhoid fever, 855.
Asiatic cholera, cholera asphyxia, 220.
Asphyxia, 432.
Asphyxia of new-born infants during uterine life, 434.
Asphyxia from anæsthesia, 435.
Asthma, 403.
Asthma, thymic, 474.
Asthma, Lobelia inflata in, 782.
Attack, liability to a second, in diphtheria, 323.
Atheroma, 463.
Atrophy of the spleen, 274.
Auscultation, 277.
Augmentation of sensibility, 618.
Aurea zizia in epileptiform diseases, 776.

B

Baryta carb. in whooping cough, 774.
Baryta carb. in asthma, 824.
Belladonna in chronic laryngitis, 828.
Belladonna in acute bronchitis, 839.
Belladonna in cough, 839.
Belladonna in erysipelas, 844.
Belladonna in chills, 848.
Bilious colic, 201.
Biliary system, diseases of the, 476.
Bituminous coal in pneumonia, 809.
Blood, fullness of, 438.

Blood, paucity of, 439.
Bleeding from the nose, 730.
Bladder, diseases of the gall, 482.
Bodies, foreign, in the larynx or trachea, 336.
Boils, 521.
Body, general view of the, 87.
Bronchia and lungs, diseases of the, 337.
Bronchitis, acute, 341.
Bronchitis, chronic, 344.
Bronchitis, summer, 351.
Bronchia, hæmorrhage in the, 366.
Bronchitis and pneumonia, Lachesis in, 780.
Bronchocele, 485.
Bright's disease, Ars. in, 774.
Bright's disease of the kidneys, 485.
Bromium in membranous croup, 835.
Bromium in catarrhal croup, 837.
Bryonia in pemphigus, 844.
Bryonia in acute rheumatism, 845.
Bryonia and Rhus in typhoid fever, 851.

C

Cancer of the tongue, 140.
Cancer of the stomach, 166.
Cancer of the mammary gland, 757.
Cancer of the womb, 758.
Cancer of the intestines, 205.
Caries of the teeth, 142.
Cavities, nasal, 269.
Catarrh, nasal, 294.

Capillary vessels, diseases of the, 464.
Calculi, renal, 497.
Calculi, urinary, 496.
Carbuncles, 522.
Carb. animalis in pneumonia, 802.
Carb. baryta, in whooping cough, 774.
Catalepsy, 655.
Catarrhal inflammation of the eyes, 707.
Cataract, 715.
Cantharis in dysentery, 787.
Causticum in laryngitis, 833.
Causticum in chronic hoarseness, 838.
Centers, diseases of the nervous, 575.
Cerebrum, hyperæmia of the, 575.
Cerebellum, hyperæmia of the, 581.
Centres, inflammation of the nervous, 590.
Cerebro-spinal meningitis, 602.
Centres, anæmia of the nervous, 604.
Centres, hæmorrhage in the nervous, 612.
Centres, induration of the nervous, 613.
Centres, accumulation of blood in the nervous, 614.
Centres, morbid formation in the nervous, 616.
Cephalalgia, 624.
Certain muscles, paralysis of, 700.
Chronic inflammation of the stomach, 163.
Chronic dysentery, 186.
Chronic laryngitis, 296.
Chronic bronchitis, 344.
Chronic form of pleurisy, 427.
Chronic ottorhœa, Alcohol in, 778.

Chronic cystitis, 495.
Cholera infantum, 196.
Cholera morbus, 219.
Cholera asphyxia, 220.
Chest, physical ex. of the, 274.
Character of the effusion in syphilis, 321.
Chicken pox, 530.
Chorea, 650.
Chorea, Ignatia in, 777.
Chlorosis, 751.
Choleroid affections, Iris vers. in, 779.
Chamomilla in cholera infantum 793.
China in dysentery, 789.
China in cholera infantum, 793.
Chamomilla in a case of protracted colic, 794.
Chelidonium in pneumonia, 811.
Change of climate for asthma, 847.
Circulation, diseases of the, 437.
Circulatory organs, diseases of the, 442.
Clinical notes and observations, 774.
Clonic spasms in pregnant women, 639.
Cognizable agents in causing disease, 49.
Colon, inflammation of the, 182.
Constipation, 198.
Colic, common, 199.
Colic, enteric, 199.
Colic, bilious, 201.
Colic, painless, 203.
Cough, whooping, 357.
Consumption, pulmonary, 410.
Continued fever, 534.
Continued fever, inflammatory, 549.
Congestive fever, non-malarious, 346.
Congestion of the cerebrum, 575.

Congestion of the spinal cord, 587.

Cord, spinal, inflammation of the, 595.

Cordes, palpitatio, 705.

Convulsions of children, 635.

Concerning the ears, 728.

Colchicum and Iris in dysentery, 788.

Colchicum in diarrhœa, 792.

Cramps in the stomach, 171.

Croup, 302.

Croup, Iodine in, 778.

Croup, diphtheritic, Kali bichromicum in, 779.

Cyanche trachealis, 302.

Cystic peritonitis, 253.

Cystitis, chronic, 495.

Cystitis, acute, 195.

D

Dance, St. Vitus, 650.

Death, modes of termination in scarlet fever, 323.

Delirium tremens, 672.

Dengue fever, 561.

Deafness, 727.

Diseases of the tongue, 138.

Diseases of the teeth, 141.

Diseases of the gums, 147.

Diseases of the throat, 149.

Diseases of the stomach, 160.

Diseases of the intestines, 175.

Diseases of the intestines, continued, 190.

Diseases of the peritoneum, 239.

Diseases of the respiratory organs, 269.

Diseases of the larynx and trachea, 288.

Diseases of the bronchia and lungs, 337.

Diseases of the pleura, 423.

Diseases of the circulation, 437.

Diseases of the circulatory organs, 442.

Diseases of the arteries, 461.

Diseases of the capillary vessels, 464.

Diseases of the glandiform, ganglions, 468.

Diseases of the spleen, 469.

Diseases of the mesenteric glands 474.

Diseases of the biliary system, 476.

Diseases of the gall bladder, 482.

Diseases of the pancreas, 483.

Diseases of the renal organs, 484.

Diseases of the kidneys, 485.

Diseases of the urinary organs continued, 509.

Diseases of the skin, 510.

Diseases, exanthematous, 524.

Diseases, febrile, 526.

Diseases of the nervous centres, 575.

Diseases supposed to have their seat in the nervous system, 618.

Diseases of the nerves, 693.

Diseases of the eye, 707.

Diseases of the ears and nose, 722.

Diseases of the membranous tympani, 724.

Diseases of the nose, 729.

Diseases of the male sexual organs, urethretis, 732.

Diseases of the female generative organs, metritis.

Disease, Arsenicum in Bright's, 774.

Diseases, Zizia aurea in epileptiform, 776.

Diphtheritic croup, Kali bi-chromicum in, 779.
Dioscorea in chronic bronchitis, 826.
Diseases which generate cardiac lesions, 862.
Diarrhœa, 190.
Diarrhœa, adipose, 237.
Diphtheria, laryngitis exudativa, 315.
Diphtheria and scarlatina, 322.
Diphtheria and syphilitic ulcer on the tonsil, 324.
Diphtheria and erysipelas, relation between, 324.
Diphtheria and scarlatina anginosa, 324.
Diabetes, 488.
Diabetes mellitis, 488.
Diabetes insipidus, 494.
Diminution or deprivation of sensibility, 624.
Distinction between diphtheria and scarlatina, 322.
Dropsy, hydrops, 260.
Dropsical affections, 323.
Dropsy of the pleura, 428.
Dropsy of the pericardium, 445.
Dropsies, Helleborus niger in, 776.
Dumb ague, 540.
Dulcamara in diarrhœa, 791.
Dysentery, 182.
Dysentery, chronic, 186.
Dysmenorrhœa, 759.
Dysentery, Gambogia in, 776.

E

Ears and nose, diseases of the, 722.
Ears, general remarks concerning the, 728.

Eczema or herpes, 519.
Eclamsia, epileptic spasms, 635.
Eclamsia in pregnant and parturient females, clonic spasms, 639.
Effusion, character of the, 321.
Emphysema of the lungs, 400.
Emphysema, inter-lobular, 402.
Embolism, 463.
Emprosthotonos, opisthotonos, tetanus and trismus, 668.
Encephalitis, 590.
Enteralgic colic, 199.
Endocarditis, 446.
Enlargement of the heart, 447.
Enlargement of the spleen, 470.
Enlargement of the liver, 477.
Epistaxis or nose bleed, 287.
Epidemic bronchitis, 341.
Epilepsy, 643.
Epistaxis, bleeding from the nose, 730.
Epileptiform diseases, Zizia aurea in, 776.
Eruption, 323.
Erysipelas and diphtheria, relations between, 324.
Erysipelas, 510.
Erythema, 514.
Eucalyptus in erysipelas, 774.
Eucalyptus in hay fever, 774.
Examination of the chest, physical, 274.
Exanthematous diseases, 524.
Eyes, diseases of the, 707.
Eyes, catarrhal inflammation of the, 707.
Eye-lids, inflammation of the, 719.
Eye-lids, stye on the, 720.
Eye-lids, inversion and eversion of the, 720.
Eye-lids granular, eczema, tarsal ophthalmia, 421.

F

Fauces, inflammation of the, 149.
Fainting fits, swooning or syncope, 450.
Febrile diseases, 534.
Fever, continued, 634.
Fever, intermittent, 536.
Fever, intermittent, 543.
Fever, congestive, non-malarious, 546.
Fever, irritative, 547.
Fever, remittent, infantile, 648.
Fever, continued inflammatory, 549.
Fever, typhus, 551.
Fever, typhoid, 554.
Fever, relapsing, 558.
Fever, yellow, 559.
Fever, dengue, 561.
Fever, spotted, cerebro-spinal meningitis, 602.
Female generative organs, diseases of the, metritis, 744.
Fever, Apis mellifica in intermittent, 774.
Fever, hay, Eucalyptus in, 774.
Fever, hay, Gelsemium in, 775.
Fever, hay, Naphthalin in, 775.
Fever, quotidian, Ignatia amara in, 777.
Ferrum met. in bronchial cough, 824.
Fluid, serous, accumulation of, in the nervous centres, 616.
Foreign bodies in the larynx and trachea, 336.
Form of pleurisy, chronic, 427.
Formations, morbid, in the nervous centres, 616.
Functions of the living human body, 95.
Fullness of the blood or plethora, 438.

G

Gangrene of the lungs, 399.
Gangrenous inflammation of the mouth, 137.
Gangrenous inflammation of the pharynx, 156.
Gastralgia, 170.
Gastrodynia, 171.
Ganglions diseases of the glandiform, 468.
Gall bladder, diseases of the, 482.
Gambogia in dysentery, 776.
General remarks concerning the ears, 728.
Generative organs, diseases of the female, metritis, 744.
Gelsemium in hay fever, 775.
Gelsemium in pneumonia, 811.
Glossitis, 138.
Glottis, œdematous inflammation of the, 299.
Glottis, spasm of the, 332.
Glottis, spasms of the, in adults, 332.
Glandiform ganglions, diseases of the, 468.
Gland, the thymus, 474.
Glands, diseases of the mesenteric, 474.
Glaucoma, 717.
Gland, cancer of the mammary, 757.
Glands, Iodine in indurated swelling of the, 779.
Goitre or bronchocele, 458.
Gout, 507.
Gonorrhœal ophthalmia, 709.
Goitre, Iodine in, 778.
Gums, diseases of the, 147.
Gums, hypertrophy of the, 147.
Gums, shrinking of the, 148.

H

Hæmorrhage from the stomach, hæmetamesis, 169.
Hæmorrhage of the intestines, 207.
Hæmorrhoids, piles, 207.
Hay fever or summer bronchitis, 351.
Hæmorrhage in the bronchia, hæmoptysis, 366.
Hæmorrhage into the lungs, 371.
Hæmaturia, 500.
Hæmorrhagical purpuras, 522.
Hæmorrhage in the nervous centers, apoplexy, 606.
Hay fever, Eucalyptus in, 774.
Hay fever, Gelsemium in, 775.
Hay fever, Naphthalin in, 775.
Hamamelis in dysentery, 787.
Hamamelis in pneumonia, 827.
Health and disease, a general view of, 40.
Heartburn, gastralgia, 170.
Heart, hypertrophy or enlargement of the, 447.
Hepatitis or inflammation of the liver, 476.
Herpes or eczema, 519.
Hectic, intermittent, 542.
Headache, cephalalgia, 624.
Headache, sick, 628.
Heart, palpitation of the, palpitatio cordis, 705.
Helleborous niger in dropsies, 776.
Heart disease, Lachesis in, 782.
Hepar sulph. in acute laryngitis, 830.
Hepar sul. in laryngitis, 833.
Hepar sul. in laryngitis, 838.
Human body, a general view of the structure of the, 87.
Hypertrophy of the gums, 147.
Hydrops, dropsy, 260.

Hypertrophy or enlargement of the heart, 447.
Hyperæmia, 464.
Hypertrophy or enlargement of the spleen, 470.
Hyperæmia of the cerebrum, or congestion, 575.
Hyperæmia of the cerebellum, or congestion, 581.
Hyperæmia of the spinal cord, or congestion, 587.
Hysteria, 650.
Hydrophobia, rabies, 667.
Hydrophobia, 668.
Hypochondriasis, hypochondria, 689.
Hypericum perforatum, for injury and laceration of the nerves, 776.

I

Ignatia amara in quotidian fever 777.
Ignatia in chorea, 777.
Ignatia in affections of the heart, 778.
Impetigo, 513.
Impetigo, 521.
Introduction, 33.
Influence of occupation and sedentary habits and study, 74.
Inflammation of the mouth, 133.
Inflammation of the tongue, 138.
Inflammation of the velum and uvula, 148.
Inflammation of the fauces or throat, 149.
Inflammation of the tonsils, 150.

Inflammation of the pharynx, pharyngitis, 151.
Inflammation of the œsophagus, 157.
Inflammation of the stomach, 160.
Intestines, diseases of the, 175.
Intestines, inflammation of the small, 176.
Inflammation of the large intestines, 180.
Inflammation of the colon, 181.
Intestines, diseases of the, continued, 190.
Intestines, perforation of the, 190.
Infantum, cholera, 196.
Intestines, obstruction of the, 199.
Intestines, cancer of the, 205.
Intestines, hæmorrhage of the, 207.
Invermination, worms, 212.
Inflammation of the peritoneum, 239.
Intestines and peritoneum, morbid productions in the, 258.
Inflammation of the larynx, 290.
Influenza or acute bronchitis, epidemic, 341.
Inflammation of the lungs, pneumonia, 373.
Inter-current pneumonia with spinal schlerosis, 389.
Inflammation, typhoid, of the lungs, typhoid pneumonia, 395.
Inter lobular emphysema, 402.
Inflammation of the pleura, typhoid, 427.
Infants during uterine life, asphyxia of new born, 434.
Intermittent pulse, 452.
Inflammation of the veins, phlebitis, 455.

Inflammation of the arteries, 461.
Inflammation, 466.
Inflammation of the liver or hepatitis, 476.
Inflammation of the kidneys, or nephritis, 485.
Inflammatory or acute rheumatism, 503.
Intermittent fever, 536.
Intermittent hectic, 542.
Infantile remittent fever, 548.
Inflammatory, continued, fever, 549.
Inflammation of the nervous centres, 590.
Inflammation of the spinal cord, myelitis, 597.
Induration of the nervous centers, 613.
Inflammation of the nerves, neuritis, 693.
Inflammation of the eyes, catarrhal, 707.
Infants, purulent ophthalmia of, 709.
Inflammation of the eye-lids, 719.
Inversion and reversion of the eye-lids, 720.
Inflammation of the mucous membrane of the tympanum, 725.
Inflammation of the nose, nasitis, 730.
Intermittent fever, Apis mellifica in, 774.
In Bright's disease, Arsenicum, 774.
In whooping cough, Baryta carb., 774.
In hay fever, Eucalyptus, 774.
Injury and laceration of the nerves, Hypericum perforatum, 776.
Iodine in goitre, 778.
Iodine in croup, 778.

Iodine in indurated swellings of the glands, 779.
Irregular ague, 541.
Irritative fevers, 547.
Iritis, 711.
Iritis, rheumatic, 712.
Iris versicolor in sick headache, 779.
Iris versicolor in choleroid affections, 779.
Iris versicolor in chronic diarrhœa, 796.
Iris versicolor in bilious diarrhœa, 789.
Isipidus diabetes, 494.

J

Jaundice, 480.

K

Kali bichromicum in diphtheritic croup, 779.
Kali bichromicum in membranous croup, 779.
Kali carbonicum in asthma, 779.
Kali hydriodicum in rheumatism, 779.
Kali bich. in laryngitis, 834.
Kali hyd. in asthma, 847.
Kali hyd. in acute muscular rheumatism, 842.
Kali hyd. in asthma, 848.
Kali hyd. in congenital asthma, 848.
Kidneys, inflammation of the, or nephritis, 485.

Kidneys, Bright's disease of the' or albuminuria, 485.

L

Large intestines, inflammation of the, 180.
Larynx and trachea, diseases of the, 288.
Larynx, inflammation of the, 290.
Laryngitis, chronic, 296.
Laryngitis exudativa, diphtheria, 315.
Larynx and trachea, morbid productions in the, 335.
Larynx and trachea, foreign bodies in the, 336.
Laceration and injury of the nerves, Hypericum perforatum, 776.
Lachesis in chronic sore throat, 780.
Lachesis in quinsy, 781.
Lachesis in bronchitis and pneumonia, 781.
Lachesis in heart disease, 782.
Laurocerasus in phthisis and pulmonalis, 782.
Lachesis in tuberculous deposits, 808.
Leg, phlegmatia dolens or milk, 455.
Lepra, 520.
Leucorrhœa, 769.
Life, period of, 321.
Liability to a second attack, 321.
Liver, inflammation of the, or hepatitis, 476.
Liver, enlargement of the, 477.
Lobular, inter, emphysema of the, 402.

Lobelia inflata in asthma, 782.
Lungs and bronchia, diseases of the, 337.
Lungs, hæmorrhage into the, 371.
Lungs, inflammation of the, pneumonia, 373.
Lungs, typhoid inflammation of the, typhoid pneumonia, 395.
Lungs, gangrene of the, 399.
Lungs, œdema of the, 400.
Lungs, emphysema of the, 400.
Lungs, tubercles in the, 407.
Lycopodium in pneumonia, 782.
Lycopodium in pneumonia, 808.
Lycopersicum esculatum in tetter, 817.

M

Materia medica and therapeutics, 101.
Malignant scarlatina, 525.
Male sexual organs, diseases of the, urethritis, 732.
Mammary gland, cancer of the, 757.
Mesenteric glands, diseases of the, 474.
Mellitus diabetes, 489.
Measles, rubeola morbili, 521.
Meningitis, cerebro-spinal, spotted fever, 602.
Mental alienation, 674.
Membrana tympani, diseases of the, 724.
Membrana tympani, perforated, 724.
Metritis, diseases of the female generative organs, 744.

Menses, suppression of the, 749.
Metrorrhagia, 769.
Menorrhagia, 764.
Membranous croup, Kali bichromicum in, 780.
Mercurius vivus for cough, 783.
Mercurius corrosivus for sore mouth, 783.
Mercurius corrosivus in dysentery, 783.
Mercurius iodatus for nasal catarrh, 783.
Mercurius dulcis, in cholera infantum, 784.
Merc. viv. in dysentery, 788.
Merc. cor. in tenesmus, 788.
Merc. viv. in typhoid fever, 833.
Milk leg or phlegmatia dolens, 455.
Morbid productions in the peritoneum and intestines,
Modes of scarlatina terminating in death, 323.
Morbid productions in the larynx and trachea, 335.
Modified small-pox or varioloid, 533.
Morbid formations in the nervous centres, 616.
Moschus in nervous prostration, 784.
Moschus in hysteria, 784.
Moschus in laryngitis, 831.
Mucous membrane of the tympanum, inflammation of the, 725.
Mucus accumulation within the tympanum, ottorrhœa, running from the ears, 726.
Muscles, paralysis of certain, or partial paralysis, 700.
Muscæ volitantes, 714.
Myelitis, inflammation of the spinal cord, 597.
Nature and division of the causes of disease, etiology, 46.

Nasal cavities, 269.

Natrum muriaticum in herpes, 784.

Naphthalin in hay fever, 775.

New born infants during uterine life, asphyxia of, 434.

Nephrites or inflammation of the kidneys, 485.

Nettle rash or urticaria, 515.

Nervous system, 563.

Nervous centers, diseases of the 575.

Nervous centers, inflammation of the, 590.

Nervous centers, anæmia of the, 604.

Nervous centers, hæmorrhage in the, apoplexy, 606.

Nervous centers, softening of the, 612.

Nervous centers, induration of the, 613.

Nervous centers, accumulation of serous fluid in the, 614.

Nervous centers, morbid formations in the, 616.

Nervous system, diseases supposed to have their seat in the, 618.

Nervous apoplexy, 654.

Nerves, diseases of the, 693.

Nerves, for injury and laceration of the, Hypericum perforatum, 776.

Neuritis, inflammation of the nerves, 693.

Neuralgia or pain in the nerves, 694.

Niger, helleborus, in dropsies, 776.

Nose bleed, epistaxis, 730.

Non-malarious congestive fever, 546.

Nose and ears, diseases of the, 722.

Nose, diseases of the, 729.

Nose, inflammation of the, nasitis, 730.

Nose, bleeding from the, epistaxis, 730.

Notes and observations, clinical, 774.

Nux juglans in noli-me-tangere, 784.

Nux juglans in scrofulous consumption, 785.

Nux moschata for headache, 786.

Nux vomica in sleeplessness, 840.

Nux vom. in acute articular rheumatism, 840.

Nux vom. in chronic rheumatism, 843.

Nux vom. in antecedent heart disease, 859.

O

Observations on diet, clothing and exercise, 60.

Observations on ablutions, baths, including the use of water as a therapeutic agent, 70.

Observations and notes, clinical, 774.

Obstruction of the intestines, 199.

Odontalgia, toothache, 699.

Œdema of the lungs, 400.

Œsophagus, diseases of the, 149.

Œsophagus, inflammation of, 157.

Œdematous inflammation of the glottis, 399.

Oleum jecoris in rheumatism, 786.

Opisthotonos, 668.

Ophthalmia, simple, 707.

Ophthalmia, purulent, 708.

Ophthalmia, purulent, of infants, 709.

Ophthalmia, gonorrhœal, 709.

Opium in coma, 786.

Organs, respiratory, diseases of the, 269.

Organs, circulatory, diseases of the, 442.

Organs, urinary, diseases of the, continued, 495.

Organs, diseases of the male sexual, urethritis, 732.

Organs, diseases of the female generative, metritis, 744.

Ossification of the arteries, 462.

Ottorrhœa, running from the ears, accumulation of mucus within the tympanum, 726.

Ottorrhœa, alcohol in chronic, 775.

P

Painters' colic, 203.

Paucity of blood, 439.

Pain in the nerves, or neuralgia, 694.

Partial paralysis or paralysis of certain muscles, 700.

Partial paralysis, 701.

Palpitation of the heart, palpitatio cordis, 705.

Pancreas, diseases of the, 483.

Perforation of the intestines, 190.

Peritoneum, diseases of the, 239.

Peritoneum, inflammation of the, 239.

Peritonitis, chronic, 242.

Peritonitis, puerperal, 244.

Peritonitis, cystic, 253.

Peritoneum and intestines, morbid productions in the, 258.

Percussion, what is, 274.

Period of life, critical, 321.

Pericardium, dropsy of the, 445.

Pectoris, angina, 448.

Perforated membrana tympani, 724.

Perversion of the sense of smell, 730.

Perverted sensibility, 621.

Perforatum Hypericum for injury and laceration of the nerves, 776.

Petroleum in hypochondria, 786.

Pemphigus, 520.

Pepsin for dyspepsia, 816.

Pharynx, diseases of the, 149.

Pharynx, inflammation of the, 151.

Pharynx, gangrenous inflammation of the, 156.

Phlebitis, inflammation of the veins, 455.

Phlegmatia dolens or milk leg, 455.

Phthisis pulmonalis, Laurocerasus in, 782.

Phosphoric acid in a case of chronic diarrhœa, 790.

Phosphorus in chronic diarrhœa, 790.

Phosphorus in pneumonia, 801.

Phosphorus in asthma, 853.

Phosphorus in typhoid fever, 856.

Phytolacca decandra in diphtheria, 811.

Phytolacca in rheumatism, 812.

Phytolacca in swelling, indura- | Purpura hæmorrhagica, 522.
tion and abscess of the mam- | Purulent ophthalmia, 708.
mary gland, 813. | Purulent ophthalmia of infants,
Physical examination of the | 709.
chest, 274. | Pulsatilla in diarrhœa, 793.
Piles, hæmorrhoids, 207. | Pulsatilla nuttiliana in irregular
Pleura, diseases of the, 423. | menstruation, 814.
Pleurisy, chronic, 427. | Pulmonary consumption, 410.
Pleura, typhoid inflammation of | Pulse, intermittent, 452.
the, 427.
Pleurodynia, 428.
Pleura, dropsy of the, 428.
Pleura, air in the, 431.
Plethora or fullness of blood,
439.

Q

Plague, the, 560.
Plumbum in dysentery, 787.
Pneumonia, inflammation of the | Quotidian fever, Ignatia amara
lungs, 373. | in, 777.
Pneumonia with inter-current | Quinsy, Lachesis in, 780.
spinal schlerosis, 389.
Pneumonia, typhoid, typhoid
inflammation of the lungs,
395.
Pneumonia and bronchitis, La- | **R**
chesis in, 782.
Pneumonia, Lycopodium in,
782. | Rash, nettle, or urticaria, 375.
Pneumonia, 795. | Rabies, hydrophobia, 667.
Pox, small, or variola, 531. | Remedies and their antidotes,
Pox, small, modified or varioloid, | 126.
533. | Remedies which may follow each
Polygonum hydropiper in amen- | other, 131.
orrhœa, 815. | Respiratory organs, diseases of
Polygonum hydropiper in the | the, 269.
treatment of ulcers, 814. | Relations between diphtheria
Prolapsus ani, 209. | and erysipelas, 324.
Principle symptoms, 321. | Renal diseases, 484.
Productions, morbid, in the la- | Renal calculi, 497.
rynx and trachea, 335. | Remittent fever, 543.
Prurigo, 510. | Remittent fever, infantile, 548.
Pregnant and parturient wom- | Relapsing fever, 558.
en, eclamsia in, clonic spasms, | Remarks concerning the ears,
639. | general, 728.
Psoriasis, 521. | Rheumatism, acute or inflama-
Psoriasis palmasis, 521. | tory, 503.
Psoriasis scrotalis, 521. | Rheumatics, iritis, 712.

Rheumatism, Kali bichromicum in, 780.

Rheum in the treatment of diarrhœa in teething children, 791.

Rhus glabrum in syphilitic ulceration, 815.

Rhus venenata in erysipelas, 815.

Rhus in typhoid fever, 849.

Rubeola, morbili measles, 527.

Running from the ears, accumulation of mucuous within the tympanum—ottorrhœa, 726.

Rumex crispus in diarrhœa, 818.

Rumex c. in croup, 849.

S

Scarlatina and diphtheria, distinction between, 322.

Scarlatina anginosa and diphtheria, 324.

Scabies, 517.

Scrotalis, psoriasis, 510.

Scorbutus, scurvy, 523.

Scurvy, scorbutus, 523.

Scarlatina simplex, 524.

Simplex scarlatina, 524.

Scarlatina anginosis, 525.

Scarlatina maligna, 525.

Serous fluid, accumulation of in the nervous centers, 614.

Sensibility, augmentation of, 618.

Sensibility, diminution or deprivation of, 620.

Sensibility perverted, 621.

Sexual organs, diseases of the male—urethritis, 732.

Second attack of diphtheria, liability to, 323.

Shrinking of the gums, 148.

Sick headache, Iris versicolor in, 779.

Simplex oppthalmia, 707.

Sick headache, 628.

Skin and its diseases, the, 510.

Small intestines, inflammation in the, 176.

Small pox or variola, 531.

Small pox, modified or varioloid, 533.

Smell, perversion of the sense of, 731.

Sore throat, Lachesis in chronic, 780.

Softening of the nervous centres, 612.

Special diseases and therapeutics, diseases of the alimentary canal, 133.

Spasm of the glottis, 334.

Spasm of the glottis in adults, 334.

Spinal schlerosis with inter-current pneumonia, 389.

Spleen, diseases of the, 469.

Spleen, hypertrophy or enlargement of the, 470.

Spleen, atrophy of the, 474.

Spinal cord, hyperæmia of the, or congestion, 587.

Spinal cord, inflammation of the, myelitis, 597.

Spasms, eclamsia, epileptic, 635.

Spasms, clonic, eclamsia, in pregnant and parturient females, 639.

Spermatorrhœa, 741.

Spigelia in disease of the heart, 819.

Spigelia in neuralgia of the face, 818.

Stomach, diseases of the, 160.

Stomach, inflammation of the, 160.

Stomach, chronic inflammation of the, 163.

Stomach, cancer of the, 166.

Stomach, hæmorrhage from the, 169.

Stomach, cramps in the, 171.

Strabismus or squinting, 718.

St. Vitus dance, chorea, 650.

Sty on the eye-lids, 720.

Stibium in pneumonia, 807.

Stannum in chronic bronchitis, 820.

Summer bronchitis or hay fever, 351.

Sulphur in chronic dysentery, 787.

Sulphur in typhoid pneumonia, 807.

Sulphur in chronic bronchitis, 823.

Sulphur in chronic rheumatism, 842.

Sulphate of Nickel in headache, 785.

Sulphate of Zinc in dysentery, 787.

Suppression of the menses, 749.

Swooning or syncope, fainting fits, 450.

Symptoms, principle, in diphtheria and croup, 321.

System, disease of the biliary, 476.

System, the nervous, 563.

System, diseases supposed to have their seat in the nervous, 618.

Syphilitic ulcer on the tonsil and diphtheria, 324.

Syphilis, 736.

T

Tarsal ophthalmia, 720.

Tartar emetic in pneumonia, 808.

Tartar emetic in croup, 835.

Tartar emetic in typhoid fever 857.

Teeth, diseases of the, 141.

Teeth, caries of the, 142.

Termination in death, modes of, diphtheria, 323.

Tetanus and trismus, 668.

The signs of health and how to denote any departure from the standard, 81.

The nasal cavities, 269.

The anginæ, 323.

The phlegmatia dolens or milk leg, 455.

The capillary vessels, diseases of, 464.

The thymus gland, 474.

The skin and its diseases, 510.

The plague, 560.

The ears, general remarks concerning, 728.

The nose, diseases of, 729.

The nervous system, 563.

The nervous centres, disease of, 575.

Throat, inflammation of the, 149.

Throat, Lachesis in chronic sore, - 780.

Thrombosis, 463.

Thymic asthma, 474.

Tympanitis, 269.

Tympani membrana, diseases of the, 724.

Tympani membrana, perforated, 724.

Tympanum, inflammation of the mucous membrane of the, 725.

Tympanum, accumulation of mucous within the, 726.

Typhoid inflammation of the lungs, 395.

Typhoid pneumonia, 395.

Typhoid inflammation of the pleura, 427.

Typhoid fever, 554.

Typhus fever, 551.
Typhus abdominalis, 553.
Tongue, diseases of, 138.
Tongue, cancer of, 140.
Toothache, 142.
Toothache odontalgia, 699.
Tonsils, inflammation of the, 150.
Tonsils, diphtheria and spyphilitic ulcer on the, 324.
Trachea and larynx, diseases of the, 288.
Trachea and larynx, morbid production in the, 335.
Trachea and larynx, foreign bodies in the, 336.
Tremens, delirium, 672.
Tusis convulsiva, 357.
Tubercle in the lungs, 407.
Tubercle, 407.

U

Ulcer, syphilitic, and diphtheria on the tonsil, 324.
Ulcers, varicose, 458.
Urinary organs, diseases of the, continued, 495.
Urinary calculi, 496.
Urticaria or nettle rash, 515.
Urethritis, diseases of the male sexual organs, 732.
Urtica urens in burns, 819.
Uterine life, asphyxia of new born infants during, 434.
Uvula, inflammation of the, 148.

V

Varicose ulcers, 456.
Varicose veins, 458.
Varicella or chicken pox, 439.
Variola or small pox, 531.
Vessels, capillary, diseases of the, 464.
Veins, inflammation of the, 455.
Velum, inflammation of the, 148.
Veratrum in diarrhœa, 792.
Veratrum viride in convulsions, 819.
Volitantes muscæ, 714.

W

Wax, accumulation of, 723.
What is percussion, 274.
Whooping cough, 357.
Whooping cough, Baryta carb. in, 774.
Womb, cancer of the, 758.
Worms, invermination, 212.

Y

Yellow fever, 559.

Z

Zizia aurea in epileptiform diseases, 776.

www.ingramcontent.com/pod-product-compliance
Lightning Source LLC
LaVergne TN
LVHW050150060326
832904LV00003B/95